ESSENTIALS OF
NEUROPSYCHIATRY
AND BEHAVIORAL
NEUROSCIENCES

SECOND EDITION

ESSENTIALS OF
NEUROPSYCHIATRY AND BEHAVIORAL NEUROSCIENCES

SECOND EDITION

Edited by

Stuart C. Yudofsky, M.D.

D.C. and Irene Ellwood Professor and Chairman,
Menninger Department of Psychiatry and Behavioral Sciences,
Baylor College of Medicine; Chairman, Department of Psychiatry,
The Methodist Hospital, Houston, Texas

Robert E. Hales, M.D., M.B.A.

Joe P. Tupin Professor and Chair,
Department of Psychiatry and Behavioral Sciences,
University of California–Davis School of Medicine;
Medical Director, Sacramento County Mental Health Services,
Sacramento, California

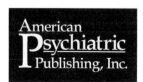

American Psychiatric Publishing, Inc.

Washington, DC
London, England

Copyright © 2010 American Psychiatric Publishing, Inc.
ALL RIGHTS RESERVED

Manufactured in the United States of America on acid-free paper

14   13   12   11   10   5   4   3   2   1

Typeset in Adobe's Revival565 and Gill Sans

American Psychiatric Publishing, Inc.
1000 Wilson Boulevard
Arlington, VA 22209-3901
www.appi.org

Library of Congress Cataloging-in-Publication Data
Essentials of neuropsychiatry and behavioral neurosciences / edited by Stuart C. Yudofsky, Robert E. Hales. — 2nd ed.
      p. ; cm.
   Rev. ed. of: Essentials of neuropsychiatry and clinical neurosciences / edited by Stuart C. Yudofsky, Robert E. Hales. c2004.
   Includes bibliographical references and index.
   ISBN 978-1-58562-376-1 (alk. paper)
   1. Neuropsychiatry. I. Yudofsky, Stuart C. II. Hales, Robert E. III. Essentials of neuropsychiatry and clinical neurosciences.
   [DNLM: 1. Mental Disorders—physiopathology. 2. Nervous System Diseases—psychology. WM 140 E784 2010]
   RC341.E84 2010
   616.8—dc22

2010001084

British Library Cataloguing in Publication Data
A CIP record is available from the British Library.

To purchase 25 to 99 copies of this or any other APPI title at a 20% discount, please contact APPI Customer Service at appi@psych.org or 800-368-5777. For purchases of 100 or more copies of the same title, please e-mail bulksales@psych.org for a price quote.

CONTENTS

CONTRIBUTORS

Liana G. Apostolova, M.D.
Assistant Professor, Department of Neurology, David Geffen School of Medicine, University of California at Los Angeles

Frank Y. Chen, M.D.
Private practice, Houston, Texas

Cheryl Corcoran, M.D., M.S.P.H.
Assistant Professor of Clinical Psychiatry, Department of Psychiatry, Columbia University College of Physicians and Surgeons, New York, New York

Jeffrey L. Cummings, M.D.
Augustus S. Rose Professor of Neurology; Professor of Psychiatry and Biobehavioral Neurosciences; Director, Mary S. Easton Center for Alzheimer's Disease Research; and Director, Deane F. Johnson Center for Neurotherapeutics, David Geffen School of Medicine, University of California at Los Angeles

Francisco Fernandez, M.D.
Professor and Chair, Department of Psychiatry and Behavioral Medicine, University of South Florida, Tampa, Florida

Ronald E. Fisher, M.D., Ph.D.
Assistant Professor, Departments of Radiology and Neuroscience, Baylor College of Medicine; Director of Nuclear Medicine, The Methodist Hospital, Houston, Texas

Michael D. Franzen, Ph.D.
Associate Professor of Psychiatry, Drexel University College of Medicine, Allegheny General Hospital, Pittsburgh, Pennsylvania

Subroto Ghose, M.D., Ph.D.
Assistant Professor of Psychiatry, University of Texas Southwestern Medical Center, Dallas, Texas

Kenneth L. Goetz, M.D.
Associate Professor, Department of Psychiatry, Drexel University College of Medicine, Pittsbugh, Pennsylvania

Brian Guinta, M.D., M.S.
Assistant Professor and Director, Neuroimmunology Laboratory, Department of Psychiatry and Behavioral Medicine, University of South Florida, Tampa, Florida

Robert E. Hales, M.D., M.B.A.
Joe P. Tupin Professor and Chair, Department of Psychiatry and Behavioral Sciences, University of California–Davis School of Medicine, Sacramento, California; Medical Director, Sacramento County Mental Health Services, and Editor-in-Chief, American Psychiatric Publishing, Inc.

Steven P. Hamilton, M.D., Ph.D.
Associate Professor, Department of Psychiatry, University of California–San Francisco

Paul E. Holtzheimer III, M.D.
Assistant Professor of Psychiatry, Emory University School of Medicine, Atlanta, Georgia

Diane B. Howieson, Ph.D.
Associate Professor of Neurology and Psychiatry, Oregon Health and Science University, Portland, Oregon

Robin A. Hurley, M.D., FANPA
Associate Professor, Departments of Psychiatry and Radiology, Wake Forest University School of Medicine, Winston-Salem, North Carolina; Clinical Associate Professor, Department of Psychiatry, Baylor College of Medicine, Houston, Texas; Acting Chief of Staff and Associate Chief of Staff for Mental Health, W. G. "Bill" Hefner VAMC, Salisbury, North Carolina; and Co-Director for Education, Mid-Atlantic MIRECC, Salisbury, North Carolina

H. Florence Kim, M.D.
Private practice, Houston, Texas

Alan J. Lerner, M.D.
Professor of Neurology, Case Western Reserve University School of Medicine; Director, Memory and Cognition Center, Neurological Institute, University Hospitals Case Medical Center, Cleveland, Ohio

Muriel D. Lezak, Ph.D.
Professor Emerita, Neurology, Oregon Health and Science University, Portland, Oregon

Mark R. Lovell, Ph.D.
Assistant Professor, Department of Orthopedic Surgery, University of Pittsburgh School of Medicine; Director, Sports Medicine Concussion Program, UPMC Center for Sports Medicine, Pittsburgh, Pennsylvania

Dolores Malaspina, M.D., M.S.P.H.
Anita Steckler and Joseph Steckler Professor of Psychiatry and Director, Institute for Severe and Persistent Illness–Research, Education and Services, New York University Medical Center, New York, New York

Helen S. Mayberg, M.D.
Professor of Psychiatry and Neurology, Emory University School of Medicine, Atlanta, Georgia

A. Kimberley McAllister, Ph.D.
Associate Professor of Neuroscience, Center for Neuroscience, University of California–Davis

David J. Meagher, M.D., M.R.C.Psych.
Consultant Psychiatrist and Director of Clinical Research, Department of Psychiatry, Midwestern Regional Hospital, Dooradoyle, Limerick, Ireland

Eric J. Nestler, M.D., Ph.D.
Nash Family Professor of Neuroscience; Chair, Department of Neuroscience; and Director, Brain Institute, Mount Sinai School of Medicine, New York, New York

Stephen C. Noctor, Ph.D.
Research Scientist, Institute for Regenerative Medicine, Department of Neurology, University of California–San Francisco

Trevor R. P. Price, M.D.
Private practice of psychiatry, Bryn Mawr, Pennsylvania

Scott L. Rauch, M.D.
Professor of Psychiatry, Harvard Medical School, Boston, Massachusetts; Chair, Partners Psychiatry and Mental Health; and President and Psychiatrist-in-Chief, McLean Hospital, Belmont, Massachusetts

Stephen Rayport, M.D., Ph.D.
Associate Professor of Clinical Neuroscience, Department of Psychiatry, Columbia University College of Physicians and Surgeons, New York, New York

David Riley, M.D.
Professor of Neurology, Case Western Reserve University; Director, Movement Disorders Center, Neurological Institute, University Hospitals Case Medical Center, Cleveland, Ohio

Robert G. Robinson, M.D.
Paul W. Penningroth Chair, Professor and Head, Department of Psychiatry, University of Iowa College of Medicine, Iowa City, Iowa

Peter P. Roy-Byrne, M.D.
Professor and Vice-Chair, Department of Psychiatry and Behavioral Sciences, University of

Washington; Director, Harborview Center for Healthcare Improvement for Addictions, Mental Illness and Medically Vulnerable Populations; and Chief of Psychiatry, Harborview Medical Center, Seattle, Washington

Scott Schobel, M.D.
Postdoctoral Clinical Fellow, Department of Psychiatry, Columbia University College of Physicians and Surgeons, New York, New York

David W. Self, Ph.D.
Associate Professor, Department of Psychiatry and Center for Basic Neuroscience, University of Texas Southwestern Medical Center, Dallas, Texas

Mujeeb U. Shad, M.D.
Assistant Professor of Psychiatry, University of Texas Southwestern Medical Center, Dallas, Texas

Jonathan M. Silver, M.D.
Clinical Professor of Psychiatry, New York University School of Medicine, New York, New York

Mark Snowden, M.D., M.P.H.
Associate Professor, Department of Psychiatry and Behavioral Sciences, University of Washington, Seattle, Washington

Sergio E. Starkstein, M.D., Ph.D.
Professor of Psychiatry and Clinical Neurosciences, University of Western Australia, Fremantle, Australia

Dan J. Stein, M.D., Ph.D.
Professor, Department of Psychiatry, University of Cape Town, Groote Schuur Hospital, Cape Town, South Africa; Mount Sinai School of Medicine, New York, New York

Katherine H. Taber, Ph.D., FANPA
Research Professor, Division of Biomedical Sciences, Virginia College of Osteopathic Medicine, Blacksburg, Virginia; Adjunct Associate Professor, Department of Physical Medicine and Rehabilitation, Baylor College of Medicine, Houston, Texas; Assistant Co-Director for Education, Mid-Atlantic MIRECC, Salisbury, North Carolina; and Research Scientist, W.G. "Bill" Hefner VAMC, Salisbury, North Carolina

Carol A. Tamminga, M.D.
Professor and Vice Chair of Clinical Research, Department of Psychiatry, University of Texas Southwestern Medical Center, Dallas, Texas

Jun Tan, M.D., Ph.D.
Associate Professor, Robert A. Silver Chair in Developmental Neurobiology, Department of Psychiatry and Behavioral Medicine, University of South Florida; Director, Jerri and Sam Rashid Laboratories, Tampa, Florida

Paula T. Trzepacz, M.D.
Senior Medical Fellow, Neurosciences Research, Lilly Research Laboratories; Clinical Professor of Psychiatry, Indiana University School of Medicine, Indianapolis, Indiana

Gary J. Tucker, M.D. (deceased)
Department of Psychiatry and Behavioral Sciences, University of Washington, Seattle, Washington

W. Martin Usrey, Ph.D.
Associate Professor of Neurology, Center for Neuroscience, University of California–Davis

Stuart C. Yudofsky, M.D.
D.C. and Irene Ellwood Professor and Chairman, Menninger Department of Psychiatry and Behavioral Sciences, Baylor College of Medicine; Chairman, Department of Psychiatry, The Methodist Hospital, Houston, Texas

DISCLOSURE OF INTERESTS

Contributors have declared all forms of support received that may represent a competing interest relative to the work republished in this volume, as follows:

Jeffrey L. Cummings, M.D. *Grants/Research Support:* Janssen. *Consultant:* Avanir, Eisai, Eli Lilly, EnVivo, Forest, Janssen, Lundbeck, Merz, Myriad, Neurochem, Novartis, Ono, Pfizer, Sanofi-Aventis, Sepracor, Takeda. *Speakers' Bureau:* Eisai, Forest, Janssen, Lundbeck, Merz, Novartis, Pfizer. *Honoraria:* Avanir, Eisai, Janssen, Forest, Lundbeck, Merz, Myriad, Neurochem, Novartis, Ono, Pfizer, Sanofi-Aventis, Sepracor, Takeda. *Board Member:* EnVivo, Myriad, Pfizer.

Paul E. Holtzheimer III, M.D. *Consultant:* Advanced Neuromodulation Systems, Inc. [ongoing], AstraZeneca, Inc. [2007], AvaCat Consulting [2009], Oppenheimer & Co. [2009], Shaw Science [2009], Tetragenex, Inc. [2008]. *Grants/ Research Support:* American Federation for Aging Research, Dana Foundation, Greenwall Foundation, Neuronetics, Inc, NARSAD, National Institute of Mental Health (K23 MH077869), National Institutes of Health Loan Repayment Program, Northstar, Inc. [2006]; Stanley Medical Research Institute; Woodruff Foundation. *Honoraria:* CME Outfitters, Inc. (Cyberonics), Cerebrio, Inc. (Boerhinger-Ingelheim) [2006]; CME LLC, Inc. (Bristol-Myers Squibb) [2007]; Letters and Sciences (Bristol-Myers Squibb) [2007, 2008], Prescott Medical Communications Group (Forest) [2007]. *Other:* Travel awards from APA Colloquium for Junior Investigators and American College of Neuropsychopharmacology.

Helen S. Mayberg, M.D. *Consultant:* St Jude Medical. *Other:* Intellectual property holder and licensor in the field of deep brain stimulation.

David J. Meagher, M.D., M.R.C.Psych. *Grants/ Research Support:* Unrestricted educational grant, AstraZeneca.

Scott L. Rauch, M.D. *Grants/Research Support:* Cephalon, Cyberonics, Medtronic Inc, Northstar. *Fellowship Support:* Pfizer. *Consultant:* Cyberonics, Novartis.

David Riley, M.D. *Honoraria:* Boehringer Ingelheim, GlaxoSmithKline.

Peter P. Roy-Byrne, M.D. *Grants/Research Support:* Forest, GlaxoSmithKline, Pfizer. *Consultant/Advisor:* Alza, Cephalon, GlaxoSmithKline, Eli Lilly, Forest, Janssen, Jazz, Pfizer, Pharmacia, Roche, Wyeth-Ayerst. *Speakers' Honoraria:* Forest, GlaxoSmithKline, Novartis, Pfizer, Pharmacia, Wyeth-Ayerst.

Mark Snowden, M.D., M.P.H. *Speakers' Bureau:* Pfizer.

Dan J. Stein, M.D., Ph.D. *Grants/Research Support or Consultancy Honoraria:* AstraZeneca, Eli Lilly, GlaxoSmithKline, Lundbeck, Orion, Pfizer, Pharmacia, Roche, Servier, Solvay, Sumitomo, Wyeth-Ayerst.

Carol A. Tamminga, M.D. *Grants/Research Support:* Bristol-Myers Squibb for Physicians Postgraduate Press monograph. *Speaker:* AstraZeneca (once). *Consultant, ad hoc:* Abbott, ARYx Therapeutics, Becker Pharma, Organon, Patterson, Balknap, Webb & Tyler for Johnson & Johnson (once), Saegis, Sumitomo. *Consultant, Drug Development:* Nupathe. *Advisory Board, Drug Development:* Acadia, Avera, Intracellular Therapies, Neurogen.

Paula T. Trzepacz, M.D. Full-time salaried employee of and shareholder in Eli Lilly and Company.

The following contributors stated that they had no competing interests relative to the work republished in this volume:

Liana G. Apostolova, M.D.
Frank Chen, M.D.
Cheryl Corcoran, M.D., M.S.P.H.
Francisco Fernandez, M.D.
Ronald E. Fisher, M.D., Ph.D.
Michael D. Franzen, Ph.D.
Subroto Ghose, M.D., Ph.D.
Kenneth L. Goetz, M.D.
Robert E. Hales, M.D., M.B.A.
Steven P. Hamilton, M.D., Ph.D.
Diane B. Howieson, Ph.D.
Robin A. Hurley, M.D.
H. Florence Kim, M.D.
Alan J. Lerner, M.D.
Muriel D. Lezak, Ph.D.
Mark R. Lovell, Ph.D.
Dolores Malaspina, M.D., M.S.P.H.
A. Kimberley McAllister, Ph.D.
Eric Nestler, M.D., Ph.D.
Stephen C. Noctor, Ph.D.
Trevor R.P. Price, M.D.
Stephen Rayport, M.D., Ph.D.
Robert G. Robinson, M.D.
Scott Schobel, M.D.
David W. Self, Ph.D.
Mujeeb U. Shad, M.D.
Jonathan M. Silver, M.D.
Sergio E. Starkstein, M.D., Ph.D.
Katherine H. Taber, Ph.D.
Jun Tan, M.D., Ph.D.
W. Martin Usrey, Ph.D.
Stuart C. Yudofsky, M.D.

FUNDAMENTALS OF CELLULAR NEUROBIOLOGY

A. Kimberley McAllister, Ph.D.

W. Martin Usrey, Ph.D.

Stephen C. Noctor, Ph.D.

Stephen Rayport, M.D., Ph.D.

Neuropsychiatric disorders are due to disordered functioning of neurons and, in particular, their synapses. Many neuropsychiatric disorders arise from aberrations in neurodevelopmental mechanisms. In the initial stages of brain development, cell-cell interactions are the dominant force in the assembly of the brain (Wichterle et al. 2002). As circuits form, individual neurons and connections are pruned on an activity-dependent basis, driven by intrinsic activity and competition for trophic factors. Neurogenesis does not stop with maturation but in fact continues in some brain regions and appears to be required for mood regulation (Santarelli et al. 2003; Warner-Schmidt and Duman 2006). With further maturation, experience becomes the dominant force in shaping neuronal connections and regulating their effi-

cacy. In the mature brain, these neurodevelopmental mechanisms are harnessed in muted form and mediate most plastic processes (Black 1995; Kandel and O'Dell 1992). Neuropsychiatric disorders arising from problems in early brain development are more likely to be intrinsically or genetically based, whereas those arising during later stages are more likely to be experience based (Toga and Thompson 2005). In senescence, neurodegenerative processes may unravel neural circuits through limiting neural plasticity.

Experience is so pivotal in fine-tuning neural connectivity that aberrant experience—particularly during critical periods in development—may give rise to or exacerbate neuropsychiatric disorders. For example, monocular occlusion or strabismus in young animals results in permanent pathologic connectivity of the visual system (Hubel et al. 1977). In humans, failure to achieve conjugate gaze in childhood results in permanent visual loss. In mice, early blockade of the serotonin transporter with fluoxetine engenders an anxious phenotype when the mice grow up (Ansorge et al. 2004). In humans, early life stress engenders greater vulnerability to depression in adult life (Caspi et al. 2003). Similar but subtler changes occur in adulthood during learning when changes in synaptic connections encode memories. Here, too, abnormal experiences may permanently alter patterns of neuronal connectivity. In the human brain, imaging studies have begun to reveal changes in regional brain activity that occur after learning and that are suggestive of changes in the strength of neuronal connections (Maguire et al. 2000; Pantev et al. 1998; Sadato et al. 1996). Some functional neuropsychiatric disorders have now been shown to have a direct impact on brain structure; for example, posttraumatic stress disorder has been associated with alterations in hippocampal size (Kitayama et al. 2005).

In this chapter, we focus first on the cellular function of neurons and then on how they develop. The accelerating pace of recent advances begins now to offer a glimmer of how therapeutic interventions to correct aberrant neuronal growth and differentiation during development and maturation, or later to normalize neuronal signaling, may translate into revolutionary treatments for neuropsychiatric disorders.

CELLULAR FUNCTION OF NEURONS

Individual neurons in the brain receive signals from thousands of neurons and, in turn, send information to thousands of others. Whereas activity in peripheral sensory neurons may represent particular bits of information, activity of networks of neurons in the central nervous system (CNS) represents integrated sensory and associational information. CNS neurons are part of dynamic cellular ensembles that shift their participation from one network to another as information is used in varied tasks. The sophistication of these networks depends on both the properties of the neurons themselves and the patterns and strength of their connections.

CELLULAR COMPOSITION OF THE BRAIN

Brain cells comprise two principal types: *neurons* and *glia*. Neurons are highly differentiated cells that are the substrate for most information processing. Neurons show considerable heterogeneity in shape and size; in fact, there are more types of neurons than types of cells in any other part of the body. Some are among the largest cells in the body, as in the case of the upper motor neurons that project to the lumbar spinal cord and have axons that are a meter or more in length; others are among the smallest cells in the body, as in the case of the granule cells of the cerebellum. Neurons are quite numerous, and they interconnect via synapses that are still more numerous. The human brain contains 10^{12}–10^{13} neurons. Each neuron forms an average of 10^3 connections, which is a minimal estimate, so the brain has on the order of 10^{15}–10^{16} synapses. In childhood and continuing throughout the life span to a more limited extent, the numbers of neurons and synapses show dramatic changes. During early development, neurogenesis can occur at a rate of up to 250,000 neurons per minute. In childhood, there is considerable refinement in neural circuits and a reduction in the number of synapses. In later life, neurodegenerative disorders produce losses in the number of neurons and synapses.

Glial cells can be divided into three classes: 1) astrocytes, 2) oligodendrocytes, and 3) microglia. *Astrocytes* have three traditional functions: they provide the scaffolding of the brain, form the blood-brain barrier, and guide neuronal migration during development. Evidence is accumulating, however, that astroglial cells are more dynamic than previously suspected and are capable of cell-cell signaling over long distances (Dani et al. 1992; Fellin and Carmignoto 2004; Murphy et al. 1993). Moreover, they can influence neuronal activity, enhance neuronal connectivity, and play critical roles in regulating neuronal excitability during normal processes as well as in disease states (Araque et al. 1999; Mennerick and Zorumski 1994; Nedergaard 1994; Pfrieger and Barres 1997). *Oligodendrocytes* produce the myelin sheath that speeds conduction of the action potential along axons. In patients with multiple sclerosis, which results from an immune attack on the principal protein of the myelin sheath, myelin basic protein, there is a failure in action potential conduction (Graham and Lantos 2002). *Microglia* are the macrophages of the brain: quiescent until activated by brain injury.

NEURONAL SHAPE

Neurons share a common organization dictated by their function, which is to receive, process, and transmit information. The great Spanish neuroanatomist Santiago Ramón y Cajal called this *dynamic polarization* (Ramón y Cajal 1894). Although neurons show a wide diversity of sizes and shapes, they generally have four well-defined regions (Figure 1–1): 1) dendrites, 2) cell body, 3) axon, and 4) synaptic specializations. Each region has distinct functions. *Dendrites* receive signals from other neurons, process and modify this information, and then convey these signals to the cell body. As in all cells, the *cell body* contains the genetic information resident in the nucleus that codes for the fabrication of the necessary elements of cellular function, as well as sites for their manufacture, processing, and transport. The *axon* makes highly specific connections and conveys information over long distances to its terminals. Finally, *synaptic specializations* comprise the active zone and synaptic terminal on the presynaptic axon and the postsynaptic density on the postsynaptic dendrite.

A neuron's shape is determined by the cytoskeleton. The cytoskeleton is composed primarily of three filamentous components: 1) microtubules, 2) neurofilaments, and 3) actin (Pigino et al. 2006). *Microtubules* are composed of tubulin subunits and form a scaffold that determines the shape of the neuron. *Neurofilaments* are the most abundant cytoskeletal components of the axon and are much more stable than microtubules. In disease, these neurofilaments are constituents of neurofibrillary tangles, characteristic of Alzheimer's disease. Finally, *actin* filaments form a dense network concentrated just under the cell membrane. Together with a large number of actin-binding proteins, this network facilitates cell motility and formation of synaptic specializations and allows for plasticity of axonal and dendritic structure (Dillon and Goda 2005). In addition to its important structural role, the cytoskeleton is essential for intracellular trafficking of proteins and organelles and facilitates the selective transport of axonal and dendritic proteins (Burack et al. 2000; Kamal and Goldstein 2002). Thus, cytoskeletal defects are likely to cause devastating neuronal damage—impairing axonal and dendritic transport and cell signaling, and eventually causing cell death (Hirokawa and Takemura 2003). Many neurodegenerative disorders are associated with defects in the trafficking of molecules or synaptic function (Cummings 2003).

NEURONAL EXCITABILITY

Neurons are capable of transmitting information because they are electrically and chemically excitable. This excitability is conferred by a number of classes of ion channels that are selectively permeable to specific ions and that are regulated by voltage (voltage-gated channels), neurotransmitter binding (ligand-gated channels), or pressure or stretch (mechanically gated channels) (reviewed in Hille 2001). In general, neuronal ion channels conduct ions across the plasma membrane at extremely rapid rates—100 million ions may pass through a single channel in a second. This large flow of current causes rapid changes in membrane potential and is the basis for the action potential, the substrate for information transfer *within* neurons, and for fast synaptic responses, the substrate for information transfer *between* neurons. Ligand-gated channels are often targets

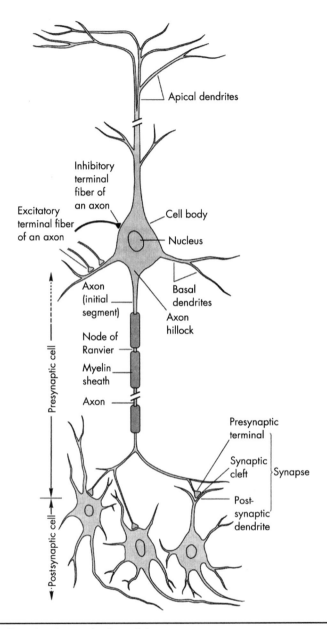

FIGURE 1–1. Functional organization of the neuron.

Neurons have distinct cellular regions subserving the input, integration, conduction, and output of information: the dendrites, cell body, axon, and synaptic specializations, respectively. Excitatory and inhibitory neurotransmitters released by other neurons induce depolarizing or hyperpolarizing current flow in dendrites. These currents converge in the cell body, and if the resulting polarization is sufficient to bring the initial segment of the axon to threshold, an action potential is initiated. The action potential travels down the axon, speeded by myelination, to reach the synaptic terminals. Axon terminals form synapses with other neurons or effector cells, renewing the cycle of information flow in postsynaptic cells. As in all cells, the cell body (or perikaryon) is also the repository of the neuron's genetic information (in the nucleus) and the principal site of macromolecular synthesis.

Source. Reprinted from Kandel ER: "Nerve Cells and Behavior," in *Principles of Neural Science*, 4th Edition. Edited by Kandel ER, Schwartz JH, Jessell TM. New York, McGraw-Hill, 2000, pp. 19–35. Copyright 2000, The McGraw-Hill Companies, Inc. Used with permission.

for psychiatric drugs, anesthetics, and neuro-toxins. As expected, diseases caused by defects in ion channels are diverse and devastating. For example, in myasthenia gravis the immune system mounts an attack on nicotinic acetylcholine receptors; in hyperkalemic periodic paralysis, muscle stiffness and weakness following exercise result from a point mutation in voltage-gated Na^+ channels; and in episodic ataxia, the generalized ataxia triggered by periods of stress results from point mutation in a delayed-rectifier voltage-gated K^+ channel (reviewed in Koester and Siegelbaum 2000).

Neurotransmitters released by one neuron at synapses activate receptors (ligand-gated channels) on dendrites of other neurons and induce ion flux across the membrane. The resulting electrical signals spread passively over some distance, often reaching the cell body in this way. In addition to passive conductances, localized regenerative mechanisms similar to those that give rise to the action potential (discussed later in this section) amplify dendritic input signals, boosting them so that they can reach the cell body (Eilers and Konnerth 1997; Magee and Carruth 1999; Yuste and Tank 1996). In the cell body, these synaptic inputs combine and, if sufficient, depolarize the initial segment of the axon, or axon hillock, which is the part of the axon closest to the cell body that has the lowest threshold for activation. When a threshold level of depolarization is reached, the action potential is initiated. The action potential, or spike, is an electrical wave that propagates down the axon. In the axon terminals, this wave triggers an influx of calcium (Ca^{2+}), which leads to exocytosis of neurotransmitters from synaptic vesicles at specialized sites called active zones. The released neurotransmitter reaches and activates closely apposed receptors in the postsynaptic density on the postsynaptic cell's dendrites. Ultimately, this information flow reaches effector cells, principally motor fibers that mediate movement and thus generate behavior.

The regenerative property of the action potential not only serves to amplify threshold potentials (its principal function in dendrites) but also confers long-distance signaling capabilities in the axon (Figure 1–2). When the membrane potential peaks under the control of the increase in Na^+ permeability, adjacent regions of the axon become sufficiently depolarized that they, in turn, are brought to threshold and generate an action potential. As successive axonal segments are depolarized, the action potential conducts at great speed down the axon. This is further enhanced by myelination, which increases the rate of conduction several fold by restricting the current flow required for action potential generation to the gaps between myelin segments, the nodes of Ranvier (see Figure 1–2). Because of its all-or-none characteristics and ability to conduct over long distances, the action potential provides a high-quality digital signaling mechanism in neurons.

Although the information that a neuron integrates comes from synaptic input, how the neuron processes that information depends on its intrinsic properties (Llinás 1988; London and Häusser 2005). Many CNS neurons have the ability to generate their own patterns of activity in the absence of synaptic input, firing either at a regular rate (pacemaker firing) or in clusters of spikes (burst firing) (McCormick and Bal 1997). This endogenous activity is driven by specialized ion channels with their own voltage and time dependence that periodically bring the initial segment of the axon to threshold. These channels can be modulated by the membrane potential of the cell or by second messenger systems. Depending on the activation of these specialized channels, neurons may profoundly change how they respond to a given synaptic input. Changes in second messenger levels may also profoundly affect the activity or response properties of neurons, lending still a greater repertoire to the functioning of individual neurons. Thus, synaptic inputs may not only evoke a response in a postsynaptic neuron, but may also shape intrinsic firing patterns, cause a cell to shift from one mode of activity to another, or modulate responses to other synaptic inputs.

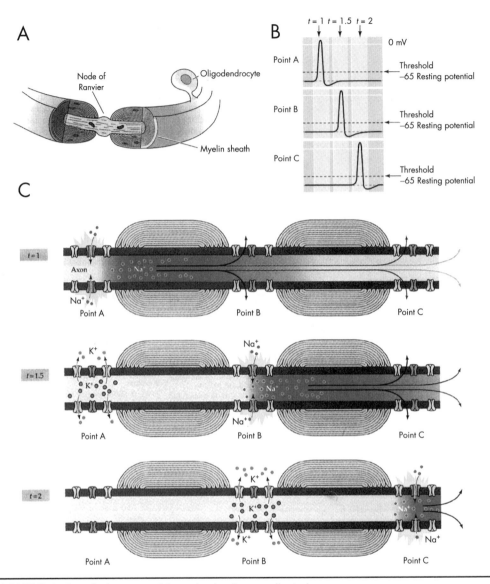

FIGURE 1–2.   Action potential conduction in a myelinated axon.

See Appendix for color version. Panel A. Schematic of a myelinated axon. Oligodendrocytes produce the insulating myelin sheath that surrounds the axon in segments. Myelination restricts current flow to the gaps between myelin segments, the nodes of Ranvier, where Na^+ channels are concentrated. The result is a dramatic enhancement of the conduction velocity of the action potential. *Panel B.* Because sodium channels are activated by membrane depolarization and also cause depolarization, they have regenerative properties. This underlies the "all-or-nothing" properties of the action potential and also explains its rapid spread down the axon. The action potential is an electrical wave; as each node of Ranvier is depolarized, it in turn depolarizes the subsequent node. *Panel C.* The Na^+ current underlying the action potential is shown in three successive images at 0.5-millisecond intervals and corresponds to the current traces in Panel B. As the action potential (*shading*) travels to the right, Na^+ channels go from closed to open to inactivated to closed. In this way, an action potential initiated at the initial segment of the axon conducts reliably to the axon terminals. Because Na^+ channels temporarily inactivate after depolarization, there is a brief refractory period following the action potential that blocks backward spread of the action potential and thus ensures reliable forward conduction.

Source.   Reprinted from Purves D, Augustine GJ, Fitzpatrick D, et al. (eds): *Neuroscience*, 3rd Edition. Sunderland, MA, Sinauer Associates, 2004, p. 64. Used with permission.

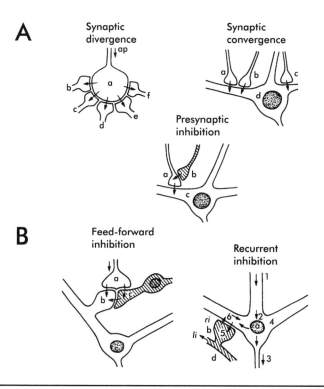

FIGURE 1–3. Modes of interneuronal communication.

Panel A. Different connection patterns dictate how information flows between neurons. In synaptic divergence, one neuron (a) may disseminate information to several postsynaptic cells (b–f) simultaneously (information flow is shown by *arrows*). Alternatively, in the case of synaptic convergence, a single neuron (d) may receive input from an array of presynaptic neurons (a–c). In presynaptic inhibition, one neuron (b) can modulate information flowing between two other neurons (from a to c) by influencing neurotransmitter release from the presynaptic neuron's terminals; this can be inhibitory (as shown) or facilitatory. *Panel B.* Neurons may modulate their own actions. In feed-forward inhibition, the presynaptic cell (a) may directly activate a postsynaptic cell (b) and at the same time modulate its effects via activation of an inhibitory cell (c), which in turn inhibits the cell (b). In recurrent inhibition, a presynaptic cell (a) activates an inhibitory cell (b) that synapses back onto the presynaptic cell (a), limiting the duration of its activity. ap = action potential; *li* = lateral inhibition; *ri* = recurrent inhibition.

Source. Adapted from Shepherd GM, Koch C: "Introduction to Synaptic Circuits," in *The Synaptic Organization of the Brain*, 3rd Edition. Edited by Shepherd GM. New York, Oxford University Press, 1990, pp. 3–31.. Used with permission.

SIGNALING BETWEEN NEURONS

Neurons communicate with one another at specialized sites of close membrane apposition called *synapses*. The prototypic axodendritic synapse connects a presynaptic axon terminal with a postsynaptic dendrite. This arrangement is typical for projection neurons that convey information from one region of the brain to another. In contrast, local circuit interneurons interact with neighboring neurons. While interneurons may make axodendritic and axosomatic connections, they can also form several other kinds of synaptic contacts that greatly increase their functional sophistication (Figure 1–3). For example, axons may synapse onto the axon terminals of other axons (*axoaxonic* connections) and modulate transmitter release by presynaptic inhibition or facilitation.

A minority of local connections are mediated by electrical synapses that do not require chemical neurotransmitters at all. Electrical synapses are formed by multisubunit channels, called *gap junctions*, that link the cytoplasm of adjacent cells (Bennett et al. 1991; Sohl et al. 2005), allowing both small molecules and ions carrying electrical signals to flow directly from one cell to another. During embryonic development, the ability to pass small molecules, including second messengers, between cells is important for the generation of morphogenic gradients (Dealy et al. 1994). During early brain development, such gradients regulate cell proliferation and establish patterns of connectivity (Kandler and Katz 1995). In the mature brain, electrical synapses act to synchronize the electrical activity of groups of neurons and mediate high-frequency transmission of signals (Bennett 1977; Brivanlou et al. 1998; Tamas et al. 2000). Glial cells are also connected by gap junctions, which link these cells into large syncytia, providing avenues for intercellular propagation of chemical signals mediated by small molecules and ions. The importance of gap junctions for glial cell function is underscored by the fact that the X-linked form of Charcot-Marie-Tooth disease results from a single mutation in a connexin gene required for formation of gap junctions between Schwann cells (reviewed in Schenone and Mancardi 1999).

Most CNS synaptic connections are mediated by chemical neurotransmitters. Although chemical synapses are slower than electrical ones, they allow for signal amplification, may be inhibitory as well as excitatory, are susceptible to a wide range of modulation, and can modulate the activities of other cells through the release of transmitters activating second messenger cascades. There are primarily two classes of neurotransmitters in the nervous system: 1) small molecule transmitters and 2) neuropeptides. In general, *small molecule transmitters* mediate fast synaptic transmission; are stored in small, clear synaptic vesicles; and include glutamate, γ-aminobutyric acid (GABA), glycine, acetylcholine, serotonin, dopamine, norepinephrine, epinephrine, and histamine. The cellular and molecular mechanisms of release of these synaptic vesicles are described in the remainder of this section. In contrast, the *neuropeptides* are a very large family of neurotransmitters that modulate synaptic transmission, are stored in large dense-core vesicles, and include somatostatin, the hypothalamic-releasing hormones, endorphins, enkephalins, and the opioids. Interestingly, small molecule transmitters and neuropeptides are often released from the same neuron and can act together on the same target (Hökfelt 1991).

Small neurotransmitter molecules are stored in small, clear, membrane-bound granules called *synaptic vesicles* (Figure 1–4). Each synaptic vesicle contains several thousand neurotransmitter molecules. When an action potential invades the presynaptic region, the depolarization activates voltage-dependent Ca^{2+} channels and triggers transmitter release (Figure 1–5). The subsequent Ca^{2+} influx raises the local Ca^{2+} concentration near the active zone, promoting synaptic vesicle fusion and neurotransmitter release via *exocytosis*. Neurotransmitter then diffuses a short distance across the synaptic cleft and binds to postsynaptic receptors. The dynamics and modulation of synaptic transmission are fundamental to alterations in synaptic connections that underlie both normal and pathologic learning and memory. In recent years, the molecular machinery involved in synaptic transmission has been increasingly clarified (Sudhof 2004). A coordinated set of proteins is involved in the positioning of vesicles at the presynaptic membrane and in controlling release by membrane fusion. The current theory for how synaptic vesicles fuse with the membrane and release neurotransmitter is called the SNARE (soluble NSF attachment protein receptor) hypothesis. Both the synaptic vesicles and the plasma membrane express proteins that mediate docking and fusion: v-SNAREs (synaptic vesicles) and t-SNAREs (plasma membrane). Vesicles are brought close to the membrane through interactions between VAMP (synaptobrevin), syntaxin, and SNAP-25. *N*-ethylmaleimide-sensitive fusion protein (NSF) then binds to the complex to facilitate fusion. Calcium influx is required to stimulate fusion, but

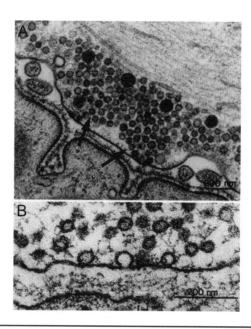

FIGURE 1–4. Synaptic ultrastructure.

Neuromuscular junctions from frog sartorius muscle were flash-frozen milliseconds after high potassium treatment to increase synaptic transmission. *Panel A.* Synaptic vesicles are clustered at two active zones (*arrows*), which are sites where vesicles fuse with the plasma membrane to release their neurotransmitter. *Panel B.* At higher magnification, and after stimulation, omega profiles of vesicles in the process of releasing their neurotransmitter are visible.

Source. Reprinted from Schwarz TL: "Release of Neurotransmitters," in *Fundamental Neuroscience*, 2nd Edition. Edited by Squire LR, Roberts JL, Spitzer NC, Zigmond MZ, McConnell SK, Bloom FE. San Diego, CA, Academic Press, 2003, pp. 197–224; original source Heuser JE: "Synaptic Vesicle Endocytosis Revealed in Quick-Frozen Frog Neuromuscular Junctions Treated With 4-Aminopyridine and Given a Single Electrical Shock." *Society for Neuroscience Symposia* 2:215–239, 1977. Copyright 1977. Used with permission.

the precise binding partner for calcium and the exact events leading to fusion remain obscure. Interestingly, several potent neurotoxins act directly on this machinery.

Neurotransmitter activity is typically limited in duration by several mechanisms that rapidly remove released neurotransmitter from the synapse. First, simple diffusion out of the synaptic cleft limits the duration of action of all neurotransmitters. Second, neurotransmitters may be enzymatically degraded; for example, acetylcholine is hydrolyzed by acetylcholinesterase bound to the postsynaptic membrane adjacent to the receptors. Finally, although the monoamine and amino acid neurotransmitters are also metabolized, they are principally removed from the synaptic cleft by

rapid reuptake mechanisms, whereby they are repackaged in synaptic vesicles or metabolized (Masson et al. 1999).

The monoamine neurotransmitter transporters, which mediate this rapid reuptake process, are the sites of action of a number of drugs and neurotoxins (Gainetdinov and Caron 2003). Prominent among these are the tricyclic antidepressants, selective serotonin reuptake inhibitors (SSRIs), the psychostimulants, and the neurotoxin 1-methyl-4-phenyl-1,2,3,6-tetrahydropyridine (MPTP). The tricyclics block serotonin and norepinephrine reuptake, while the SSRIs, as their name suggests, block serotonin reuptake. Other newer antidepressants block feedback inhibition of release, thereby increasing synaptic serotonin

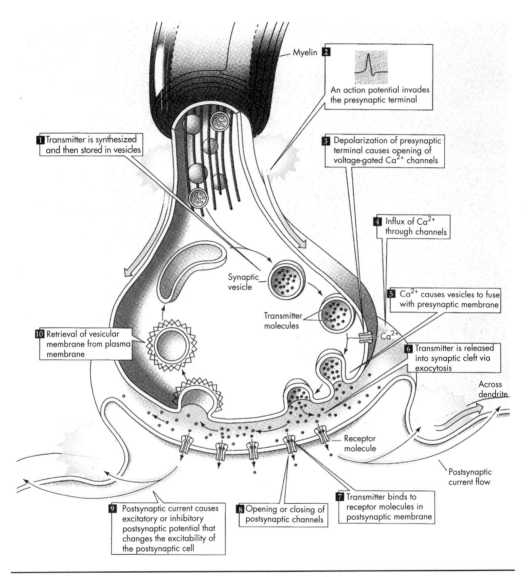

Myelin 2

An action potential invades
the presynaptic terminal

1 Transmitter is synthesized
and then stored in vesicles

3 Depolarization of presynaptic
terminal causes opening of
voltage-gated Ca^{2+} channels

4 Influx of Ca^{2+}
through channels

Synaptic
vesicle

5 Ca^{2+} causes vesicles to fuse
with presynaptic membrane

Transmitter
molecules

Ca^{2+}

10 Retrieval of vesicular
membrane from plasma
membrane

6 Transmitter is released
into synaptic cleft via
exocytosis

Across
dendrite

Receptor
molecule

Postsynaptic
current flow

9 Postsynaptic current causes
excitatory or inhibitory
postsynaptic potential that
changes the excitability of
the postsynaptic cell

8 Opening or closing of
postsynaptic channels

7 Transmitter binds to
receptor molecules in
postsynaptic membrane

FIGURE 1–5.   Steps in synaptic transmission at a chemical synapse.

See Appendix for color version. Essential steps in the process of synaptic transmission are numbered.

Source. Reprinted from Purves D, Augustine GJ, Fitzpatrick D, et al. (eds): *Neuroscience*, 3rd Edition. Sunderland, MA, Sinauer Associates, 2004, p. 97. Used with permission.

levels. Cocaine prevents dopamine and serotonin reuptake, whereas amphetamine both slows reuptake of dopamine and serotonin and induces dopamine release (Ramamoorthy and Blakely 1999; Sulzer et al. 2005). Molecular studies have also suggested that cocaine binding and dopamine reuptake occur at separate sites on the transporter, suggesting the possibility that cocaine action could be successfully

blocked without impeding normal reuptake (Lin et al. 2000). Mice lacking the dopamine transporter show a profound persistence of synaptic dopamine, so they appear as if they are permanently on psychostimulants (Giros et al. 1996); psychostimulants have no effect on these animals, confirming that the dopamine transporter is critical to the action of these drugs. MPTP is taken up by the dopamine transporter selectively; once in dopamine neurons, it increases oxidative stress, leading to the demise of the neurons and behaviorally to parkinsonism (Pifl et al. 1996).

RAPID POSTSYNAPTIC RESPONSES

The action of a neurotransmitter depends on the properties of the postsynaptic receptors to which it binds. Postsynaptic receptors activated by neurotransmitter fall into two classes: 1) ionotropic and 2) metabotropic (discussed below). Ionotropic receptors are directly linked to an ion channel; these receptors undergo a conformational change upon neurotransmitter binding that opens the channel. This results in either depolarization, giving rise to an excitatory postsynaptic potential, or hyperpolarization, giving rise to an inhibitory postsynaptic potential.

In the CNS, glutamate receptors mediate most fast excitatory transmission; GABA and glycine are the most common inhibitory neurotransmitters.

GLUTAMATE RECEPTORS

Excitatory postsynaptic potentials are mediated by two classes of ionotropic glutamate receptors: NMDA (*N*-methyl-D-aspartate) receptors and non-NMDA, or AMPA (α-amino-3-hydroxy-5-methylisoxazole-4–propionic acid), receptors (Hassel and Dingledine 2006). NMDA receptors depolarize cells by opening channels that principally allow Ca^{2+} to enter the cell. The most striking property of NMDA receptors is that the ion channel is usually blocked by Mg^{2+} at membrane potentials more negative than about –40 mV (MacDermott et al. 1986; Nowak et al. 1984). As a result, at the resting potential of most neurons, the NMDA receptor channel is occluded. For current to flow through NMDA channels, glutamate must bind to the receptor and the membrane must be depolarized simultaneously to displace the Mg^{2+}. This dual requirement underlies the unique role of NMDA receptors in processes as varied as synaptogenesis, learning and memory, and even cell death. NMDA receptors are also likely to be critical for proper

mental functioning. NMDA receptor hypofunction has been implicated as a pathogenic mechanism in schizophrenia (Coyle 2006).

The non-NMDA glutamate receptors are further divided into AMPA receptors and kainate receptors on the basis of their affinities for these glutamate analogues. AMPA receptors are formed from combinations of subunits GluR1 to GluR4, and kainate receptors are formed from combinations of GluR5 to GluR7 plus KA1 and KA2. Non-NMDA receptors generally gate channels that allow cations to cross the membrane. Neurons that express such Ca^{2+}-permeable AMPA receptors may be particularly vulnerable to excitotoxic cell death in disease states such as amyotrophic lateral sclerosis (Van Den Bosch et al. 2006). Ca^{2+}-permeable AMPA receptors mediate non-NMDA-dependent long-term potentiation, which has been implicated in anxiety states (Mahanty and Sah 1998).

GABA RECEPTORS

Inhibitory postsynaptic potentials in the brain are mediated primarily by GABA receptors (Olsen and Betz 2006). Several classes of GABA receptors have been identified. $GABA_A$ receptors are ionotropic receptors that form Cl^--selective channels and mediate fast synaptic inhibition in the brain. $GABA_B$ receptors are metabotropic receptors that tend to be slower acting and play a modulatory role; they are often found on presynaptic terminals, where they inhibit transmitter release. $GABA_A$ receptors are members of the nicotinic acetylcholine receptor superfamily. The $GABA_A$ receptor-channel complex is composed of a mixture of five subunits from α, β, γ, and ρ families.

GABA receptors are the targets of several potent psychiatric drugs. Benzodiazepines bind to a recognition site formed by the α and γ subunits. The $α_1$ subunits mediate the sedating effects of benzodiazepines and are targeted selectively by the newer-generation soporifics such as zolpidem, while the $α_2$ subunits mediate the anxiolytic effects. The clinical actions of benzodiazepines, along with two other classes of CNS-depressant drugs, barbiturates and anesthetic steroids, as well as ethanol, seem to be related to their ability to bind to $GABA_A$ receptors and to enhance $GABA_A$ receptor currents (Yamakura et al. 2001). Although they engage distinct mechanisms, each of these drugs enhances GABAergic transmission, accounting for their shared properties as anticonvulsants. In fact, they may directly counteract a GABA deficit due to a reduction in GABA transporter numbers in epileptogenic cortex that may be etiological in epilepsy (During et al. 1995).

METABOTROPIC RECEPTORS

Longer-term modulatory effects are generally mediated by metabotropic receptors (Greengard 2001). These non-channel-linked receptors regulate cell function via activation of G proteins that couple to second messenger cascades. In fact, the majority of neurotransmitters and neuromodulators exert their effects through binding to G protein receptors. G protein–linked receptors are so named because they couple to intracellular guanosine triphosphate (GTP)–binding regulatory proteins. G proteins are formed from a complex of three membrane-bound proteins ($G_{\alpha\beta\gamma}$); when the receptor is activated, the α subunit (G_α) binds GTP and dissociates from a complex of the β and γ subunits ($G_{\beta\gamma}$). Both G_α and $G_{\beta\gamma}$ may go on to trigger subsequent events. Activated G proteins have a life span of seconds to minutes.

G proteins are the first link in signaling cascades that either directly activate protein kinases—enzymes that phosphorylate cellular proteins (Walaas and Greengard 1991)—or raise intracellular Ca^{2+} and indirectly activate kinases (Ghosh and Greenberg 1995). Proteins undergo conformational changes when they are phosphorylated that may lead to either their activation or inactivation. Proteins affected may include membrane channels, cytoskeletal elements, and transcriptional regulators of gene expression. In this way, modulatory actions mediated by second messengers control most cellular processes.

The slower actions of metabotropic receptors are responsible for altering neuronal excitability and the strength of synaptic connections, often reinforcing neural pathways involved in learning (Bailey and Kandel 2004). Activation of these receptors generally does not directly change the membrane potential at all. Rather, receptor binding activates second messenger cascades that can dramatically alter the response properties of other receptors. Most profoundly, second messengers may translocate to the nucleus, where they may control gene expression, exerting longer-term changes in cell function via the activation of genes in a temporal sequence (Girault and Greengard 2004). Many long-term adaptations, such as those induced by psychotropic agents, appear to be mediated by adaptations in metabotropic receptor signaling. For instance, the antidepressant effects of SSRIs are not due to the immediate surge in serotonin associated with the blockade of the serotonin reuptake transporter, but rather to longer-term adaptations in signaling mediated by $5\text{-}HT_{1A}$ and $5\text{-}HT_{2A}$ serotonin receptors (Blier and Abbott 2001). Dopaminergic actions in cortex, implicated in the modulation of working memory (Goldman-Rakic et al. 2000), also result in long-term adaptations in cortical signaling (Seamans and Yang 2004).

As these G protein–coupled receptors are the targets of many therapeutic and abused drugs, understanding their regulation is of paramount clinical importance. Major advances have been made in defining the mechanisms mediating the downregulation of G protein–coupled receptors (Tsao and von Zastrow 2000). Receptor downregulation is generally induced by prolonged activation of receptors, leading to receptor internalization. Determining the mechanisms of G protein receptor downregulation may identify targets for development of new classes of drugs useful for the therapeutic manipulation of G protein receptor signaling.

ORGANIZATION OF POSTSYNAPTIC RECEPTORS AT SYNAPSES

Most neurotransmitter receptors are clustered at postsynaptic sites closely apposed to the presynaptic terminal. Several laboratories have made remarkable progress in identifying the molecular components of the postsynaptic scaffold that holds synaptic receptors in place (Figure 1–6) (Lee and Sheng 2000; O'Brien et al. 1998). One of the most abundant proteins in the postsynaptic density is PSD-95. PSD-95 is a cytoplasmic protein that contains three domains important for protein binding, called *PDZ domains*. These domains of PSD-95 bind to the NMDA receptor, to the Shaker K^+ channel, and to cell adhesion proteins called *neuroligins*. In contrast, AMPA receptors bind a distinct PDZ domain protein called GRIP, and metabotropic glutamate receptors interact with HOMER. PDZ proteins in general are believed to cluster neurotransmitter receptors and other important components of the synapse at the postsynaptic density and to localize signaling complexes important for synaptic plasticity to these receptors (Kennedy and Ehlers 2006).

SYNAPTIC MODULATION IN LEARNING AND MEMORY

Learning and memory require both short- and long-term changes at synapses. In addition to rapid signals, neurotransmitters activate second messenger systems that profoundly increase the range of responses a neuron shows to synaptic input. Second messengers activate kinases that both amplify and prolong signals by phosphorylating other proteins. Phosphorylated proteins remain active—often for a much longer period than agonist remains bound to receptor—until they are dephosphorylated by protein phosphatases. Because second messengers trigger numerous cellular functions, activation of a single receptor may trigger a coordinated cellular response involving several systems. This may include activity-dependent modulation of genomic transcription, leading to enduring changes in cellular function.

LONG-TERM POTENTIATION

Since the pioneering observations more than 50 years ago on patient H.M., who following bilateral hippocampal resection was no longer able to encode memories, studies of memory have focused on the circuitry of the hippocampus (Lynch 2004). This focus was further strengthened, more than 30 years ago, by the discovery that brief high-frequency stimulation of hippocampal pathways leads to long-term potentiation (LTP) of synaptic connections (Bliss and Lomo 1973). In intact animals, LTP may last for days to weeks, and so has come to be seen as the crucial synaptic process underlying memory formation. In the hippocampus, each of the three major synaptic circuits shows LTP, with distinct but shared mechanisms. At the most studied synapse, the Schaffer collateral synapse made by the projections of CA3 onto CA1 pyramidal neurons (Figure 1–7), LTP is initiated by Ca^{2+} influx into the postsynaptic neuron via NMDA receptors. Although glutamate released by CA3 neurons acts on NMDA and AMPA receptors, only high-frequency firing activates sufficient numbers of AMPA receptors to depolarize the postsynaptic membrane, relieve the voltage-dependent Mg^{2+} block of the NMDA receptor, and allow Ca^{2+} influx, initiating LTP (Blitzer et al. 2005). Because NMDA receptor activation requires both binding of neurotransmitter and postsynaptic depolarization, the NMDA receptor provides molecular coincidence detection, requiring that alterations in synaptic strength involve coordinated pre- and postsynaptic activity.

The influx of Ca^{2+} into the postsynaptic CA3 neuron activates Ca^{2+}/calmodulin-dependent protein kinase II (CaMKII), which mediates the phosphorylation of AMPA receptors, increasing their sensitivity (Lisman et al. 2002). CaMKII is capable of autophosphorylation and locks itself in an active catalytic state. This provides a molecular basis for early LTP. Ca^{2+} also activates calcineurin (PP2b), a phosphatase, which modulates PP1, which in turn can dephosphorylate CaMKII and block LTP. Calcineurin's action is modulated by cAMP, which acting through protein kinase A blocks PP1 activity (Blitzer et al. 1998). This pathway, which is activated by catecholamines and Ca^{2+}, serves a gating function. Dopamine acting via D_1 receptors is required for late LTP (Huang and Kandel 1995).

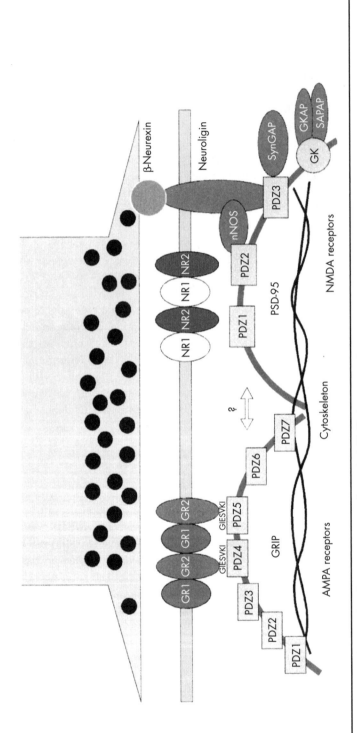

FIGURE 1–6.   Some of the molecular components of a typical CNS glutamatergic synapse.

α-Amino-3-hydroxy-5-methylisoxazole-4-propionic acid (AMPA) receptor subunits are tethered to GRIP through PDZ domain interactions, and the N-methyl-D-aspartate (NMDA) receptor subunits are bound to PSD-95. Both GRIP and PSD-95 also interact with the cytoskeleton, providing a protein scaffold for glutamate receptors in the postsynaptic density. This scaffold may regulate the dynamic, activity-dependent insertion or removal of glutamate receptors from CNS synapses. GIESVKI = the amino acids critical for binding GR2 to PDZ4 and PDZ5; nNOS = neuronal nitric oxide synthase.

Source.   Reprinted from O'Brien RJ, Lau LF, Huganir RL: "Molecular Mechanisms of Glutamate Receptor Clustering at Excitatory Synapses." *Current Opinion in Neurobiology* 8:364–369, 1998. Copyright 1998. Used with permission from Elsevier.

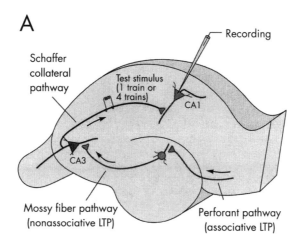

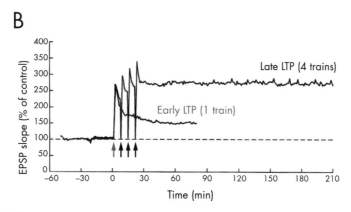

FIGURE 1–7.   Long-term potentiation (LTP) in the hippocampus.

Panel A. A brain slice preparation from the rodent hippocampus is shown with the postsynaptic recording electrode in a CA1 pyramidal cell and a presynaptic stimulating electrode (coil) on the Schaffer collateral pathway axon of a CA3 pyramidal cell. *Panel B.* Stimulating the Schaffer collateral pathway at low frequency (once a minute) causes the CA3 axon terminals to release glutamate, which evokes a stable excitatory response (measured as the rising slope of the excitatory postsynaptic potential, EPSP; the control response is normalized to 100%). A single tetanus (*gray arrow*, 100 stimuli in 1 second) evokes early LTP, which is weak and lasts on the order of an hour. In contrast, with four tetani (*gray and black arrows*), the postsynaptic response is dramatically increased. Late LTP lasts for over 24 hours, as would be required for a synaptic mechanism encoding long-term memory.

Source. Adapted from Kandel ER: "Cellular Mechanisms of Learning and the Biological Basis of Individuality," in *Principles of Neural Science*, 4th Edition. Edited by Kandel ER, Schwartz JH, Jessell TM. New York, McGraw-Hill, 2000, pp. 1247–1279. Copyright 2000, The McGraw-Hill Companies, Inc. Used with permission.

LTP is composed of at least two phases: early and late LTP. Early LTP lasts for the first 3 hours after induction and does not require protein synthesis. In contrast, late LTP lasts for several hours and requires both gene transcription and protein translation. Late LTP involves activation of CaMKII, production of cAMP, and activation of gene transcription through a cAMP-response element binding protein (CREB)–dependent process. LTP can also stimulate the growth of new synaptic connections. Such changes are likely to underlie the more permanent synaptic alterations necessary for learning and memory (Bailey and Kandel 2004). In early LTP, synaptic strengthening occurs postsynaptically via increased sensitivity of existing AMPA receptors. As memory is encoded in late LTP, AMPA receptors are inserted into functionally silent synapses, and altogether new postsynaptic structures develop (Lisman et al. 2002). In particular, *silent* synapses—synapses that contain only NMDA receptors before induction of LTP—may be activated by activity-dependent insertion of new AMPA receptors. Increases in AMPA receptor function at previously silent synapses after LTP-inducing stimuli also mediate long-term plasticity. Relatively subtle changes in AMPA receptor trafficking are crucial, as has been shown in the amygdala for fear conditioning (Rumpel et al. 2005).

Whereas the *induction* of LTP is postsynaptic and depends on Ca^{2+} and the activation of CaMKII, the *expression* of LTP involves coordinated pre- and postsynaptic changes. Recordings from single synapses have shown that the expression of LTP is associated with an increase in the numbers of synaptic vesicles released (Bolshakov et al. 1997).

How is the strengthening of synapses by LTP kept in check? Hippocampal synapses also show long-term depression (LTD), which involves a similar array of mechanisms activated by low-frequency synaptic activation (Anwyl 2006). LTD may be mediated by a decrease in neurotransmitter release and/or a decrease in postsynaptic responsiveness due to lowered numbers or sensitivity of glutamate receptors. Thus, through a dynamic balance between LTP and LTD, memories of irrelevant information may be eliminated and lasting memories finetuned. The regulation of synaptic strength appears to be controlled in the hippocampus by the predominant theta rhythm. Stimulation at the theta frequency produces LTP, whereas stimulation that is slower or specifically associated with the troughs of the rhythm produces LTD (Huerta and Lisman 1996). Possibly alterations in brain rhythms, implicated in several neuropsychiatric disorders (Behrendt and

Young 2004; Spencer et al. 2004), act in part via modulation of synaptic plasticity.

DEVELOPMENT OF NEURONS

NEUROGENESIS

The human nervous system is the most complex organ system in vertebrates and contains a greater variety of cell types than is found in any other organ. Remarkably, the diversity of cell types that regulate every aspect of our lives is accomplished during a brief span of development, encompassing just 3–4 months in humans. It is therefore not surprising that this critical period of gestation is sensitive to interference through environmental factors and pathogens, as well as genetic mutations. For example, extrinsic factors such as alcohol exposure have been shown to decrease neuronal production, and in severe cases to produce microcephaly and mental retardation (Miller 1989). In addition, mutations in the doublecortin gene dramatically interfere with neocortical development, resulting in epilepsy and in severe cortical malformations such as lissencephaly (des Portes et al. 1998; Gleeson et al. 1998).

The principal cell types in the brain, neurons and glia, are generated in two proliferative zones that line the ventricular system during development, after which they migrate into the overlying cortical mantle. Each proliferative zone comprises a different class of progenitor cells. The ventricular zone (VZ), which is adjacent to the ventricular lumen during CNS development, consists primarily of *radial glial cells* (Rakic 1971). Radial glia are bipolar cells with a soma located in the VZ, a long, thin ascending process that often contacts the pial surface of the developing brain (Misson et al. 1988), and a short descending process that contacts the ventricular lumen. A second proliferative zone, the subventricular zone (SVZ), appears just above the VZ at the onset of neurogenesis in many CNS regions (Boulder Committee 1970). SVZ progenitor cells are generated by VZ precursor cells but have distinguishing features. SVZ cells are multipolar, they do not maintain contact with the pial and ventricular surfaces as do radial glial cells, and they divide away from the ventricular lumen (Takahashi et al. 1995).

Radial glial cells are present along the entire axis of the developing CNS (Ramón y Cajal 1911), raising the possibility that they might be universal neural progenitor cells. When neurogenesis is complete, radial glial cells migrate away from the proliferative zones into the cortical mantle and transform into mature astrocytes in several brain regions (Schmechel and Rakic 1979). Individual radial glial cells can generate neurons before transforming into astrocytes (Noctor et al. 2004). Astrocytes remain capable of division in the postnatal brain and, interestingly, can generate neurons in specific regions of the adult brain such as the hippocampus (Doetsch et al. 1999; Seri et al. 2001). Identification and characterization of these important progenitor cells has led to identification of a potential source of cells for replacement strategies in the treatment of neurodegenerative disorders.

A number of factors, including neurotransmitter substances, growth factors, and even hormones, are present in proliferative regions of the brain and are known to regulate cell division in the developing and adult brain. For example, it has been shown that the classical neurotransmitters GABA and glutamate differentially regulate proliferation in the ventricular and subventricular zones during neocortical development (Haydar et al. 2000; LoTurco et al. 1995). Proliferative VZ radial glial cells are coupled to one another through connexin gap junction channels (LoTurco and Kriegstein 1991). New evidence indicates that waves of Ca^{2+} activity in radial glial cells are transmitted through connexin channels (gap junctions) and may be instrumental in regulating the proliferation of radial glial cells and thereby neurogenesis (Weissman et al. 2004). These and many other varied factors thus work in conjunction to regulate the proliferative behavior of progenitor cells during specific stages of brain development.

MIGRATION

Neurons in the adult brain are organized into complex, intricately interconnected groups of nuclei and laminae. One of the remarkable aspects of brain development is that neurons are not born in their final locations. Instead, neurons are generated in proliferative zones surrounding the ventricular lumen and then must migrate substantial distances, as long as 7,000 µm or more, to reach their destination. Despite the complexity of the task, this feat is achieved with such regularity and precision that there is little variation in the architectonic pattern of brain structures from one person to the next, and even between species. In the developing neocortex, cortical neurons are generated in an inside-out sequence such that the deepest layers of the cerebral cortex form first, and subsequent waves of migrating neurons traverse the established layers as they migrate into the cortical mantle. Thus, as development proceeds, neurons must migrate progressively longer distances and through increasing numbers of cortical cells. Migration relies on cell-cell adhesion ligand molecules that signal between the radial glial fibers and migrating neurons (Hatten 1990). Neuronal migration is also regulated by a number of extracellular signaling molecules, such as neurotransmitter substances acting through the NMDA receptor (Komuro and Rakic 1993) and reelin protein acting through its constituent receptor molecules (Tissir and Goffinet 2003).

Different forms of migration have been identified in other regions of the developing brain, such as the tangential migration of interneurons from the ganglionic eminences of the ventral telencephalon into the dorsal telencephalon. Interneurons do not appear to migrate along radial glial fibers during their journey from the ventral into the dorsal telencephalon. But it has yet to be determined whether they rely on cellular guides, such as developing axonal pathways in the intermediate zone of the developing cortex, or rather are guided solely along gradients of chemoattractive and repulsive factors (Marin and Rubenstein 2003). Despite differences in the forms of migration, each appears to rely on a shared set of intracellular molecules that are involved in the extension of leading processes and the transportation of cellular structures such as the nucleus (Feng and Walsh 2001). Neuronal migration is thus a complex interplay between the migrating cell and its environment that relies on intracellular machinery as well as extrinsic signaling factors. Given the complexity of this task, it is not surprising that a number of nervous system malformations have been identified that result from defects in neuronal migration (Feng and Walsh 2001). These range from severe brain malformations such as lissencephaly to periventricular nodular heterotopia to more moderate cases involving small ectopic clusters of neurons. In each case, varying proportions of neurons fail to migrate to their proper destinations. Afflicted individuals present with mental retardation in severe cases. Mild malformations are often associated with epilepsy. The lifelong impact of these neurological disorders on affected individuals and families cannot be overstated and necessitates further research for the root causes of these conditions.

SYNAPSE FORMATION

Once neurons migrate to their proper position in the brain, they stop moving and start differentiating. Axons extend sometimes extremely long distances to connect to their appropriate targets, thereby forming the nerves that subserve all neurological and psychiatric function. When an axonal growth cone reaches a target cell, a complex series of interactions commences, ultimately resulting in the formation of a synapse. Although there is still much to be learned about the formation of synapses in the CNS, the basic process of synaptogenesis at the neuromuscular junction (NMJ; the synapse between a motor neuron and a muscle cell) has been well described (Figure 1–8). Both the motor neuron and the muscle cell have the necessary molecular machinery prefabricated before synapse formation (Sanes and Lichtman 1999). The motor neuron growth cone functions like a protosynapse, showing activity-

dependent neurotransmitter release. Non-innervated postsynaptic cells have transmitter receptors distributed over much of their surface, and within minutes of initial contact, a rudimentary form of synaptic transmission begins. Over subsequent days, connections become stronger and stabilize as the growth cone matures into a presynaptic terminal, gathering the cellular elements necessary for focused release of neurotransmitter at active zones. In parallel, the postsynaptic cell concentrates receptors at the site of contact, removing them from other regions, and over the course of days it develops postsynaptic specializations.

Although there are many differences between the NMJ and CNS synapses, the general principles of synapse formation appear to be conserved. As at the NMJ, presynaptic and postsynaptic proteins are present in axons and dendrites, respectively, of CNS neurons prior to synapse formation. Pre- and postsynaptic proteins are transported in multi-protein-containing transport vesicles that are mobile before synapse formation (Washbourne et al. 2004; Ziv and Garner 2004). These mobile transport vesicles accumulate rapidly at new sites of contact between CNS neurons. Axodendritic contact is followed within minutes by the rapid and simultaneous recruitment of synaptic vesicles and NMDA receptors to new synapses (Washbourne et al. 2002). This early recruitment of NMDA receptors, but not AMPA receptors, to new synapses has been described in multiple systems; the resulting synapses are electrically "silent" until AMPA receptors are inserted (Isaac 2003). In the hours following contact, scaffolding proteins such as PSD-95 are also recruited to nascent synapses by as yet unknown mechanisms (Kim and Sheng 2004).

In order for synapses to form so quickly, specific contacts between axons and dendrites must initiate intracellular signals that lead to rapid recruitment of pre- and postsynaptic proteins. In general, there are three major classes of signals that regulate synapse formation: adhesion molecules, diffusible molecules, and molecules secreted from glial cells (McAllister 2007). Recent studies have begun to pro-

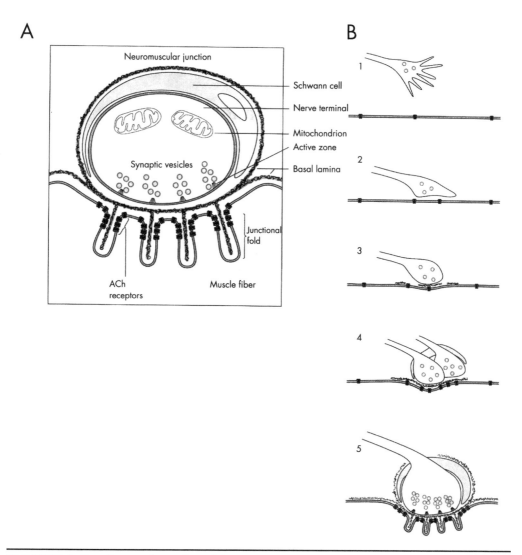

FIGURE 1–8. Synapse formation of the neuromuscular junction (NMJ).

Panel A. Schematic view of the molecular components of a typical neuromuscular junction. At a mature NMJ, the presynaptic terminal is separated from the postsynaptic muscle cell by the synaptic cleft. Synaptic vesicles filled with acetylcholine (ACh) are clustered at active zones, where they can fuse with the plasma membrane upon depolarization to release their transmitter into the synaptic cleft. Ach receptors are found postsynaptically, and glial cells called Schwann cells surround the synaptic terminal. *Panel B.* Stages in the formation of the NMJ: 1) An isolated growth cone from a motor neuron is guided to the muscle by axon guidance cues. 2) The first contact is an unspecialized physical contact. 3) However, synaptic vesicles rapidly cluster in the axon terminal, Ach receptors start to cluster under the forming synapse, and a basal lamina is deposited in the synaptic cleft. 4) As development proceeds, multiple motor neurons innervate each muscle. 5) Over time, however, all but one of the axons are eliminated through an activity-dependent process, and the remaining terminal matures.

Source. Reprinted from Sanes JR, Jessell TM: "The Formation and Regeneration of Synapses," in *Principles of Neural Science,* 4th Edition. Edited by Kandel ER, Schwartz JH, Jessell TM. New York, McGraw-Hill, 2000, pp. 1087–1114. Copyright 2000, The McGraw-Hill Companies, Inc. Used with permission.

vide strong evidence that a lack, or abnormal expression, of synaptogenic molecules may cause neurodevelopmental disorders. For example, intense interest has recently been focused on the possibility that mutations in one or more of the genes that encode the neuroligin/β-neurexin cell adhesion pair may contribute to some forms of autism (Chih et al. 2004). The second class of synaptogenic molecules is diffusible molecules—brain-derived neurotrophic factor (BDNF) and members of the Wnt and TGF-β families (Salinas 2005). Less is known about how and when, after initial contact, these molecules influence the recruitment of synaptic proteins to new contacts. Finally, the role of glial cells in regulating synapse formation has been an area of recent intense research (Allen and Barres 2005). Glial cells potently influence synapse formation and function through the secretion of thrombospondins, cholesterol, and cytokines. In sum, although this field is making remarkably rapid progress in identifying synaptogenic molecules, there is not yet a clear understanding of how these many molecules interact to initiate synapse formation. Moreover, little is known about the molecular mechanisms of synapse stabilization or elimination in the CNS—processes that are critical for learning and memory and that are likely to give rise to connectional deficits in neurodegenerative disorders.

NEURONAL MATURATION AND SURVIVAL

In many areas of the vertebrate nervous system, neurons are initially produced in excess. To survive, neurons must receive an adequate supply of one or more trophic factors produced by their target neurons. Competition for limited supplies of these factors ensures that surviving neurons will be correctly connected and that the number of neurons will be matched to the size of the target. In general, cells deprived of neurotrophic factors undergo apoptosis, a genetically programmed form of cell death characterized by cytoplasmic shrinkage, chromatin condensation, and degradation of DNA

into oligonucleosomal fragments (Edwards et al. 1991). Apoptosis is an active process that requires RNA and protein synthesis (Oppenheim et al. 1991; Scott and Davies 1990). Data are accumulating to support the remarkable hypothesis that apoptosis is the default program for most cells and that widespread cell suicide is prevented only by the continual presence of survival signals that suppress the intrinsic cell death program (Raff et al. 1993).

The molecular events that underlie apoptosis are likely to include an array of initiators, mediators, and inhibitors, but several common features are emerging. There is evidence that reactive oxygen species can trigger apoptosis in neurons (Greenlund et al. 1995), and *Bcl-2* may prevent apoptosis by suppressing free radical production (Hockenbery et al. 1990; Kane et al. 1993). This hypothesis has led to attempts to use antioxidants and inhibitors of free radical production as therapeutic agents in several neurodegenerative diseases, trauma, and stroke. For example, superoxide dismutase (a free-radical scavenger) protects neurons from ischemic injury. Transgenic mice that overexpress superoxide dismutase have smaller infarcts after arterial occlusion (Kinouchi et al. 1991). Mutations in the Cu/Zn superoxide dismutase gene are associated with certain forms of familial amyotrophic lateral sclerosis, suggesting that oxygen radicals may be responsible for motor neuron degeneration in patients with this disease (Rosen et al. 1993).

EXPERIENCE-DEPENDENT SYNAPTIC REFINEMENT

Normal sensory experience is essential to the maturation of neural connections in both the peripheral and central nervous systems. Sensory experience shapes the development of many diverse brain regions during a specific time window during development called the *critical period*. The process of synaptic refinement becomes clinically significant as it continues to be important throughout the life span, providing mechanisms for activity-dependent modification of neuronal structure and connectivity that may be the basis for learning, memory, and forgetting.

The cellular and molecular mechanisms underlying activity-dependent synaptic refinement are just beginning to be elucidated. Many of these mechanisms are remarkably similar to the cellular mechanisms that underlie learning and memory in the adult brain. In the visual system, geniculate afferents are believed to undergo segregation into ocular dominance (OD) columns based on a Hebbian learning rule (Hebb 1949), whereby neurons that fire together are selectively strengthened. This rule predicts that neurons that fire synchronously will strengthen their synapses, whereas asynchronous firing will weaken synapses. LTP and LTD are attractive candidates for mediating the process of OD column formation (Bear and Rittenhouse 1999). In addition to activity, molecular signals such as the neurotrophins may also act to selectively strengthen coincidentally active synapses (Huberman and McAllister 2002). Finally, in recent years, a critical role for inhibitory neurons in mediating activity-dependent changes in circuitry has been revealed.

NEUROTROPHIC AND NEUROTOXIC ACTIONS OF NEUROTRANSMITTERS

Neurotransmitters themselves may have trophic or toxic roles in the shaping of neurons and their interconnections (Lipton and Kater 1989). Excitatory neurotransmitters such as glutamate trigger Ca^{2+} influx that controls the progress of growth cones. Local intracellular levels of Ca^{2+} act within a narrow window. When levels are low, growth cones are quiescent; when levels rise, growth cones begin to move. Above a certain level, however, further elevations of Ca^{2+} arrest growth and cause retraction or destruction of neuronal processes (al-Mohanna et al. 1992). This can be countered by inhibitory neurotransmitters as well as by provision of neurotrophic factors (Kater et al. 1989; Mattson and Kater 1989).

Higher levels of glutamate produce excitotoxicity, perhaps reflecting the pathologic functioning of these developmental signaling systems (Kater et al. 1989). Alternatively, excitotoxicity may have a normal function in regulating cell numbers and connectivity. Excitotoxicity appears to be mediated acutely by the entry of Na^+ through AMPA channels. This leads to neuronal swelling (resulting in brain edema). Sustained Ca^{2+} entry through NMDA receptor channels causes a delayed mode of excitotoxicity that kills neurons, probably by activation of intracellular proteases and/or generation of free radicals (Arundine and Tymianski 2003; Choi 1994; Dawson et al. 1994).

Excitotoxicity figures prominently in neuronal loss in strokes, status epilepticus, hypoglycemia, and head trauma (Choi and Rothman 1990). These brain insults are linked in that all lead to neuronal depolarization, which results in excessive electrical activity, evoking excessive increases in glutamate release. In each case, elevated levels of extracellular glutamate are present in experimental models, and their cytopathology can be mimicked by intracerebral injections of excitatory amino acids. The same neurons spared in these disease states are also less affected in the experimental models, probably because they have fewer excitatory amino acid receptors. Injured neurons show increased intracellular levels of Ca^{2+}, and excitatory amino acid antagonists, particularly those blocking NMDA receptors or channels, prevent or dramatically reduce neuronal loss in these conditions.

Similarities between other neuropsychiatric disorders and idiopathic neurodegenerative disorders suggest a pervasive role for excitotoxic mechanisms (Arundine and Tymianski 2003). Intriguingly, a growing body of findings implicates excitotoxic mechanisms in the pathology of Huntington's disease. The neuropathology of Huntington's disease is mimicked by the injection of excitatory amino acids, and the same classes of striatal neurons are spared in both cases (Wexler et al. 1991).

PERSPECTIVES

Brain development is not determined merely by cell-autonomous genetic programs but is instead highly interactive, depending on complex hierarchies of signaling factors operating to progressively restrict cell fate. Once cells have achieved a specific phenotype and have arrived at an appropriate location, competition for survival factors provides another opportunity for environmental influence over developmental outcome. The cellular development of the brain is therefore not strictly lineage dependent, but rather involves a remarkable degree of interactive signaling. In many brain areas, pruning of exuberant synaptic contacts on an activity-dependent basis is yet another example of a mechanism by which experience can refine structural aspects of brain development. One consequence of these developmental mechanisms is that no two outcomes will be exactly the same, even in a case of twins with identical genetic makeup. Another consequence is the potential for pathologic disruption of normal development by physical, chemical, or infectious agents in the fetal or neonatal period.

It is becoming increasingly clear that the adult brain retains a significant degree of plasticity throughout life and that changes in cortical organization can be induced by behaviorally important, temporally coincident sensory inputs (Buonomano and Merzenich 1998). Behavioral training of adult owl monkeys in discrimination of the temporal features of a tactile stimulus can alter the spatial and temporal response properties of cortical neurons. When adult owl monkeys are rewarded for responding to a 30-Hz tactile stimulation of one finger, there is a progressive increase in the area of somatosensory cortex over which neurons respond to the 30-Hz stimulation. The kinds of changes that take place in the organization of somatosensory cortex also occur in primary auditory cortex. Owl monkeys trained for several weeks to discriminate small differences in the frequency of sequentially presented tones demonstrate progressive improvement in performance with training. At the end of the training period, the amount of cortex responding to behaviorally relevant frequencies is increased. In control studies with equivalent stimulation procedures in which stimuli are unattended, no

significant representational changes are recorded. Thus, attended, rewarded behaviors can induce changes in the organization of primary sensory cortex that are correlated with an improvement in perceptual acuity. These experiments begin to suggest ways in which life experiences, including psychotherapy (Etkin et al. 2005), can potentially modify cortical function and alter perception or behavior.

These plastic changes appear to share a common molecular language that is first expressed during development involving activity-dependent mechanisms. Neural activity is essential to activity-dependent synaptic refinement, LTP, LTD, and excitotoxicity (Bailey et al. 2000; Brown et al. 1990; Choi and Rothman 1990; Constantine-Paton et al. 1990; Lipton and Kater 1989). The key player is the NMDA receptor, which requires both agonist binding and depolarization for activation. This appears to be the essential requirement for pairing specificity, a mode of synaptic plasticity initially postulated by Hebb (1949), whereby simultaneous activation of presynaptic and postsynaptic elements strengthens connections. Simultaneously, correlation of presynaptic activity with postsynaptic inhibition may selectively weaken connections (Reiter and Stryker 1988). The Ca^{2+} influx mediated by the NMDA receptor may trigger changes in the strength of synapses, in time leading to more permanent structural changes in synapse number. At higher levels, Ca^{2+} may arrest the growth of neurites, cause their retraction, or selectively lesion the susceptible cell.

Many neuropsychiatric disorders no doubt play out in this context. To consider a few examples, most of which have already been mentioned, striatal degeneration in Huntington's disease appears to be due to the overproduction of huntingtin, a synaptic vesicle–associated protein (DiFiglia et al. 1995) that among a multiplicity of actions may trigger NMDA receptor–mediated excitotoxicity (Rego and de Almeida 2005). In Parkinson's disease, a selective loss of dopaminergic neurons in the substantia nigra may be the delayed result of a viral process, lesioning by dopaminergic neurotoxins exemplified by MPTP, or a deficiency in BDNF or glia cell line–derived neurotrophic factor, both of which may be essential for the survival of dopaminergic neurons (Cardoso et al. 2005). In Alzheimer's disease, the loss of cholinergic neurons may result from a deficiency or perhaps aberrant handling of nerve growth factor once it is taken up by neurons in the basal forebrain (Pereira et al. 2005). Clearly, elucidation of the cellular and molecular events that occur during normal brain development, maturation, and aging, as well as those that underlie neuropsychiatric disorders, will greatly enhance approaches to their treatment and prevention.

Perhaps the most exciting and revolutionary possible intervention to treat neuropsychiatric diseases is the potential use of stem cells to repair the damaged brain (Lee et al. 2000). Despite tremendous efforts by the neuroscience community during the last century, there are currently no feasible therapies for repairing the damaged adult human brain. Clearly, treatment of many neuropsychiatric diseases would be greatly enhanced if new neurons could be added to a particular damaged brain region and stimulated to differentiate into the appropriate neuronal type and to form appropriate connections. There are currently two approaches to achieving this goal. First, pluripotent stem cells are being used, with increasing success, to repopulate damaged brain regions. For example, adult rats with symptoms similar to Parkinson's disease can regain function after implantation of dopaminergic neurons created in vitro from fetal rat neuronal precursors (Studer et al. 1998). Second, newly discovered intrinsic repair mechanisms in the adult brain are being studied for their therapeutic potential. Neurogenesis has been discovered in several regions of the adult brain, including the dentate gyrus of the hippocampal formation (Fuchs and Gould 2000). These neurons migrate within the brain regions, differentiate, and form functional connections. Moreover, experience, learning, and physical exercise enhance neuronal proliferation in the adult (Fuchs and Gould 2000; Kempermann et

al. 2004). The discovery of neurogenesis in the adult brain suggests that the adult brain may have intrinsic mechanisms for repair that could be manipulated to treat neurodegenerative disorders (Kozorovitskiy and Gould 2003; Lie et al. 2004). As the mechanisms of neuropsychiatric disorders are resolved at the cellular and molecular levels, and the tremendous potential of stem cell research is harnessed, it is likely that revolutionary treatments for many neuropsychiatric diseases will be forthcoming.

RECOMMENDED READINGS

Cummings JL: Toward a molecular neuropsychiatry of neurodegenerative diseases. Ann Neurol 54:147–154, 2003

Graham D, Lantos P: Greenfield's Neuropathology, 7th Edition. London, Arnold, 2002

Kandel ER, Schwartz JH, Jessell TM: Principles of Neural Science, 4th Edition. New York, McGraw-Hill, 2000

Siegel GJ, Albers RW, Brady S, et al: Basic Neurochemistry: Molecular, Cellular and Medical Aspects, 7th Edition. New York, Elsevier, 2006

REFERENCES

Allen NJ, Barres BA: Signaling between glia and neurons: focus on synaptic plasticity. Curr Opin Neurobiol 15:542–548, 2005

al-Mohanna FA, Cave J, Bolsover SR: A narrow window of intracellular calcium concentration is optimal for neurite outgrowth in rat sensory neurones. Brain Res Dev Brain Res 70:287–290, 1992

Ansorge MS, Zhou M, Lira A, et al: Early life blockade of the 5-HT transporter alters emotional behavior in adult mice. Science 306:879–881, 2004

Anwyl R: Induction and expression mechanisms of postsynaptic NMDA receptor-independent homosynaptic long-term depression. Prog Neurobiol 78:17–37, 2006

Araque A, Parpura V, Sanzgiri RP, et al: Tripartite synapses: glia, the unacknowledged partner. Trends Neurosci 22:208–215, 1999

Arundine M, Tymianski M: Molecular mechanisms of calcium-dependent neurodegeneration in excitotoxicity. Cell Calcium 34:325–337, 2003

Bailey C, Kandel E: Synaptic growth and the persistence of long-term memory: a molecular perspective, in The Cognitive Neurosciences, 3rd Edition. Edited by Gazzaniga MS. Cambridge, MA, MIT Press, 2004, pp 647–663

Bailey CH, Giustetto M, Huang YY, et al: Is heterosynaptic modulation essential for stabilizing Hebbian plasticity and memory? Nat Rev Neurosci 1:11–20, 2000

Bear MF, Rittenhouse CD: Molecular basis for induction of ocular dominance plasticity. J Neurobiol 41:83–91, 1999

Behrendt RP, Young C: Hallucinations in schizophrenia, sensory impairment, and brain disease: a unifying model. Behav Brain Sci 27:771–830, 2004

Bennett MVL: Electrical transmission: a functional analysis and comparison to chemical transmission, in Handbook of Physiology, Vol I: The Nervous System. Bethesda, MD, American Physiological Society, 1977, pp 357–416

Bennett MVL, Barrio LC, Bargiello TA, et al: Gap junctions: new tools, new answers, new questions. Neuron 6:305–320, 1991

Black IB: Trophic interactions and brain plasticity, in The Cognitive Neurosciences. Edited by Gazzaniga MS. Cambridge, MA, MIT Press, 1995, pp 9–17

Blier P, Abbott FV: Putative mechanisms of action of antidepressant drugs in affective and anxiety disorders and pain. J Psychiatry Neurosci 26:37–43, 2001

Bliss TV, Lomo T: Long-lasting potentiation of synaptic transmission in the dentate area of the anaesthetized rabbit following stimulation of the perforant path. J Physiol 232:331–356, 1973

Blitzer RD, Connor JH, Brown GP, et al: Gating of CaMKII by cAMP-regulated protein phosphatase activity during LTP. Science 280:1940–1942, 1998

Blitzer RD, Iyengar R, Landau EM: Postsynaptic signaling networks: cellular cogwheels underlying long-term plasticity. Biol Psychiatry 57:113–119, 2005

Bolshakov VY, Golan H, Kandel ER, et al: Recruitment of new sites of synaptic transmission during the cAMP-dependent late phase of LTP at CA3-CA1 synapses in the hippocampus. Neuron 19:635–651, 1997

Boulder Committee: Embryonic vertebrate central nervous system: revised terminology. Anat Rec 166:257–261, 1970

Brivanlou IH, Warland DK, Meister M: Mechanisms of concerted firing among retinal ganglion cells. Neuron 20:527–539, 1998

Brown TH, Kairiss EW, Keenan CL: Hebbian synapses: biophysical mechanisms and algorithms. Annu Rev Neurosci 13:475–511, 1990

Buonomano DV, Merzenich MM: Cortical plasticity: from synapses to maps. Annu Rev Neurosci 21:149–186, 1998

Burack MA, Silverman MA, Banker G: The role of selective transport in neuronal protein sorting. Neuron 26:465–472, 2000

Cardoso SM, Moreira PI, Agostinho P, et al: Neurodegenerative pathways in Parkinson's disease: therapeutic strategies. Curr Drug Targets CNS Neurol Disord 4:405–419, 2005

Caspi A, Sugden K, Moffitt TE, et al: Influence of life stress on depression: moderation by a polymorphism in the 5-HTT gene. Science 301:386–389, 2003

Chih B, Afridi SK, Clark L, et al: Disorder-associated mutations lead to functional inactivation of neuroligins. Hum Mol Genet 13:1471–1477, 2004

Choi DW: Calcium and excitotoxic neuronal injury. Ann N Y Acad Sci 747:162–171, 1994

Choi DW, Rothman SM: The role of glutamate neurotoxicity in hypoxic-ischemic neuronal death. Annu Rev Neurosci 13:171–182, 1990

Constantine-Paton M, Cline HT, Debski E: Patterned activity, synaptic convergence, and the NMDA receptor in developing visual pathways. Annu Rev Neurosci 13:129–154, 1990

Coyle JT: The neurochemistry of schizophrenia, in Basic Neurochemistry: Molecular, Cellular and Medical Aspects, 7th Edition. Edited by Siegel GJ, Albers RW, Brady S, et al. Burlington, MA, Elsevier Academic, 2006, pp 875–885

Cummings JL: Toward a molecular neuropsychiatry of neurodegenerative diseases. Ann Neurol 54:147–154, 2003

Dani JW, Chernjavsky A, Smith SJ: Neuronal activity triggers calcium waves in hippocampal astrocyte networks. Neuron 8:429–440, 1992

Dawson TM, Zhang J, Dawson VL, et al: Nitric oxide: cellular regulation and neuronal injury. Prog Brain Res 103:365–369, 1994

Dealy CN, Beyer EC, Kosher RA: Expression patterns of mRNAs for the gap junction proteins connexin43 and connexin42 suggest their involvement in chick limb morphogenesis and specification of the arterial vasculature. Dev Dyn 199:156–167, 1994 des Portes V, Pinard JM, Billuart P, et al: A novel CNS gene required for neuronal migration and involved in X-linked subcortical laminar heterotopia and lissencephaly syndrome. Cell 92:51–61, 1998

DiFiglia M, Sapp E, Chase K, et al: Huntingtin is a cytoplasmic protein associated with vesicles in human and rat brain neurons. Neuron 14:1075–1081, 1995

Dillon C, Goda Y: The actin cytoskeleton: integrating form and function at the synapse. Annu Rev Neurosci 28:25–55, 2005

Doetsch F, Caille I, Lim DA, et al: Subventricular zone astrocytes are neural stem cells in the adult mammalian brain. Cell 97:703–716, 1999

During MJ, Ryder KM, Spencer DD: Hippocampal GABA transporter function in temporal-lobe epilepsy. Nature 376:174–177, 1995

Edwards SN, Buckmaster AE, Tolkovsky AM: The death programme in cultured sympathetic neurones can be suppressed at the posttranslational level by nerve growth factor, cyclic AMP, and depolarization. J Neurochem 57:2140–2143, 1991

Eilers J, Konnerth A: Dendritic signal integration. Curr Opin Neurobiol 7:385–390, 1997

Etkin A, Pittenger C, Polan HJ, et al: Toward a neurobiology of psychotherapy: basic science and clinical applications. J Neuropsychiatry Clin Neurosci 17:145–158, 2005

Fellin T, Carmignoto G: Neurone-to-astrocyte signalling in the brain represents a distinct multifunctional unit. J Physiol 559:3–15, 2004

Feng Y, Walsh CA: Protein-protein interactions, cytoskeletal regulation and neuronal migration. Nat Rev Neurosci 2:408–416, 2001

Fuchs E, Gould E: Mini-review: in vivo neurogenesis in the adult brain: regulation and functional implications. Eur J Neurosci 12:2211–2214, 2000

Gainetdinov RR, Caron MG: Monoamine transporters: from genes to behavior. Annu Rev Pharmacol Toxicol 43:261–284, 2003

Ghosh A, Greenberg ME: Calcium signaling in neurons: molecular mechanisms and cellular consequences. Science 268:239–247, 1995

Girault JA, Greengard P: Principles of signal transduction, in Neurobiology of Mental Illness, 2nd Edition. Edited by Charney DS, Nestler EJ. New York, Oxford University Press, 2004, pp 41–65

Giros B, Jaber M, Jones SR, et al: Hyperlocomotion and indifference to cocaine and amphetamine in mice lacking the dopamine transporter. Nature 379:606–612, 1996

Gleeson JG, Allen KM, Fox JW, et al: Doublecortin, a brain-specific gene mutated in human X-linked lissencephaly and double cortex syndrome, encodes a putative signaling protein. Cell 92:63–72, 1998

Goldman-Rakic PS, Muly EC 3rd, Williams GV: D(1) receptors in prefrontal cells and circuits. Brain Res Brain Res Rev 31:295–301, 2000

Graham D, Lantos P: Greenfield's Neuropathology, 7th Edition. London, Arnold, 2002

Greengard P: The neurobiology of slow synaptic transmission. Science 294:1024–1030, 2001

Greenlund LJ, Deckwerth TL, Johnson E Jr: Superoxide dismutase delays neuronal apoptosis: a role for reactive oxygen species in programmed neuronal death. Neuron 14:303–315, 1995

Hassel B, Dingledine R: Glutamate, in Basic Neurochemistry: Molecular, Cellular and Medical Aspects, 7th Edition. Edited by Siegel GJ, Albers RW, Brady S, et al. Burlington, MA, Elsevier Academic, 2006, pp 267–290

Hatten ME: Riding the glial monorail: a common mechanism for glial-guided neuronal migration in different regions of the developing mammalian brain. Trends Neurosci 13:179–184, 1990

Haydar TF, Wang F, Schwartz ML, et al: Differential modulation of proliferation in the neocortical ventricular and subventricular zones. J Neurosci 20:5764–5774, 2000

Hebb DO: The Organization of Behavior: A Neuropsychological theory. New York, Wiley, 1949

Hille B: Ion Channels of Excitable Membranes, 3rd Edition. Sunderland, MA, Sinauer Associates, 2001

Hirokawa N, Takemura R: Biochemical and molecular characterization of diseases linked to motor proteins. Trends Biochem Sci 28:558–565, 2003

Hockenbery D, Nunez G, Milliman C, et al: Bcl-2 is an inner mitochondrial membrane protein that blocks programmed cell death. Nature 348:334–336, 1990

Hökfelt T: Neuropeptides in perspective: the last ten years. Neuron 7:867–879, 1991

Huang YY, Kandel ER: D1/D5 receptor agonists induce a protein synthesis-dependent late potentiation in the CA1 region of the hippocampus. Proc Natl Acad Sci U S A 92:2446–2450, 1995

Hubel DH, Wiesel TN, LeVay S: Plasticity of ocular dominance columns in monkey striate cortex. Philos Trans R Soc Lond B Biol Sci 278:377–409, 1977

Huberman AD, McAllister AK: Neurotrophins and visual cortical plasticity. Prog Brain Res 138:39–51, 2002

Huerta PT, Lisman JE: Low-frequency stimulation at the troughs of theta-oscillation induces long-term depression of previously potentiated CA1 synapses. J Neurophysiol 75:877–884, 1996

Isaac JT: Postsynaptic silent synapses: evidence and mechanisms. Neuropharmacology 45:450–460, 2003

Kamal A, Goldstein LS: Principles of cargo attachment to cytoplasmic motor proteins. Curr Opin Cell Biol 14:63–68, 2002

Kandel ER, O'Dell TJ: Are adult learning mechanisms also used for development? Science 258:243–245, 1992

Kandler K, Katz LC: Neuronal coupling and uncoupling in the developing nervous system. Curr Opin Neurobiol 5:98–105, 1995

Kane DJ, Sarafian TA, Anton R, et al: Bcl-2 inhibition of neural death: decreased generation of reactive oxygen species. Science 262:1274–1277, 1993

Kater SB, Mattson MP, Guthrie PB: Calcium-induced neuronal degeneration: a normal growth cone regulating signal gone awry (?). Ann N Y Acad Sci 568:252–261, 1989

Kempermann G, Wiskott L, Gage FH: Functional significance of adult neurogenesis. Curr Opin Neurobiol 14:186–191, 2004

Kennedy MJ, Ehlers MD: Organelles and trafficking machinery for postsynaptic plasticity. Annu Rev Neurosci 29:325–362, 2006

Kim E, Sheng M: PDZ domain proteins of synapses. Nat Rev Neurosci 5:771–781, 2004

Kinouchi H, Epstein CJ, Mizui T, et al: Attenuation of focal cerebral ischemic injury in transgenic mice overexpressing CuZn superoxide dismutase. Proc Natl Acad Sci U S A 88:11158–11162, 1991

Kitayama N, Vaccarino V, Kutner M, et al: Magnetic resonance imaging (MRI) measurement of hippocampal volume in posttraumatic stress disorder: a meta-analysis. J Affect Disord 88:79–86, 2005

Koester J, Siegelbaum S: Propagated signaling: the action potential, in Principles of Neural Science, 4th Edition. Edited by Kandel ER, Schwartz JH, Jessell TM. New York, McGraw-Hill, 2000, pp 167–169

Komuro H, Rakic P: Modulation of neuronal migration by NMDA receptors. Science 260:95–97, 1993

Kozorovitskiy Y, Gould E: Adult neurogenesis: a mechanism for brain repair? J Clin Exp Neuropsychol 25:721–732, 2003

Lee SH, Sheng M: Development of neuron-neuron synapses. Curr Opin Neurobiol 10:125–131, 2000

Lee SH, Lumelsky N, Studer L, et al: Efficient generation of midbrain and hindbrain neurons from mouse embryonic stem cells. Nat Biotechnol 18:675–679, 2000

Lie DC, Song H, Colamarino SA, et al: Neurogenesis in the adult brain: new strategies for central nervous system diseases. Annu Rev Pharmacol Toxicol 44:399–421, 2004

Lin Z, Wang W, Uhl GR: Dopamine transporter tryptophan mutants highlight candidate dopamine- and cocaine-selective domains. Mol Pharmacol 58:1581–1592, 2000

Lipton SA, Kater SB: Neurotransmitter regulation of neuronal outgrowth, plasticity and survival. Trends Neurosci 12:265–270, 1989

Lisman J, Schulman H, Cline H: The molecular basis of CaMKII function in synaptic and behavioural memory. Nat Rev Neurosci 3:175–190, 2002

Llinás R: The intrinsic electrophysiological properties of mammalian neurons: insights into central nervous system function. Science 242:1654–1664, 1988

London M, Häusser M: Dendritic computation. Annu Rev Neurosci 28:503–532, 2005

LoTurco JJ, Kriegstein AR: Clusters of coupled neuroblasts in embryonic neocortex. Science 252:563–566, 1991

LoTurco JJ, Owens DF, Heath MJS, et al: GABA and glutamate depolarize cortical progenitor cells and inhibit DNA synthesis. Neuron 15:1287–1298, 1995

Lynch MA: Long-term potentiation and memory. Physiol Rev 84:87–136, 2004

MacDermott AB, Mayer ML, Westbrook GL, et al: NMDA-receptor activation increases cytoplasmic calcium concentration in cultured spinal cord neurones. Nature 321:519–522, 1986

Magee JC, Carruth M: Dendritic voltage-gated ion channels regulate the action potential firing mode of hippocampal CA1 pyramidal neurons. J Neurophysiol 82:1895–1901, 1999

Maguire EA, Gadian DG, Johnsrude IS, et al: Navigation-related structural change in the hippocampi of taxi drivers. Proc Natl Acad Sci U S A 97:4398–4403, 2000

Mahanty NK, Sah P: Calcium-permeable AMPA receptors mediate long-term potentiation in interneurons in the amygdala. Nature 394:683–687, 1998

Marin O, Rubenstein JL: Cell migration in the forebrain. Annu Rev Neurosci 26:441–483, 2003

Masson J, Sagn C, Hamon M, et al: Neurotransmitter transporters in the central nervous system. Pharmacol Rev 51:439–464, 1999

Mattson MP, Kater SB: Excitatory and inhibitory neurotransmitters in the generation and degeneration of hippocampal neuroarchitecture. Brain Res 478:337–348, 1989

McAllister AK: Dynamic aspects of CNS synapse formation. Annu Rev Neurosci 30:425–450, 2007

McCormick DA, Bal T: Sleep and arousal: thalamocortical mechanisms. Annu Rev Neurosci 20:185–215, 1997

Mennerick S, Zorumski CF: Glial contributions to excitatory neurotransmission in cultured hippocampal cells. Nature 368:59–62, 1994

Miller MW: Effects of prenatal exposure to ethanol on neocortical development, II: cell proliferation in the ventricular and subventricular zones of the rat. J Comp Neurol 287:326–338, 1989

Misson JP, Edwards MA, Yamamoto M, et al: Identification of radial glial cells within the developing murine central nervous system: studies based upon a new immunohistochemical marker. Brain Res Dev Brain Res 44:95–108, 1988

Murphy TH, Blatter LA, Wier WG, et al: Rapid communication between neurons and astrocytes in primary cortical cultures. J Neurosci 13:2672–2679, 1993

Nedergaard M: Direct signaling from astrocytes to neurons in cultures of mammalian brain cells. Science 263:1768–1771, 1994

Noctor SC, Martinez-Cerdeno V, Ivic L, et al: Cortical neurons arise in symmetric and asymmetric division zones and migrate through specific phases. Nat Neurosci 7:136–144, 2004

Nowak L, Bregestovski P, Ascher P, et al: Magnesium gates glutamate-activated channels in mouse central neurones. Nature 307:462–465, 1984

O'Brien RJ, Lau LF, Huganir RL: Molecular mechanisms of glutamate receptor clustering at excitatory synapses. Curr Opin Neurobiol 8:364–369, 1998

Olsen R, Betz H: GABA and glycine, in Basic Neurochemistry: Molecular, Cellular and Medical Aspects, 7th Edition. Edited by Siegel GJ, Albers RW, Brady S, et al. Burlington, MA, Elsevier Academic, 2006, pp 291–301

Oppenheim A, Altuvia S, Kornitzer D, et al: Translation control of gene expression. J Basic Clin Physiol Pharmacol 2:223–231, 1991

Pantev C, Oostenveld R, Engelien A, et al: Increased auditory cortical representation in musicians. Nature 392:811–814, 1998

Pereira C, Agostinho P, Moreira PI, et al: Alzheimer's disease-associated neurotoxic mechanisms and neuroprotective strategies. Curr Drug Targets CNS Neurol Disord 4:383–403, 2005

Pfrieger FW, Barres BA: Synaptic efficacy enhanced by glial cells in vitro. Science 277:1684–1687, 1997

Pifl C, Giros B, Caron MG: The dopamine transporter: the cloned target site of parkinsonism-inducing toxins and of drugs of abuse. Adv Neurol 69:235–238, 1996

Pigino G, Kirkpatrick L, Brady S: The cytoskeleton of neurons and glia, in Basic Neurochemistry: Molecular, Cellular and Medical Aspects, 7th Edition. Edited by Siegel GJ, Albers RW, Brady S, et al. Burlington, MA, Elsevier Academic, 2006, pp 123–137

Raff MC, Barres BA, Burne JF, et al: Programmed cell death and the control of cell survival: lessons from the nervous system. Science 262:695–700, 1993

Rakic P: Guidance of neurons migrating to the fetal monkey neocortex. Brain Res 33:471–476, 1971

Ramamoorthy S, Blakely RD: Phosphorylation and sequestration of serotonin transporters differentially modulated by psychostimulants. Science 285:763–766, 1999

Ramón y Cajal S: Les nouvelles idées sur la structure du système nerveux chez l'homme et chez les vertébrés [New ideas on the structure of the nervous system in man and in vertebrates]. Paris, C. Reinwald, 1894

Ramón y Cajal S: Histologie du système nerveux de l'homme et des vertébrés [Histology of the nervous system in man and in vertebrates]. Paris, Maloine, 1911

Rego AC, de Almeida LP: Molecular targets and therapeutic strategies in Huntington's disease. Curr Drug Targets CNS Neurol Disord 4:361–381, 2005

Reiter HO, Stryker MP: Neural plasticity without postsynaptic action potentials: less-active inputs become dominant when kitten visual cortical cells are pharmacologically inhibited. Proc Natl Acad Sci USA 85:3623–3627, 1988

Rosen DR, Siddique T, Patterson D, et al: Mutations in Cu/Zn superoxide dismutase gene are associated with familial amyotrophic lateral sclerosis. Nature 362:59–62, 1993

Rumpel S, LeDoux J, Zador A, et al: Postsynaptic receptor trafficking underlying a form of associative learning. Science 308:83–88, 2005

Sadato N, Pascual-Leone A, Grafman J, et al: Activation of the primary visual cortex by Braille reading in blind subjects. Nature 380:526–528, 1996

Salinas PC: Signaling at the vertebrate synapse: new roles for embryonic morphogens? J Neurobiol 64:435–445, 2005

Sanes JR, Lichtman JW: Development of the vertebrate neuromuscular junction. Annu Rev Neurosci 22:389–442, 1999

Santarelli L, Saxe M, Gross C, et al: Requirement of hippocampal neurogenesis for the behavioral effects of antidepressants. Science 301:805–809, 2003

Schenone A, Mancardi GL: Molecular basis of inherited neuropathies. Curr Opin Neurol 12:603–616, 1999

Schmechel DE, Rakic P: A Golgi study of radial glial cells in developing monkey telencephalon: morphogenesis and transformation into astrocytes. Anat Embryol 156:115–152, 1979

Scott SA, Davies AM: Inhibition of protein synthesis prevents cell death in sensory and parasympathetic neurons deprived of neurotrophic factor in vitro. J Neurobiol 21:630–638, 1990

Seamans JK, Yang CR: The principal features and mechanisms of dopamine modulation in the prefrontal cortex. Prog Neurobiol 74:1–58, 2004

Seri B, García-Verdugo JM, McEwen BS, et al: Astrocytes give rise to new neurons in the adult mammalian hippocampus. J Neurosci 21:7153–7160, 2001

Sohl G, Maxeiner S, Willecke K: Expression and functions of neuronal gap junctions. Nat Rev Neurosci 6:191–200, 2005

Spencer KM, Nestor PG, Perlmutter R, et al: Neural synchrony indexes disordered perception and cognition in schizophrenia. Proc Natl Acad Sci U S A 101:17288–17293, 2004

Studer L, Tabar V, McKay RDG: Transplantation of expanded mesencephalic precursors leads to recovery in parkinsonian rats. Nature Neurosci 1:290–295, 1998

Sudhof TC: The synaptic vesicle cycle. Annu Rev Neurosci 27:509–547, 2004

Sulzer D, Sonders MS, Poulsen NW, et al: Mechanisms of neurotransmitter release by amphetamines: a review. Prog Neurobiol 75:406–433, 2005

Takahashi T, Nowakowski RS, Caviness VS Jr: Early ontogeny of the secondary proliferative population of the embryonic murine cerebral wall. J Neurosci 15:6058–6068, 1995

Tamas G, Buhl EH, Lorincz A, et al: Proximally targeted GABAergic synapses and gap junctions synchronize cortical interneurons. Nat Neurosci 3:366–371, 2000

Tissir F, Goffinet AM: Reelin and brain development. Nat Rev Neurosci 4:496–505, 2003

Toga AW, Thompson PM: Genetics of brain structure and intelligence. Annu Rev Neurosci 28:1–23, 2005

Tsao P, von Zastrow M: Downregulation of G protein-coupled receptors. Curr Opin Neurobiol 10:365–369, 2000

Van Den Bosch L, Van Damme P, Bogaert E, et al: The role of excitotoxicity in the pathogenesis of amyotrophic lateral sclerosis. Biochim Biophys Acta 1762:1068–1082, 2006

Walaas SI, Greengard P: Protein phosphorylation and neuronal function. Pharmacol Rev 43:299–349, 1991

Warner-Schmidt JL, Duman RS: Hippocampal neurogenesis: opposing effects of stress and antidepressant treatment. Hippocampus 16:239–249, 2006

Washbourne P, Bennett JE, McAllister AK: Rapid recruitment of NMDA receptor transport packets to nascent synapses. Nat Neurosci 5:751–759, 2002

Washbourne P, Liu XB, Jones EG, et al: Cycling of NMDA receptors during trafficking in neurons before synapse formation. J Neurosci 24:8253–8264, 2004

Weissman TA, Riquelme PA, Ivic L, et al: Calcium waves propagate through radial glial cells and modulate proliferation in the developing neocortex. Neuron 43:647–661, 2004

Wexler NS, Rose EA, Housman DE: Molecular approaches to hereditary diseases of the nervous system: Huntington's disease as a paradigm. Annu Rev Neurosci 14:503–529, 1991

Wichterle H, Lieberam I, Porter JA, et al: Directed differentiation of embryonic stem cells into motor neurons. Cell 110:385–397, 2002

Yamakura T, Bertaccini E, Trudell JR, et al: Anesthetics and ion channels: molecular models and sites of action. Annu Rev Pharmacol Toxicol 41:23–51, 2001

Yuste R, Tank DW: Dendritic integration in mammalian neurons, a century after Cajal. Neuron 16:701–716, 1996

Ziv NE, Garner CC: Cellular and molecular mechanisms of presynaptic assembly. Nat Rev Neurosci 5:385–399, 2004

2

THE NEUROPSYCHOLOGICAL EVALUATION

Diane B. Howieson, Ph.D.
Muriel D. Lezak, Ph.D.

Neuropsychologists assess brain function by making inferences from an individual's cognitive, sensorimotor, emotional, and social behavior. During the early history of neuropsychology, these assessments were often the most direct measure of brain integrity in persons who did not have localizing neurological signs and symptoms and who had problems confined to higher mental functions (Hebb 1942; Teuber 1948). Neuropsychological measures are useful diagnostic indicators of brain dysfunction for many conditions and will remain the major diagnostic modality for some (Bigler 1999; Farah and Feinberg 2000; Lezak et al. 2004; Mesulam 2000; Petersen et al. 2001). However, methods for determining brain structure and function have become increasingly accurate in recent decades (e.g., Kamitani and Tong 2005). Advances in quantitative and functional neuroimaging have enriched our understanding of pathological disturbances of the brain (Aine 1995; Damasio

and Damasio 2003; J.M. Levin et al. 1996; Menon and Kim 1999; Stern and Silbersweig 2001; Tilak Ratnanather et al. 2004). It is even possible to produce precisely placed, reversible "lesions" to study how the remainder of the brain functions without a designated cortical area (Deouell et al. 2003; Grafman and Wassermann 1999; V. Walsh and Rushworth 1999). These developments have allowed a shift in the focus of neuropsychological assessment from the diagnosis of possible brain damage to a better understanding of specific brain-behavior relations and the psychosocial consequences of brain damage.

INDICATIONS FOR A NEUROPSYCHOLOGICAL EVALUATION

Patients referred to a neuropsychologist for assessment typically fall into one of three groups. The first, and probably largest, group consists of patients with known brain disorders. The more common neurological disorders are cerebrovascular disorders, developmental disorders, traumatic brain injury, Alzheimer's disease and related dementing disorders, progressive diseases primarily involving subcortical structures (e.g., Parkinson's disease, multiple sclerosis, Huntington's chorea), tumors, seizures, and infections. Psychiatric disorders also may be associated with brain dysfunction; chief among them are schizophrenia, obsessive-compulsive disorder, and depression.

A neuropsychological evaluation can be useful in defining the nature and severity of the associated behavior and emotional problems. The assessment provides information about patients' cognition, personality characteristics, social behavior, emotional status, and adaptation to their conditions. Patients' potential for independent living and productive activity can be inferred from these data. Information about their behavioral strengths and weaknesses provides a foundation for treatment planning, vocational training, competency determination, and counseling for both patients and their families (Bennett and Raymond 2003; Diller 2000; Kalechstein et al. 2003; Sloan and Ponsford 1995).

The second group of patients is composed of persons with a known risk factor for brain disorder in whom a change in behavior might be the result of such a disorder. In these cases, a neuropsychological evaluation might be used both to provide evidence of brain dysfunction and to describe the nature and severity of problems.

In the third group, brain disease or dysfunction may be suspected when a person's behavior changes without an identifiable cause: that is, the patient has no known risk factors for brain disorder, so this possible diagnosis is based on exclusion of other diagnoses. The most common application of the neuropsychological evaluation of older adults without obvious risk factors for brain disease—other than age—is for early detection of progressive dementia, such as Alzheimer's disease (Howieson et al. 1997;

Knopman and Selnes 2003; Kramer et al. 2003; Rentz and Weintraub 2000). Most persons have symptoms associated with dementia for at least 1 year before they see a health care provider, because the problems initially are minor and easily attributed to factors such as aging, a concurrent illness, or recent emotional stress. The progression of these symptoms is insidious, especially because many patients have "good" as well as "bad" days during the early stages of a dementing disorder. Neuropsychological assessment is useful in evaluating whether problems noted by the family or the individual are age-related, are attributable to other factors such as depression, or are suggestive of early dementia. During the past decade, human immunodeficiency virus (HIV) infection and the complications of drug abuse have been added as conditions that can produce an insidious dementia in younger persons (Dore et al. 2003; I. Grant et al. 1995; Kelly et al. 1996; Rogers and Robbins 2003).

Another clinical condition that produces no clinical clues for brain damage except for a change in behavior is the so-called silent stroke. Without obvious sensory, motor, or speech problems, a stroke may go undetected yet produce persistent behavioral alterations. Silent strokes can produce subtle cognitive impairment (Armstrong et al. 1996; Pohjasvaara et al. 1999; W.P. Schmidt et al. 2004); a series of small strokes may generate an insidious dementia over time (O'Connell et al. 1998; Vermeer et al. 2003). Silent strokes and white matter hyperintensities observed on magnetic resonance imaging scans (Nebes et al. 2001) and cerebrovascular risk factors (Mast et al. 2005) of elderly persons also may be associated with depression. Exposure to environmental toxins also can result in common patterns of neuropsychological impairment (Morrow et al. 2001; Reif et al. 2003).

In cases with no known explanation for mental deterioration, it becomes important to search for possible risk factors or other reasons for brain disease through history taking, the physical examination, laboratory tests, and interviews with the patient's family or close associates. Should this search produce no basis for the mental deterioration, a diagnostic neuropsychological study can be useful. The neuropsychological examination of persons with or without known risk factors for brain damage is diagnostically useful if it identifies cognitive or behavioral deficits, particularly if these deficits occur in a meaningful pattern. A pattern is considered meaningful when it is specific to one or only a few diagnoses, such as a pattern of cognitive disruption suggestive of a lateralized or focal brain lesion.

Neuropsychological signs and symptoms that are possible indicators of a pathological brain disorder are presented in Table 2–1. Confidence in diagnoses based on neuropsychological evidence will be greater when risk factors for brain dysfunction exist or the patient shows signs and symptoms of brain dysfunction than when neuropsychological diagnoses rely solely on exclusion of other diagnoses.

One of the greatest challenges for a neuropsychologist is to determine whether patients with psychiatric illness show evidence of an underlying neurological disorder. Many psychiatric patients without neurological disease have cognitive disruptions and behavioral or emotional aberrations. Cognitive impairment is highly prevalent in schizophrenia (Heinrichs and Zakzanis 1998; Hill et al. 2001), particularly for attention, processing speed, memory, problem solving, cognitive flexibility, and organizational and planning abilities (Goldman et al. 1996). Because considerable heterogeneity exists for symptoms of schizophrenia (Binks and Gold 1998; Goldstein et al. 1998; Seaton et al. 2001), some patients appear cognitively normal (Allen et al. 2003; Palmer et al. 1997). Obsessive-compulsive disorders are often accompanied by mild cognitive impairment. Areas of difficulty may include nonverbal memory, use of strategies, visuospatial skills, and selected executive functions (Deckersbach et al. 2000; Greisberg and McKay 2003; Mataix-Cols et al. 1999; Savage et al. 2000; K.D. Wilson 1998). Both schizophrenia and obsessive-compulsive behavior have been linked to dysfunction of frontal subcortical circuits (Ab-

bruzzese et al. 1995; Chamberlain et al. 2005), and temporal lobe structures also have been implicated (Adler et al. 2000; Post 2000).

Depressed patients often underperform on measures of speed of processing, mental flexibility, and executive function compared with control subjects (Veiel 1997; Weiland-Fiedler et al. 2004). Memory impairment occurs less consistently (Basso and Bornstein 1999b; Boone et al. 1995; Palmer et al. 1996), and memory performance may be intact even when memory complaints are present (Dalgleish and Cox 2000; Kalska et al. 1999). Cognitive deficits, including memory, are more common in depressed patients with psychotic features than in those with no psychotic features (Basso and Bornstein 1999a; McKenna et al. 2000). Compared with control subjects, euthymic bipolar patients may have difficulty with attention, memory, abstraction (Denicoff et al. 1999; Quraishi and Frangou 2002), and executive functions (Ferrier et al. 1999; Malhi et al. 2004). The degree of cognitive impairment appears to be related to the number of prior depressive episodes (Denicoff et al. 1999; Van Gorp et al. 1998). Although several psychological explanations have been proposed to explain cognitive deficits in mood disorders, such as self-focused rumination associated with dysphoria (Hertel 1998), underlying structural and functional abnormalities have been reported in the neural pathways that modulate mood (Ali et al. 2000; Caetano et al. 2004; Liotti and Mayberg 2001; Neumeister et al. 2005; Strakowski et al. 1999).

Conversely, neurological diseases can present with prominent psychiatric features (Cummings 1999; Lezak et al. 2004). Confabulations associated with undiagnosed brain lesions, such as Korsakoff's syndrome, may be misinterpreted as a psychotic illness (Benson et al. 1996). An assortment of delusional misidentification syndromes have been associated with neurological diseases (Feinberg and Roane 2003). Hallucinations may be an early feature of Lewy body dementia and may occur with Parkinson's disease, Alzheimer's disease, other neurodegenerative diseases, stroke, epi-

TABLE 2–1.　Neuropsychological signs and symptoms that may indicate a pathological brain process

Functional class	Symptoms and signs
Speech and language	Dysarthria Dysfluency Marked change in amount of speech output Paraphasias Word-finding problems
Academic skills	Alterations in reading, writing, calculating, and number abilities Frequent letter or number reversals
Thinking	Perseveration of speech Simplified or confused mental tracking, reasoning, and concept formation
Motor	Weakness or clumsiness, particularly if lateralized Impaired fine motor coordination (e.g., changes in handwriting) Apraxias Perseveration of action components
Memory[a]	Impaired recent memory for verbal or visuospatial material or both Disorientation
Perception	Diplopia or visual field alterations Inattention (usually left-sided) Somatosensory alterations (particularly if lateralized) Inability to recognize familiar stimuli (agnosia)
Visuospatial abilities	Diminished ability to perform manual skills (e.g., mechanical repairs and sewing) Spatial disorientation Left-right disorientation Impaired spatial judgment (e.g., angulation of distances)
Emotions[b]	Diminished emotional control with temper outburst and antisocial behavior Diminished empathy or interest in interpersonal relationships Affective changes Irritability without evident precipitating factors Personality change
Comportment[b]	Altered appetites and appetitive activities Altered grooming habits (excessive fastidiousness or carelessness) Hyperactivity or hypoactivity Social inappropriateness

[a]Many emotionally disturbed persons complain of memory deficits, which most typically reflect the person's self-preoccupation, distractibility, or anxiety rather than a dysfunctional brain. Thus, memory complaints in themselves do not necessarily warrant neuropsychological evaluation.
[b]Some of these changes are most likely to be neuropsychologically relevant in the absence of depression, although they can also be mistaken for depression.

lepsy, migraine, and toxic-metabolic encephalopathies (Tekin and Cummings 2003).

Although neuropsychological assessment provides a measure of the type and degree of cognitive disorder, it often cannot specify the cause of the disturbance. Cognitive deficits appearing in an adult patient who previously functioned well and has no history of psychiatric illness or recent stress should raise suspicions of a neurological disorder.

THE ASSESSMENT PROCESS

Interview and observation provide the data of neuropsychological evaluations. The interview is the basic component of the evaluation (Lezak et al. 2004; Luria 1980; Sbordone 2000). Its main purposes are to elicit the patient's and family's complaints, understand the circumstances in which these problems occur, and evaluate the patient's attitude toward these problems. Understanding the range of the patient's complaints, as well as which ones the patient views as most troublesome, contributes to the framework on which the assessment and recommendations are based. A thorough history of complaints and pertinent background is essential.

The presenting problems and the patient's attitude toward them also may provide important diagnostic information. Patients with certain neuropsychological conditions lack awareness of their problems or belittle their significance (Markova and Berrios 2000; Prigatano and Schacter 1991). Many patients with right hemisphere stroke, Alzheimer's disease, or frontal lobe damage are unaware of or unable to appreciate the problems resulting from their brain injury. In the extreme form of right hemisphere stroke, some patients with hemiplegia are unable to comprehend that the left side of their body is part of them, let alone that they cannot use it. In a more muted form, many patients with dementia attribute their memory problems to aging and minimize their significance (see Strub and Black 2000). Conversely, patients, families, or caregivers sometimes attribute problems to brain damage when a careful history suggests otherwise.

The interview provides an opportunity to observe the patient's appearance, attention, speech, thought content, and motor abilities and to evaluate affect, appropriateness of behavior, orientation, insight, and judgment. The interview can provide information about the patient's premorbid intellectual ability and personality, occupational and school background, social situation, and ability to use leisure time.

The tests used by neuropsychologists are simply standardized observational tools that, in many instances, have the added advantage of providing normative data to aid in interpreting the observations. Various assessment approaches are available, but they all have in common the goals of determining whether the patient shows evidence of brain dysfunction, identifying the nature of problems detected, and determining which functions have been preserved and, thus, what are the patient's cognitive strengths.

Cognitive performance is only one aspect of an assessment. A full evaluation of the individual assesses emotional and social characteristics as well. Many patients with brain injuries experience changes in personality, mood, or ability to control emotional states (Gainotti 2003; Heilman et al. 2003; Ochoa et al. 2003) and problems with social relationships (Dikmen et al. 1996; Lezak 1988a). Depression is a common and sometimes serious complication of brain disease. An unusually high incidence of depression occurs with certain neurodegenerative disorders, such as Parkinson's disease and Huntington's disease (Brandstadter and Oertel 2003; Levy et al. 1998; Rickards 2005). Other neurological diseases in which depression is common are tumors (particularly those of the orbitofrontal and temporoparietal cortex), multiple sclerosis, Wilson's disease, HIV encephalopathy, Alzheimer's disease, vascular dementia, and Lewy body dementia (Cummings 1994). At least 30% of stroke patients experience depression at some time (Paradiso et al. 1997; Pohjasvaara et al. 1998; Singh et al. 2000). Factors that appear to determine the presence of depression include the location of the brain injury and its recency, the degree of disability, and the patient's level of social activity (Gustafson et al. 1995; Robinson 1998). In some cases, these changes may be secondary to cognitive impairment (Andersen et al. 1995). Patients who have had a right hemisphere stroke may show impaired processing of emotional material and complex social situations, which leads to interpersonal problems (Lezak 1994). Although the history and observers' reports will inform the examiner of changes in these characteristics, current emotional status and personality also can be evaluated by standard psychological questionnaires and inventories (Gass 1992; Lezak et al. 2004).

As computers have become valuable aids in many fields, there has been increasing interest in using computerized testing procedures (Bleiberg et al. 2000; De Luca et al. 2003; Fowler et al. 1997; Tornatore et al. 2005; Wild et al. 2008). This technology offers the possibility of obtaining test data under highly standardized conditions with minimal time expenditure by the examiner. These features make it valuable in circumstances when many individuals need to be screened for potential problems. Computers also have timing and scoring features and can plot the data graphically. In addition, computer programs are available in some cases for interpreting test responses.

THE NATURE OF NEUROPSYCHOLOGICAL TESTS

An important component of neuropsychological evaluations is psychological testing, in which an individual's cognitive and often emotional status and executive functioning are assessed with standardized formats. Neuropsychological assessment differs from psychological assessment in its basic assumptions. The latter compares the individual's responses with normative data from a sample of healthy individuals taking the same test (Lezak et al. 2004; Urbina 2004). The neuropsychological assessment of adults relies on comparisons between the patient's current level of functioning and the known or estimated level of premorbid functioning according to demographically similar individuals and current performance on tests of functions less likely to be affected by brain disorders. Thus, much of clinical neuropsychological assessment involves *intraindividual* comparisons of the abilities and skills under consideration.

Most tests of cognitive abilities are designed with the expectation that only very few persons will obtain a perfect score and that most scores will cluster in a middle range. For these tests, scores are conceptualized as continuous variables. The scores of many persons taking the test can be plotted as a distribution curve. Most scores on tests of complex learned behaviors fall into a characteristic bell-shaped curve called a normal distribution curve (Figure 2–1). The statistical descriptors of the curve are the *mean*, or average score; the degree of spread of scores about the mean, expressed as the *standard deviation;* and the *range*, or the distance from the highest to the lowest scores.

The level of competence in different cognitive functions as well as other behaviors varies from individual to individual and also within the same individual at different times. This variability also has the characteristics of a normal curve, as in Figure 2–1. Because of the normal variability of performance on cognitive tests, any single score can be considered only as representative of a normal performance range and must not be taken as a precise value. For example, the statistical properties of a score at the 75th percentile (the equivalent of a scaled score of 12 on a test in the Wechsler Intelligence Scale [WIS] battery) must be understood as likely representing a range of scores from the 50th to the 90th percentile. For this reason, many neuropsychologists are reluctant to report scores, but rather describe their findings in terms of ability levels (Table 2–2).

An individual's score is compared with the normative data, often by calculating a standard or z score, which describes the individual's performance in terms of statistically regular distances (i.e., standard deviations). In this framework, scores within ±0.66 standard deviation are considered average because 50% of a normative sample scores within this range. The z scores are used to describe the probability that a deviant response occurs by chance or because of an impairment. A performance in the below average direction that is greater than two standard deviations from the mean is usually described as falling in the impaired range, because 98% of the normative sample taking the test achieve better scores.

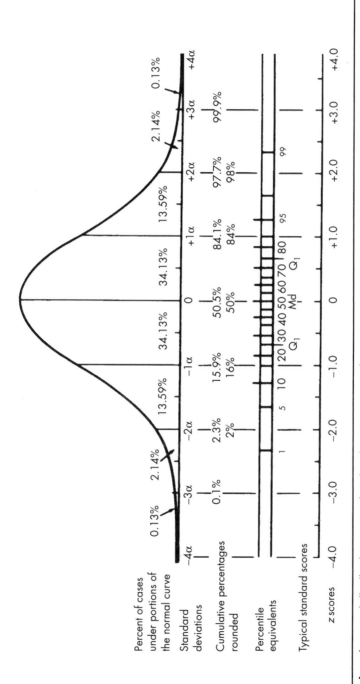

FIGURE 2–1. A normal distribution curve, showing the percentage of cases between −4 standard deviations (−σ) and +4 standard deviations (+σ).

The average range is defined as −0.6 to +0.6 standard deviation or the 25th to the 75th percentile.

Source. Adapted from the Test Service Bulletin of The Psychological Corporation, 1955.

TABLE 2–2.   Ability test classifications expressed as deviations from the mean calculated from the normative sample

z Score range	Percentile	Classification
>+2.0	98–100	Very superior
+1.3 to +2.0	91–97	Superior
+0.67 to +1.3	75–90	High average
–0.66 to +0.66	26–74	Average
–0.67 to –1.3	10–25	Low average
–1.3 to –2.0	3–9	Borderline
<–2.0	0–2	Defective

Psychological tests should be constructed to satisfy both reliability and validity criteria (Urbina 2004). The *reliability* of a test refers to the consistency of test scores when the test is given to the same individual at different times or with different sets of equivalent items. Because perfect reliability cannot be achieved for any test, each individual score represents a range of variability, which narrows to the degree that the reliability of the test approaches the ideal (Anastasi and Urbina 1997). Tests have *validity* when they measure what they purport to measure. If a test is designed to measure an attentional disorder, then patient groups known to have attention deficits should perform more poorly on the test than should persons from the population at large. Tests also should be constructed with large normative samples of individuals with similar demographic characteristics, particularly for age and education (Heaton et al. 2003; Steinberg and Bieliauskas 2005).

Some psychological tests detect subtle deficits better than do others. A simple signal detection test of attention, such as crossing out all the letter *A*'s on a page, is a less sensitive test of attention than is a divided attention task, such as crossing out all letters *A* and *C*. Tests involving complex tasks, such as problem solving requiring abstract thinking and cognitive flexibility, are more sensitive for reflecting brain dysfunction than many other cognitive tests because a wide variety of brain disorders can easily disrupt performance on them. How-

ever, other factors such as depression, anxiety, medicine side effects, and low energy level due to systemic illness also may disrupt cognition on these sensitive tests. Therefore, they are sensitive to cognitive disruption but not specific to one type of cognitive disturbance. The specificity of a test in detecting a disorder depends on the overlap between the distributions of the scores for persons who are intact and persons who have the disorder (Figure 2–2). The less overlap there is, the better the test can differentiate normal and abnormal performances. A test that is highly specific, such as the Token Test (Boller and Vignolo 1966; De Renzi and Vignolo 1962), which assesses language comprehension, produces few abnormal test scores in nonaphasic persons; that is, few false positive findings. However, for such a test, false negative results (i.e., that an impaired patient has normal findings) will be considerable because many persons with brain disorders have good language comprehension. Many neuropsychological tests offer a tradeoff between sensitivity and specificity.

Indications of brain dysfunction come from qualitative features of the patient's performance as well as from test scores (Lezak et al. 2004; Malloy et al. 2003; Pankratz and Taplin 1982). There are many ways of failing a test, and a poor score does not tell us the means that produced the end (K.W. Walsh 1987). Occasionally, a patient gives a "far out" response to a question. The examiner asks the patient to repeat the question and, often in this

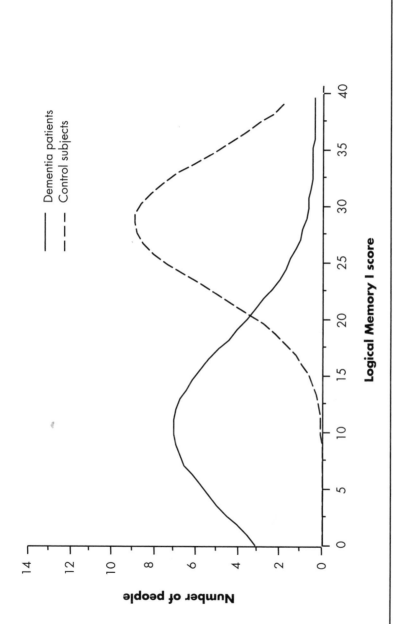

FIGURE 2–2. Distribution of test scores by a group with mild dementia and age-matched control subjects on the Wechsler Memory Scale–Revised Logical Memory I, a story-recall test.

Scores ranging from 15 to 39 occurred in both groups, whereas scores below 15 occurred in only the dementia group. The smaller the areas of overlapping curves, the higher the test specificity.

circumstance, finds that the patient has misunderstood the question or instruction rather than lacked the ability to produce a correct response. Some features of behavioral disturbance are best recognized by the manner in which the patient approaches the testing situation or behaves with the examiner. Brain-injured patients are prone to problems with short attention span, distractibility, impulsivity, poor self-monitoring, disorganization, irritability, perplexity, and suspiciousness.

INTERPRETATION: PRINCIPLES AND CAUTIONS

The interpretation of test performance is based on an assumption that the patient is expected to perform in a particular way on tasks; deviations from expectation require evaluation (Lezak 1986; Lezak et al. 2004). Most healthy people perform within a statistically definable range on cognitive tests, and this range of performance levels is considered to be characteristic of healthy people. Deviations below this expected range raise the question of an impairment. A person may have scores in the high average range on many tests except for low average performance in one functional area.

The assumption of deficit is valid in most instances in which one score or a set of scores falls significantly below expectations, although a few persons show an unusual variability on cognitive tasks (Lezak et al. 2004). Multiple measures involving similar or related abilities increase the reliability of findings. Thus, if a deviant score occurs on one task, other tests requiring similar skills are used to determine whether the deviant finding persists across tasks. If so, the finding is considered reliable. If similar tasks do not elicit a deviant performance, either the finding was spurious or the additional tasks varied in important features that did not involve the patient's problem area. The need to have multiple measures of many cognitive functions is the reason that some neuropsychological examinations may be lengthy.

Interpretation of test performances also must take into account demographic variables. In the estimates of premorbid ability levels necessary for making intraindividual comparisons, patients' educational and occupational background, sex, and race must be considered along with their level of test performance (Lezak et al. 2004; Vanderploeg et al. 1996). In cases in which educational level may not represent premorbid ability, reading level is often used as a best indicator (Manly et al. 2004). The more severely impaired the patients, the more unlikely it is that they will be performing at premorbid levels on any of the tests. This increases the examiner's reliance on demographic and historical data to estimate premorbid functioning. Some tests are fairly resistant to disruption by brain damage and may offer the best estimates of premorbid ability. Good examples are fund of information and reading vocabulary tests, such as the National Adult Reading Test (NART; Nelson 1982), and a revision for American English, the North American Adult Reading Test (NAART; Spreen and Strauss 1998).

For meaningful interpretations of neuropsychological test performance, examiners not only rely on many tests but also search for a performance pattern (test scores plus qualitative features) that makes neuropsychological sense. Because there are few pathognomonic findings in neuropsychology (or in most other branches of medical science for that matter) (Hertzman et al. 2001; Sox et al. 1988), a performance pattern often can suggest several diagnoses. For example, a cluster of documented deficits including slowed thinking and mild impairment of concentration and memory is a nonspecific finding associated with several conditions: very mild dementia, a mild postconcussion syndrome, mild toxic encephalopathy, depression, and fatigue, to name a few. Other patterns may be highly specific for certain conditions. The finding of left-sided neglect and visuospatial distortions is highly suggestive of brain dysfunction and specifically occurs with right hemisphere damage. For many neuropsychological conditions, typical deficit patterns are known, allowing the examiner to evaluate the patient's performances in light of these known patterns for a possible match.

MAJOR TEST CATEGORIES

In this section, we present a brief review of tests used for assessment of major areas of cognition and personality. Many useful neuropsychological tests are not described in this summary. Please refer to *Neuropsychological Assessment*, 4th Edition (Lezak et al. 2004), for a relatively complete review and to *A Compendium of Neuropsychological Tests*, 3rd Edition (Strauss et al. 2006), for more detailed normative data on many frequently used tests.

MENTAL ABILITY

The most commonly used set of tests of general intellectual function of adults in the Western world is contained in the various versions and translations of the WIS (Wechsler 1997a, 2008). These batteries of brief tests provide scores on a variety of cognitive tasks covering a range of skills. Each version was originally developed as an "intelligence" test to predict academic and vocational performance of neurologically intact adults by giving an IQ (intelligence quotient) score, which is based on the mean performance on the tests in this battery. The entire test battery may provide the bulk of the tests included in a neuropsychological examination. The individual tests were designed to assess relatively distinct areas of cognition, such as arithmetic, abstract thinking, and visuospatial organization, and thus are differentially sensitive to dysfunction of various areas of the brain. Therefore, these tests are often used to screen for specific areas of cognitive deficits. Many experienced neuropsychologists use and interpret these tests discretely, administering only those deemed relevant for each patient and treating the findings as they treat data obtained from individually developed tests.

When given to neuropsychologically impaired persons, the summary IQ scores can be very misleading because individual test scores lowered by specific cognitive deficits, when averaged in with scores relatively unaffected by the brain dysfunction, can result in IQ scores associated with ability levels that represent neither the severity of deficits nor the patient's residual competencies (Lezak 1988b). For example, a patient with a visuospatial deficit consisting of an inability to appreciate the structure of visual patterns would have difficulty performing the Block Design test, which requires copying pictured designs with blocks. When such a patient performs well above average on other tests, a summation of all the scores would both hide the important data and be lower than the other test scores in the battery would warrant. Therefore, neuropsychologists focus on the pattern of the Wechsler scores rather than the summed or average performance on all the tests in the battery.

LANGUAGE

Lesions to the hemisphere dominant for speech and language, which is the left hemisphere in 95%–97% of right-handed persons and 60%–70% of left-handed ones (Corballis 1991; Strauss and Goldsmith 1987), can produce any of a variety of disorders of symbol formulation and use—the aphasias (Spreen and Risser 2003). Although many aphasiologists argue against attempting to classify all patients into one of the standard aphasia syndromes because of so many individual differences, persons with aphasia tend to be grouped according to whether the main disorder is in language comprehension (receptive aphasia), expression (expressive aphasia), repetition (conduction aphasia), or naming (anomic aphasia). Many comprehensive language assessment tests are available, such as the Multilingual Aphasia Examination (Benton and Hamsher 1989). Comprehensive aphasia test batteries are best administered by speech pathologists or other clinicians with special training in this field. These batteries usually include measures of spontaneous speech, speech comprehension, repetition, naming, reading, and writing.

Test selection may be based on whether the information is to be used for diagnostic, prognostic, or rehabilitation purposes. For example, the Boston Diagnostic Aphasia Examination, 3rd Edition (Goodglass et al. 2000), might be selected as an aid for treatment planning because of its wide scope and sensitivity to different aphasic characteristics. The Porch Index of Communicative Ability (Porch 1981) best measures treatment progress because of its sensitivity to small changes in performance. A language screening examination is the Bedside Evaluation Screening Test, 2nd Edition (West et al. 1998). This approximately 20-minute examination provides measures of comprehension, talking, and reading.

ATTENTION AND MENTAL TRACKING

A frequent consequence of brain disorders is slowed mental processing and impaired ability for focused behavior (Duncan and Mirsky 2004; Leclercq and Zimmermann 2002). Damage to the brain stem or diffuse damage involving the cerebral hemispheres, especially the white matter interconnections, can produce a variety of attentional deficits. Attentional deficits are very common in neuropsychiatric disorders. Most neuropsychological assessments will include measures of these abilities. The Wechsler scales contain several relevant tests. Digit Span measures attention span or short-term memory for numbers in two ways: forward and backward digit repetition. Backward digit repetition is a more demanding task because it requires concentration and mental tracking plus the short-term memory component. It is not uncommon for moderately to severely brain-damaged patients to perform poorly on only the backward repetition portion of this test. Because Digits Forward and Digits Backward measure different functions, assessment data for each should be reported separately. Digit Symbol also requires concentration plus motor and mental speed for successful performance. The patient must accurately and rapidly code numbers into symbols. The Arithmetic test in the Wechsler battery is very sensitive to attentional disorders because it requires short-term auditory memory and rapid mental juggling of

arithmetic problem elements. Poor performance on this test must be evaluated for the nature of the failures. Another commonly used measure of concentration and mental tracking is the Trail Making Test (Armitage 1946). In the first part of this test (Part A), the patient is asked to draw rapidly and accurately a line connecting in sequence a random display of numbered circles on a page. The level of difficulty is increased in the second part (Part B) by having the patient again sequence a random display of circles, this time alternating numbers and letters (Figure 2–3). This test requires concentration, visual scanning, and flexibility in shifting cognitive sets (Cicerone and Azulay 2002). It shares with many attention tests vulnerability to other kinds of deficits such as motor slowing, which could be based on peripheral factors such as nerve or muscle damage, and diminished visual acuity.

In cases of subtle brain injury, assessment sensitivity can be increased by selecting a more difficult measure of concentration and mental tracking in which material must be held in mind while information is manipulated for the performance of complex cognitive activities such as comprehension, learning, and reasoning. The ability to hold information in mind while performing a mental task is called *working memory* (Baddeley 1994). As such, working memory requires attention and short-term memory. The Self-Ordered Pointing Task (Petrides and Milner 1982; Strauss et al. 2006) instructs patients to point to one item in a set ranging from 6 to 18 varied items. On each trial, in which the positions of the items are randomly changed, patients are told to point to a different item than they previously pointed to, and then another, until they have pointed to all the items. The successful performance of this working memory task depends on keeping in mind which items have already been eliminated. Another example of a difficult attentional task is the Paced Auditory Serial Addition Task (PASAT; Gronwall 1977; Gronwall and Sampson 1974). The patient is required to add consecutive pairs of numbers rapidly under an interference condition. As numbers are

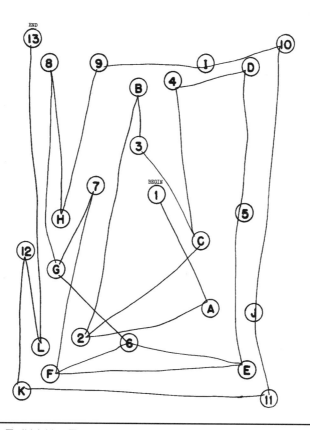

FIGURE 2–3.   Trail Making Test (Armitage 1946) Part B performance by a 61-year-old man with normal pressure hydrocephalus.

Two types of errors are shown: erroneous sequencing (1→A→2→C) and failure to alternate between numbers and letters (D→5→E→F).

presented at a fixed rate, the patient must always add the last two numbers presented and ignore the number that represents the last summation. For example, if the numbers "3–5–2–7" are presented, the patient must respond "8" after the number 5, and then "7" after the number 2, and then "9." It is a difficult test of divided attention because of the strong tendency to add the last number presented to the last summation. The level of difficulty can be heightened by speeding up the rate of presentation of numbers. The PASAT is among those tests that are most sensitive to attentional disorders (Cicerone and Azulay 2002). However, because most persons taking this test, even those who achieve good scores, believe that they have done poorly, its negative effect on a patient's mood and test-taking atti-

tude must be taken into account before selecting it (Feldner et al. 2006).

MEMORY

Memory is another cognitive function that is frequently impaired by brain disorders. Many diffuse brain injuries produce general impairments in abilities for new learning and retention. Many focal brain injuries also produce memory impairment; left hemisphere lesions are most likely to produce primarily verbal memory deficits, whereas visuospatial memory impairments tend to be associated with right hemisphere lesions (Abrahams et al. 1997; Ojemann and Dodrill 1985; Wagner et al. 1998), although not all visuospatial tests show a right hemisphere advantage (Raspall et al. 2005). Memory impairment often is a prominent feature of herpes encephalitis, Huntington's chorea, Korsakoff's syndrome, hypoxia, closed head injury, and a variety of neurological degenerative diseases such as Alzheimer's disease (Baddeley et al. 2002; Bauer et al. 2003; Mayes 2000).

In most cases of brain injury, memory for information learned before the injury is relatively preserved compared with new learning. For this reason, many patients with memory impairment will perform relatively well on tests of fund of information or recall of remote events. However, amnestic disorders can produce a retrograde amnesia, with loss of memory extending weeks, months, or years before the onset of the injury. Electroconvulsive therapy also can produce retrograde amnesia (Squire et al. 1975). The retrograde amnesia of Huntington's chorea or Korsakoff's syndrome can go back for decades (Butters and Miliotis 1985; Cermak 1982). In rare cases, a patient will have retrograde amnesia without significant anterograde amnesia; that is, new learning ability remains intact (Kapur et al. 1996; Reed and Squire 1998). Isolated retrograde amnesia may include amnesia for autobiographical events (Della Sala et al. 1993; Evans et al. 1996; Kapur 1997; Levine et al. 1998). However, cases of isolated amnesia for personal identity often have a psychogenic cause (Hodges 1991).

The Wechsler Memory Scale batteries (Wechsler 1987, 1997b) are the most commonly used set of tests of new learning and retention in the United States. These batteries are composed of a variety of tests measuring free recall or recognition of both verbal and visual material. In addition, these tests include measures of recall of personal information and attention, concentration, and mental tracking. Several of the tests provide measures of both immediate and delayed (approximately 30 minutes) recall.

Other memory tests frequently used include word-list learning tasks, such as the Rey Auditory Verbal Learning Test (Lezak et al. 2004; Rey 1964; M. Schmidt 1996) and the California Verbal Learning Test (Delis et al.

1986, 2000), and visuospatial tasks, such the Complex Figure Test (Mitrushina et al. 2005; Osterrieth 1944; Rey 1941; Strauss et al. 2006).

PERCEPTION

Perception in any of the sensory modalities can be affected by brain disease. Perceptional inattention (sometimes called neglect) is one of the major perceptual syndromes because it occurs frequently with focal brain damage (Bisiach and Vallar 1988; Heilman et al. 2000b; Lezak 1994; Rafal 2000). This phenomenon involves diminished or absent awareness of stimuli in one side of personal space by a patient with an intact sensory system. Unilateral inattention is often most prominent immediately after acute-onset brain injury such as stroke. Most commonly seen is left-sided inattention associated with right hemisphere lesions.

Several techniques can be used to detect unilateral inattention. Visual inattention can be assessed by using a Line Bisection Test (Schenkenberg et al. 1980), in which the patient is asked to bisect a series of uneven lines on a page, or by using a cancellation task requiring the patient to cross out a designated symbol distributed among other similar symbols over a page (Haeske-Dewick et al. 1996; Mesulam 2000). A commonly used test for tactile inattention is the Face-Hand Test (G. Berg et al. 1987; Smith 1983). With eyes closed, the patient is instructed to indicate when points on the face (cheeks) or hands or both are touched by the examiner. Each side is touched singly and then in combination with the other side, such as left cheek and right hand. The patient should have no difficulty reporting a single point of stimulation. Failure to report stimulation to one side when both sides are stimulated is referred to as *tactile inattention* or *double simultaneous extinction*.

Another important area of perceptual assessment is recognition of familiar visual stimuli. Although the syndromes are rare and often occur independently of one another, a brain injury can produce an inability to recognize visually familiar objects (visual object agnosia) or faces (prosopagnosia) (Barton et al. 2004; Bauer and Demery 2003; McCarthy and Warrington 1990). Assessment involves testing the recognition—often in the form of naming—of real objects or representations of objects, sometimes in a masked or distorted form. For facial recognition, "same or different" questions have been used. The WIS batteries include a perceptual task in which the subject must identify missing features of drawings of familiar objects.

PRAXIS

Many patients with left hemisphere damage have at least one form of apraxia, and apraxia is common in progressed stages of Alzheimer's disease, Parkinson's disease, Pick's disease, and progressive supranuclear palsy (Dobigny-Roman et al. 1998; Fukui et al. 1996; Leiguarda et al. 1997). Apraxic patients' inability to perform a desired sequence of motor activities is not the result of motor weakness. Rather, the deficit is in planning and carrying out the required activities (De Renzi et al. 1983; Heilman et al. 2000a; Jason 1990) and is associated with disruption of neural representations for extrapersonal (e.g., spatial location) and intrapersonal (e.g., hand position) features of movement (Haaland et al. 1999). Tests for apraxia assess the patient's ability to reproduce learned movements of the face or limbs. These learned movements can include the use of objects (usually pantomime use of objects) and gestures (Goodglass et al. 2000; Rothi et al. 1997; Strub and Black 2000) or sequences of movements demonstrated by the examiner (Christensen 1979; Haaland and Flaherty 1984).

CONSTRUCTIONAL ABILITY

Although constructional problems were once considered a form of apraxia, more recent analysis has shown that the underlying deficits involve impaired appreciation of one or more aspects of spatial relationships. These can include distortions in perspective, angulation, size, and distance judgment. Thus, unlike apraxia, the problem is not an inability to organize a motor response for drawing lines or

assembling constructions but rather misperceptions and misjudgments involving spatial relationships. Neuropsychological assessments may include any of a number of measures of visuospatial processing. Patients may be asked to copy geometric designs, such as the Complex Figure (Mitrushina et al. 2005; Osterrieth 1944; Rey 1941; Strauss et al. 2006). The WIS battery includes constructional tasks involving copying pictured designs with blocks and assembling puzzle pieces (Wechsler 1997a, 2009). Lesions of the posterior cerebral cortex are associated with the greatest difficulty with constructions, and right hemisphere lesions produce greater deficits than do left hemisphere lesions (Benton and Tranel 1993).

CONCEPTUAL FUNCTIONS

Tests of concept formation measure aspects of thinking that include reasoning, abstraction, and problem solving. Conceptual dysfunction tends to occur with serious brain injury regardless of site. Most neuropsychological tests require that simple conceptual functioning be intact. For example, reasoning skills are required for the successful performance of most WIS tests: Comprehension assesses commonsense verbal reasoning and interpretation of proverbs; Similarities measures ability to make verbal abstractions by asking for similarities between objects or concepts; Arithmetic involves arithmetic problem solving; Picture Completion requires perceptual reasoning; Picture Arrangement examines sequential reasoning for thematic pictures; Block Design and Object Assembly test visuospatial analysis and synthesis, respectively; and Matrix Reasoning depends on pattern, spatial, and numerical relationships as well as verbal components.

Other commonly used tests of concept formation include the Category Test (Halstead 1947), the Wisconsin Card Sorting Test (WCST; E.A. Berg 1948; D.A. Grant and Berg 1948; Spreen and Strauss 1998), and the California Sorting Test (Hartman et al. 2004). These tests measure concept formation, hypothesis testing, problem solving, flexibility of thinking, and short-term memory. The Category Test presents patterns of stimuli and requires the patient to figure out a principle or concept that is true for each item within the set based on feedback about the correctness of each response. The patient is told that the correct principle may be the same for all sets or different for each set. For example, the correct principle in one set is position (first, second, etc.) of the stimulus on the page, whereas for another, it is the number of items on the page.

The WCST is similar to the Category Test in requiring the patient to figure out a principle that is true for items within a set. This test differs in several ways. One of the main ways is that without warning the patient, the examiner changes the correct principle as the test proceeds. Therefore, the patient must figure out independently that a shift in principles has occurred and act accordingly. The California Sorting Test asks patients to sort cards with multiple features into sets with common features and to repeat the sorting with as many new sorting criteria as possible.

Tests of conceptualization and reasoning illustrate some of the interpretation problems inherent in most neuropsychological tests because they require complex mental activity. Thus, patients with recent memory disorders and those who are highly distractible may be able to solve the conceptual problems presented by these tests but fail because of inability to keep the correct solution in mind.

EXECUTIVE FUNCTIONS

Executive functions include abilities to formulate a goal, to plan, to carry out goal-directed plans effectively, and to monitor and self-correct spontaneously and reliably (Lezak 1982). Open-ended tests that permit the patient to decide how to perform the task and when it is complete are difficult tasks for many patients with frontal lobe or diffuse brain injuries (Lezak 1982; Luria 1980). Yet the abilities these tasks test are essential for fulfilling most adult responsibilities and maintaining socially appropriate conduct. The Tower of London (Shallice 1982) and Tower of Hanoi tests also assess planning and foresight, as disks are

moved from stack to stack to reach a stated goal. Patients with frontal lobe lesions have particular difficulty with planning tests (Carlin et al. 2000; Goel and Grafman 1995). Other tasks that rely heavily on planning for successful completion are multistep tasks calling for decision-making or priority-setting abilities. Few neuropsychological tests are specifically designed to assess these aspects of behavior, yet many complex tasks depend on this analysis. An exception is a set of real-world tasks developed for this purpose called the Behavioural Assessment of the Dysexecutive Syndrome (B.A. Wilson et al. 1996), which has been shown to bring out problems with flexibility, planning, and priority setting in patients with brain injury (Norris and Tate 2000), or schizophrenia (Krabbendam et al. 1999).

Adaptive behavior often requires changing behavior according to new demands. The WCST also measures adaptive decision making in that the patient must be able to recognize the changed sorting principle and adjust his or her responses accordingly. Many patients with dorsolateral frontal lobe lesions recognize that a change has occurred but either are slow or never alter their responses according to the new demands (Stuss et al. 2000).

Inertia presents one of the most difficult assessment problems for neuropsychologists. Few open-ended tests measure initiation or ability to carry out purposeful behavior. By their very nature, most tests are structured and require little initiation by the patient (Lezak 1982). Examples of less structured tests include the Tinker Toy Test, in which the patient decides what to build and how to design it (Bayless et al. 1989; Lezak 1982). Because there are few rules, the patient's level of productivity on this task typically reflects his or her level of productivity in the real world (Lezak et al. 2004).

PERSONALITY AND EMOTIONAL STATUS

Numerous questionnaires have been devised to measure symptoms of physical and emotional distress of patients with neurological or medical problems (Fischer et al. 2004; Lezak 1989). As examples, the Neurobehavioral Rating Scale (H.S. Levin et al. 1987) is an examiner-rated measure of problems commonly associated with traumatic brain injury, and the Mayo-Portland Adaptability Inventory provides for ratings from clinicians, the patient, and the patient's family members (Malec et al. 2000).

Many tests devised to measure psychological distress or psychiatric illness have been used with persons with brain disorders. The Symptom Checklist–90—Revised (SCL-90-R; Derogatis 1983) is a self-report of symptoms associated with psychiatric disorders when they occur at high frequency levels. The Minnesota Multiphasic Personality Inventory (MMPI; Dahlstrom et al. 1975; Hathaway and McKinley 1951; Welsh and Dahlstrom 1956) and the revised version, the MMPI-2 (Butcher 1989; Butcher and Pope 1990; Butcher et al. 1989), have been used extensively with patients with brain disorders (Chelune et al. 1986; Dahlstrom et al. 1975; Mueller and Girace 1988). In general, these patients tend to have elevated MMPI and MMPI-2 profiles, which may reflect the relatively frequent incidence of emotional disturbance (Filskov and Leli 1981), patients' accurate reporting of symptoms and deficits (Lezak et al. 2004), or their compromised ability to read or understand the test questions. Elevations on scales Hs ("Hypochondriasis"), Hy ("Hysteria"), and Sc ("Schizophrenia") are common because many "neurological" symptoms appear on these scales (Cripe 1999; Gass 1992; Gass and Apple 1997; Lachapelle and Alfano 2005). The interpretation of data from persons with brain disorders must take into account the contributions of neurological symptoms, the patient's emotional reactions to the condition, and the patient's premorbid personality.

Many attempts have been made to use the MMPI to differentiate diagnoses of psychiatric and neurological illness. Results generally have been unsatisfactory, probably due to the extreme variety of brain disorders and their associated problems (Glassmire et al. 2003; Lezak et al. 2004). It is not surprising that the MMPI also has been an inefficient instrument for localizing cerebral lesions (Lezak et al. 2004).

Neuropsychologists are frequently asked to evaluate "psychological overlay" or functional complaints. The diagnostic problem occurs because some individuals may be financially motivated to establish injuries related to work or accidents for which financial compensation may be sought. In addition, some individuals receive emotional or social rewards for invalidism, leading to malingering and functional disabilities. It is difficult to establish with complete certainty that a person's complaints are functional. To add to the complexity of the diagnosis, patients with established brain injury sometimes embellish their symptoms, wittingly or unwittingly, so that the range of problems may represent a combination of true deficits and exaggeration. The clinician usually must search for a combination of factors that would support or discredit a functional diagnosis (Lezak et al. 2004). General factors include evidence of inconsistency in history, reporting of symptoms, or test performance; the individual's emotional predisposition; the probability of secondary gain; and the patient's emotional reactions to his or her complaints, such as the classic *la belle indifférence*.

TREATMENT AND PLANNING

Examination findings are used to assess an individual's strengths and weaknesses and to formulate treatment interventions (Christensen and Uzzell 2000; Lezak 1987; Raskin and Mateer 1999; B.A. Wilson et al. 2002). Clinical interventions vary according to the individual's specific needs. Many patients with brain disorders have primary or secondary emotional problems for which psychotherapy or counseling is advisable. However, brain-injured patients frequently have problems that require special consideration. Foremost among these problems are cognitive rigidity, impaired learning ability, and diminished self-awareness, any one of which may limit the patient's adaptability and capacity to benefit from rehabilitation.

Therefore, neuropsychological evaluations provide important information about treatment possibilities and strategies. The evaluation is also used to consider patients' capability for independence in society and their educational or vocational potential.

RECOMMENDED READINGS

Heilman K, Valenstein E (eds): Clinical Neuropsychology, 4th Edition. New York, Oxford University Press, 2003

Lezak M, Howieson D, Loring D: Neuropsychological Assessment, 4th Edition. New York, Oxford University Press, 2004

REFERENCES

Abbruzzese M, Bellodi L, Ferri S, et al: Frontal lobe dysfunction in schizophrenia and obsessive-compulsive disorder: a neuropsychological study. Brain Cogn 27:202–212, 1995

Abrahams S, Pickering A, Polkey CE, et al: Spatial memory deficits in patients with unilateral damage to the right hippocampal formation. Neuropsychologia 35:11–24, 1997

Adler CM, McDonough-Ryan P, Sax KW, et al: fMRI of neuronal activation with symptom provocation in unmedicated patients with obsessive compulsive disorder. J Psychiatr Res 34:317–324, 2000

Aine CJ: A conceptual overview and critiques of functional neuroimaging techniques in humans, I: MRI/FMRI and PET. Crit Rev Neurobiol 9:229–309, 1995

Ali SO, Denicoff KD, Altshuler LL, et al: A preliminary study of the relation of neuropsychological performance to neuroanatomic structures in bipolar disorder. Neuropsychiatry Neuropsychol Behav Neurol 13:20–28, 2000

Allen DN, Goldstein G, Warnick E: A consideration of neuropsychologically normal schizophrenia. J Int Neuropsychol Soc 9:56–63, 2003

Anastasi A, Urbina S: Psychological Testing. Upper Saddle River, NJ, Prentice-Hall, 1997

Andersen G, Vestergaard K, Ingemann-Nielsen M, et al: Risk factors for post-stroke depression. Acta Psychiatr Scand 92:193–198, 1995

Armitage SG: An analysis of certain psychological tests used for the evaluation of brain injury. Psychol Monogr (No 277) 60:1–48, 1946

Armstrong FD, Thompson RJ Jr, Wang W, et al: Cognitive functioning and brain magnetic resonance imaging in children with sickle cell disease. Neuropsychology Committee of the Cooperative Study of Sickle Cell Disease. Pediatrics 97:864–870, 1996

Baddeley A: Working memory: the interface between memory and cognition, in Memory Systems 1994. Edited by Schacter DL, Tulving E. Cambridge, MA, MIT Press, 1994, pp 351–367

Baddeley A, Kopelman M, Wilson B (eds): The Handbook of Memory Disorders, 2nd Edition. West Sussex, England, Wiley, 2002

Barton JJ, Cherkasova MV, Press DZ, et al: Perceptual functions in prosopagnosia. Perception 33:939–956, 2004

Basso MR, Bornstein RA: Neuropsychological deficits in psychotic versus nonpsychotic unipolar depression. Neuropsychology 13:69–75, 1999a

Basso MR, Bornstein RA: Relative memory deficits in recurrent versus first-episode major depression on a word-list learning task. Neuropsychology 13:557–563, 1999b

Bauer R, Demery J: Agnosia, in Clinical Neuropsychology. Edited by Heilman K, Valenstein E. New York, Oxford University Press, 2003, pp 236–295

Bauer R, Grande L, Valenstein E: Amnesic disorders, in Clinical Neuropsychology. Edited by Heilman K, Valenstein E. New York, Oxford University Press, 2003, pp 495–573

Bayless JD, Varney NR, Roberts RJ: Tinker Toy Test performance and vocational outcome in patients with closed head injuries. J Clin Exp Neuropsychol 11:913–917, 1989

Bennett T, Raymond M: Utilizing neuropsychological assessment in disability determination and rehabilitation planning, in Handbook of Forensic Neuropsychology. Edited by Horton AJ, Hartlage L. New York, Springer, 2003, pp 237–257

Benson DF, Djenderedjian A, Miller BL, et al: Neural basis of confabulation. Neurology 46:1239–1243, 1996

Benton AL, Hamsher KD: Multilingual Aphasia Examination. Iowa City, IO, AJA Associates, 1989

Benton AL, Tranel D: Visuoperceptual, visuospatial, and visuoconstructive disorders, in Clinical Neuropsychology. Edited by Heilman KM, Valenstein E. New York, Oxford University Press, 1993, pp 461–497

Berg EA: A simple objective test for measuring flexibility in thinking. J Gen Psychol 39:15–22, 1948

Berg G, Edwards DR, Danzinger WL, et al: Longitudinal change in three brief assessments of SDAT. J Am Geriatr Soc 35:205–212, 1987

Bigler ED: Neuroimaging in mild TBI, in The Evaluation and Treatment of Mild Traumatic Brain Injury. Edited by Varney NR, Roberts RJ. Hillsdale, NJ, Erlbaum, 1999, pp 63–80

Binks SW, Gold JJ: Differential cognitive deficits in the neuropsychology of schizophrenia. Clin Neuropsychol 12:8–20, 1998

Bisiach E, Vallar G: Hemineglect in humans, in Handbook of Neuropsychology, Vol 1. Edited by Boller F, Grafman J. Amsterdam, The Netherlands, Elsevier, 1988, pp 195–222

Bleiberg J, Kane RL, Reeves DL, et al: Factor analysis of computerized and traditional tests used in mild brain injury research. Clin Neuropsychol 14:287–294, 2000

Boller F, Vignolo LA: Latent sensory aphasia in hemisphere-damaged patients: an experimental study with the Token Test. Brain 89:815–831, 1966

Boone KB, Lesser IM, Miller BL, et al: Cognitive functioning in older depressed outpatients: relationship of presence and severity of depression to neuropsychological test scores. Neuropsychology 9:390–398, 1995

Brandstadter D, Oertel WH: Depression in Parkinson's disease. Adv Neurol 91:371–381, 2003

Butcher JN: User's Guide for the MMPI-2 Minnesota Report: Adult Clinical System. Minneapolis, MN, National Computer Systems, 1989

Butcher JN, Pope KS: MMPI-2: a practical guide to clinical, psychometric, and ethical issues. Independent Practitioner 10:20–25, 1990

Butcher JN, Dahlstrom WG, Graham JR, et al: Minnesota Multiphasic Personality Inventory (MMPI-2): Manual for Administration and Scoring. Minneapolis, University of Minnesota Press, 1989

Butters J, Miliotis P: Amnesic disorders, in Clinical Neuropsychology, 2nd Edition. Edited by Heilman KM, Valenstein E. New York, Oxford University Press, 1985, pp 403–451

Caetano SC, Hatch JP, Brambilla P, et al: Anatomical MRI study of hippocampus and amygdala in patients with current and remitted major depression. Psychiatry Res 132:141–147, 2004

Carlin D, Bonerba J, Phipps M, et al: Planning impairments in frontal lobe dementia and frontal lobe lesion patients. Neuropsychologia 38:655–665, 2000

Cermak LS (ed): Human Memory and Amnesia. Hillsdale, NJ, Erlbaum, 1982

Chamberlain SR, Blackwell AD, Fineberg NA, et al: The neuropsychology of obsessive compulsive disorder: the importance of failures in cognitive and behavioural inhibition as candidate endophenotypic markers. Neurosci Biobehav Rev 29:399–419, 2005

Chelune GJ, Ferguson W, Moehle K: The role of standard cognitive and personality tests in neuropsychological assessment, in Clinical Application of Neuropsychological Test Batteries. Edited by Incagnoli T, Goldstein G, Golden CJ. New York, Plenum, 1986, pp 75–119

Christensen A-L: Luria's Neuropsychological Investigation Test, 2nd Edition. Copenhagen, Denmark, Munksgaard, 1979

Christensen A-L, Uzzell B (eds): International Handbook of Neuropsychological Rehabilitation. Dordrecht, The Netherlands, Kluwer Academic Publishers, 2000

Cicerone K, Azulay J: Diagnostic utility of attention measures in postconcussion syndrome. Clin Neuropsychol 16:280–289, 2002

Corballis MC: The Lopsided Ape. New York, Oxford University Press, 1991

Cripe LI: Use of the MMPI with mild closed head injury, in The Evaluation and Treatment of Mild Traumatic Brain Injury. Edited by Varney NR, Roberts RJ. Hillsdale, NJ, Erlbaum, 1999, pp 291–314

Cummings JL: Depression in neurologic diseases. Psychiatr Ann 24:525–531, 1994

Cummings JL: Principles of neuropsychiatry: towards a neuropsychiatric epistemology. Neurocase 5:181–188, 1999

Dahlstrom WG, Welsh GS, Dahlstrom LE: An MMPI Handbook, Vol 1: Clinical Interpretation, Revised. Minneapolis, University of Minnesota Press, 1975

Dalgleish R, Cox SG: Mood and memory, in Memory Disorders in Psychiatric Practice. Edited by Berrios GE, Hodges JR. New York, Cambridge University Press, 2000, pp 34–46

Damasio H, Damasio A: The lesion method in behavioral neurology and neuropsychology, in Behavioral Neurology and Neuropsychology. Edited by Feinberg T, Farah M. New York, McGraw-Hill, 2003, pp 71–84

Deckersbach T, Otto MW, Savage CR, et al: The relationship between semantic organization and memory in obsessive-compulsive disorder. Psychother Psychosom 69:101–107, 2000

Delis DC, Kramer JH, Kaplan E, et al: California Verbal Learning Test. San Antonio, TX, Psychological Corporation, 1986

Delis DC, Kaplan E, Kramer JH, et al: California Verbal Learning Test, 2nd Edition (CVLT-II) Manual. San Antonio, TX, Harcourt Brace, 2000

Della Sala S, Laiacona M, Spinnler H, et al: Autobiographical recollection and frontal damage. Neuropsychologia 31:823–839, 1993

De Luca CR, Wood SJ, Anderson V, et al: Normative data from the CANTAB, I: development of executive function over the lifespan. J Clin Exp Neuropsychol 25:242–254, 2003

Denicoff KD, Ali SO, Mirsky AF, et al: Relationship between prior course of illness and neuropsychological functioning in patients with bipolar disorder. J Affect Disord 56:67–73, 1999

Deouell L, Ivry R, Knight R: Electrophysiologic methods and transcranial magnetic stimulation in behavioral neurology and neuropsychology, in Behavioral Neurology and Neuropsychology. Edited by Feinberg T, Farah M. New York, McGraw-Hill, 2003, pp 105–134

De Renzi E, Vignolo LA: The Token Test: a sensitive test to detect disturbances in aphasics. Brain 85:665–678, 1962

De Renzi E, Faglioni P, Lodesani M, et al: Performance of left brain–damaged patients on imitation of single movements and motor sequences. Cortex 19:333–343, 1983

Derogatis LR: Symptom Checklist–90—Revised (SCL-90-R). Towson, MD, Clinical Psychometric Research, 1983

Dikmen S, Machamer J, Savoie T, et al: Life quality outcome in head injury, in Neuropsychological Assessment of Neuropsychiatric Disorders, 2nd Edition. Edited by Grant I, Adams KM. New York, Oxford University Press, 1996, pp 552–576

Diller L: Poststroke rehabilitation practice guidelines, in International Handbook of Neuropsychological Rehabilitation. Edited by Christensen A-L, Uzzell BP. New York, Kluwer Academic/Plenum, 2000, pp 167–182

Dobigny-Roman N, Dieudonne-Moinet B, Verny M, et al: Ideomotor apraxia test: a new test of imitation of gestures for elderly people. Eur J Neurol 5:571–578, 1998

Dore GJ, McDonald A, Li Y, et al: Marked improvement in survival following AIDS dementia complex in the era of highly active antiretroviral therapy. AIDS 17:1539–1545, 2003

Duncan C, Mirsky A: The Attention Battery for Adults: a systematic approach to assessment, in Comprehensive Handbook of Psychological Assessment, Vol 1: Intellectual and Neuropsychological Assessment. Edited by Goldstein G, Beers S, Hersen M. Hoboken, NJ, Wiley, 2004, pp 263–276

Evans JJ, Breen EK, Antoun N, et al: Focal retrograde amnesia for autobiographical events following cerebral vasculitis: a connectionist account. Neurocase 2:1–11, 1996

Farah MJ, Feinberg TE (eds): Patient-Based Approaches to Cognitive Neuroscience. Cambridge, MA, MIT Press, 2000

Feinberg T, Roane D: Misidentification syndromes, in Behavioral Neurology and Neuropsychology. Edited by Feinberg T, Farah M. New York, McGraw-Hill, 2003, pp 373–381

Feldner MT, Leen-Feldner EW, Zvolensky MJ, et al: Examining the association between rumination, negative affectivity, and negative affect induced by a paced auditory serial addition task. J Behav Ther Exp Psychiatry 37:171–187, 2006

Ferrier IN, Stanton BR, Kelly TP, et al: Neuropsychological function in euthymic patients with bipolar disorder. Br J Psychiatry 175:246–251, 1999

Filskov SB, Leli DA: Assessment of the individual in neuropsychological practice, in Handbook of Clinical Neuropsychology. Edited by Filskov SB, Boll TJ. New York, Wiley-Interscience, 1981, pp 545–576

Fischer J, Hannay J, Loring D, et al: Observational methods, rating scales, and inventories, in Neuropsychological Assessment. Edited by Lezak M, Howieson D, Loring D. New York, Oxford University Press, 2004, pp 698–737

Fowler KS, Saling MM, Conway EL, et al: Computerized neuropsychological tests in the early detection of dementia: prospective findings. J Int Neuropsychol Soc 3:139–146, 1997

Fukui T, Sugita K, Kawamura M, et al: Primary progressive apraxia in Pick's disease: a clinicopathologic study. Neurology 47:467–473, 1996

Gainotti G: Emotional disorders in relation to unilateral brain damage, in Behavioral Neurology and Neuropsychology. Edited by Feinberg T, Farah M. New York, McGraw-Hill, 2003, pp 725–734

Gass CS: MMPI-2 interpretation of patients with cerebrovascular disease: a correction factor. Arch Clin Neuropsychol 7:17–27, 1992

Gass CS, Apple C: Cognitive complaints in closed-head injury: relationship to memory test performance and emotional disturbance. J Clin Exp Neuropsychol 19:290–299, 1997

Glassmire DM, Kinney DI, Greene RL, et al: Sensitivity and specificity of MMPI-2 neurologic correction factors: receiver operating characteristic analysis. Assessment 10:299–309, 2003

Goel V, Grafman J: Are the frontal lobes implicated in "planning" functions? Interpreting data from the Tower of Hanoi. Neuropsychologia 33:623–642, 1995

Goldman RS, Axelrod BN, Taylor SF: Neuropsychological aspects of schizophrenia, in Neuropsychological Assessment of Neuropsychiatric Disorders. Edited by Grant I, Adams KM. New York, Oxford University Press, 1996, pp 504–528

Goldstein G, Allen DN, Seaton BE: A comparison of clustering solutions for cognitive heterogeneity in schizophrenia. J Int Neuropsychol Soc 4:353–362, 1998

Goodglass H, Kaplan E, Barresi B: Boston Diagnostic Aphasia Examination, 3rd Edition. Philadelphia, PA, Lippincott Williams & Wilkins, 2000

Grafman J, Wassermann E: Transcranial magnetic stimulation can measure and modulate learning and memory. Neuropsychologia 37:159–167, 1999

Grant DA, Berg EA: A behavioral analysis of degree of reinforcement and ease of shifting to new responses on a Weigl-type card-sorting problem. J Exp Psychol 38:404–411, 1948

Grant I, Heaton RK, Atkinson JH: Neurocognitive disorders in HIV-1 infection. HNRC Group. HIV Neurobehavioral Research Center. Curr Top Microbiol Immunol 202:11–32, 1995

Greisberg S, McKay D: Neuropsychology of obsessive-compulsive disorder: a review and treatment implications. Clin Psychol Rev 23:95–117, 2003

Gronwall DMA: Paced auditory serial-addition task: a measure of recovery from concussion. Percept Mot Skills 44:367–373, 1977

Gronwall DMA, Sampson H: The Psychological Effects of Concussion. Auckland, New Zealand, University Press, 1974

Gustafson Y, Nilsson I, Mattsson M, et al: Epidemiology and treatment of post-stroke depression. Drugs Aging 7:298–309, 1995

Haaland KY, Flaherty D: The different types of limb apraxia made by patients with left vs. right hemisphere damage. Brain Cogn 3:370–384, 1984

Haaland KY, Harrington DL, Kneight RT: Spatial deficits in ideomotor limb apraxia: a kinematic analysis of aiming movements. Brain 122:1169–1182, 1999

Haeske-Dewick HC, Canavan AG, Homberg V: Directional hyperattention in tactile neglect within grasping space. J Clin Exp Neuropsychol 18:724–732, 1996

Halstead WC: Brain and Intelligence. Chicago, IL, University of Chicago Press, 1947

Hartman M, Nielsen C, Stratton B: The contributions of attention and working memory to age differences in concept identification. J Clin Exp Neuropsychol 26:227–245, 2004

Hathaway SR, McKinley JC: The Minnesota Multiphasic Personality Inventory Manual, Revised. New York, Psychological Corporation, 1951

Heaton RK, Taylor M, Manly J: Demographic effects and use of demographically corrected norms with the WAIS-III and WMS-III, in Clinical Interpretation of the WAIS-III and WMS-III. Edited by Tulsky D, Saklofske D. San Diego, CA, Academic Press, 2003, pp 181–210

Hebb DO: The effect of early and late brain injury upon test scores, and the nature of adult intelligence. Proc Am Philo Soc 85:275–292, 1942

Heilman KM, Watson RT, Rothi LJG: Disorders of skilled movement, in Patient-Based Approaches to Cognitive Neuroscience. Edited by Farah MJ, Feinberg TE. Cambridge, MA, MIT Press, 2000a, pp 335–343

Heilman KM, Watson RT, Valenstein E: Neglect, I: clinical and anatomic issues, in Patient-Based Approaches to Cognitive Neuroscience. Edited by Farah MJ, Feinberg TE. Cambridge, MA, MIT Press, 2000b, pp 115–123

Heilman K, Blonder L, Bowers D, et al: Emotional disorders associated with neurological diseases, in Clinical Neuropsychology. Edited by Heilman K, Valenstein E. New York, Oxford University Press, 2003, pp 447–478

Heinrichs RW, Zakzanis KK: Neurocognitive deficit in schizophrenia: a quantitative review of the evidence. Neuropsychology 12:426–445, 1998

Hertel PT: Relation between rumination and impaired memory in dysphoric moods. J Abnorm Psychol 107:166–172, 1998

Hertzman PA, Clauw DJ, Duffy J, et al: Rigorous new approach to constructing a gold standard for validating new diagnostic criteria, as exemplified by the eosinophilia-myalgia syndrome. Arch Intern Med 161:2301–2306, 2001

Hill SK, Ragland JD, Gur RC, et al: Neuropsychological differences among empirically derived clinical subtypes of schizophrenia. Neuropsychology 15:492–501, 2001

Hodges JR: Transient Amnesia: Clinical and Neuropsychological Aspects. London, WB Saunders, 1991

Howieson DB, Dame A, Camicioli R, et al: Cognitive markers preceding Alzheimer's dementia in the healthy oldest old. J Am Geriatr Soc 45:584–589, 1997

Jason GW: Disorders of motor function following cortical lesions: review and theoretical considerations, in Cerebral Control of Speech and Limb Movements. Edited by Hammond GR. Amsterdam, The Netherlands, Elsevier, 1990, pp 141–168

Kalechstein AD, Newton TF, van Gorp WG: Neurocognitive functioning is associated with employment status: a quantitative review. J Clin Exp Neuropsychol 25:1186–1191, 2003

Kalska H, Punamaki RL, Makinen-Belli T, et al: Memory and metamemory functioning among depressed patients. Appl Neuropsychol 6:96–107, 1999

Kamitani Y, Tong F: Decoding the visual and subjective contents of the human brain. Nat Neurosci 8:679–685, 2005

Kapur N: How can we best explain retrograde amnesia in human memory disorder? Memory 5:115–129, 1997

Kapur N, Scholey K, Moore E, et al: Long-term retention deficits in two cases of disproportionate retrograde amnesia. J Cogn Neurosci 8:416–434, 1996

Kelly MD, Grant I, Heaton RK: Neuropsychological findings in HIV infection and AIDS, in Neuropsychological Assessment of Psychiatric Disorders. Edited by Grant I, Adams KM. New York, Oxford University Press, 1996, pp 403–422

Knopman D, Selnes O: Neuropsychology of dementia, in Clinical Neuropsychology. Edited by Heilman K, Valenstein E. New York, Oxford University Press, 2003, pp 574–616

Krabbendam L, de Vugt ME, Derix MM, et al: The behavioural assessment of the dysexecutive syndrome as a tool to assess executive functions in schizophrenia. Clin Neuropsychol 13:370–375, 1999

Kramer JH, Jurik J, Sha SJ, et al: Distinctive neuropsychological patterns in frontotemporal dementia, semantic dementia, and Alzheimer disease. Cogn Behav Neurol 16:211–218, 2003

Lachapelle DL, Alfano DP: Revised Neurobehavioral Scales of the MMPI: sensitivity and specificity in traumatic brain injury. Appl Neuropsychol 12:143–150, 2005

Leclercq M, Zimmermann P (eds): Applied Neuropsychology of Attention: Theory, Diagnosis, and Rehabilitation. New York, Psychology Press, 2002

Leiguarda RC, Pramstaller PP, Merello M, et al: Apraxia in Parkinson's disease, progressive supranuclear palsy, multiple system atrophy and neuroleptic-induced parkinsonism. Brain 120:75–90, 1997

Levin HS, High WM, Goethe KE, et al: The Neurobehavioral Rating Scale assessment of behavioural sequelae of head injury by the clinician. J Neurol Neurosurg Psychiatry 50:183–193, 1987

Levin JM, Ross MH, Harris G, et al: Applications of dynamic susceptibility contrast magnetic resonance imaging in neuropsychiatry. Neuroimage 4:S147–162, 1996

Levine B, Black SE, Cabeza R, et al: Episodic memory and the self in a case of isolated retrograde amnesia. Brain 121:1951–1973, 1998

Levy ML, Cummings JL, Fairbanks LA, et al: Apathy is not depression. J Neuropsychiatry Clin Neurosci 10:314–319, 1998

Lezak MD: The problem of assessing executive functions. Int J Psychol 17:281–297, 1982

Lezak MD: An individual approach to neuropsychological assessment, in Clinical Neuropsychology. Edited by Logue PE, Schear JM. Springfield, IL, Charles C Thomas, 1986, pp 29–49

Lezak MD: Assessment for rehabilitation planning, in Neuropsychological Rehabilitation. Edited by Meier M, Benton AL, Diller L. Edinburgh, UK, Churchill Livingstone, 1987, pp 41–58

Lezak MD: Brain damage is a family affair. J Clin Exp Neuropsychol 10:111–123, 1988a

Lezak MD: IQ: R.I.P. J Clin Exp Neuropsychol 10:351–361, 1988b

Lezak MD: Assessment of psychosocial dysfunctions resulting from head trauma, in Assessment of the Behavioral Consequences of Head Trauma, Vol 7: Frontiers of Clinical Neuroscience. Edited by Lezak MD. New York, Alan R Liss, 1989, pp 113–144

Lezak MD: Domains of behavior from a neuropsychological perspective: the whole story, in Integrative Views of Motivation, Cognition, and Emotion. Nebraska Symposium on Motivation. Edited by Spaulding WD. Lincoln, University of Nebraska Press, 1994, pp 23–55

Lezak M, Howieson D, Loring D: Neuropsychological Assessment, 4th Edition. New York, Oxford University Press, 2004

Liotti M, Mayberg HS: The role of functional neuroimaging in the neuropsychology of depression. J Clin Exp Neuropsychol 23:121–136, 2001

Luria AR: Higher Cortical Functions in Man, 2nd Edition. New York, Basic Books, 1980

Malec JF, Moessner AM, Kragness M, et al: Refining a measure of brain injury sequelae to predict postacute rehabilitation outcome: rating scale analysis of the Mayo-Portland Adaptability Inventory. J Head Trauma Rehabil 15:670–682, 2000

Malhi GS, Ivanovski B, Szekeres V, et al: Bipolar disorder: it's all in your mind? The neuropsychological profile of a biological disorder. Can J Psychiatry 49:813–819, 2004

Malloy P, Belanger H, Hall S, et al: Assessing visuoconstructional performance in AD, MCI and normal elderly using the Beery Visual-Motor Integration Test. Clin Neuropsychol 17:544–550, 2003

Manly JJ, Byrd DA, Touradji P, et al: Acculturation, reading level, and neuropsychological test performance among African American elders. Appl Neuropsychol 11:37–46, 2004

Markova IS, Berrios GE: Insight into memory deficits, in Memory Disorders in Psychiatric Practice. Edited by Berrios GE, Hodges JR. New York, Cambridge University Press, 2000, pp 34–46

Mast BT, Azar AR, Murrell SA: The vascular depression hypothesis: the influence of age on the relationship between cerebrovascular risk factors and depressive symptoms in community dwelling elders. Aging Ment Health 9:146–152, 2005

Mataix-Cols D, Junque C, Sanchez-Turet M, et al: Neuropsychological functioning in a subclinical obsessive-compulsive sample. Biol Psychiatry 45:898–904, 1999

Mayes AR: Selective memory disorders, in The Oxford Handbook of Memory. Edited by Tulving E, Craik FIM. Oxford, UK, Oxford University Press, 2000, pp 427–440

McCarthy RA, Warrington EK: Cognitive Neuropsychology: A Clinical Introduction. San Diego, CA, Academic Press, 1990

McKenna PJ, McKay AP, Laws K: Memory in functional psychosis, in Memory Disorders in Psychiatric Practice. Edited by Berrios GE, Hodges JR. New York, Cambridge University Press, 2000, pp 234–267

Menon RS, Kim SG: Spatial and temporal limits in cognitive neuroimaging with fMRI. Trends Cogn Sci 3:207–216, 1999

Mesulam M-M: Principles of Behavioral and Cognitive Neurology, 2nd Edition. New York, Oxford University Press, 2000

Mitrushina M, Boone K, Razani J, et al: Handbook of Normative Data for Neuropsychological Assessment, 2nd Edition. New York, Oxford University Press, 2005

Morrow L, Muldoon S, Sandstrom D: Neuropsychological sequelae associated with occupational and environmental exposure to chemicals, in Medical Neuropsychology. Edited by Tarter R, Butters M, Beers S. New York, Kluwer Academic/Plenum Press, 2001, pp 199–246

Mueller SR, Girace M: Use and misuse of the MMPI, a reconsideration. Psychol Rep 63:483–491, 1988

Nebes RD, Vora IJ, Meltzer CC, et al: Relationship of deep white matter hyperintensities and apolipoprotein E genotype to depressive symptoms in older adults without clinical depression. Am J Psychiatry 158:878–884, 2001

Nelson HE: The National Adult Reading Test (NART): Test Manual. Windsor, UK, UK:NFER-Nelson, 1982

Neumeister A, Wood S, Bonne O, et al: Reduced hippocampal volume in unmedicated, remitted patients with major depression versus control subjects. Biol Psychiatry 57:935–937, 2005

Norris G, Tate RL: The Behavioural Assessment of the Dysexecutive Syndrome (BADS): ecological, concurrent and construct validity. Neuropsychol Rehabil 10:33–45, 2000

Ochoa E, Erhan H, Feinberg T: Emotional disorders in relation to nonfocal brain damage, in Behavioral Neurology and Neuropsychology. Edited by Feinberg T, Farah M. New York, McGraw-Hill, 2003, pp 735–742

O'Connell JE, Gray CS, French JM, et al: Atrial fibrillation and cognitive function: case-control study. J Neurol Neurosurg Psychiatry 65:386–389, 1998

Ojemann GA, Dodrill CB: Verbal memory deficits after left temporal lobectomy for epilepsy. J Neurosurg 62:101–107, 1985

Osterrieth PA: Le test de copie d'une figure complexe. Archives de Psychologie 30:206–356, 1944

Palmer BW, Boone KB, Lesser IM, et al: Neuropsychological deficits among older depressed patients with predominantly psychological or vegetative symptoms. J Affect Disord 41:17–24, 1996

Palmer BW, Heaton RK, Paulsen JS, et al: Is it possible to be schizophrenic yet neuropsychologically normal? Neuropsychology 11:437–446, 1997

Pankratz LD, Taplin JD: Issues in psychological assessment, in Critical Issues, Developments, and Trends in Professional Psychology. Edited by McNamara JR, Barclay AG. New York, Praeger, 1982, pp 115–151

Paradiso S, Ohkubo T, Robinson RG: Vegetative and psychological symptoms associated with depressed mood over the first two years after stroke. Int J Psychiatry Med 27:137–157, 1997

Petersen RC, Stevens JC, Ganguli M, et al: Practice parameter: early detection of dementia: mild cognitive impairment (an evidence-based review). Report of the Quality Standards Subcommittee of the American Academy of Neurology. Neurology 56:1133–1142, 2001

Petrides M, Milner B: Deficits on subject-ordered tasks after frontal- and temporal-lobe lesions in man. Neuropsychologia 20:249–262, 1982

Pohjasvaara T, Leppavuori A, Siira I, et al: Frequency and clinical determinants of poststroke depression. Stroke 29:2311–2317, 1998

Pohjasvaara T, Mantyla R, Aronen HJ, et al: Clinical and radiological determinants of prestroke cognitive decline in a stroke cohort. J Neurol Neurosurg Psychiatry 67:742–748, 1999

Porch BE: Porch Index of Communicative Ability: Manual. Austin, TX, Pro-Ed, 1981

Post RM: Neural substrates of psychiatric syndromes, in Principles of Behavioral and Cognitive Neurology. Edited by Mesulam M-M. New York, Oxford University Press, 2000, pp 406–438

Prigatano GP, Schacter DL (eds): Awareness of Deficit After Brain Injury. New York, Oxford University Press, 1991

Quraishi S, Frangou S: Neuropsychology of bipolar disorder: a review. J Affect Disord 72:209–226, 2002

Rafal RD: Neglect II: cognitive neuropsychological issues, in Patient-Based Approaches to Cognitive Neuroscience. Edited by Farah MJ, Feinberg TE. Cambridge, MA, MIT Press, 2000, pp 115–123

Raskin SA, Mateer CA: Neuropsychological Management of Mild Traumatic Brain Injury. New York, Oxford University Press, 1999

Raspall T, Donate M, Boget T, et al: Neuropsychological tests with lateralizing value in patients with temporal lobe epilepsy: reconsidering material-specific theory. Seizure 14: 569–576, 2005

Reed JM, Squire LR: Retrograde amnesia for facts and events: findings from four new cases. J Neurosci 18:3943–3954, 1998

Reif JS, Burch JB, Nuckols JR, et al: Neurobehavioral effects of exposure to trichloroethylene through a municipal water supply. Environ Res 93:248–258, 2003

Rentz DM, Weintraub S: Neuropsychological detection of early probable Alzheimer's disease, in Early Diagnosis of Alzheimer's Disease. Edited by Scinto LFM, Daffner KR. Totowa, NJ, Humana Press, 2000, pp 169–189

Rey A: L'examen psychologique dans les cas d'encephalopathie traumatique. Archives de Psychologie 28:286–340, 1941

Rey A: L'examen clinique en psychologie. Paris, France, Presses Universitaires de France, 1964

Rickards H: Depression in neurological disorders: Parkinson's disease, multiple sclerosis, and stroke. J Neurol Neurosurg Psychiatry 76 (suppl 1):i48–i52, 2005

Robinson RG: The Clinical Neuropsychiatry of Stroke. New York, Cambridge University Press, 1998

Rogers R, Robbins T: The neuropsychology of chronic drug abuse, in Disorders of Brain and Mind. Edited by Ron M, Robbins T. New York, Cambridge University Press, 2003, pp 447–467

Rothi LJG, Raymer AM, Heilman KM: Limb praxis assessment, in Apraxia: The Neuropsychology of Action. Edited by Rothi LJG, Heilman KM. Hove, UK, Psychology Press, 1997, pp 61–73

Savage CR, Deckersbach T, Wilhelm S, et al: Strategic processing and episodic memory impairment in obsessive compulsive disorder. Neuropsychology 14:141–151, 2000

Sbordone RJ: The assessment interview in clinical neuropsychology, in Neuropsychological Assessment in Clinical Practice. Edited by Groth-Marnat G. New York, Wiley, 2000, pp 94–126

Schenkenberg T, Bradford DC, Ajax ET: Line bisection and unilateral visual neglect in patients with neurologic impairment. Neurology 30:509–517, 1980

Schmidt M: Rey Auditory Verbal Learning Test (RAVLT): A Handbook. Los Angeles, CA, Western Psychological Services, 1996

Schmidt WP, Roesler A, Kretzschmar K, et al: Functional and cognitive consequences of silent stroke discovered using brain magnetic resonance imaging in an elderly population. J Am Geriatr Soc 52:1045–1050, 2004

Seaton BE, Goldstein G, Allen DN: Sources of heterogeneity in schizophrenia: the role of neuropsychological functioning. Neuropsychol Rev 11:45–67, 2001

Shallice T: Specific impairments of planning. Philos Trans R Soc Lond B Biol Sci 298:199–209, 1982

Singh A, Black SE, Herrmann N, et al: Functional and neuroanatomic correlations in poststroke depression: the Sunnybrook Stroke Study. Stroke 31:637–644, 2000

Sloan S, Ponsford J: Assessment of cognitive difficulties following TBI, in Traumatic Brain Injury: Rehabilitation for Everyday Adaptive Living. Edited by Ponsford J. Hillsdale, NJ, Erlbaum, 1995, pp 65–101

Smith A: Clinical psychological practice and principles of neuropsychological assessment, in Handbook of Clinical Psychology: Theory, Research and Practice. Edited by Walker CE. Homewood, IL, Dorsey Press, 1983, pp 445–500

Sox HC, Blatt MA, Higgins MC, et al: Medical Decision Making. Boston, MA, Butterworth, 1988

Spreen O, Risser AH: Assessment of Aphasia. New York, Oxford University Press, 2003

Spreen O, Strauss E: A Compendium of Neuropsychological Tests, 2nd Edition. New York, Oxford University Press, 1998

Squire LR, Slater PC, Chase PM: Retrograde amnesia: temporal gradient in very long-term memory following electroconvulsive therapy. Science 187:77–79, 1975

Steinberg B, Bieliauskas L: Introduction to the special edition: IQ-based MOANS norms for multiple neuropsychological instruments. Clin Neuropsychol 19:277–279, 2005

Stern E, Silbersweig DA: Advances in functional neuroimaging methodology for the study of brain systems underlying human neuropsychological function and dysfunction. J Clin Exp Neuropsychol 23:3–18, 2001

Strakowski SM, Del Bello MP, Sax KW, et al: Brain magnetic resonance imaging of structural abnormalities in bipolar disorder. Arch Gen Psychiatry 56:254–260, 1999

Strauss E, Goldsmith SM: Lateral preferences and performance on non-verbal laterality tests in a normal population. Cortex 23:495–503, 1987

Strauss E, Sherman E, Spreen O: A Compendium of Neuropsychological Tests: Administration, Norms, and Commentary, 3rd Edition. New York, Oxford University Press, 2006

Strub RL, Black FW: The Mental Status Examination in Neurology. Philadelphia, PA, FA Davis, 2000

Stuss DT, Levine B, Alexander MP, et al: Wisconsin Card Sorting Test performance in patients with focal frontal and posterior brain damage: effects of lesion location and test structure on separable cognitive processes. Neuropsychologia 38:388–402, 2000

Tekin S, Cummings JL: Hallucinations and related conditions, in Clinical Neuropsychology. Edited by Heilman K, Valenstein E. New York, Oxford University Press, 2003, pp 479–494

Teuber H-L: Neuropsychology, in Recent Advances in Diagnostic Psychological Testing. Edited by Harrower MR. Springfield, IL, Charles C Thomas, 1948, pp 30–52

Tilak Ratnanather J, Wang L, Nebel MB, et al: Validation of semiautomated methods for quantifying cingulate cortical metrics in schizophrenia. Psychiatry Res 132:53–68, 2004

Tornatore JB, Hill E, Laboff JA, et al: Self-administered screening for mild cognitive impairment: initial validation of a computerized test battery. J Neuropsychiatry Clin Neurosci 17:98–105, 2005

Urbina S: Essentials of Psychological Testing. New York, Wiley, 2004

Vanderploeg RD, Schinka JA, Axelrod BN, et al: Estimation of WAIS-R premorbid intelligence: current ability and demographic data used in a best-performance fashion. Psychol Assess 8:404–411, 1996

Van Gorp WG, Altshuler L, Theberge DC, et al: Cognitive impairment in euthymic bipolar patients with and without prior alcohol dependence: a preliminary study. Arch Gen Psychiatry 55:41–46, 1998

Veiel HO: A preliminary profile of neuropsychological deficits associated with major depression. J Clin Exp Neuropsychol 19:587–603, 1997

Vermeer SE, Prins ND, den Heijer T, et al: Silent brain infarcts and the risk of dementia and cognitive decline. N Engl J Med 348:1215–1222, 2003

Wagner AD, Poldrack RA, Eldridge LL, et al: Material-specific lateralization of prefrontal activation during episodic encoding and retrieval. Neuroreport 9:3711–3717, 1998

Walsh KW: Neuropsychology, 2nd Edition. Edinburgh, UK, Churchill Livingstone, 1987

Walsh V, Rushworth M: A primer of magnetic stimulation as a tool for neuropsychology. Neuropsychologia 37:125–135, 1999

Wechsler D: Wechsler Memory Scale—Revised Manual. San Antonio, TX, Psychological Corporation, 1987

Wechsler D: WAIS-III: Administration and Scoring Manual. San Antonio, TX, Psychological Corporation, 1997a

Wechsler D: WMS-III: Administration and Scoring Manual. San Antonio, TX, Psychological Corporation, 1997b

Wechsler D: Wechsler Adult Intelligence Scale—Fourth Edition (WAIS-IV) Technical and Interpretative Manual. San Antonio, TX, Pearson, 2008

Wechsler D: Wechsler Memory Scale—Fourth Edition (WAIS-IV) Technical and Interpretive Manual. San Antonio, TX, Pearson, 2009

Weiland-Fiedler P, Erickson K, Waldeck T, et al: Evidence for continuing neuropsychological impairments in depression. J Affect Disord 82:253–258, 2004

Welsh GS, Dahlstrom WG (eds): Basic Readings on the MMPI in Psychology and Medicine. Minneapolis, University of Minnesota Press, 1956

West JF, Sands E, Ross-Swain D: Bedside Evaluation Screening Test, 2nd Edition. Austin, TX, Pro-Ed, 1998

Wild K, Howieson D, Webbe F, et al: Status of computerized cognitive testing in aging: a systematic review. Alzheimers Dement 4:428–437, 2008

Wilson BA, Alderman N, Burgess PW, et al: Behavioural Assessment of the Dysexecutive Syndrome. Bury St Edmunds, England, Thames Valley Test Co, 1996

Wilson BA, Evans JJ, Keohane C: Cognitive rehabilitation: a goal-planning approach. J Head Trauma Rehabil 17:542–555, 2002

Wilson KD: Issues surrounding the cognitive neuroscience of obsessive-compulsive disorder. Psychon Bull Rev 5:161–172, 1998

3

CLINICAL AND FUNCTIONAL IMAGING IN NEUROPSYCHIATRY

Robin A. Hurley, M.D.
Ronald E. Fisher, M.D., Ph.D.
Katherine H. Taber, Ph.D.

Modern medicine has embraced technology in almost every field. Although it is slightly more challenging to adapt the marvels of engineering and physics to emotion and behavior, psychiatry has seen the influence. Neuropsychiatry, as a subspecialty, developed to assess and treat cognitive or emotional disturbances caused by brain dysfunction. This concept could not have evolved without the influence of brain imaging, engineering, and physics. In the short time span of one century, imaging technology advanced from a primitive skull X ray to real-time pictures of brain changes as we perform a task or feel an emotion such as sadness or happiness. Cutting-edge imaging contributions are found not only in the diagnostic arena but also in estimating the course of illness and the expected treatment response and in the development of new neurotransmitter-specific medications.

Currently, brain imaging is divided into two categories: structural and functional (Table 3–1). *Structural imaging* is defined as information regarding the physical appearance of the brain that is independent of thought, neuronal or motor activity, or mood. Computed tomography (CT) and magnetic resonance imaging (MRI) are the standard tools. *Functional imaging* of the brain measures changes related to neuronal activity. The most common functional imaging techniques use indirect measures, such as blood flow, metabolism, and oxygen extraction. Functional imaging techniques currently used in clinical practice include single-photon emission computed tomography (SPECT), positron emission tomography (PET), and magnetic resonance spectroscopy (MRS). Other functional imaging techniques under development for clinical use or for research include functional magnetic resonance imaging (fMRI),

TABLE 3–1.   Brain imaging modalities

Type of imaging	Parameter measured
Anatomical and pathological	
Computed tomography (CT)	Tissue density
Magnetic resonance imaging (MRI)	Many properties of tissue (T1 and T2 relaxation times, spin density, magnetic susceptibility, water diffusion, blood flow)
Functional (resting brain activity, brain activation, neurotransmitter receptors)	
Positron emission tomography (PET)	Radioactive tracers in blood or tissue
Single-photon emission computed tomography (SPECT)	Radioactive tracers in tissue
Xenon-enhanced computed tomography (Xe/CT)	Xenon concentration in blood
Functional magnetic resonance imaging (fMRI)	Deoxyhemoglobin levels in blood
Magnetoencephalography (MEG)	Magnetic fields induced by neuronal discharges
Magnetic resonance spectroscopy (MRS)	Metabolite concentrations in tissue

xenon-enhanced computed tomography (Xe/CT), and magnetoencephalography (MEG).

In the first section of this chapter, we review structural imaging concepts and basic technologies; we then discuss the functional techniques most used in psychiatric patients and conclude with a brief discussion of functional neuroanatomy and an imaging atlas. We do not summarize the imaging findings of all neuropsychiatric diseases or all of the potential research applications. We do, however, review the basics of how and why to image and how to understand the findings; thus, this chapter provides the reader with a knowledge base for using neuroimaging in clinical practice.

GENERAL PRINCIPLES OF STRUCTURAL IMAGING

Early studies in the 1980s promoted the limited use of CT scanning in psychiatric patients only after focal neurological findings had been developed (Larson et al. 1981). Studies in the late 1980s and 1990s encouraged a broader use of diagnostic CT in psychiatric patients (Beres-

ford et al. 1986; Kaplan et al. 1994; Rauch and Renshaw 1995; Weinberger 1984). With the advent of utilization review and cost containment in the late 1990s, once again more narrow criteria were proposed that recommended use of CT only when reversible pathology was suspected (Branton 1999; Erhart et al. 2005). Diagnostic imaging has advanced considerably in the last decade, with multiple new brain imaging techniques coming into common clinical use. In addition, our understanding of functional anatomy, as it relates to psychiatric conditions, has increased enormously. A study of nondemented psychiatric patients found that treatment was changed in 15% of patients as a result of imaging examinations (Erhart et al. 2005). Clinical indications for neuroimaging include sustained confusion or delirium, subtle cognitive deficits, unusual age at symptom onset or evolution, atypical clinical findings, and abrupt personality changes with accompanying neurological signs or symptoms (Erhart et al. 2005; Hurley et al. 2002). In addition, neuroimaging is recommended following poison or toxin exposures (including significant alcohol abuse) and brain injuries of any kind (traumatic or "organic") (Table 3–2). The information obtained from brain imaging studies may assist with differential diagnosis, alter a treatment plan, and inform prognosis.

PRACTICAL CONSIDERATIONS

Ordering the Examination

The neuroradiologist needs very clear clinical information on the imaging request form (not just "rule out pathology" or "new-onset mental status changes"). If a lesion is suspected in a particular location, the neuroradiologist should be informed of this or given enough clinical data for selection of the best imaging method and parameters to view suspicious areas. The clinician should ask the neuroradiologist about any special imaging techniques that may enhance visualization of the limbic circuits (see subsection "Common Pulse Sequences" later in this chapter). The neuroradiologist and technical staff also need information on the patient's current condition (e.g., delirious, psychotic, easily agitated, paranoid). This may eliminate difficulties with patient management during the scan.

Contrast-Enhanced Studies

When ordering a CT or an MRI scan, the physician can request that an additional set of images be gathered after intravenous administration of a contrast agent. This process, although different physical principles are used for CT and MRI (see later sections for full discussion), is required for identification of lesions that are the same signal intensity as surrounding brain tissue. Contrast agents travel in the vascular system and normally do not cross into the brain parenchyma because they cannot pass through the blood-brain barrier. The blood-brain barrier is formed by tight junctions in the capillaries that serve as a structural barrier and function like a plasma membrane. The ability of a substance to pass through these junctions depends on several factors, including the substance's affinity for plasma proteins, its lipophilic nature, and its size. (An excellent

TABLE 3–2. Indications for imaging
Diagnosis or medical condition
Traumatic brain injury
Significant alcohol abuse
Seizure disorders with psychiatric symptoms
Movement disorders
Autoimmune disorders
Eating disorders
Poison or toxin exposure
Delirium
Clinical signs and symptoms
Dementia or cognitive decline
New-onset mental illness after age 50
Initial psychotic break
Presentation at an atypical age for diagnosis
Focal neurological signs
Catatonia
Sudden personality changes

review of the physiology of the blood-brain barrier and the basics of contrast enhancement can be found in Sage et al. 1998.)

In some disease processes, the blood-brain barrier is broken or damaged. As a result, contrast agents can diffuse into brain tissue. Pathological processes in which the blood-brain barrier is disrupted include autoimmune diseases, infections, and tumors. Contrast enhancement also can be useful in the case of vascular abnormalities (such as arteriovenous malformations and aneurysms), although the contrast agent remains intravascular. When ordering the imaging procedure, the psychiatrist should be mindful to request a study with contrast enhancement if one of the above disease states is suspected.

Patient Preparation

The psychiatrist should always explain the procedure to the patient shortly beforehand, being mindful to mention the loud noises of the scanner (MRI), the tightly enclosing imaging coil (MRI) (Figure 3–1A), and the requirement for absolute immobility during the test (MRI and CT). If the psychiatrist suspects that the patient may become agitated or be unable to remain still for the length of the examination, then sedation may be necessary. A clinician may select a regimen that he or she is familiar and comfortable with. We have found that for patients with agitation and psychosis, a sedating antipsychotic with lorazepam 1–2 mg intramuscularly 30 minutes before scanning usually works well in a physically healthy nongeriatric adult.

Understanding the Scan

The psychiatrist should review the scan and radiology report with the neuroradiologist. It is important to remember that the radiographic view places the patient's right on the reader's left and the patient's left on the reader's right. The first points to observe on a scan are the demographics: the hospital name; the date; the scanner number; and the patient's name, age, sex, and identification number. It is also important to note whether the scan was done with or without contrast enhancement. If an MRI scan has been obtained, the weighting parameters are important. The locations of these factors on CT and MRI scans are illustrated later in the chapter. Next, the psychiatrist should ask the neuroradiologist to point out the normal anatomical markers and any pathology observed on the films. Prior understanding of the limbic system anatomy is essential; this anatomy is reviewed later in the chapter.

WHAT CAN BE LEARNED FROM STRUCTURAL IMAGING?

Soon after the advent of CT and MRI, scientists began to image patients with psychotic and mood disorders, hoping to demonstrate concrete proof that these illnesses are indeed brain disorders and not conditions of "weak personalities" or "poor parenting." Initial studies in the classic conditions of bipolar disorder, major depression, and schizophrenia met with disappointing results—with, at most, nonspe-

cific findings that occur in many disease states (e.g., ventricular enlargement or generalized atrophy). As neuropsychiatry matures, so has the knowledge that can be attained from structural images. Researchers studying conditions such as cerebral vascular accidents, ruptured aneurysms, traumatic brain injury, and multiple sclerosis were among the first to document that psychiatric symptoms do occur as a result of brain injury; that emotion, memory, and thought processing happen by way of tracts or circuits (Mega and Cummings 1994); and that indeed many patients do have subtle lesions that account for their symptoms. Not only has this information led to a further understanding of brain function, but it has provided prognostic information for patients and has led to treatment plan changes (Diwadkar and Keshavan 2002; Erhart et al. 2005; Gupta et al. 2004; Symms et al. 2004).

COMPUTED TOMOGRAPHY

The first computed tomographic image, obtained in 1972, required 9 days to collect the data and more than 2 hours to process it on a mainframe computer (Orrison and Sanders 1995). The multiple detector scanners of today can capture multiple slices in less than one half second, with the entire brain scanned in about 5 seconds.

Technical Considerations

Standard two-dimensional CT. Like a conventional radiograph, CT uses an X-ray tube as a source of photons. When a conventional radiograph is acquired, the photons directly expose X-ray film. When a CT image is acquired, the photons are collected by detectors. The latest-generation CT scanners split the X-ray beam and add multiple detectors, allowing collection of multiple slices simultaneously ("multislice scanners"). These data are relayed to a computer that places the data in a two-dimensional grid to form the image (Rauch and Renshaw 1995). Many hospitals now display and store the resultant images digitally via a picture archiving and communication system, although some still print to X-ray film (De

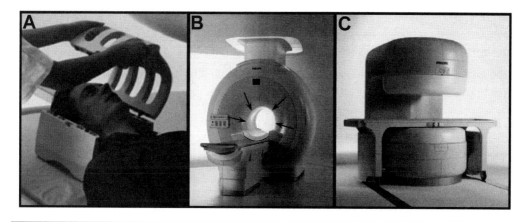

FIGURE 3–1. Magnetic resonance (MR) scanner designs.

The head coil used in magnetic resonance imaging fits rather snugly, which can be difficult for some patients (*A*). Openings have been included in modern head coils to improve patient tolerance. The traditional MR scanner is an enclosing tunnel (*B, arrows*). Open designs are gaining in popularity (*C*).

Source. Pictures courtesy of Phillips Medical Systems.

Backer et al. 2004a, 2004b). CT scans deliver a radiation dose of about 5 rads to the lens of the eye. A minimum of 200 rads is thought to be necessary to induce cataracts, but many patients receive multiple scans, and pediatric patients are more sensitive than are adults (Hopper et al. 2001). To avoid even this small dose of radiation to the lens of the eye, some institutions use a line drawn between the orbit and the external auditory meatus (referred to as the *orbitomeatal line*) as the inferior boundary of brain CT scans, thereby avoiding most of the exposure to the lens. The dose to the brain is about 7 rads in adults and about 10 rads in infants; although this amount was long believed to be quite safe, some controversy has arisen regarding data suggesting a possible long-term decrease in cognitive function following this level of radiation to the brain in infants (Hall et al. 2004). Although no appreciable radiation is deposited outside the head, a lead apron is often placed over the abdomen of a pregnant woman during a head CT scan.

The patient lies on a table that is advanced between acquisition of each CT slice. To acquire each CT slice, a beam of photons rotates around the head. As the photons pass through the head, some are absorbed by the tissues of

the head. Detectors located opposite the beam source measure the attenuation of the photons. Thus, the CT images of the brain record tissue density as measured by the variable attenuation of X-ray photons. High-density tissues such as bone appear white, indicating an almost complete absorption of the X rays (high attenuation). Air has the lowest rate of attenuation (or absorption of radiation) and appears black. The appearance of other tissues is given in Table 3–3.

Modern CT scanners generate brain images with slice thickness typically in the 2.5- to 5.0-mm range. The slice thickness of a CT image is an important variable in clinical scanning. Thinner slices allow visualization of smaller lesions. However, the thinnest sections have less contrast (i.e., the signal intensity difference between gray and white matter is less) because the signal-to-noise ratio is lower. It also takes longer to complete the examination because more slices must be acquired. Thus, there is more chance of patient motion degrading the images. Thicker sections (or slices) have greater contrast, but smaller lesions may be missed. Also, the incidence of artifacts is greater as a result of increased volume averaging (averaging of two adjacent, but very differ-

TABLE 3–3.   Relative grayscale appearance on a noncontrast computed tomography scan

Tissue	Appearance
Bone	White
Calcified tissue	White
Clotted blood	White[a]
Gray matter	Light gray
White matter	Medium gray
Cerebrospinal fluid	Nearly black
Water	Nearly black
Air	Black

[a]Becomes isointense to brain as clot ages approximately 1–2 weeks.

ent, parts of the brain within a single CT slice). This is particularly true in the base of the skull, and this may obscure brain stem and mesial temporal structures.

Three-dimensional CT (single-slice and multislice helical CT). As CT imaging became an integral part of medical diagnostics, faster and more advanced technologies were invented. The 1990s brought the clinical introduction of helical (spiral) CT, in which the detector rotates continuously around the patient during scanning (Figure 3–1C). This is much faster than the older "scan—stop—move the table and reset the detector—scan again" sequence used for standard two-dimensional CT (Figure 3–1B). Even more recently, multiple-detector helical CT scanners have come into clinical use; they produce multiple slices as multiple detectors rotate together around the patient. Sixty-four-slice (64-detector) scanners are now clinically available. These allow for extremely rapid imaging, the most important advantage of which is capturing contrast flowing through arteries, thereby creating superb CT angiograms, which are likely to replace most traditional invasive diagnostic angiography in the near future (Willmann and Wildermuth 2005). On all CT scanners, two-

dimensional images are obtained, from which reconstructions in coronal or sagittal planes can be made in a few minutes, if desired. Three-dimensional reconstructions can also be done.

Initially, single-slice helical CT was principally useful in body scanning. It had limited use in the brain because of skull thickness (i.e., it produced grainy images that did not discriminate between gray and white matter very well) (Bahner et al. 1998; Coleman and Zimmerman 1994). Applications for the head included evaluations of pediatric patients (thinner cranium), adult carotid stenosis, aneurysms, arteriovenous malformations, and vessel occlusions in acute stroke and as a tool for intravenous angiography (Coleman and Zimmerman 1994; Kuszyk et al. 1998; Schwartz 1995). The newest helical CT scanners provide images of similar quality to the standard single-slice CT and are now the standard of care for brain CT imaging (Kuntz et al. 1998).

Contrast Agents

The administration of intravenous iodinated contrast medium immediately before obtaining a CT scan greatly improves the detection of many brain lesions that are isodense on noncontrast CT. Contrast agents are useful when a breakdown of the blood-brain barrier occurs. Under normal circumstances, the blood-brain barrier does not allow passage of contrast medium into the extravascular spaces of the brain. When a break in this barrier occurs, the contrast agent enters the damaged area and collects in or around the lesion. The *increased* density of the contrast agent will appear as a white area on the scan. Without a companion noncontrast CT scan, preexisting dense areas (calcified or hemorrhagic) might be mistaken for contrast-enhanced lesions. In difficult cases, a double dose of contrast agent may be used to improve detection of lesions with minimal blood-brain barrier impairment. Contrast agents, when administered as a fast bolus, can also be used to measure several aspects of cerebral perfusion, including cerebral blood flow, cerebral blood volume, and mean transit time (Halpin 2004).

Currently, there are two types of iodinated CT contrast agents: ionic or high osmolality and nonionic or low osmolality. Both types are associated with allergic reactions, and contraindications for both exist. Allergic reactions to contrast agents are defined by two types in two time frames: anaphylactoid or nonanaphylactoid (chemotoxic) and immediate or delayed (Detre and Alsop 2005; Federle et al. 1998; Jacobs et al. 1998; Oi et al. 1997; Yasuda and Munechika 1998). Anaphylactoid reactions include hives, rhinitis, bronchospasm, laryngeal edema, hypotension, and death. Chemotoxic reactions include nausea, vomiting, warmth or pain at the injection site, hypotension, tachycardia, and arrhythmias (Cohan et al. 1998; Federle et al. 1998; Mortele et al. 2005). Immediate reactions occur within 1 hour of injection; delayed reactions, within 7 days but usually within 24 hours. The overall mortality rate from any contrast dye is reported to be 1 per 100,000. Data suggest that ionic contrast reactions occur at a rate of 4%–12% (most commonly mild) and nonionic reactions occur at a rate of 1%–3% (Cochran 2005; Cochran et al. 2002). One study reviewed approximately 20,000 contrast-enhanced CT examinations and found the rate of mild and moderate ionic dye reactions to be 2.2% and 0.08%, respectively, with 0.59% mild and 0.05% moderate with the nonionic (Valls et al. 2003).

The ionic agents are significantly less expensive, but they are less often used because of the greater risk of allergic reactions. The American College of Radiology standards recommend the use of nonionic dye in patients with histories of significant contrast media reactions; any previous serious allergic reaction to any material; asthma; sickle cell disease; diabetes; renal insufficiency (creatinine ≥1.5 mg/dL); cardiac diseases; inability to communicate; geriatric age; or other debilitating health problems (including myasthenia gravis, multiple myeloma, and pheochromocytoma) (Cohan et al. 1998; Halpern et al. 1999; Konen et al. 2002). Patients who are receiving dialysis or who have histories of milder reactions to shellfish require the use of nonionic dyes when contrast CT is unavoidable. The older ionic agents are not used in these patients.

Extravasation (leakage of the contrast dye at the injection site) is generally a mild problem associated with some stinging or burning. However, in infrequent cases, patients have developed tissue ulceration or necrosis. If a patient has had a previous episode of extravasation, then nonionic dye should be used because it is associated with fewer reactions.

Other areas of caution include patients with histories of anaphylaxis. These patients should be considered for other types of imaging rather than contrast-enhanced CT. If contrast-enhanced CT is necessary, then premedication with steroids and antihistamines and the use of nonionic dye are recommended. Metformin, an oral antihyperglycemic agent, must be withheld before iodinated dye is given. It can be restarted after 48 hours with laboratory evidence of normal renal function. Metformin can cause lactic acidosis, especially in patients with a history of renal or hepatic dysfunction, alcohol abuse, or cardiac disease (Cohan et al. 1998).

MAGNETIC RESONANCE IMAGING

In 1946, the phenomenon of nuclear magnetic resonance was discovered. The discovery led to the development of a powerful new technique for studying matter by using radio waves together with a static magnetic field. This development, combined with other important insights and emerging technologies in the 1970s, led to the first magnetic resonance image of a living patient. By the 1980s, commercial MRI scanners were becoming more common. Although the physics that make MRI possible are complex, a grasp of the basic principles will help the clinician understand the results of the imaging examination and explain this procedure to anxious patients.

Physical Principles

Reconstructing an image. Clinical MRI is based on manipulating the small magnetic field around the nucleus of the hydrogen atom (proton), a major component of water in soft tissue. To make a magnetic resonance image of a patient's soft tissues, the patient must be placed inside a large magnet. The strength of the magnet is measured in teslas (T). A high-field clinical system has a field strength of 1.5 or 3.0 T. (More powerful systems are often used in research settings.) A mid-field system is generally 0.5 T, and low-field units range from 0.1 to 0.5 T (Scarabino et al. 2003).

The magnetic field of the MRI scanner slightly magnetizes the hydrogen atoms in the body, changing their alignment. The stronger the magnetic field, the more magnetized the hydrogen atoms in tissue become and the more signal they will produce. The stronger signal available with 1.5-T and 3.0-T systems allows images of higher resolution to be collected. Some patients feel uncomfortable or frankly claustrophobic while lying inside these huge enclosing magnets (Figure 3–1B). Open-design magnets are now available that help the patient feel less confined (Figure 3–1C) (Scarabino et al. 2003). These are increasingly popular, constituting an estimated 40% of sales in the last 5 years, although the image quality is lower than in closed systems (Moseley et al. 2005).

To create a magnetic resonance image, the patient is placed in the center of the magnetic resonance scanner's powerful magnetic field. This strong magnetic field (usually 1.5 or 3.0 T) is always on and is perfectly uniform across the patient. The nuclei of the hydrogen atoms in the patient's body possess tiny magnetic fields, which instantly align with the strong magnetic field of the scanner. A series of precisely calculated radio frequency (RF) pulses is then applied. The hydrogen nuclei absorb this RF energy, which causes them to temporarily lose their alignment with the strong magnetic field. They gradually relax back into magnetic alignment, releasing the absorbed energy in a characteristic temporal pattern, depending on the nature of the tissue containing the hydrogen atoms. This electromagnetic energy is detected by the same coils used to generate the RF pulses and is converted into an electrical signal that is sent to a computer. For some body re-

gions, such as the brain or knee, a coil is placed directly around the body region to improve delivery and reception of the electromagnetic pulses and signals. The scanner's computer converts these signals into a spatial map, the magnetic resonance image. The final output is a matrix consisting of a three-dimensional image composed of many small blocks, or voxels. The voxel size on a 1.5-T scan of the brain is variable but approximately 1 mm on each side.

Creation of a magnetic resonance image requires the application of small magnetic field gradients across the patient in addition to the constant, more powerful field. This allows the scanner to tell which part of the body is emitting what signal. The magnetic field gradients needed to acquire the image are created by huge coils of wire embedded in the magnet. These are driven with large-current audio amplifiers similar to those used for musical concerts. The current in these coils must be switched on and off very rapidly. This causes the coils to vibrate and creates loud noises during the scan that may occasionally distress the unprepared patient, although patients are always given earplugs, which greatly dampen the noise.

Common pulse sequences. The combination of RF and magnetic field pulses used by the computer to create the image is called the *pulse sequence*. Pulse sequences have been developed that result in images sensitive to different aspects of the hydrogen atom's behavior in a high magnetic field. Thus, each image type contains unique information about the tissue. A pulse sequence is repeated many times to form an image.

The pulse sequence used most commonly in clinical MRI is the *spin echo* sequence. Most centers now use a faster variant of this sequence, the *fast spin echo*. These pulse sequences emphasize different tissue properties by varying two factors. One is the time between applying each repetition of the sequence, referred to as the *repetition time* or *time to recovery* (TR). The other is the time at which the receiver coil collects signal after the RF pulses have been given. This is called the *echo time* or *time until the echo* (TE). Images collected using a short TR and short TE are most heavily influenced by the T1 relaxation times of the tissues and so are called *T1 weighted*. Traditionally, this type of image is considered best for displaying anatomy because there are sharply marginated boundaries between the gray matter of the brain (medium gray), the white matter of the brain (very light gray), and cerebrospinal fluid (CSF) (black). Images collected using a long TR and a long TE are most heavily influenced by the T2 relaxation times of the tissues and so are called *T2 weighted*. Boundaries between the gray matter of the brain (medium gray), the white matter of the brain (dark gray), and CSF (white) are more blurred than on T1-weighted images. This type of image is best for displaying pathology, which most commonly appears bright, often similar in intensity to CSF. A very useful variant on the T2-weighted scan, called a *fluid-attenuated inversion recovery* (FLAIR) image, allows the intense signal from CSF to be nullified (CSF appears dark). This makes pathology near CSF-filled spaces much easier to see (Arakia et al. 1999; Bergin et al. 1995; Brant-Zawadzki et al. 1996; Rydberg et al. 1994). FLAIR improves identification of subtle lesions, making it useful for neuropsychiatric imaging. A summary of the expected imaging appearance of various tissues on commonly used types of magnetic resonance images is given in Table 3–4. The appearance of the brain is illustrated in Figure 3–2.

The next most commonly used pulse sequence in clinical imaging is the *gradient echo* sequence. In this type of image acquisition, a gradient-reversing RF pulse is used to generate the echo. This technique is very sensitive to anything in the tissue causing magnetic field inhomogeneity, such as hemorrhage or calcium. These images are sometimes called *susceptibility weighted* because differences in magnetic susceptibility between tissues cause localized magnetic field inhomogeneity and signal loss. As a result, gradient echo images have artifacts at the interfaces between tissues with very different magnetic susceptibility, such as bone and brain. The artifacts at the skull base are sometimes severe. A more recently developed method of MRI that is finding increasing clinical use is diffusion-weighted imaging. Diffusion-weighted MRI is sensitive to the speed of water diffusion and may be able to visualize areas of ischemic stroke in the critical first few hours after onset (Huisman 2003; Kuhl et al. 2005; Mascalchi et al. 2005; Nakamura et al. 2005; Symms et al. 2004). It is also showing potential in the imaging of other conditions, such as hypoglycemic encephalopathy, infection, neurodegenerative conditions, traumatic brain injury, and metabolic diseases (Jung et al. 2005; Mascalchi et al. 2005; Symms et al. 2004).

New pulse sequences. Two pulse sequences that are sensitive to other aspects of tissue state are being tested for clinical work. Magnetization transfer imaging is sensitive to interactions between free protons (unbound water in tissue) and bound protons (water bound to macromolecules such as those in myelin membranes) (Hanyu et al. 1999; Tanabe et al. 1999). It may be able to differentiate white matter lesions from different causes and thus provide insight into pathological processes (Filippi and Rocca 2004; Hanyu et al. 1999; Hurley et al. 2003; Symms et al. 2004; Tanabe et al. 1999). Diffusion tensor imaging is a more complex version of diffusion-weighted imaging (Dong et al. 2004; Kubicki et al. 2002; Sundgren et al. 2004; Taber et al. 2002b; Taylor et al. 2004). A set of images is collected that allows calculation of a multidimensional matrix (the diffusion tensor) that describes the diffusional speed in each direction for every voxel in the image. The speed of diffusion is similar in all directions in gray matter (isotropic diffusion) but is faster parallel to axons in white matter (anisotropic diffusion). This technique is sensitive to many processes that alter diffusion, including ischemia and gliosis. It can be used to identify areas of pathology or damage, such as those that occur in multiple sclerosis or following traumatic brain injury. It also has potential for studying very subtle structural changes, such as altered brain connectivity in neuropsychiatric disorders. Another promising

TABLE 3–4. Relative grayscale values present in tissues visible on magnetic resonance imaging scans (non-contrast-enhanced)

| Tissue | T1-weighted | Spin echo pulse sequences | |
		T2-weighted	FLAIR
Bone	Black	Black	Black
Calcified tissue	Variable, usually gray	Variable, usually gray	Variable, usually gray
Gray matter	Medium gray	Medium gray	Medium gray
White matter	Light gray	Dark gray	Dark gray
Cerebrospinal fluid	Black	White	Black
Water	Black	White	Black
Air	Black	Black	Black
Pathology (excluding blood)	Gray	White	White
Blood			
Acute	Dark gray	Black	Black
Subacute	White	White	White

Note. FLAIR = fluid-attenuated inversion recovery.

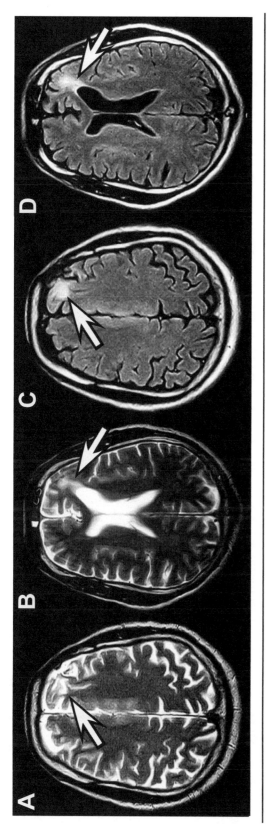

FIGURE 3–2. Appearance of the brain imaged with T2 weighting and with FLAIR.

Comparison of axial T2-weighted (T2W) and fluid-attenuated inversion recovery (FLAIR) magnetic resonance imaging (MRI) in a 36-year-old man who presented for admission with nausea, vomiting, and hyponatremia. Two days later, the patient was agitated, sexually inappropriate, and wandering incoherently. Neuropsychiatric workup revealed status epilepticus. Subsequent MRI demonstrated a previous left frontal traumatic brain injury (*arrows*). Although the injury is visible on T2W images (*A, B*), the extent of the injury is much more easily appreciated on the FLAIR images (*C, D*).

new magnetic resonance technique provides a method for imaging of cerebral blood flow by "tagging" water molecules in the carotid arteries with RF pulses (arterial spin labeling), which changes the signal intensity of the blood as it flows up into the brain (Detre and Alsop 2005). This technique has great potential because it does not require administration of a contrast agent or exposure to any form of radiation. In the future, a combination of some of these newer methods of MRI may provide important information for differential diagnosis.

Contrast Agents

The first experimental contrast-enhanced magnetic resonance image was made in 1982 using a gadolinium complex, gadolinium diethylenetriamine penta-acetic acid (Gd-DTPA), now called gadopentetate dimeglumine. Six years later, gadopentetate dimeglumine was approved as an intravenous contrast agent for human clinical MRI scans (Wolf 1991). Metal ions such as gadolinium are quite toxic to the body if they are in a free state. To make an MRI contrast agent, the metal ion is attached to a very strong ligand (such as DTPA) that prevents any interaction with surrounding tissue. This allows the gadolinium complex to be excreted intact by the kidneys. Several gadolinium-based contrast agents are currently in common use for brain imaging, including gadopentetate dimeglumine (Magnevist, Berlex Laboratories), gadodiamide (Omniscan, Nycomed Amersham), gadoteridol (ProHance, Bracco Diagnostics), gadobenate dimeglumine (MultiHance, Bracco Diagnostics), and gadoversetamide (OptiMARK, Tyco Healthcare/Mallinckrodt Inc) (Baker et al. 2004; Kirchin and Runge 2003; Runge 2001; Shellock and Kanal 1999). These agents are administered intravenously, whereupon they distribute to the vascular compartment and then diffuse throughout the extracellular compartment (Mitchell 1997).

Gadolinium is a metal ion that is highly paramagnetic, with a natural magnetic field 657 times greater than that of the hydrogen atom. Unlike the iodinated contrast agents used in CT, the currently used clinical MRI

contrast agents are not imaged directly. Rather, the presence of the contrast agent changes the T1 and T2 properties of hydrogen atoms (protons) in nearby tissue (Runge et al. 1997). Like CT contrast agents, MRI contrast agents do not enter the brain under normal conditions, because they cannot pass through the blood-brain barrier. When the blood-brain barrier is damaged, these agents accumulate in tissue around the breakdown. The effect of this accumulation is most easily seen on a T2-weighted scan. It results in an increase in signal (seen as a white or bright area; illustrated in Figure 3–3) (Runge et al. 1997). As in CT, cerebral blood flow can be assessed if images are acquired very quickly after administration of a contrast agent (this technique is variously called dynamic susceptibility contrast, first-pass perfusion MRI, or bolus perfusion MRI) (Latchaw 2004; Sunshine 2004).

On a worldwide basis, 30%–40% of MRI studies include contrast enhancement (Shellock and Kanal 1999). The total incidence of adverse side effects appears to be less than 3%–5%, with any single type of side effect occurring in fewer than 1% of patients (Kirchin and Runge 2003; Runge 2001; Runge et al. 1997; Shellock and Kanal 1999). Immediate reactions at the injection site include warmth or a burning sensation, pain, and local edema. Delayed reactions (including erythema, swelling, and pain) appear 1–4 days after the injection. Immediate systemic reactions include nausea (sometimes vomiting) and headache. Anaphylactoid reactions have been reported, particularly in patients with a history of allergic respiratory disease. The incidence of these reactions appears to be somewhere between 1 and 5 in 500,000. These agents can be used even in a patient with severe renal disease, provided he or she has some renal output. This allows contrast-enhanced MRI scans to be obtained in dialysis patients. The presence of some of these contrast agents (Omniscan, OptiMARK) has been reported to interfere with colorimetric assays for serum calcium, resulting in an incorrect diagnosis of hypocalcemia in 15% of patients in one study (Kirchin and Runge 2003). (For a more extensive review of the biosafety

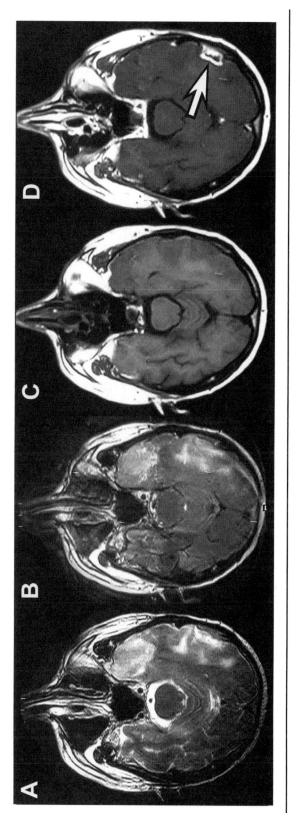

FIGURE 3–3. Improved visualization of pathology with T2-weighted imaging and use of a contrast agent.

Some types of pathology are much more easily visualized following administration of a contrast agent. A 69-year-old man presented with acute confusion after having experienced a generalized tonic-clonic seizure. Sequential magnetic resonance imaging revealed a left temporal mass, most probably an astrocytoma (infiltrating type). The tumor is more easily seen on T2-weighted (A) and FLAIR (B) images than on T1-weighted images (C). Following contrast administration (D), an area of blood-brain barrier breakdown within the tumor becomes visible (*arrow*).

aspects of MRI contrast agents, see Shellock and Kanal 1999.) Many new MRI contrast agents are under development (Bulte 2004). As new contrast agents become available for MRI of the brain, the range of applications in neuropsychiatry may well expand.

Safety and Contraindications

To date, there appear to be no permanent hazardous effects from short-term exposure to magnetic fields and RF pulses generated in clinical MRI scanners (Price 1999; Shellock and Crues 2004). Volunteers scanned in systems with higher field strength (4 T) have reported effects including headache, dizziness, and nausea (Shellock 1991). With very intense gradients, it is possible to stimulate peripheral nerves directly, but this is not a concern at clinical field strengths (Bourland et al. 1999; Hoffmann et al. 2000; Shellock and Crues 2004).

There are, however, important contraindications to the use of MRI (see Table 3–5 for summary). The magnetic field can damage electrical, mechanical, or magnetic devices implanted in or attached to the patient. Pacemakers can be damaged by programming changes, possibly inducing arrhythmias. Currents can develop within the wires, leading to burns, fibrillation, or movement of the wires or the pacemaker unit itself. Cochlear implants, dental implants, magnetic stoma plugs, bone-growth stimulators, and implanted medication-infusion pumps can all be demagnetized or injure the patient by movement during exposure to the scanner's magnetic field. In addition, metallic implants, shrapnel, bullets, or metal shavings within the eye (e.g., from welding) can conduct a current and/or move, injuring the eye. All of these devices distort the magnetic resonance image locally and may decrease diagnostic accuracy. Metallic objects near the magnet can be drawn into the magnet at high speed, injuring the patient or staff (Price 1999; Shellock 1991, 2002; Shellock and Crues 2004).

Although there is no evidence of damage to the developing fetus, most authorities recommend caution. Judgment should be exercised when considering MRI of a pregnant woman. When possible, express written consent might be obtained from the patient, especially in the first trimester (Shellock 1991; Shellock and Crues 2004; Shellock and Kanal 1991; Wilde et al. 2005). Difficulties also have been encountered when a patient requires physiological monitoring during the procedure. Several manufacturers have developed MRI-compatible respirators and monitors for blood pressure and heart rate. If these are not available, then the standard monitoring devices must be placed at least 8 feet from the magnet. Otherwise, the readout may be altered or the devices may interfere with obtaining the MRI scan.

MRI VERSUS CT

The choice of imaging modality should be based on the anatomy and/or pathology that one desires to view (see Table 3–5). CT is used as an inexpensive screening examination. Also, a few conditions are best viewed with CT, including calcification, acute hemorrhage, and any bone injury, because these pathologies are not yet reliably imaged with MRI. However, in the vast majority of cases, MRI is the preferred modality. The anatomical detail is much better, more types of pathology are visible, and the brain can be imaged in any plane of section. For example, subcortical lesions are consistently better visualized with MRI because of the greater gray-white contrast and the ability to image in planes other than axial. Thus, most temporal lobe structures, especially the hippocampal formation and amygdala, are most easily evaluated with the coronal and sagittal planes of section rather than axial. Demyelination resulting from poison exposure or autoimmune disease (such as multiple sclerosis) is also better visualized with MRI, especially when many small lesions are present. MRI does not produce the artifacts from bone that are seen with CT, so all lesions near bone (e.g., brain stem, posterior fossa, pituitary, hypothalamus) are better visualized on MRI.

TABLE 3–5. Factors considered when choosing computed tomography (CT) or magnetic resonance imaging (MRI) examination

Clinical considerations	CT	MRI
Availability	Universal	Limited
Sensitivity	Good	Superior
Resolution	1.0 mm	1.0 mm
Average examination time	4–5 minutes	30–35 minutes
Plane of section	Axial only	Any plane of section
Conditions for which it is the preferred procedure	Screening examination Acute hemorrhage Calcified lesions Bone injury	All subcortical lesions Poison or toxin exposure Demyelinating disorders Eating disorders Examination requiring anatomical detail, especially temporal lobe or cerebellum Any condition best viewed in nonaxial plane
Contraindications	History of anaphylaxis or severe allergic reaction (contrast-enhanced CT) Creatinine ≥1.5 mg/dL (contrast-enhanced CT) Metformin administration on day of scan (contrast-enhanced CT)	Any magnetic metal in the body, including surgical clips and sutures Implanted electrical, mechanical, or magnetic devices Claustrophobia History of welding (requires skull films before MRI) Pregnancy (legal contraindication)
Medicare reimbursement per scan without contrast medium	~$240	~$540
Medicare reimbursement with and without contrast medium[a]	~$380	~$1,150

[a]A scan without contrast medium is always acquired before the contrast-enhanced scan.

GENERAL PRINCIPLES OF FUNCTIONAL IMAGING

Functional brain imaging techniques provide several ways of assessing brain physiology. Regional cerebral blood flow (rCBF) and regional cerebral metabolic rate (rCMR) are the most broadly used measures (SPECT and PET). These both provide an indirect measure of brain activity. Neuronal activity consumes oxygen and metabolites and induces vasodilation of the nearby muscular arterioles, leading to a prompt increase in blood flow. A close coupling occurs between neuronal activity, rCBF, and rCMR, although the increase in blood flow, for unknown reasons, is more than is necessary to supply the increased demand for oxygen and glucose.

If acquired under resting conditions, both rCMR and rCBF provide a way to assess the baseline functional state of brain areas. Many of these techniques can also be used during performance of a mental or physical task designed to activate specific neuronal pathways or structures. This allows brain activity under specific cognitive or affective conditions to be measured. Pharmacological challenges are also used. Neuronal activity can be directly assessed during activation tasks via measures of electrical activity (electroencephalography [EEG]) or magnetic activity (MEG). In addition, functional imaging techniques are available to measure various neurotransmitter receptor systems and regional brain metabolites. These techniques have been immensely helpful in laboratory study of multiple aspects of cognitive and emotional functioning, including learning, memory, emotional regulation, control of attention, and modulation of behavior. Differences between specific patient groups and healthy individuals have provided important insights into functional impairments that occur in some psychiatric diseases. There are many research studies of common psychiatric conditions such as major depressive disorder, schizophrenia, obsessive-compulsive disorder, and attention-deficit/hyperactivity disorder. Results have been quite variable; thus, clinical applications of functional imaging have been limited by the translation of this understanding to the individual patient.

Unlike structural imaging, functional imaging is dynamic and state-dependent. Many factors can influence scan results of a particular individual on a particular day. Thus, its penetrance into the clinical arena has been slower to evolve. Functional imaging is particularly useful for identification of "hidden" lesions, areas that are dysfunctional but do not look abnormal on structural imaging. Evaluation of the resting state also has shown potential for prediction of treatment response in some conditions. In general, patients whose clinical symptoms do not fit the classic historical picture for the working diagnosis should be considered for some form of functional imaging.

NUCLEAR BRAIN IMAGING: PET AND SPECT

Both PET and SPECT involve intravenous injection of a radioactive compound that distributes in the brain and emits (indirectly, in the case of PET) photons that are detected and used to form an image. The tracer is a molecule whose chemical properties determine its distribution in the body (e.g., fluorodeoxyglucose [FDG] distributes in cells in proportion to their glucose metabolic rate) and which contains one radioactive atom, called a *radionuclide*. Depending on what compound was injected, the distribution of radioactivity indicates regional blood flow, metabolism, number of available neurotransmitter receptors, and so forth. Regional cerebral metabolism and cerebral perfusion are tightly linked under most physiological and pathophysiological conditions (Raichle 2003). Both types of imaging studies provide very similar functional information. It is important to note that, in principle, almost any cellular function can be imaged by synthesizing a radioactive compound that crosses the blood-brain barrier and binds to a component of the relevant cellular machinery. For example, this has already been accomplished for adenylyl cyclase, protein kinase C, more than a dozen neurotransmitter receptors and transporters, and many other components of cellular biochemistry and physiology. Although these tracers are most useful in research, clinical applications for some are under development.

Practical Considerations

Ordering the examination. The nuclear medicine physician needs very clear clinical information on the imaging request form (not just "rule out pathology" or "new-onset mental status changes"). If a lesion is suspected in a particular location, this should be noted. The imaging physician and technical staff also need information on the patient's current condition (e.g., delirious, psychotic, easily agitated, paranoid). This may eliminate difficulties with patient management during tracer administration or scanning.

Patient preparation. The psychiatrist should always explain the procedure to the patient shortly beforehand, being mindful to mention the requirement for absolute immobility during the approximately 30 minutes of scanning. Nuclear cameras are not nearly as confining as magnetic resonance scanners are and very rarely cause claustrophobic reactions. Nonetheless, the scanning table is quite hard and can be uncomfortable for patients with back pain; pain medication may be worthwhile in some patients. If the psychiatrist suspects that the patient may become agitated or be unable to remain still for the length of the examination, then sedation may be necessary. Because of unknown effects on cerebral activity and blood flow, antianxiety medications and other sedative medications are best given after the tracer distribution in the brain has become fixed. This occurs approximately 5–10 minutes after injection for SPECT and 20–30 minutes after injection for PET. Such medications can be critical to achieving a successful scan in selected patients. A clinician may select a regimen that he or she is familiar and comfortable with. We have found that for patients with agitation and psychosis, a sedating antipsychotic with lorazepam 1–2 mg intramuscularly 30

minutes before scanning usually works well in a physically healthy nongeriatric adult. During imaging, the head is generally held still with support from a head-holder attachment on the imaging table, sometimes with additional support from light taping.

In preparation for scanning, an intravenous line is inserted, and the patient is placed in a quiet and darkened room. Ten to 20 minutes later, a technologist enters the room quietly and injects the radioactive tracer. This procedure allows for decreased visual and auditory stimulation during tracer uptake. The patient typically remains in the room for 30–60 minutes, although the darkness and quiet are essential only during the tracer uptake period. For clinical SPECT, uptake occurs within 1–2 minutes of injection; for clinical PET, uptake requires 20–30 minutes. During the uptake period, the tracer distributes and is trapped in the tissue of interest. Theoretically, the patient could be imaged immediately following the uptake period. Image quality is improved, however, if one waits at least 30 minutes for tracer washout from adjacent facial and scalp areas, decreasing background activity. The patient is then transported to the scanner, where he or she will lie on the imaging table for about 30 minutes for the scan. If clinically necessary, scanning can be delayed for up to about 4 hours, although tracer activity in the brain is gradually decreasing from radioactive decay, resulting in gradually worsening image quality.

Understanding the scan. Cerebral blood flow and cerebral metabolism are high in gray matter where synapses and cell bodies are located. They are lower in white matter, composed of axons. Thus, tracer uptake is high in cellular areas, such as the thalami, basal ganglia, and cortex, and lower in white matter. Consequently, SPECT and PET are not good for evaluating white matter diseases.

The psychiatrist should review the images and radiology report with the nuclear medicine physician. It is important to remember that the radiographic view places the patient's right on the reader's left and the patient's left on the reader's right. After confirmation of patient identification, the psychiatrist should ask the nuclear medicine physician to point out normal anatomical markers and any pathology observed on the images. Note that PET and SPECT scans are always interpreted as digital images. Reasonable copies can be printed on photographic paper. However, paper reproductions are often quite suboptimal for image interpretation. Images printed on X-ray film are rarely diagnostically useful and should be avoided. Three-dimensional renderings are sometimes available.

SINGLE-PHOTON EMISSION COMPUTED TOMOGRAPHY

Technical Considerations

As noted earlier, SPECT, like PET, is based on imaging the distribution of a radiotracer injected into the blood. As the radiotracer decays, it emits a photon. This is detected by a gamma camera and used by the computer to reconstruct a tomographic image, similar to the procedure for standard CT (see section "Computed Tomography" earlier in this chapter for a more extensive description of technique) (Warwick 2004). Attenuation correction for brain SPECT is estimated with a computer algorithm that assumes an ellipsoid shape of the head and constant water-density tissue attenuation. Although these assumptions are not entirely accurate, they provide a reasonable attenuation correction without the need for delivering X rays within the scanner (such SPECT-CT scanners are now commercially available).

Resolution is heavily dependent on the age and sophistication of the equipment. Older systems had limited detectors and produced lower-quality images. "Triple-head" cameras developed in the 1990s provide the best images because they acquire more counts and can be positioned very close to the patient's head. Unfortunately, the commercial market for SPECT cameras is dominated by cardiac and oncological applications, and triple-head cameras are no longer sold. Most modern SPECT cameras have a theoretical resolution of about 6–7 mm. In practice, the shoulders physically prevent the camera heads from being positioned close enough to the patient's head, reducing clinical resolution to about 1–1.3 cm (Van Heertum et al. 2004).

The two SPECT tracers approved for clinical use in the United States are [^{99m}Tc]-HMPAO (Ceretec; d,l-hexamethylpropyleneamine oxime) and [^{99m}Tc]-ECD (Neurolite; ethyl cysteinate dimer). Both provide very comparable measures of cerebral blood flow (perfusion), with regional uptake roughly proportional to flow. Uptake occurs during the first 1–2 minutes after injection. After that, the tracer is "fixed" in the brain. These are lipophilic compounds that diffuse across the blood-brain barrier and into neurons and glia, where they are converted into hydrophilic compounds that cannot diffuse out of the cell. Abnormalities in intracellular esterase or glutathione metabolism, in neurons or glia, might lead to SPECT abnormalities independent of blood flow changes. In fact, evidence suggests that most tracer uptake, at least for HMPAO, may be in glial cells rather than in neurons (Slosman et al. 2001). It must be remembered that the uptake of tracer does not have to be within neurons to be useful. Uptake is used as an indirect indicator of neuronal electrochemical activity. Even if the uptake is mainly in glia, it has been shown to clearly reflect local cerebral blood flow, which is tightly linked to neuronal activity (Magistretti and Pellerin 1996).

Although several differences between these two tracers have been described (Inoue et al. 2003), the two remain very comparable in terms of their clinical utility. A previously used perfusion tracer, [^{123}I]-IMP (iodoamphetamine), is no longer commercially available in the United States and is infrequently used elsewhere. SPECT tracers are commonly available for imaging the dopamine transporter (DAT) in Europe and Asia, but this technique has not been approved by the U.S. Food and Drug Administration (Warwick 2004).

Safety and Contraindications

The only contraindication to a nuclear medicine scan is pregnancy, and even this is only a relative indication. If the brain scan can be postponed until after delivery, a small radiation dose to the fetus can be avoided. Although very rarely necessary, the study could be performed in uncommon situations in which the scan result is critical. It is important to recognize that the tracers used in all diagnostic nuclear medicine examinations are at 1,000 to 1 million times too low a concentration to have any pharmacological effects or allergenic side effects (other than placebo effects). These tracers disappear by radioactive decay, so renal and hepatic function are irrelevant. The radiation dose to the patient as a result of a nuclear brain scan is comparable to that of a CT scan and is generally considered to be without long-term consequences, although some controversy over this issue has arisen (see discussion in subsection "Standard Two-Dimensional CT" earlier in this chapter).

POSITRON EMISSION TOMOGRAPHY

Technical Considerations

PET is based on imaging the distribution of a short-lived radioactive tracer (radiotracer) that has been introduced into the bloodstream (Cherry 2001; Fahey 2002; Paans et al. 2002; Turner and Jones 2003; Van Heertum et al. 2004). Several positron-emitting radionuclides are available for incorporation into tracers, but virtually all current clinical PET tracers use fluorine 18 (^{18}F). The most important PET tracer is [^{18}F]-FDG, which provides a map of glucose metabolism.

Positrons are released as the radiotracer decays. These travel a very short distance in tissue (about a millimeter on average for fluorine 18) before encountering an electron, and the two mutually annihilate. The mass of the two particles is converted into pure energy in the form of two high-energy photons. These travel away from each other in a straight line at the speed of light (line of response). Most of these photon pairs pass through the body and strike detectors on opposite sides of the scanner nearly simultaneously. The PET scanner recognizes when two photons have struck the ring simultaneously (annihilation coincidence detection) and estimates the site of origin of the photons as lying somewhere on a path between the two involved detectors. The object to be imaged (the head) is surrounded by several parallel rings containing thousands of these detector pairs. By combining the results of millions of such coincidence detection events, the scanner's computer can generate a high-resolution image of the distribution of radiotracer in the body, with areas of relatively high concentration appearing as "hot spots" in the image.

PET scanners contain retractable septa made of lead or tungsten between detector rings. These septa reduce detection of photons that have changed direction while in the body (such scattered photons exit the body at a location that causes the scanner to miscalculate their sites of origin). The septa allow imaging in one plane at a time, a two-dimensional acquisition. This mode is preferred on some scanner systems for whole-body imaging. The septa can be removed to yield a higher count rate. This is called three-dimensional acquisition and is much faster than two-dimensional acquisition because of the higher count rate. The increase in scattered photons striking the detector and the increase in random counts that also occur when the septa are removed can be reasonably well corrected with various software algorithms. Most centers prefer a three-dimensional acquisition for brain PET scanning. It allows a high-quality brain PET scan to be acquired in as little as 6–8 minutes. A comparable two-dimensional brain scan would take approximately 15–20 minutes. The theoretical limit for spatial resolution is about 2.5 mm (Turner and Jones 2003), whereas the resolution of clinical PET is on the order of 4–5 mm.

The only approved PET tracer for clinical use in the United States is [^{18}F]-FDG. It is taken up into cells similarly to glucose and undergoes metabolism to FDG-6-phosphate. It does not undergo further metabolism and is trapped within these cells, providing a measure of cerebral metabolic activity (rCMR glucose). Glucose uptake in PET images is likely to reside predominantly in glial cells, which convert glucose into lactate and provide the lactate to neurons as a key energy source for neurons (Magistretti and Pellerin 1996). It must be remembered that the uptake of tracer does not have to be within neurons: uptake is used as an indirect indicator of neuronal electrochemical activity. Even if the uptake is mainly in glia, it has been shown to clearly reflect local cerebral glucose metabolism, which is tightly linked to neuronal activity.

Safety and Contraindications

The safety considerations and contraindications are the same as for SPECT (see prior section).

CLINICAL APPLICATIONS

SPECT Versus PET

Nuclear brain imaging is coming into increasing use for the clinical evaluation and case formulation of psychiatric patients. These techniques can contribute to differential diagnosis, assist treatment planning, and provide information for prognostic decisions. PET has the advantages of higher spatial resolution and true attenuation correction (nearly eliminating attenuation artifacts). SPECT has the advantages of being more widely available, less expensive (approximately $1,200 for SPECT vs. approximately $1,800 for PET), and reimbursable for most conditions. Reimbursement for brain PET in the United States is currently limited to distinguishing frontotemporal dementia from Alzheimer's disease, doing presurgical evaluation of intractable epilepsy (seizure focus localization), and distinguishing radiation necrosis from recurrent brain tumors. SPECT imaging is considered a standard clinical investigative tool for neuropsychiatric evaluation. However, PET scanners are rapidly becoming more commonplace, and reimbursement for other indications is likely to occur in the near future. The old requirement

for an on-site cyclotron has been obviated by the establishment of numerous commercial cyclotrons throughout the United States, many of which can deliver an ^{18}F tracer (110-minute half-life) great distances by airplane. Virtually any hospital in the United States with a PET scanner can have [^{18}F]-FDG delivered to it relatively inexpensively. Tracers that utilize carbon 11 (20-minute half-life), oxygen 15 (2-minute half-life), or nitrogen 13 (10-minute half-life) require an on-site cyclotron facility. Common nuclear medicine findings in selected clinical conditions are discussed in the following subsections.

Primary Dementias

Dementia is the most common clinical reason for nuclear brain imaging. Scanning is particularly helpful in the evaluation of patients with atypical clinical presentations. It is expected to play a more significant role as better treatment options become available for different etiologies. For Alzheimer's disease, bilateral, symmetrical posterior temporoparietal decreased perfusion or metabolism is the classic pattern (Figure 3–4B and C). However, this is seen in approximately one-third of the patients with Alzheimer's disease. Frequently, the abnormalities are asymmetrical and may initially involve only temporal or parietal cortex. As the disease progresses, the frontal (and occasionally occipital) lobes become involved, with decreased perfusion (Figure 3–4D). Uptake in the subcortical structures, primary visual cortex, and primary sensorimotor cortex is usually preserved even in late-stage disease. The defects are always diffuse, over a large area of cortex, and easily recognizable as neurodegenerative in origin, although not necessarily specific to Alzheimer's disease.

Clinical SPECT and PET findings in dementia with Lewy bodies (DLB) overlap those of Alzheimer's disease, although the abnormalities in DLB are more likely to be asymmetrical and to involve the occipital cortex (Figure 3–5A). DAT imaging has shown more promise in distinguishing the two entities. The loss of dopamine neurons is significant in DLB, result-

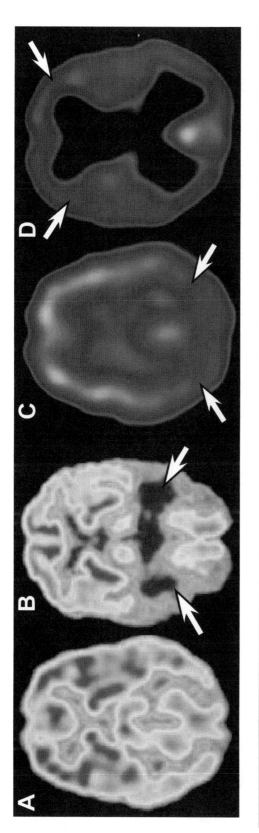

FIGURE 3–4. Diagnostic use of functional imaging in Alzheimer's disease.

See Appendix for color version. Functional imaging is very useful in diagnosis of Alzheimer's disease. Positron emission tomography (PET) imaging of cerebral metabolism in a normal individual shows high uptake of [18F]-fluorodeoxyglucose (FDG) (indicated by *orange-red*) throughout the cerebral cortex (*A*). Uptake is reduced (indicated by *blue*) regionally, usually symmetrically (*arrows*), in patients with Alzheimer's disease (*B*). Similarly, regional cerebral blood flow, imaged here using single-photon emission computed tomography (SPECT), is decreased in posterior temporoparietal cortex in early Alzheimer's disease (*C*, *arrows*). As the disease progresses, frontal lobe involvement is common (*D*, *arrows*).

Source. Images (*A*) and (*B*), pictures courtesy of CTI Molecular Imaging, Inc.

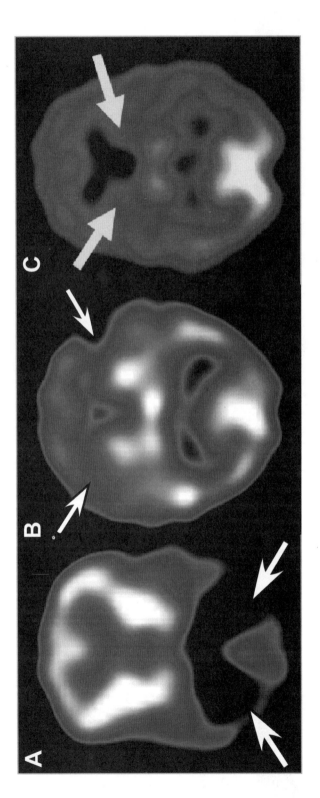

FIGURE 3–5.   Functional imaging for differential diagnosis of dementia.

See Appendix for color version. Functional imaging is also useful in differential diagnosis of dementia. A common finding in dementia with Lewy bodies is decreased perfusion in occipital cortex (*A, arrows*). A common finding in frontotemporal dementia (e.g., Pick's disease) is decreased perfusion in frontal and temporal cortex (*B, arrows*). A characteristic finding early in Huntington's disease is decreased perfusion in the basal ganglia, particularly caudate (*C, arrows*). All images are single-photon emission computed tomography (SPECT).

ing in striking abnormalities in the striatum in these patients compared with those who have Alzheimer's disease (Walker et al. 2002).

SPECT or PET scanning shows reduced perfusion of the frontal and/or anterior temporal cortex (usually bilaterally) in frontotemporal dementia (e.g., Pick's disease), which is usually readily distinguished from Alzheimer's disease and DLB (Figure 3–5B). Parkinson's disease patients often develop dementia that may be etiologically distinct from DLB, but the SPECT and PET appearance has not been well characterized and likely overlaps significantly with both Alzheimer's disease and DLB. Clinical SPECT and PET imaging in Creutzfeldt-Jakob disease identify large areas of severely reduced perfusion. These are usually symmetrical. This appearance overlaps with Alzheimer's disease and DLB, so clinical correlation is needed. Sequential SPECT and PET scans (performed about 2 months apart) often show dramatic progression (Taber et al. 2002a). In Huntington's disease, SPECT and PET imaging show characteristic reduced perfusion to the basal ganglia, especially the head of the caudate, often early in the course of the illness (Figure 3–5C). Nuclear imaging is quite sensitive and reasonably specific but is rarely used for diagnosis (diagnosis is made very accurately by sequence analysis of the Huntington's disease gene). It may be useful in predicting progression of disease (Hurley et al. 1999). As dementia progresses, many patients develop large regions of reduced cortical perfusion or metabolism on SPECT and PET in a pattern similar to that for other neurodegenerative diseases.

Epilepsy

SPECT and PET are used along with MRI and EEG in patients with medically refractory seizures to determine the optimum site for stereotaxic placement of depth electrodes. The implanted electrodes, in turn, usually provide the definitive localization of the seizure focus and the boundaries of the tissue to be surgically resected. Nuclear medicine examinations are performed either in the presence of seizure activity (ictal examination, blood flow

increased in the focus) or in the absence of seizure activity (interictal examination, blood flow decreased in the focus). Ictal examinations can only be performed with SPECT because it has rapid tracer uptake (seizures tend to last only a few minutes). This provides an accurate picture of cerebral blood flow as it was during the seizure. Ictal imaging is the better method but requires that the tracer be injected at the beginning of a seizure, less than 1 minute after onset. This necessitates that the patient be admitted to a surveillance room with EEG and videotape monitoring. The tracer is kept in a syringe attached to the patient's intravenous line. When EEG confirms onset of a seizure, tracer is immediately injected. Most centers now perform both ictal and interictal studies on every patient, looking for regions that are hot on the ictal scan but normal or cold on the interictal scan. Sensitivity and accuracy of emission tomographic imaging have been reported to be approximately 80% (Henry and Van Heertum 2003). However, most studies include large numbers of patients with seizure foci easily determined from structural lesions on MRI or by EEG. In practice, nuclear imaging is needed primarily in patients with normal MRI results and nonlocalizing or equivocal EEG findings. Accuracy of SPECT and PET in this subset of patients is likely much lower, although fewer data are available.

Vascular Disease

Although multi-infarct dementia is commonly diagnosed by structural imaging, the pattern of SPECT and PET abnormalities is often quite distinctive, with multiple moderate-sized perfusion defects that have well-defined boundaries. Small vessel disease (e.g., Binswanger's disease) is not associated with a specific SPECT or PET pattern, although basal ganglia and frontal cortex lesions often have been reported (Hurley et al. 2000). Areas of cerebral infarction are easily identified on clinical SPECT, but it is rarely clinically useful in this regard. In acute stroke, the essential information that is needed from neuroimaging is whether the stroke is hemorrhagic prior to initiating thrombolytic therapy. CT scanning is much quicker to obtain and is quite accurate in this regard. SPECT is superior to CT and MRI in predicting outcome of acute stroke and defining the size of viable but at-risk tissue but not sufficiently so to warrant routine clinical use (Barthel et al. 2001; Guadagno et al. 2003). Areas of compromised vascular reserve (partially occluded vessels), which often appear normal on a resting SPECT scan, can be visualized on a SPECT scan performed following intravenous injection of acetazolamide. Acetazolamide raises blood carbon dioxide levels, causing normal arterioles to dilate. Arterioles distal to an arterial stenosis or obstruction are already fully dilated as a physiological compensatory mechanism and cannot dilate further in response to acetazolamide. Brain regions supplied by such arterioles thus appear relatively hypoperfused, compared with normal tissue, on a postacetazolamide SPECT perfusion scan, indicating decreased vascular reserve. Such findings are thought to predict impending ischemic events that may warrant therapeutic intervention (e.g., carotid endarterectomy), although well-controlled studies with long-term clinical follow-up are not available (Marti-Fabregas et al. 2001).

Traumatic Brain Injury

Many studies have reported that SPECT is more sensitive than CT or MRI for traumatic brain injury. SPECT often shows abnormal findings (areas of reduced perfusion) in symptomatic patients even when structural imaging shows negative results (Anderson et al. 2005). It must always be borne in mind, however, that many nonimpaired subjects have some limited areas of mildly reduced perfusion. Patient motion during imaging also can produce abnormalities. False-positive studies are an important concern because almost any abnormality, even relatively small or mild ones, would have to be called positive in the scenario of traumatic brain injury. Perhaps the most useful result at this time is that a few studies have indicated that a negative (normal) brain SPECT result

after mild traumatic brain injury predicts an excellent long-term neurological outcome (Anderson et al. 2005; Bonne et al. 2003).

SPECT AND PET: IMAGING NEUROTRANSMITTER SYSTEMS

Radioligands that bind to neurotransmitter receptors have been developed to image multiple neurotransmitter systems. The same principles of radioligand development for SPECT and PET imaging can be applied to almost any type of synapse in the brain. Examples of available radioligands include dopamine and serotonin receptors and transporters, acetylcholine (muscarinic and nicotinic) receptors, histamine receptors, γ-aminobutyric acid type A (GABA$_A$) receptors, adenosine receptors, and opiate receptors. SPECT and PET imaging of neurotransmitter systems have shown promise for clinical applications. In particular, radioligands for the dopamine system have been very widely studied and are already in clinical use in Europe and Asia.

DATs are located on presynaptic terminals. They serve to transport dopamine from the synaptic space back into the terminal. This halts the action of the transmitter (thereby preparing the synapse for the next electrochemical message) and recycles it. Many ligands have been developed that bind to DATs. All are analogues of cocaine. Cocaine's mechanism of action is to bind to and inhibit the closely related transporters for dopamine, norepinephrine, and serotonin. Molecules structurally similar to cocaine have been developed for imaging that are more specific for the DAT. Activity on SPECT DAT scans is mainly in the striatum, consistent with the known high density of dopamine synapses in this region. SPECT yields a good semiquantitative estimate of DAT density. The primary clinical use of SPECT DAT imaging is in the diagnostic evaluation of early Parkinson's disease, for which it has been shown in repeated studies to be quite sensitive and specific (Benamer et al. 2003; Leenders 2003). DAT SPECT is already in routine clinical use in Europe and Asia for this purpose. A normal DAT SPECT result in a patient with early parkinsonian symptoms suggests that classic Parkinson's disease is not present. Possible alternative diagnoses include vascular Parkinson's disease, essential tremor, drug-induced parkinsonism, and somatization disorder. DAT SPECT sometimes has positive results in asymptomatic siblings who go on to develop Parkinson's disease. Imaging of the postsynaptic D_2 receptor, another approach to assessing the dopaminergic system, is normal in Parkinson's disease and reduced in multiple system atrophy (Kim et al. 2002; Knudsen et al. 2004). This is an emerging application in Europe. PET imaging of $[^{18}F]$-6-fluoro-L-dopa (F-DOPA) also may be useful.

CONCLUSION: SPECT AND PET IN NEUROPSYCHIATRY

In summary, perfusion SPECT and glucose metabolism PET find their primary use in the diagnostic workup of patients with dementia. Both types of imaging produce reasonably high diagnostic accuracy in distinguishing Alzheimer's disease from frontotemporal dementia (currently the only reimbursable indication for brain PET in dementia) and in distinguishing neurodegenerative disease from other causes of dementia and from pseudodementia. PET is generally superior to SPECT because of higher resolution and better attenuation correction. It is more expensive and less widely available than SPECT, but both of these issues are rapidly improving. Both modalities have a clearly defined role in the preoperative evaluation of patients with medically refractory epilepsy, with ictal perfusion SPECT showing the best results. Both tests are sensitive and reasonably specific for vascular disease, but a specific clinical role has yet to be defined. Acetazolamide stress perfusion SPECT shows promise for determining clinical significance of borderline vascular obstructions and for selecting patients who need intervention. Clinical benefit for these potential indications, however, has yet to be proven. Both modalities are very sensitive in detecting neuronal injury in patients with mild traumatic brain injuries. However, false positive scans are a concern, and the clinical significance of positive scans in patients with brain trauma has yet

to be fully determined. The routine clinical application of nuclear imaging to patients with mood disorders, attention-deficit/hyperactivity disorder, schizophrenia, obsessive-compulsive disorder, or other psychiatric disorders has been disappointing, despite numerous abnormalities reported in research studies. Perhaps more promising in these disorders is the use of neurotransmitter SPECT and PET. Such studies, particularly DAT SPECT, have already shown excellent accuracy and clinical utility in patients with movement disorders, especially Parkinson's disease and related disorders. Imaging of receptors and transporters may eventually play an important role in the diagnosis and management of many neuropsychiatric illnesses.

FUNCTIONAL MAGNETIC RESONANCE IMAGING

fMRI is based on the modulation of image intensity by the oxygenation state of blood. Deoxygenated hemoglobin (deoxyhemoglobin) is highly paramagnetic. It distorts the local magnetic field in its immediate vicinity. This causes a loss of magnetic resonance signal, particularly on gradient echo and other susceptibility-weighted pulse sequences. Thus, it is a natural magnetic resonance contrast agent. Image intensity is dependent on the local balance between oxygenated and deoxygenated hemoglobin. This is the origin of the acronym BOLD (blood oxygen level dependent) for the fMRI technique (Taber et al. 2003; Turner and Jones 2003).

An area of brain suddenly becomes more active when it is participating in a cognitive task. The increase in local blood flow is larger than is required to meet the activity-related increase in oxygen consumption. As a result, the venous blood becomes slightly *more* oxygenated. This decrease in local deoxyhemoglobin concentration causes a slight (1%–5%) increase in signal intensity in the activated area of brain on the magnetic resonance image. The change is too small to see by eye. It is measured by comparing signal intensity under a baseline (resting or control) condition with the signal intensity under an activated condition. Unlike PET or SPECT, all fMRI measures depend on comparison of two conditions (e.g., baseline and activated).

Activations will be seen in many areas when a subject performs a task in a scanner. Defining and creating a baseline state for comparison can be a considerable challenge. Ideally, the subject is scanned under two conditions that differ only in the cognitive function under study. For example, to identify the brain regions involved in verbal short-term memory, the subject might be scanned while viewing words projected onto a screen and then clicking with a mouse on those recently seen (test scan). For comparison, the same subject might be scanned while viewing words and clicking on all words beginning with a particular letter (control scan). When the areas of activity on the control scan are subtracted from the areas of activity on the test scan, the remaining areas of activation should primarily reflect verbal short-term memory. However, if a brain area of interest is abnormally active under the baseline (control) condition, further activation may not be measurable, resulting in an apparent absence of activation when the image sets are analyzed.

A problem with the most commonly used fMRI methods is presence of susceptibility-related artifacts in areas of magnetic field inhomogeneity, such as the interfaces between brain, bone, and air. Thus, regions of importance to neuropsychiatry adjacent to bone, such as the orbitofrontal cortex and the inferior temporal region, may be difficult to assess. It is also important to differentiate areas of increased signal within activated tissue itself from increased signal in the veins that drain the activated area. Motion artifacts can also be a problem. Any movement (minor head movement, respiration, speech-related movement) can create spurious areas of activation and mask areas of true activation. Head restraints and post processing are both important in this regard (Bizzi et al. 1993; Desmond and Annabel Chen 2002; Matthews and Jezzard 2004; Taber et al. 2003; Turner and Jones 2003).

fMRI has several advantages over other methods of imaging brain activity. Most impor-

tant, it is totally noninvasive and requires no ionizing radiation or radiopharmaceuticals. Minimal risk makes it appropriate for use in both children and adults and for use in longitudinal studies requiring multiple scanning sessions for each subject. High-resolution structural images are acquired in the same session, providing much better localization of areas of interest than is possible with PET or SPECT. In addition, most clinical MRI scanners can be modified without great expense to enable fMRI. However, fMRI is neither simple nor easy to implement and analyze, which may limit its clinical usefulness. At present, it should be considered a research technique.

The most common application of fMRI is in the field of cognitive neuroscience with psychiatrically healthy volunteers. However, interest in using fMRI to assess patients with neurological and/or neuropsychiatric disorders is increasing. Evaluation of brain function, recovery, and reorganization (adaptive plasticity, compensatory recruitment) after stroke is a promising potential area for its use (Cao et al. 1998; Marshall et al. 2000; Matthews and Jezzard 2004; Pineiro et al. 2002). It also may be of value prior to surgical brain resection in patients with epilepsy or brain tumors for definition of the exact boundaries of the primary motor areas and for lateralization of language function. The language area is now identified with the Wada test. The Wada test is both invasive and expensive, so this will be an important clinical application for fMRI if validation studies support its use (Desmond and Annabel Chen 2002; Matthews and Jezzard 2004). Preliminary studies found amygdala hyperactivity in depression, which normalized with antidepressant treatment (Sheline et al. 2001). Abnormalities in prefrontal and parietal cortex activity while performing cognitive tasks have been reported in patients with schizophrenia (Holmes et al. 2005; Menon et al. 2001). Studies also have been done in substance abuse populations (Garavan et al. 2000). Identification of early (perhaps even preclinical) disease may be possible, as indicated by differences in activation to a memory task in patients who later developed Alzheimer's disease and abnormalities of activation during a semantic categorization task in asymptomatic apolipoprotein ε4 carriers (who are genetically at risk to develop Alzheimer's disease) (Bookheimer et al. 2000; Lind et al. 2006). Evaluation of the effects of genetic polymorphisms on information processing and emotional function as measured by fMRI (imaging genomics) is of increasing interest (Hariri et al. 2002). However, development of standardized protocols and comparison groups will be critical for clinical use (Desmond and Annabel Chen 2002).

It is important to note that all of the previously mentioned studies averaged data from multiple patients and compared these data with averaged data from control subjects to find general differences in brain activity. These are all research experiments designed to probe the pathophysiology of a disease. They do not yet provide a useful diagnostic or prognostic test for an individual clinical patient. Data from individual subjects, however, are increasingly appearing in fMRI reports. With carefully designed and analyzed studies, it is quite possible that fMRI will eventually be applied clinically in specialized centers. As mentioned previously, implementation and analysis of fMRI require considerable expertise. This technique is unlikely to become a routine hospital procedure in the near future.

NORMAL IMAGING ANATOMY

It is essential for the practicing psychiatrist to have a basic understanding of the cortical and subcortical anatomy involved in thought, memory, and emotion if he or she is to use information gathered from imaging. This includes sufficient knowledge to identify these structures on neuroimaging in the various planes of section. In addition, the psychiatrist must have the ability to identify clinical scenarios that warrant imaging investigation for lesions (e.g., traumatic brain injury, stroke, poison and toxin exposure).

In this section, we present an introductory overview of the functional neuroanatomy of executive function, memory, and emotion, as well as clinical examples and references for further reading. An illustration of the key subcortical structures is given in Figure 3–6. These structures are color-coded within the axial imaging atlas to promote understanding (Figures 3–7 through 3–9). It is important to realize that in many cases, lesions within these structures are best viewed in the coronal and sagittal planes of section—thus, MRI is often preferable to CT. In addition, both T2-weighted sagittal and FLAIR sequences may provide details of lesions not seen on other sequences. However, the attending physician may need to specifically request these pulse sequences before imaging. This atlas and the accompanying brief descriptive material can not only familiarize the clinician with normal imaging anatomy pertinent to a psychiatrist but also serve as a base for more in-depth study. The cranial nerves, motor pathways, and peripheral sensory tracts are not discussed.

Thought, memory, and emotion are believed to occur by way of complicated circuits or networks of interconnected areas of brain. Lesions at any point in a circuit can potentially give rise to identical symptoms (Burruss et al. 2000; Dalgleish 2004; Taber et al. 2004; Tekin and Cummings 2002). The reader should be mindful that although the larger brain structures are mentioned in the following discussion, any lesion along the small tracts between regions can also produce similar deficits. A comprehensive review of these circuits is beyond the scope of this chapter. With the advent of graphic programs and computer technology, many three-dimensional models are available that make these circuits easier to understand. The major neuropsychiatric symptoms associated with damage to various subcortical structures are summarized in the following subsections. These summaries were derived from a more comprehensive review, which can be consulted for more detail (Naumescu et al. 1999).

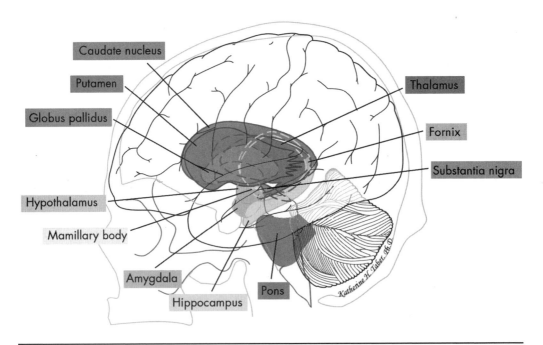

FIGURE 3–6.   This cartoon of a lateral view of the brain and skull shows the approximate positions and configurations of the major subcortical structures.

See Appendix for color version. The colors assigned in this figure are used in the axial atlas (Figures 3–7 through 3–9) to facilitate structure identification.

CEREBRAL CORTEX

The largest division of the human brain is the cerebral cortex. Anatomists divide the cerebral cortex into either four or five lobes. All recognize the frontal, temporal, parietal, and occipital lobes. Some consider the limbic lobe a fifth lobe; others consider it to be contained within the temporal and frontal lobes and diencephalon (see Figures 3–7 through 3–9).

BASAL GANGLIA

The basal ganglia are a group of small, interconnected subcortical nuclei made up of the caudate nucleus, putamen, globus pallidus, claustrum, subthalamus, and substantia nigra (see Figures 3–8 and 3–9). The caudate nucleus and putamen are often called the *corpus striatum*, and the globus pallidus and putamen are called the *lentiform nucleus*. Together, the structures of the basal ganglia are familiar to psychiatrists from disorders such as Huntington's chorea

and Parkinson's disease or as the targets of many poison and toxin exposures. These nuclei serve a key role as a site for bringing emotion, executive function, motivation, and motor activity together. Many input and output circuits traverse these areas, including the three frontal lobe circuits of dorsolateral, orbitofrontal, and anterior cingulate gyrus (Burruss et al. 2000; Tekin and Cummings 2002; Tisch et al. 2004). Lesions within these structures result in syndromes of hypokinetic or hyperkinetic movements as well as cognitive and emotional dysfunction. The basal ganglia contain significant acetylcholine, dopamine, GABA, and neuropeptide projections. The dopaminergic projections have been pharmacological targets for schizophrenia and Parkinson's disease.

Caudate Nucleus

The caudate nuclei are **C**-shaped structures, each having a head, body, and tail. They arch to follow the walls of the lateral ventricles and

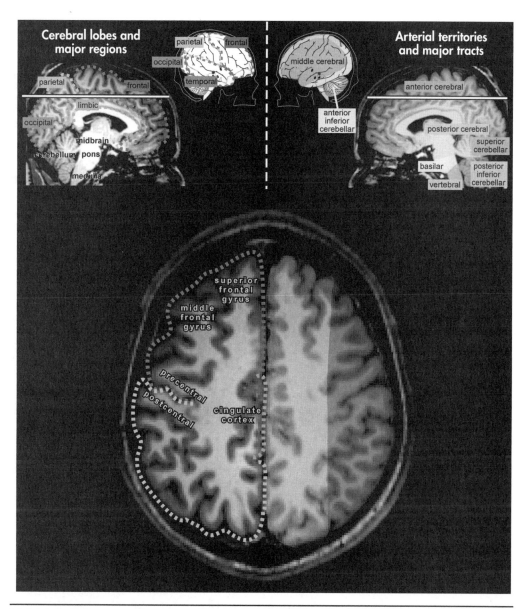

FIGURE 3–7. T1-weighted axial magnetic resonance image (MRI) with major tracts (*right side*) and brain regions (*left side*) labeled.

See Appendix for color version. Major subcortical structures are color-coded to match Figure 3–6. Vascular territories (*right side*) and lobes (*left side*) are color-coded to match the key.

Source. MRI courtesy of Phillips Medical Systems. Atlas section used with permission of Veterans Health Administration Mid-Atlantic Mental Illness Research, Education, and Clinical Center.

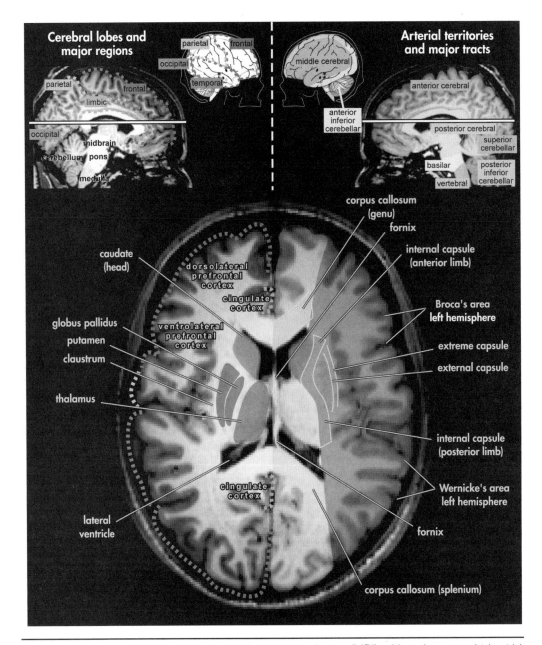

FIGURE 3–8. T1-weighted axial magnetic resonance image (MRI) with major tracts (*right side*) and brain regions (*left side*) labeled.

See Appendix for color version. Major subcortical structures are color-coded to match Figure 3–6. Vascular territories (*right side*) and lobes (*left side*) are color-coded to match the key.

Source. MRI courtesy of Phillips Medical Systems. Atlas section used with permission of Veterans Health Administration Mid-Atlantic Mental Illness Research, Education, and Clinical Center.

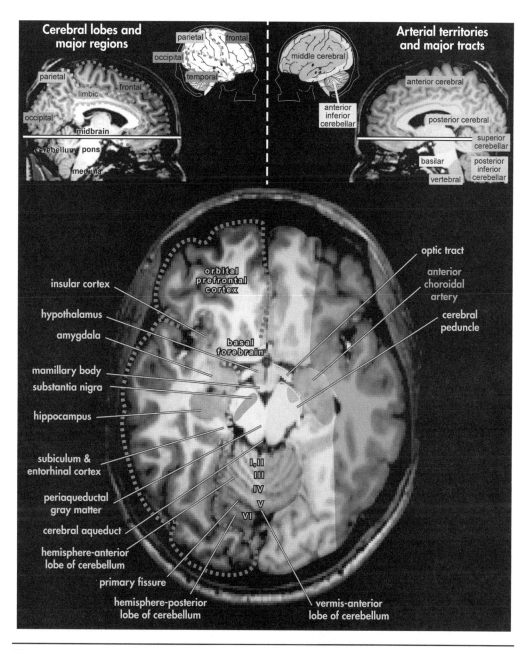

FIGURE 3–9. T1-weighted axial magnetic resonance image (MRI) with major tracts (*right side*) and brain regions (*left side*) labeled.

See Appendix for color version. Major subcortical structures are color-coded to match Figure 3–6. Vascular territories (*right side*) and lobes (*left side*) are color-coded to match the key.

Source. MRI courtesy of Phillips Medical Systems. Atlas section used with permission of Veterans Health Administration Mid-Atlantic Mental Illness Research, Education, and Clinical Center.

terminate into the amygdaloid nuclei bilaterally (see Figure 3–8). The caudate nucleus and putamen together are thought of as the input nuclei receiving projections from the cerebral cortex, thalamus, and substantia nigra pars compacta. The major outputs for the caudate nucleus and putamen are the globus pallidus and substantia nigra pars reticulata. Neuropsychiatric symptoms of damage to the caudate nucleus are numerous and can be divided into behavioral, emotional, memory, language, and other symptoms. More commonly reported deficits include disinhibition, disorganization, executive dysfunction, apathy, depression, memory loss, atypical aphasia, psychosis, personality changes, and predisposition for delirium.

Putamen

The putamen is the most lateral of the basal ganglia structures. It is separated from the caudate nucleus by the anterior limb of the internal capsule (see Figure 3–8). The putamen and the caudate nucleus are considered input nuclei. See the preceding "Caudate Nucleus" subsection for afferent and efferent projections. Neuropsychiatric symptoms of lesions to the putamen include primarily language and behavioral deficits (e.g., atypical aphasia, obsessive-compulsive traits, executive dysfunction). However, hemineglect, depression, and memory loss have been reported.

Globus Pallidus

The globus pallidus lies medial to the putamen and has two divisions (internal and external) (see Figure 3–8). The globus pallidus is functionally considered an output nucleus. Primary output is to the subthalamus and thalamus via GABAergic pathways. (For a further discussion of the afferent and efferent connections of the globus pallidus, see Crossman 1995.) Neuropsychiatric symptoms of lesions to the globus pallidus include primarily emotional and other types (e.g., anxiety, depression, apathy, psychosis, and central pain). Other less often reported symptoms include amnesia and cognitive deficits.

Substantia Nigra

The substantia nigra nuclei of the midbrain are dark because they contain melanin. They are divided into the pars compacta and the pars reticulata. The first sends dopaminergic projections to the caudate nucleus and putamen. The latter receives input from the striatum and sends efferents to the thalamus, subthalamus, and reticular formation (see Figures 3–6 and 3–9). Reported neuropsychiatric symptoms of lesions to the substantia nigra include primarily behavioral and emotional deficits (e.g., apraxia, ataxia, aggression, and depression), with less frequent reports of memory and cognitive deficits.

LIMBIC SYSTEM

The term *limbic system* is most often used to describe the areas of brain involved in the production of emotion, memory, or aggression (Dalgleish 2004; Morgane and Mokler 2006). Originally suggested by Broca (*"le grand lobe limbique"*), the name is purely descriptive of the anatomical location of these structures (*limbus* means "border," and these structures border the neocortex). Papez suggested that these areas are important for memory and emotion, rather than just smell as had been previously believed. MacLean applied the name "limbic system" to the circuit of Papez, reasoning that these structures are placed to integrate signals from the external and internal worlds (Figure 3–10). Commonly, these structures are divided into an outer and an inner lobe. The outer lobe is composed of the cingulate, subcallosal, parahippocampal, and uncal cortices. The inner lobe consists of the paraterminal gyrus, the indusium griseum (supracallosal gyrus), and the hippocampal complex. Other areas closely associated with these and often considered part of the limbic system include the mamillary bodies and parts of the thalamus. Some authors also include other areas, such as the orbitofrontal cortex and hypothalamus. (See Mega et al. 1997 for an excellent review of the anatomical and phylogenetic development of the limbic system.)

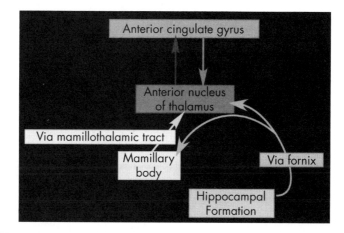

FIGURE 3–10.   Schematic diagram of the emotion and memory circuit of Papez.

Hippocampal Formation and Parahippocampal Cortex

The hippocampal formation and parahippocampal cortex (or gyrus) are collectively considered to be the "memory structures." They function in essence to form and direct the storage of memories. The parahippocampus extends from the cingulate cortex to the amygdala. The main body of the hippocampal formation extends from the crus of the fornix to the amygdala located in the medial temporal lobe. The fornix is the major fiber tract of the hippocampal formation (see Figures 3–6 and 3–8). Neuropsychiatric symptoms of lesions to the hippocampal formation are primarily memory deficits. These include anterograde and retrograde amnesia, inability to form new memories, and temporally graded amnesia.

The fornix is made up of afferent and efferent hippocampal fibers. It forms from the fibers (fimbria) that course on the ventricular surface of the hippocampus. The fimbria become the crus of the fornix. The crus join to form the body of the fornix. The body then passes between the lateral ventricles in the septum pellucidum. The body divides around the anterior commissure to form the anterior (precommissural) and posterior (postcommissural) columns of the fornix. Neuropsychiatric symptoms of lesions to the fornix are memory deficits and overlap those following damage to the hippocampal formation. They include impaired recent memory, syndrome of transitory amnesia, and long-term anterograde amnesia.

Amygdala

The amygdala lies at the juncture of the tail of the caudate nucleus and the anteriormost ends of the parahippocampus and hippocampus. It sends projections to the basal forebrain and striatum via the anterior portion of the ventral amygdalofugal pathway. The caudal portion of this pathway carries the projection from the amygdala to the thalamus. The amygdala also sends projections to the hypothalamus via both the stria terminalis and the ventral amygdalofugal pathway. A component continues on to the midbrain and brain stem (see Figures 3–6 and 3–9). Neuropsychiatric symptoms of lesions to the amygdala are primarily behavioral and emotional. They include passivity or aggression, hypersexuality, hyperorality, hyperphagia, decreased fear, anxiety or startle, and decreased link between emotion and memory.

Mamillary Body

The mamillary bodies are two small round nuclei that lie in the posterior portion of the diencephalon. They receive afferents from the hippocampus and send efferents to the brain stem and thalamus (see Figures 3–6 and 3–9). The mamillothalamic tract is the projection from the mamillary bodies to the anterior nucleus of the thalamus. Neuropsychiatric symptoms of lesions to the mamillary body or its tract are primarily memory deficits and psychosis. Confabulation and anterograde memory loss are most common.

Thalamus

The thalamus is medial to the caudate nucleus and putamen and lateral to the third ventricle. The superior and medial portions contain the anterior nucleus, medial dorsal nucleus, and lateral dorsal nucleus (see Figures 3–6 and 3–8) (Taber et al. 2004). These nuclei have intimate interconnections with the limbic system. Damage to the medial portion of the left thalamus is associated with deficits in language, verbal intellect, and verbal memory. Damage to the right is associated with deficits in visuospatial and nonverbal intellect and visual memory. Medial thalamus may be important for temporal aspects of memory. Bilateral damage is associated with severe memory impairment ("thalamic amnesia") as well as dementia. The memory deficits may result from destruction of the tracts (mamillothalamic tract, amygdalofugal tract) connecting these thalamic nuclei with limbic structures. Damage to the anterior and medial thalamus can also result in disturbances of autonomic functions, mood, and the sleep-wake cycle.

HYPOTHALAMUS

The hypothalamus lies ventral to the thalamus around the third ventricle. It has projections to and from the orbitofrontal cortex, the limbic circuits, the thalamus, the reticular formation, and the autonomic and endocrine systems. Thus, it is a key structure in bridging internal homeostasis and the outside environment (see Figures 3–6 and 3–9). Behavioral, emotional, and memory symptoms as well as other deficits are associated with damage to the hypothalamus. Examples of commonly reported symptoms are aggression, violence, anorexia, depression, impaired short-term memory, dementia, gelastic seizures, and altered sleep-wake cycle.

PONS

The pons lies in the posterior fossa between the midbrain and the medulla oblongata. It contains nuclei and tracts that are necessary for arousal (reticular formation) and affective stability (see Figure 3–6). The raphe nuclei (found at the midline along the entire brain stem) send serotonergic projections to structures throughout the brain, including the thalamus, hippocampus, basal ganglia, and frontal cortex. The locus coeruleus is also found in the pons. It sends noradrenergic projections to the limbic system, hypothalamus, thalamus, cerebellum, and cerebral cortex. Neuropsychiatric symptoms of pontine lesions include behavioral, emotional, language, memory, and other deficits. Commonly reported deficits include disinhibition, disturbed sleep-wake cycles, anxiety, depression, emotional lability, cognitive deficits, central pain, personality changes, and psychosis.

CEREBELLUM

The cerebellum lies ventral to the temporal and occipital lobes and the pons, surrounding the fourth ventricle (see Figure 3–9). In addition to its extensive connections with the motor system, the cerebellum projects (via the thalamus) to cingulate, dorsomedial prefrontal, and dorsolateral prefrontal cortices (Middleton and Strick 2000, 2001; Schmahmann and Pandya 1997a, 1997b; Taber et al. 2005). Recent work indicates that cerebellar lesions, particularly to the posterior cerebellum and vermis, can result in a range of cognitive and emotional deficits, including executive dysfunction, visual-spatial deficits, personality changes, and linguistic abnormalities (Konarski et al. 2005; Rapoport et al. 2000; Schmahmann 2004; Taber et al. 2005; Turner and Schiavetto 2004).

RECOMMENDED READINGS

Anderson KE, Taber KH, Hurley RA: Functional imaging, in Textbook of Traumatic Brain Injury. Edited by Silver JM, McAllister TW, Yudofsky SC. Washington, DC, American Psychiatric Publishing, 2005, pp 107–133

Dalgleish T: The emotional brain. Nat Rev Neurosci 5:583–589, 2004

Erhart SM, Young AS, Marder SR, et al: Clinical utility of magnetic resonance imaging radiographs for suspected organic syndromes in adult psychiatry. J Clin Psychiatry 66:968–973, 2005

Gupta A, Elheis M, Pansari K: Imaging in psychiatric illness. Int J Clin Pract 58:850–858, 2004

Schmahmann JD: Disorders of the cerebellum: ataxia, dysmetria of thought, and the cerebellar cognitive affective syndrome. J Neuropsychiatry Clin Neurosci 16:367–378, 2004

Tekin S, Cummings JL: Frontal-subcortical neuronal circuits and clinical neuropsychiatry—an update. J Psychosom Res 53:647–654, 2002

REFERENCES

Anderson KE, Taber KH, Hurley RA: Functional imaging, in Textbook of Traumatic Brain Injury. Edited by Silver JM, McAllister TW, Yudofsky SC. Washington, DC, American Psychiatric Publishing, 2005, pp 107–133

Arakia Y, Ashikaga R, Fujii K, et al: MR fluid-attenuated inversion recovery imaging as routine brain T2-weighted imaging. Eur J Radiol 32:136–143, 1999

Bahner MLRW, Zuna I, Engenhart-Cabillic R, et al: Spiral CT vs incremental CT: is spiral CT superior in imaging of the brain? Eur Radiol 8:416–420, 1998

Baker JF, Kratz LC, Stevens GR, et al: Pharmacokinetics and safety of the MRI contrast agent gadoversetamide injection (Optimark) in healthy pediatric subjects. Invest Radiol 39:334–339, 2004

Barthel H, Hesse S, Dannenberg C, et al: Prospective value of perfusion and X-ray attenuation imaging with single-photon emission and transmission computed tomography in acute cerebral ischemia. Stroke 32:1558–1597, 2001

Benamer HT, Oerel WH, Patterson J, et al: Prospective study of presynaptic dopaminergic imaging in patients with mild parkinsonism and tremor disorders, 1: baseline and 3-month observations. Mov Disord 18:977–984, 2003

Beresford TP, Blow FC, Hall RCW, et al: CT scanning in psychiatric inpatients: clinical yield. Psychosomatics 27:105–112, 1986

Bergin PS, Fish DR, Shorvon SD, et al: Magnetic resonance imaging in partial epilepsy: additional abnormalities shown with the fluid attenuate inversion recovery (FLAIR) pulse sequence. J Neurol Neurosurg Psychiatry 58:439–443, 1995

Bizzi A, Righini A, Turner R, et al: MR of diffusion slowing in global cerebral ischemia. AJNR Am J Neuroradiol 14:1347–1354, 1993

Bonne O, Gilboa A, Louzoun Y, et al: Cerebral blood flow in chronic symptomatic mild traumatic brain injury. Psychiatry Res 124:141–152, 2003

Bookheimer SY, Strojwas MH, Cohen MS, et al: Patterns of brain activation in people at risk for Alzheimer's disease. N Engl J Med 343:450–456, 2000

Bourland JD, Nyenhuis JA, Schaefer DJ: Physiologic effects of intense MR imaging gradient fields. Neuroimaging Clin N Am 9:363–377, 1999

Branton T: Use of computerized tomography by old age psychiatrists: an examination of criteria for investigation of cognitive impairment. Int J Geriatr Psychiatry 14:567–571, 1999

Brant-Zawadzki M, Atkinson D, Detrick M, et al: Fluid-attenuated inversion recovery (FLAIR) for assessment of cerebral infarction. Stroke 27:1187–1191, 1996

Bulte JW: MR contrast agents for molecular and cellular imaging (editorial). Curr Pharm Biotechnol 5(1):483, 2004

Burruss JW, Hurley RA, Taber KH, et al: Functional neuroanatomy of the frontal lobe circuits. Radiology 214:227–230, 2000

Cao Y, D'Olhaberriague L, Vikingstad EM, et al: Pilot study of functional MRI to assess cerebral activation of motor function after poststroke hemiparesis. Stroke 29:112–122, 1998

Cherry S: Fundamentals of positron emission tomography and applications in preclinical drug development. J Clin Pharmacol 41:482–491, 2001

Cochran ST: Anaphylactoid reactions to radiocontrast media. Curr Allergy Asthma Rep 5:28–31, 2005

Cochran ST, Bomyea K, Sayre JW: Trends in adverse events after IV administration of contrast media. AJR Am J Roentgenol 178:1385–1388, 2002

Cohan RH, Matsumoto JS, Quaglianao PV: ACR Manual on Contrast Media, 4th Edition. Reston, VA, American College of Radiology, 1998

Coleman LT, Zimmerman RA: Pediatric craniospinal spiral CT: current applications and future potential. Semin Ultrasound CT MR 15:148–155, 1994

Crossman AR: Neuroanatomy: An Illustration Colour Text. Edinburgh, Scotland, Churchill Livingstone, 1995, p 69

Dalgleish T: The emotional brain. Nat Rev Neurosci 5:583–589, 2004

De Backer AI, Mortele KJ, De Keulenaer BL: Considerations for planning and implementation. JBR-BTR 87:241–246, 2004a

De Backer AI, Mortele KJ, De Keulenaer BL: Picture archiving and communication system—part one: filmless radiology and distance radiology. JBR-BTR 87:234–241, 2004b

Desmond JE, Annabel Chen SH: Ethical issues in the clinical application of fMRI: factors affecting the validity and interpretation of activations. Brain Cogn 50:482–497, 2002

Detre JA, Alsop DC: Arterial spin labeled perfusion magnetic resonance imaging, in Imaging of the Nervous System. Edited by Latchaw RE, Kucharczyk J, Moseley ME. Philadelphia, PA, Elsevier Mosby, 2005, pp 323–331

Diwadkar VA, Keshavan MS: Newer techniques in magnetic resonance imaging and their potential for neuropsychiatric research. J Psychosom Res 53:677–685, 2002

Dong Q, Welsh RC, Chenevert TL, et al: Clinical applications of diffusion tensor imaging. J Magn Reson Imaging 19:6–18, 2004

Erhart SM, Young AS, Marder SR, et al: Clinical utility of magnetic resonance imaging radiographs for suspected organic syndromes in adult psychiatry. J Clin Psychiatry 66:968–973, 2005

Fahey FH: Data acquisition in PET imaging. J Nucl Med Technol 30:39–40, 2002

Federle MP, Willis LL, Swanson DP: Ionic versus nonionic contrast media: a prospective study of the effect of rapid bolus injection on nausea and anaphylactoid reaction. J Neurol Sci 22:341–345, 1998

Filippi M, Rocca MA: Magnetization transfer magnetic resonance imaging in the assessment of neurological diseases. J Neuroimaging 14:303–313, 2004

Garavan H, Pankiewicz J, Bloom A, et al: Cue-induced cocaine craving: neuroanatomical specificity for drug users and drug stimuli. Am J Psychiatry 157:1789–1798, 2000

Guadagno JV, Calautti C, Baron JC: Progress in imaging stroke: emerging clinical applications. Br Med Bull 65:145–157, 2003

Gupta A, Elheis M, Pansari K: Imaging in psychiatric illness. Int J Clin Pract 58:850–858, 2004

Hall P, Adami HO, Trichopoulos D, et al: Effect of low doses of ionising radiation in infancy on cognitive function in adulthood: Swedish population based cohort study. BMJ 328:19, 2004

Halpern JD, Hopper KD, Arredondo MG, et al: Patient allergies: role in selective use of nonionic contrast material. Radiology 199:359–362, 1999

Halpin SF: Brain imaging using multislice CT: a personal perspective. Br J Radiol 77:S20–S26, 2004

Hanyu H, Asano T, Sakurai H, et al: Magnetization transfer ratio in cerebral white matter lesions of Binswanger's disease. J Neurol Sci 1:87–89, 1999

Hariri AR, Mattay VS, Tessitore A, et al: Serotonin transporter genetic variation and the response of the human amygdala. Science 297:400–403, 2002

Henry TR, Van Heertum RL: Positron emission tomography and single photon emission computed tomography in epilepsy care. Semin Nucl Med 33:88–104, 2003

Hoffmann A, Faber SC, Werhahn KJ, et al: Electromyography in MRI—first recordings of peripheral nerve activation caused by fast magnetic field gradients. Magn Reson Med 43:534–539, 2000

Holmes AJ, MacDonald A 3rd, Carter CS, et al: Prefrontal functioning during context processing in schizophrenia and major depression: an event-related fMRI study. Schizophr Res 76:199–206, 2005

Hopper KD, Neuman JD, King SH, et al: Radioprotection to the eye during CT scanning. AJNR Am J Neuroradiol 22:1194–1198, 2001

Huisman TAGM: Diffusion-weighted imaging basic concepts and application in cerebral stroke and head trauma. Eur Radiol 13:2283–2297, 2003

Hurley RA, Jackson EF, Fisher RE, et al: New techniques for understanding Huntington's disease. J Neuropsychiatry Clin Neurosci 11:173–175, 1999

Hurley RA, Tomimoto H, Akiguchi I, et al: Binswanger's disease: an ongoing controversy. J Neuropsychiatry Clin Neurosci 12:301–304, 2000a

Hurley RA, Hayman LA, Taber KH: Clinical imaging in neuropsychiatry, in The American Psychiatric Publishing Textbook of Neuropsychiatry and Clinical Neurosciences, 4th Edition. Edited by Yudofsky SC, Hales RE. Washington, DC, American Psychiatric Publishing, 2002, pp 245–283

Hurley RA, Ernst T, Khalili K, et al: Identification of HIV associated progressive multifocal leukoencephalopathy: magnetic resonance imaging and spectroscopy. J Neuropsychiatry Clin Neurosci 15:1–6, 2003

Inoue E, Nakagawa M, Goto R, et al: Regional differences between 99mTC-ECD and 99mTc-HMPAO SPET in perfusion changes with age and gender in healthy adults. Eur J Nucl Med Mol Imaging 30:489–497, 2003

Jacobs JE, Birnbaum BA, Langlotz CP: Contrast media reactions and extravasation: relationship to intravenous injection rates. Radiology 209:411–416, 1998

Jung SL, Kim BS, Lee KS, et al: Magnetic resonance imaging and diffusion-weighted imaging changes after hypoglycemic coma. J Neuroimaging 15:193–196, 2005

Kaplan H, Sadock B, Grebb J: The brain and behavior, in Kaplan and Sadock's Synopsis of Psychiatry: Behavioral Sciences Clinical Psychiatry, 7th Edition. Edited by Kaplan H, Sadock BJ, Graff JA. Baltimore, MD, Williams & Wilkins, 1994, pp 112–125

Kim YJ, Ishise M, Ballinger JR, et al: Combination of dopamine transporter and D2 receptor SPECT in the diagnostic evaluation of PD, MSA, and PSP. Mov Disord 17:303–312, 2002

Kirchin MA, Runge VM: Contrast agents for magnetic resonance imaging safety update. Top Magn Reson Imaging 14:426–435, 2003

Knudsen GM, Karlsborg M, Thomsen G, et al: Imaging of dopamine transporters and D_2 receptors in patients with Parkinson's disease and multiple system atrophy. Eur J Nucl Med Mol Imaging 31:1631–1638, 2004

Konarski JZ, McIntyre RS, Grupp LA, et al: Is the cerebellum relevant in the circuitry of neuropsychiatric disorders? J Psychiatry Neurosci 30:178–186, 2005

Konen E, Konen O, Katz M, et al: Are referring clinicians aware of patients at risk from intravenous injection of iodinated contrast media? Clin Radiol 57:132–135, 2002

Kubicki M, Westin CF, Maier SE, et al: Uncinate fasciculus findings in schizophrenia: a magnetic resonance diffusion tensor imaging study. Am J Psychiatry 159:813–820, 2002

Kuhl CK, Textor J, Gleseke J, et al: Acute and subacute ischemic stroke at high-field-strength (3.0.T) diffusion-weighted MR imaging: intraindividual comparative study. Radiology 234:509–516, 2005

Kuntz R, Skalej M, Stefanou A: Image quality of spiral CT versus conventional CT in routine brain imaging. Eur J Radiol 26:235–240, 1998

Kuszyk BS, Beauchamp NJ, Fishman EK: Neurovascular applications of CT angiography. Semin Ultrasound CT MR 19:394–404, 1998

Larson EB, Mack LA, Watts B, et al: Computed tomography in patients with psychiatric illnesses: advantage of a "rule-in" approach. Ann Intern Med 95:360–364, 1981

Latchaw RE: Cerebral perfusion imaging in acute stroke. J Vasc Interv Radiol 15(1 pt 2):S29–S46, 2004

Leenders KL: Significance of non-presynaptic SPECT tracer methods in Parkinson's disease. Mov Disord 18:S39–S42, 2003

Lind J, Persson J, Ingvar M, et al: Reduced functional brain activity response in cognitively intact apolipoprotein E epsilon4 carriers. Brain 129:1240–1248, 2006

Magistretti PL, Pellerin L: The contribution of astrocytes to the 18F-2-deoxyglucose signal in PET activation studies. Mol Psychiatry 1:445–452, 1996

Marshall RS, Perera GM, Lazar RM, et al: Evolution of cortical activation during recovery from corticospinal tract infarction. Stroke 31:656–661, 2000

Marti-Fabregas JA, Catafau AM, Mari C, et al: Cerebral perfusion and haemodynamics measured by SPET in symptom-free patients with transient ischaemic attack: clinical implications. Eur J Nucl Med 28:1828–1835, 2001

Mascalchi M, Filippi M, Floris R, et al: Diffusion-weighted MR of the brain: methodology and clinical application. Radiol Med (Torino) 109:155–197, 2005

Matthews PM, Jezzard P: Functional magnetic resonance imaging. J Neurol Neurosurg Psychiatry 75:6–12, 2004

Mega MS, Cummings JL: Frontal-subcortical circuits and neuropsychiatric disorders. J Neuropsychiatry Clin Neurosci 6:358–370, 1994

Mega MS, Cummings JL, Salloway S, et al: The limbic system: an anatomic, phylogenetic, and clinical perspective [see comments]. J Neuropsychiatry Clin Neurosci 9:315–330, 1997

Menon V, Anagnoson RT, Mathalon DH, et al: Functional neuroanatomy of auditory working memory in schizophrenia: relation to positive and negative symptoms. Neuroimage 13:433–446, 2001

Middleton FA, Strick PL: Basal ganglia and cerebellar loops: motor and cognitive circuits. Brain Res Rev 31:236–250, 2000

Middleton FA, Strick PL: Cerebellar projections to the prefrontal cortex of the primate. J Neurosci 21:700–712, 2001

Mitchell DG: MR imaging contrast agents—what's in a name? J Magn Reson Imaging 7:1–4, 1997

Morgane PJ, Mokler DJ: The limbic brain: continuing resolution. Neurosci Biobehav Rev 30:119–125, 2006

Mortele KJ, Olivia MR, Ondategui S, et al: Universal use of nonionic iodinated contrast medium for CT: evaluation of safety in a large urban teaching hospital. AJR Am J Roentgenol 184:31–34, 2005

Moseley ME, Sawyer-Glover A, Kucharczyk J: Magnetic resonance imaging principles and techniques, in Imaging of the Nervous System. Edited by Latchaw RE, Kucharczyk J, Moseley ME. Philadelphia, PA, Elsevier Mosby, 2005, pp 3–30

Nakamura H, Yamada K, Kizu O, et al: Effect of thin-section diffusion-weighted MR imaging on stroke diagnosis. AJNR Am J Neuroradiol 26:560–565, 2005

Naumescu I, Hurley RA, Hayman LA, et al: Neuropsychiatric symptoms associated with subcortical brain injuries. Int J Neuroradiol 5:51–59, 1999

Oi H, Yamazaki H, Matsushita M: Delayed vs. immediate adverse reactions to ionic and nonionic low-osmolality contrast media. Radiat Med 15:23–27, 1997

Orrison WW Jr, Sanders JA: Clinical brain imaging: computerized axial tomography and magnetic resonance imaging, in Functional Brain Imaging. Edited by Orrison WW Jr, Lewine JD, Sanders JA, et al. St Louis, MO, Mosby-Year Book, 1995, pp 97–144

Paans AMJ, van Waarde A, Elsinga PH, et al: Positron emission tomography: the conceptual idea using a multidisciplinary approach. Methods 27:195–207, 2002

Pineiro R, Pendlebury S, Johansen-Berg H, et al: Altered hemodynamics responses in patients after subcortical stroke measured by functional MRI. Stroke 33:103–109, 2002

Price RR: The AAPM/RSNA physics tutorial for residents: MR imaging safety consideration. Radiological Society of North America. Radiographics 19:1641–1651, 1999

Raichle ME: Functional brain imaging and human brain function. J Neurosci 23:3959–3962, 2003

Rapoport M, van Reekum R, Mayberg H: The role of the cerebellum in cognition and behavior: a selective review. J Neuropsychiatry Clin Neurosci 12:193–198, 2000

Rauch S, Renshaw PF: Clinical neuroimaging in psychiatry. Harv Rev Psychiatry 2:297–312, 1995

Runge VM: Safety of magnetic resonance contrast media. Top Magn Reson Imaging 12:309–314, 2001

Runge VM, Lawrence RM, Wells JW: Principles of contrast enhancement in the evaluation of brain diseases: an overview. J Magn Reson Imaging 7:5–13, 1997

Rydberg JN, Hammond CA, Grimm RC, et al: Initial clinical experience in MR imaging of the brain with a fast fluid-attenuated inversion-recovery pulse sequence. Radiology 193:173–180, 1994

Sage MR, Wilson AJ, Scroop R: Contrast media and the brain: the basis of CT and MR imaging enhancement. Neuroimaging Clin N Am 8:695–707, 1998

Scarabino T, Nemore F, Giannatempo GM, et al: 3.0 T Magnetic resonance in neuroradiology. Eur J Radiol 48:154–164, 2003

Schmahmann JD: Disorders of the cerebellum: ataxia, dysmetria of thought, and the cerebellar cognitive affective syndrome. J Neuropsychiatry Clin Neurosci 16:367–378, 2004

Schmahmann JD, Pandya DN: Anatomic organization of the basilar pontine projections from prefrontal cortices in rhesus monkey. J Neurosci 17:438–458, 1997a

Schmahmann JD, Pandya DN: The cerebrocerebellar system. Int Rev Neurobiol 41:31–60, 1997b

Schwartz RB: Helical (spiral) CT in neuroradioliogic diagnosis. Radiol Clin North Am 33:981–995, 1995

Sheline YI, Barch DM, Donnelly JM, et al: Increased amygdala response to masked emotional faces in depressed subjects resolves with antidepressant treatment: an fMRI study. Biol Psychiatry 50:651–658, 2001

Shellock FG: Bioeffects and safety considerations, in Magnetic Resonance Imaging of the Brain and Spine. Edited by Atlas SW. New York, Raven, 1991, pp 87–107

Shellock FG: Magnetic resonance safety update 2002: implants and devices. J Magn Reson Imaging 16:485–496, 2002

Shellock FG, Crues JV: MR procedures: biologic effects, safety, and patient care. Radiology 232:635–652, 2004

Shellock FG, Kanal E: Policies, guidelines, and recommendations for MR imaging safety and patient management. SMRI Safety Committee. J Magn Reson Imaging 1:97–101, 1991

Shellock FG, Kanal E: Safety of magnetic resonance imaging contrast agents. J Magn Reson Imaging 10:477–484, 1999

Slosman DO, Ludwig C, Zerarka S, et al: Brain energy metabolism in Alzheimer's disease: 99mTc-HMPAO SPECT imaging during verbal fluency and role of astrocytes in the cellular mechanism of 99mTc-HMPAO retention. Brain Res Brain Res Rev 36:230–240, 2001

Sundgren PC, Dong Q, Gomez-Hasssan DM, et al: Diffusion tensor imaging of the brain: review of clinical applications. Neuroradiology 46:339–350, 2004

Sunshine JL: CT, MR imaging, and MR angiography in the evaluation of patients with acute stroke. J Vasc Interv Radiol 15:S47–S55, 2004

Symms M, Jäger HR, Schmierer K, et al: A review of structural magnetic resonance neuroimaging. J Neurol Neurosurg Psychiatry 75:1235–1244, 2004

Taber KH, Cortelli P, Staffen W, et al: Expanding the role of imaging in prion disease. J Neuropsychiatry Clin Neurosci 14:371–376, 2002a

Taber KH, Pierpaoli C, Rose SE, et al: The future for diffusion tensor imaging in neuropsychiatry. J Neuropsychiatry Clin Neurosci 14:1–5, 2002b

Taber KH, Rauch SL, Lanius RA, et al: Functional magnetic resonance imaging: application to post traumatic stress disorder. J Neuropsychiatry Clin Neurosci 15:125–129, 2003

Taber KH, Wen C, Khan A, et al: The limbic thalamus. J Neuropsychiatry Clin Neurosci 16:127–132, 2004

Taber KH, Strick PL, Hurley RA: Rabies and the cerebellum: new methods for tracing circuits in the brain. J Neuropsychiatry Clin Neurosci 17:133–139, 2005

Tanabe JL, Ezekeil F, Jagust WJ, et al: Magnetization transfer ratio of white matter hyperintensities in subcortical ischemic vascular dementia. AJNR Am J Neuroradiol 20:839–844, 1999

Taylor WD, Hsu E, Krishnan KRR, et al: Diffusion tensor imaging: background, potential, and utility in psychiatric research. Biol Psychiatry 55:201–207, 2004

Tekin S, Cummings JL: Frontal-subcortical neuronal circuits and clinical neuropsychiatry—an update. J Psychosom Res 53:647–654, 2002

Tisch S, Silberstein P, Limousin-Dowsey P, et al: The basal ganglia: anatomy, physiology, and pharmacology. Psychiatr Clin North Am 27:757–799, 2004

Turner R, Jones T: Techniques for imaging neuroscience. Br Med Bull 65:3–20, 2003

Turner R, Schiavetto A: The cerebellum in schizophrenia: a case of intermittent ataxia and psychosis—clinical, cognitive, and neuroanatomical correlates. J Neuropsychiatry Clin Neurosci 16:400–408, 2004

Valls C, Andria E, Sanchez A, et al: Selective use of low-osmolality contrast media in computed tomography. Eur Radiol 13:2000–2005, 2003

Van Heertum RL, Greenstein EA, Tikofsky RS: 2-Deoxy-fluoroglucose-positron emission tomography imaging of the brain: current clinical applications with emphasis on the dementias. Semin Nucl Med 34:300–312, 2004

Walker Z, Costa DC, Walker RW, et al: Differentiation of dementia with Lewy bodies from Alzheimer's disease using a dopaminergic presynaptic ligand. J Neurol Neurosurg Psychiatry 73:134–140, 2002

Warwick JM: Imaging of brain function using SPECT. Metab Brain Dis 19:113–123, 2004

Weinberger DR: Brain disease and psychiatric illness: when should a psychiatrist order a CAT scan? Am J Psychiatry 141:1521–1527, 1984

Wilde JP, Rivers AW, Price DL: A review of the current use of magnetic resonance imaging in pregnancy and safety implication for the fetus. Prog Biophys Mol Biol 87:335–353, 2005

Willmann JK, Wildermuth S: Multidetector-row CT angiography of upper- and lower-extremity peripheral arteries. Eur Radiol 15:D3–D98, 2005

Wolf GL: Paramagnetic contrast agents for MR imaging of the brain, in MR and CT Imaging of the Head, Neck, and Spine. Edited by Latchaw RE. St Louis, MO, Mosby-Year Book, 1991, pp 95–108

Yasuda M, Munechika H: Delayed adverse reaction to nonionic monomeric contrast enhanced media. Invest Radiol 33:1–5, 1998

4

EPIDEMIOLOGICAL AND GENETIC ASPECTS OF NEUROPSYCHIATRIC DISORDERS

Dolores Malaspina, M.D., M.S.P.H.
Cheryl Corcoran, M.D., M.S.P.H.
Scott Schobel, M.D.
Steven P. Hamilton, M.D., Ph.D.

The last decade has witnessed a revolution in our understanding of the etiology of many neuropsychiatric disorders. Advances in statistical genetics, genetic epidemiology, and molecular biology have provided new insights and avenues for conducting genetic and epidemiological studies and for analyzing gene-environment interactions. The recent sequencing of the human genome now sets the stage for even greater progress in the coming years. In this chapter, we first focus on the methods of genetic epidemiology and then review some of the recent findings of these disciplines in the study of neuropsychiatric disorders.

EPIDEMIOLOGICAL STUDIES

Epidemiology is based on the fundamental assumption that factors causal to human disease can be identified through the systematic examination of different populations, or of subgroups

The authors thank Jessica MacDonald, Kristin Van Heertum, and Caitlin Warinsky for their assistance in the preparation of this chapter.

within a population, in different places or at different times (Hennekens and Buring 1987). Epidemiological research may be viewed as a directed series of questions:

- What is the frequency of a disorder?
- Are there subgroups in which the disorder is more frequent?
- What specific risk factors are associated with the disorder?
- Are these risk factors consistently and specifically related to the disorder?
- Does exposure to these factors precede the development of disease?

A variety of epidemiological strategies have been developed to address these questions.

MEASURES OF DISEASE FREQUENCY

Measures of disease frequency serve as the basis for formulating and testing etiological hypotheses because they permit a comparison of frequencies between different populations or among individuals within a population with particular exposures or characteristics. The two measures of disease frequency used most often are *prevalence* and *incidence*. The former refers to the number of existing cases of a disease at a given point in time as a proportion of the total population. The latter refers to the number of new cases of a disease during a given period as a proportion of the total population at risk. The two measures are interrelated: the prevalence of a disease depends on both its incidence and its duration. One can compare two populations with and without a factor suspected of contributing to the development of disease through the calculation of the ratio of disease frequency in the two populations; this is known as the *relative risk*.

Disease incidence can be defined in several ways. *Risk* refers to the probability that an individual will develop a disease over a specified time, and thus can vary from zero (no risk) to one (an individual will develop the disease). A common difficulty in long-term studies is that subjects become lost to follow-up, thus distorting the risk estimate upward if the subject

remains disease-free or downward if the subject develops the disease. The alternative measure of incidence, called the *rate*, is used to address this problem. The rate is the instantaneous measure of individuals newly developing the disease in relation to the number of subjects who remain at risk (i.e., new cases per person-years of follow-up).

DESCRIPTIVE STUDIES

Descriptive studies contribute to formulating etiological hypotheses by showing a statistical association between exposure to specific risk factors and occurrence of the disease in single individuals or groups of individuals. Descriptive studies are conducted when little is known about the occurrence or antecedents of a disease. Hypotheses regarding risk factors then may emerge from studying several characteristics of affected individuals (e.g., sex, age, birth cohort), their place of residence, or the timing of their exposure. Descriptive studies, however, cannot be used to test etiological hypotheses; they lack adequate comparison groups, making it difficult to determine the specificity of exposure to the disease, and they are cross-sectional, making it difficult to determine the temporal relation between an exposure and the development of disease.

ANALYTIC STUDIES

An analytic study commences when enough is known about a disease that specific a priori hypotheses can be examined. Such etiological hypotheses may be tested through various analytic strategies. In a prospective cohort study, information is obtained about exposure status to selected variables at the time the study begins. New cases of illness are then identified from among those who did and those who did not have the exposure to the selected variables. This contrasts with retrospective cohort studies, in which prior exposure status is established on the basis of available information, usually obtained from available documentation and/or subject interviews. Disease incidence is determined from the time chosen by the investigator until the defined end point of the study.

Case–control studies begin with the designation of disease status, and then past exposure to a risk factor is compared in those individuals who have a disease (case subjects) and in the appropriate control subjects. Procedures for matching control subjects to case subjects involve attempting to control for confounding variables and other biases.

BIRTH COHORT STUDIES

Another important type of epidemiological study is the birth cohort study, in which all individuals born in a certain location at a certain time are followed up. Correlations between hypothetical causes and disease expression can then be explored.

GENETIC STUDIES

Genetic research is concerned with identifying inherited factors that contribute to the development of disease. It, too, may be conceptualized as a directed series of questions:

- Is the disorder familial?
- Is it inherited?
- What is being inherited in the disorder; that is, what constitutes predisposition to the disorder, and what are the earliest manifestations of such predisposition?
- What additional ("epigenetic") variables increase or decrease the chances of genetically predisposed individuals developing the disorder?
- How is the disorder inherited?
- Where and what are the abnormal genes conferring genetic risk?
- What are the molecular and, ultimately, the pathological consequences of these abnormal genes?

A variety of genetic strategies have been developed to address these questions

FAMILY, TWIN, AND ADOPTION STUDIES

Family studies are a type of relative-risk study in which patterns of disease distributions within families are examined and the variability of the disease within families is compared with the variability between families. These studies may show an elevated risk for an illness in first-degree relatives of an affected individual in comparison with that in the general population (Table 4–1), but they cannot distinguish whether this elevated risk is due primarily to shared genetic or environmental factors.

Twin studies can further be used to resolve the genetic contribution to a disorder. Although they are exposed to the same familial environment, monozygotic (MZ) and dizygotic (DZ) twin pairs differ in their genetic endowment (sharing 100% and 50% of their genes, respectively). Thus, when genetic factors are important in etiology, the MZ and DZ co-twins of probands differ in their risk for the disorder. As a result, the comparison of relative concordance rates for MZ and DZ twins is an index of the disorder's heritability, or the proportion of variability that can be attributed to genetic, as opposed to environmental and other random, variables. It is still conceivable that environmental as well as genetic differences may influence the relative risk of diseases in MZ and DZ twins.

Adoption studies offer still another strategy for disentangling genetic and environmental influences, and they are particularly useful for the study of psychiatric disorders, in which cultural influences might otherwise allow for vertical transmission of behaviors. There are several types of adoption studies. In the adoptee study method, offspring separated at birth from their affected mothers are compared with the adopted-away offspring of control mothers. This can be considered a special form of cohort study. Cross-fostering studies examine adoptees whose biological parents are without illness and contrast the rates of illness in those reared by affected and unaffected adoptive parents. In the adoptee's family method, the biological relatives of affected adoptees are matched with the biological relatives of control adoptees, and their rates of illness are compared. Such studies are examples of the case–control paradigm.

TABLE 4–1. Relative risk for neuropsychiatric disorders

Disease	Population prevalence per 100,000	Morbid risk in first-degree relatives (%)	Relative risk (%)
Narcolepsy	10–100	30–50	5,000
Huntington's disease	19	50	2,630
Wilson's disease	10	25	2,500
Parkinson's disease	133	8.3	62.4
Autism	50–100	2–4	45–90
Bipolar disorder	500–1,500	8	16
Schizophrenia	900	12.8	14.2
Panic disorder	2,700	31	10
Obsessive-compulsive disorder	1,000–2,000	10	4.5
Alzheimer's disease	7,700	14.4	1.9
Prion diseases	<0.1	?	?

HIGH-RISK STUDIES

The high-risk approach represents another form of cohort study. Individuals who are at genetic risk for a disorder (e.g., those with affected parents) are followed up prospectively, from early in life through the period of maximum risk for the disorder. This strategy permits the identification of features that are of primary pathogenic significance to the disorder, in contrast to those that are secondary to the illness or to its treatment. Moreover, by contrasting characteristics of at-risk individuals who go on to develop the disorder with characteristics of those who do not, this strategy allows for the identification of additional genetic and environmental influences that contribute to disease expression.

IDENTIFYING MODE OF INHERITANCE

Even when family, twin, and adoption studies suggest a role for genetic factors, they say nothing of which, or even how many, genes are involved. Single-gene mutations are inherited in a mendelian dominant, recessive, or sex-linked manner. They can produce thousands of

monogenic disorders, many of which affect mental functioning, but any particular monogenic disorder is rare, and common diseases are likely to be *polygenic*—representing the combined small effects of many genes (Figure 4–1). Even with genetic liability, environmental influences may be necessary for an illness to be expressed.

Segregation analysis tests explicit models about the inheritance of disease genes on existing family data by comparing the distribution of illness observed in family members with that predicted by a given genetic hypothesis. The detection of mendelian ratios in a sibship can provide support for single-locus inheritance of the genes that confer susceptibility to a disease. Segregation analysis also can be conducted in other pedigree structures, including complex genealogies, to test models of inheritance from single-gene to polygenic inheritance. Segregation analysis (of nuclear family data) allows estimation of model parameters (such as gene frequency and penetrance) by treating each family as a separate observation (Kidd 1981). Its power is limited because it assumes that the same genetic disorder is present in all families. Pedigree analysis, on the other hand, examines

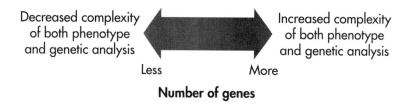

FIGURE 4–1.   Complex genetic risk.

The number of genes involved in a phenotype is theorized to be directly related to both the complexity of the phenotype and the difficulty of genetic analysis.

Source.   Reprinted from Gottesman II, Gould TD: "The Endophenotype Concept in Psychiatry: Etymology and Strategic Intentions." *American Journal of Psychiatry* 160:636–645, 2003. Used with permission.

more (multigenerational) relationships and is less likely to result in a type I error (a falsely attributed relation to disease) but is more likely to result in a type II error (an overlooked relation to disease) because an individual pedigree may manifest an idiosyncratic form of the disorder. Examination of *multiplex* sibships, in which two or more sibs are affected, represents a compromise approach.

COMPLEX DISORDERS

Genetic causation can range from a point mutation in single genes to polygenic causes that entail epistasis (interaction) among the several genes involved and/or environmental factors. Many, if not all, of the neuropsychiatric disorders have a complex pattern of inheritance. Qualities of complex disorders include the following:

- An unknown mode of inheritance
- Incomplete penetrance, wherein additional genetic or environmental factors may be necessary for the final expression of the disorder
- Epistasis, whereby the disorder may result from the interaction of several major genes
- Variable expressivity, in which a single form of the disorder may have several phenotypic expressions, making it difficult to define who is affected
- Diagnostic instability, such that a subject's affection status may change over time

- Etiological heterogeneity, under which an ordinarily genetic syndrome may have sporadic (environmentally produced) forms— known as *phenocopies*—as well as a variety of genetic forms resulting from disruption in several different genes—a condition known as *nonallelic heterogeneity*

The enormous growth in elucidating the genetics of some neuropsychiatric disorders in the last decade is chiefly the result of recent advances in statistical methods and molecular approaches designed to overcome these complexities.

LINKAGE ANALYSIS

Linkage analysis, also called positional cloning, is a strategy for isolating a gene of unknown structure or function based on its chromosomal location. It is based on establishing, within pedigrees, the coinheritance of the disorder with identifiable genetic markers of known chromosomal location. Mendel's second law (the law of independent assortment) implies that the disease gene, and hence the disorder, will not be consistently coinherited with a marker allele derived from a different chromosome. Moreover, even if the disease and marker alleles originally lie on the same parental chromosome (are *syntenic*), they may become separated during gametogenesis through the process of recombination or crossing over, wherein genetic material on homolo-

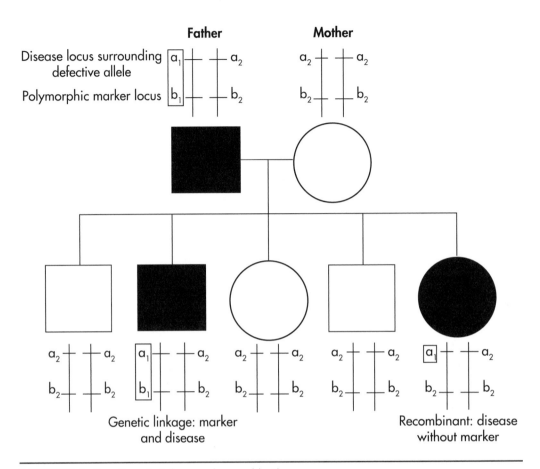

FIGURE 4–2. Genetic linkage and recombination.

Depicted is a hypothetical family (*circles = females; squares = males*) segregating an autosomal dominant disease. The disease locus a (containing either the defective allele a_1 or its normal counterpart a_2) lies close to a polymorphic marker locus b (containing marker alleles b_1 and b_2). The father is affected by the disease (*top filled square*) and is heterozygous at both the disease and the marker loci. The mother is unaffected (*top unfilled circle*) and is homozygous at both loci. Because the disease and marker loci are genetically linked (i.e., they lie near one another), crossing over rarely occurs between them. Most children who inherit the disease allele, a_1, will also receive the b_1 allele from their mothers. Occasionally, a recombination event will occur in the father, and he will transfer a chromosome bearing the b_2 marker allele along with the disease allele (as has occurred in the daughter represented by the circle labeled "recombinant").

Source. Adapted from Rieder RO, Kaufmann CA: "Genetics," in *The American Psychiatric Press Textbook of Psychiatry*, 2nd Edition. Edited by Talbott JA, Hales RE, Yudofsky SC. Washington, DC, American Psychiatric Press, 1994, pp. 35–79. Used with permission.

gous chromosomes is exchanged (Figure 4–2). These rearranged chromosomes are ultimately passed on to the offspring.

Disease genes are mapped to the human chromosomes with linkage maps of the human genome. These maps were constructed according to DNA polymorphisms, the numerous loci in the genome that vary in sequence among in-

dividuals, which can be identified by simple laboratory techniques. Types of polymorphisms that are used for genetic studies originally included restriction fragment length polymorphisms, which result from a mutation in a restriction enzyme site (Botstein et al. 1980), and later included variable-number tandem repeat sequences (Nakamura et al. 1987).

Both forms of these polymorphisms are typically found in noncoded regions of DNA. Single-nucleotide polymorphisms (SNPs) are also used in genetic studies (Wang et al. 1998). SNPs are DNA sequence variations that occur when a single nucleotide (A, T, C, or G) in the genome sequence is altered. SNPs can be in noncoding regions or in genes that affect disease susceptibility or drug response, and are becoming the marker of choice for genetic studies, given that they are the most common form of variation in the human genome.

When the polymorphism and disease gene are close to each other on the chromosome, there is a low chance of their being separated by recombination at meiosis (i.e., they are linked). The probability that a disease and marker allele will recombine depends on their distance from each other. In fact, the frequency with which the two alleles recombine (the recombination rate, or θ [theta]) can be used as a measure of the distance between their respective loci: 1% recombination is synonymous with a genetic distance of 1 centimorgan (cM) and roughly corresponds to a physical distance of 10^6 base pairs (bp) of DNA.

If disease and marker alleles lie near one another, crossing over will occur only rarely and parental gametes will be overrepresented. The disease and marker loci are then said to be *linked*. Statistical support for linkage is obtained by examining the cosegregation of disease and marker phenotypes within a pedigree, determining the likelihood (Z) of achieving the observed distribution of phenotypes given estimates for the recombination fraction, θ, ranging from 0.00 to 0.50 (the latter representing no linkage), and calculating the odds ratio [defined as the ratio $Z(\theta)/Z(\theta=0.50)$], that is, the relative likelihood of there being linkage versus no linkage. This odds ratio depends on the particular genetic parameters chosen in determining the likelihood. These parameters include the mode of inheritance, the frequency of the disease allele, and the probability of the disease given the presence of 0, 1, or 2 disease alleles. To the extent that evidence for linkage depends on such parameters, likelihood-based calcula-

tions are referred to as *parametric* linkage analyses. By convention, the odds ratio is expressed as its base 10 logarithm and is known as a *lod score*. In this way, the linkage data from several pedigrees can be pooled and their respective contributions added to obtain a combined probability of linkage. Also by convention, when the lod score at the best estimate of θ (defined as that estimate yielding the highest lod score) is greater than $+3$, linkage is confirmed; when it is less than -2, linkage is rejected for the data set supported for that set of pedigrees.

The thousands of DNA markers that encompass the genetic map of the entire genome can be used to complete the "whole genome" search for disease genes. When markers are examined that have been systematically drawn from throughout the genome, they may suggest linkage between a disorder and specific chromosomal regions. Conversely, they may reject linkage to these regions, thereby contributing to an *exclusion map* for the disorder. Markers from several regions may be examined concurrently; such a simultaneous search of the genome may detect multiple loci that contribute to a disorder. Notably, because several loci are tested as candidates with whole genome scans, P values must be made lower than 0.05 to reject the null hypothesis.

It is worth emphasizing that *linkage* refers to the two loci and not to their associated alleles. Even if crossing over is rare and certain allele pairs are disproportionately represented within any given pedigree, recombination does occasionally occur and eventually results in a more random distribution of allele combinations within the population at large. Thus, linkage of two loci does not necessarily imply an association of specific disease and marker phenotypes in the general population. An exception occurs when disease and marker loci lie so near to each other that it takes many generations for the allele combinations to equilibrate. For example, if the two loci are separated by 1 cM, it will take 69 generations, or about 2,000 years, until the frequency of an allele combination goes halfway to its equilibrium value (Ott 1985).

NONPARAMETRIC APPROACHES

Genetic linkage studies have been successful in identifying genes that have a large effect on illness risk. But such studies are problematic when several genes of small effect cause a disorder, as is true in most psychiatric conditions. It is also difficult to find enough large families with members who are willing to take part in the study. In addition, when the mode of inheritance is unknown, then many different models and assumptions must be applied to the data, leading to significant statistical problems.

Nonparametric analyses represent alternative methods for evaluating genetic linkage. These studies can be conducted without making assumptions about the mode of inheritance. One commonly used nonparametric approach is the *affected sib-pair* strategy (McCarthy et al. 1998). This method compares siblings who are definitely affected or unaffected, so the boundary of the condition does not need to be defined. It examines the frequency with which two siblings, both affected with the disorder of interest, share 0, 1, or 2 alleles coinherited from a common ancestor at the locus of interest; such alleles are said to be *identical by descent*. Under the null hypothesis of no linkage, these frequencies are 1/4, 1/2, and 1/4, respectively. Statistically significant deviations from this distribution of frequencies suggest linkage.

Association studies can examine if a particular DNA polymorphism is associated with a disorder by comparing unrelated affected and unaffected individuals. Association studies can even identify genes of very small effect or those that participate in gene-environment interactions, and may provide stronger statistical power than traditional linkage approaches (Risch and Merikangas 1996). A candidate gene study is a type of association study. Hypothesis-dependent candidate genes (those nominated by neurobiological clues to disease pathogenesis) and hypothesis-independent candidate genes (those put forward without regard to pathogenic hypotheses) may be explored. A method that is widely used to test candidate genes is allelic association, also called *linkage disequilibrium*. It can be used when most of the individuals with the disease are descended from a common ancestor in whom the disease mutation originated. Different allele frequencies will be found between individuals with the disease and the general population for markers that are very close to the disease gene. Methods have now been developed for testing association between hundreds of thousands of markers across the genome and phenotypes of interest. Figure 4–3 shows the theoretical risk of disease conferred by the assumption of allelic heterogeneity of additive effect of rare alleles versus that of multiple common interacting alleles. Figure 4–4 shows the genetic risk of schizophrenia as inferred in family studies of the disorder. Note the similarity of the curve produced by the family study data to that of the multiple common interacting alleles model shown in Figure 4–3.

ANTICIPATION, IMPRINTING, AND MITOCHONDRIAL INHERITANCE

A clinical phenomenon called *anticipation*, wherein the age at onset of disease decreases and the severity of disease increases in successive generations, has been recognized for many decades. With the discovery of expanding trinucleotide repeats in the early 1990s (Richards and Sutherland 1992), a convincing molecular mechanism was provided for this phenomenon. The phenomenon is now well described for several neuropsychiatric disorders, including myotonic dystrophy, fragile X syndrome, and Huntington's disease (HD), and there has been some evidence for anticipation in schizophrenia and bipolar disorder. Differences in the offspring's liability for illness due to the sex of the transmitting parent may be the result of genomic imprinting (Langlois 1994) or of mitochondrial inheritance. Genomic imprinting is the selective methylation of inherited chromosomes. Methylation affects the likelihood that genes will be transcribed and that correlating proteins will be made.

MOLECULAR APPROACHES

Once linkage analysis has implicated a particular chromosomal region in the etiology of

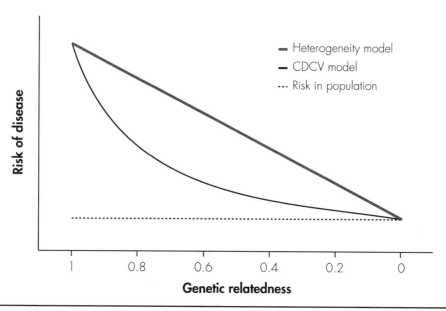

FIGURE 4–3.   The common disease/common variant model.

The risk of disease as a function of genetic relatedness to affected individuals is shown. Two hypothetical common diseases are considered (*black and gray lines*), each having the same monozygotic risk and the same underlying risk in the population (*dashed line*). For the disease represented by the gray line, the risk of disease falls linearly with decreased genetic relatedness, consistent with disease heterogeneity, owing to the reduction in the number of shared rare alleles—the disease heterogeneity model. For the disease indicated by the black line, the fall in risk as a function of genetic relatedness is more rapid, as can occur when multiple common interacting alleles contribute to disease—an example of the common disease/common variant (CDCV) model.

Source.   Reprinted from Wang WY, Barratt BJ, Clayton DG, et al.: "Genome-Wide Association Studies: Theoretical and Practical Concerns." *Nature Reviews Genetics* 6:109–118, 2005. Copyright 2005, Macmillan Magazines, Ltd. Used with permission.

a disorder, a variety of molecular genetic approaches may be used for identifying the disease gene and its pathological consequences. Thus, markers in linkage disequilibrium with, and thus in close proximity to, the disease gene may be identified. Genetic markers flanking the disease gene also may be recognized, thereby defining the minimal genetic region containing the disease gene. Overlapping cytogenetic anomalies producing the disease may then narrow this minimal genetic region. Alternatively, a more refined location for the putative disease locus may be provided by multilocus marker *haplotypes* surrounding the locus in genetically isolated populations (through a strategy known as *shared segment mapping*). The sequencing of the gene requires advanced gene sequencing and analytic technology. Specific molecular abnormalities (insertions, deletions, and base substitutions) within the disease gene then may be discovered, and research then focuses on determining how the genetic malfunction causes disease. Genetically modified animals, particularly mice, which breed rapidly, have been used to study human genetics. Introducing the normal or disease gene into appropriate in vitro and in vivo model systems may determine the pathological consequences of the disease mutation (Figure 4–5).

Although there are no clear animal models for human psychiatric diseases, certain traits that vary continuously (and are likely polygenic) can be studied with quantitative trait loci analysis (Flint et al. 2005).

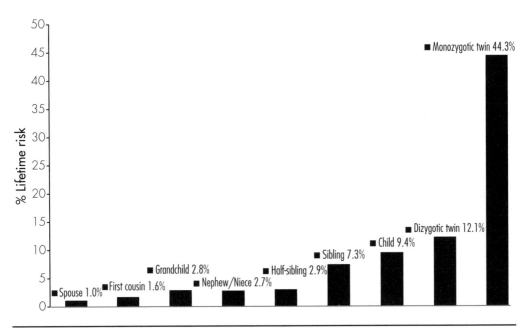

FIGURE 4–4. Family rates of schizophrenia.

Source. Data from McGue and Gottesman 1991.

HUMAN GENOME

The sequencing of the human genome provides an enormous technical advance for the understanding of human disease (Collins et al. 2003). A draft sequence map of about 90% of the DNA in the human genome was completed in 2000 (International Human Genome Sequencing Consortium 2001; Venter et al. 2001), and the "finished" sequence (2.85 billion nucleotides, representing 99% of the euchromatic genome) was reported several years later (International Human Genome Sequencing Consortium 2004). The initial analysis supports the existence of approximately 20,000–25,000 genes in the human genome. This estimate is similar to that for other mammals and only somewhat larger than that of metazoan model system genomes, such as those of the fruit fly *Drosophila melanogaster* (Adams et al. 2000) and nematode *Caenorhabditis elegans* (*C. elegans* Sequencing Consortium 1998). Allied mammalian sequencing projects in the mouse (Mouse Genome Sequencing Consortium 2002), rat (Rat Genome Sequencing Project Consortium 2004), dog (Lindblad-Toh et al. 2005), and

chimpanzee (Chimpanzee Sequencing and Analysis Consortium 2005) have been carried out, with more under way. Sequences from diverse mammals such as the rabbit, elephant, armadillo, tenrec, and hedgehog will assist in understanding the evolution of the mammalian lineage. The frog, chicken, and several species of fish have also been sequenced and will provide information about vertebrate evolution. The large amount of data from vertebrate species will provide much useful information in terms of comparative genomics. For example, highly conserved sequences not coding for proteins that are shared across the vertebrate phylogeny may suggest important regulatory functions (Boffelli et al. 2004; Dermitzakis et al. 2003).

A particularly interesting component of the effort to sequence the human genome was the discovery of vast numbers of genetic variants in the form of SNPs. These single base changes (e.g., an "A" is substituted by a "G") in genomic sequence occur every few hundred base pairs throughout the genome. Some occur in all human populations, reflecting their ancient age, whereas others occur in individual

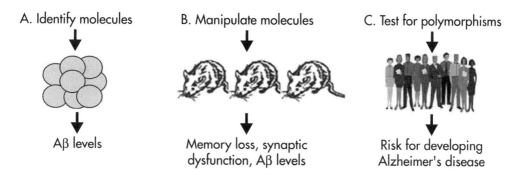

FIGURE 4–5. Alzheimer's disease genetic research strategy.

The candidate molecule (*A*), or the molecular pathway to which it belongs, can be manipulated in animal models using transgenic technologies (*B*). In the case of Alzheimer's disease, this manipulation should phenocopy the behavioral, electrophysiological, and biochemical phenotype of Alzheimer's disease. Genomic screens can be performed in humans, testing whether polymorphisms in the molecular pathway increase the risk of Alzheimer's disease (C).

Source. Reprinted from Lewandowski NM, Small SA: "Brain Microarray: Finding Needles in Molecular Haystacks." *The Journal of Neuroscience* 25:10341–10346, 2005. Used with permission.

populations, evidence of a more recent origin. It is estimated that 10 million of these variants occur within the genome. Some occur in functional regions of genes, often altering gene function, but the vast majority occur in intronic regions or in areas between genes and are less likely to have a biological effect. Given their density, SNPs are useful markers for linkage and association studies (Martin et al. 2000). The discovery that SNPs that are close to one another are often inherited in blocks of low genetic diversity led to the idea that analyzing a select set of these SNPs would allow researchers to analyze a large segment of the genome without having to examine all DNA variation while attempting to map diseases in humans (Gabriel et al. 2002; Johnson et al. 2001). The International HapMap Project was initiated to understand the patterns of DNA variation across major human populations (International HapMap Consortium 2003). This project genotyped some 5.8 million SNPs in 270 persons from Utah; Nigeria; Tokyo, Japan; and Beijing, China, and found patterns of genetic diversity common to all populations, as well as those unique to each group (International HapMap Consortium 2005). These freely available data can be used by investiga-

tors to identify genetic determinants of common diseases and has led to reports of association to genes for age-related macular degeneration and Parkinson's disease (PD) (Klein et al. 2005; Maraganore et al. 2005). The prospect of using these tools for discovery of genes for many of the disorders described in this chapter is reasonable.

BASAL GANGLIA DISEASE

HUNTINGTON'S DISEASE

In 1872, George Huntington described a familial illness he found in his Long Island, New York, practice: it was characterized by dance-like movements and "insanity." The illness appeared in midlife, afflicted men and women equally, did not skip generations, and led to early death. In 1908, the famed physician William Osler described HD as having an autosomal dominant mode of inheritance with complete penetrance: he noted that affected individuals usually had an affected parent, and conversely, approximately one-half of the offspring of affected parents were themselves affected. As early as 1932, Vessie noted that HD was prevalent throughout the world. Over the ensuing century, HD has been more completely described and its mutant gene and gene product identified, isolated, and well studied.

HD is characterized by progressive dementia, chorea, and psychiatric symptoms. The mean age at onset is about 40 years, but its symptoms can occur as early as age 2 and as late as age 80–90. HD usually causes death within 15–20 years of onset (Margolis and Ross 2003). In about 10% of the individuals with HD, the onset of symptoms occurs before age 20 (Gusella et al. 1993). Juvenile-onset HD or the "Westphal variant" is characterized by akinesia and rigidity instead of chorea, as well as a more rapid and severe course of illness.

Psychiatric symptoms occur in 70%–80% of the patients (Harper 1996) and can include a change in personality, paranoia, psychosis, and depression. About 40% of the patients develop a mood disorder; 25% of these have bipolar disorder (Peyser and Folstein 1990). Mood disorder may antedate other symptoms by 2–20 years (Folstein et al. 1983). In HD, the suicide rate is estimated to be as high as 12% (Harper 1996).

HD has an overall prevalence of 5–10 cases per 100,000 worldwide, making it the most common neurodegenerative disorder (Landles and Bates 2004). However, prevalence has been found to be higher in some places because of a large concentration of affected families; for example, the prevalence is more than 100 per 100,000 in a specific region of Venezuela (Wexler et al. 2004).

The age at onset of HD is variable and depends on the sex and the age at onset of the transmitting parent. Anticipation, which means that each successive generation tends to develop HD at an earlier age than did the previous one, occurs and is most striking with paternal inheritance. Many individuals with early-onset disease inherit the HD gene from their father and show anticipation—that is, a significantly earlier age at onset compared with their father (Ridley et al. 1988)—whereas many individuals with late-onset disease inherit the gene from their mother.

With the advent of genetic testing, it became possible to stratify at-risk relatives into gene-positive and gene-negative subgroups. A well-designed longitudinal study with multiple comparisons showed no cognitive differences between these two groups, suggesting that factors other than genetic susceptibility to HD account for differences in cognition between nominally at-risk persons and healthy control subjects (Giordani et al. 1995). However, genetic testing enables study of putative preclinical HD: asymptomatic gene carriers have declines in putamen volume (Harris et al. 1999) and mean annual striatal loss of dopamine receptors (Andrews et al. 1999) intermediate between HD patients and gene-negative at-risk individuals.

Genetics

HD is transmitted in an autosomal dominant fashion. Heterozygous inactivation of the HD gene as a result of chromosomal translocation is not associated with an abnormal phenotype (Ambrose et al. 1994).

In 1983, the gene responsible for HD was mapped to the short arm of chromosome 4 by the use of a linked polymorphic marker (Gusella et al. 1983). This evidence made it possible to detect HD allele carriers presymptomatically and also confirmed that HD is truly a dominant genetic condition (Myers et al. 1989; Wexler et al. 1987). Ten years later, in 1993, the genetic abnormality responsible for HD was identified as a CAG trinucleotide-repeat expansion in the first exon of a novel gene (Huntington Disease Collaborative Research Group 1993). No other known mutations in this gene cause the HD phenotype. The gene, *IT15*, is located on 4p16.3; it spans approximately 210 kilobases, comprises 67 exons, and encodes two messenger RNA (mRNA) species with a predicted protein product of 348 kilodaltons (kDa), known as huntingtin (see the following subsection, "Huntingtin").

The explanation for the "parental origin effect" became clear when the HD gene was identified and cloned and its nature of mutation understood. Age at onset was found to be inversely related to the length of trinucleotide repeats in the gene (Figure 4–6) (Margolis and

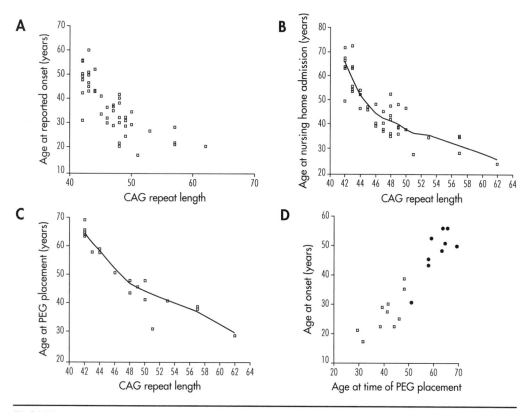

FIGURE 4–6. CAG repeats in Huntington's disease.

(*A*) Relationship between CAG repeat length and age at onset of Huntington's disease (HD). CAG repeat length is inversely correlated with age at onset of HD; $r = -0.77$. (*B*) Relationship between CAG repeat length and age at nursing home admission. CAG repeat length is inversely correlated with age at nursing home admission; $r = -0.81$. (*C*) Relationship between CAG repeat length and age at percutaneous endoscopic gastrostomy (PEG) placement. CAG repeat length is inversely correlated with age at PEG placement; $r = -0.91$. (*D*) Relationship between age at onset of HD and age at PEG placement, stratified by the median CAG repeat length. *Boxes* represent individuals with CAG repeat length > 46. *Filled circles* represent individuals with CAG repeat length ≤ 46. In a regression model, both age at onset ($P = 0.001$) and CAG repeat length ($P = 0.001$)+ were associated with age at PEG placement.

Source. Reprinted from Marder K, Sandler S, Lechich A, et al.: "Relationship Between CAG Repeat Length and Late-Stage Outcomes in Huntington's Disease." *Neurology* 59:1622–1624. Used with permission.

Ross 2003). The sex of the transmitting parent is a major factor influencing the trinucleotide expansion (Telenius et al. 1993). CAG repeats tend to expand modestly from one generation to the next but can double in length when passed from father to child. These dramatic expansions occur during spermatogenesis; examination of sperm DNA shows variation in trinucleotide repeat length among individual sperm (Leeflang et al. 1995; MacDonald et al. 1993). CAG expansions likely propagate

through the formation of stable hairpin structures and mismatched duplexes during gametogenesis (Mariappan et al. 1998).

The CAG repeat is highly polymorphic in the general population and ranges from 6 to 35 copies (Margolis and Ross 2003); 99% of people have fewer than 30 repeats. Individuals with HD, however, have more than 39 repeats and a median of 44 repeats (Kremer et al. 1994). Almost all individuals (>99%) with a clinical diagnosis of HD have CAG trinucleotide expansion of the HD gene. Adult-onset HD (ages 35–55) is associated with 40–50 CAG repeats; juvenile-onset HD is associated with repeat lengths of more than 64 CAG units. Spontaneous HD occurs when trinucleotide repeats expand beyond a threshold length of about 37 copies. Individuals with 36–39 repeats may or may not develop HD (Margolis and Ross 2003).

Multiple studies have shown that the CAG repeat size and the age at onset of HD are inversely correlated but that for a given repeat size, there is a wide range of onset ages. Thus, the use of repeat size to predict the age at onset is not particularly useful (Gusella et al. 1993). This suggests the influence of as yet unknown genetic, environmental, and stochastic modifying factors, as does the fact that individuals with 36–39 CAG repeats may develop the disease late in life or not at all. CAG repeat lengths also are associated with the age at onset of psychiatric symptoms and the presence of intranuclear inclusions but not with disease duration, which is invariably 15–20 years. The CAG expansion within the HD gene is thus a highly sensitive and specific marker for the inheritance of the HD mutation (Kremer et al. 1994). Rapid and accurate diagnosis can be made with polymerase chain reaction–based tests, even in utero (Alford et al. 1996).

Huntingtin.   The HD gene codes for huntingtin, a protein that bears no significant similarity to any known protein. Its known functions include transcriptional regulation, intracellular transport, and protection against neuronal apoptosis, and it is also involved in the endosome-lysosome pathway (Landles and Bates 2004). It is highly conserved across species and is expressed broadly across the organism during all stages of development. It is found in the cell body, nucleus, dendrites, and nerve terminals of neurons as well as in mitochondria, Golgi apparatus, and endoplasmic reticulum (Landles and Bates 2004). Homozygous inactivation of huntingtin in mouse models was found to be lethal: embryos did not develop organs and died before embryonic

day 8.5. Neuropathological analysis of these embryos showed apoptotic cell death in the embryonic ectoderm (Duyao et al. 1995), thus confirming huntingtin's involvement in prevention of neuronal apoptosis (Figure 4–7).

In another investigation (Mangiarini et al. 1996), a mouse model with a transgene of the huntingtin gene with 115–150 CAG repeats yielded a phenotype that included progressive involuntary stereotypies, tremors, seizures, reduction in brain and body weight, and early death. These mice did not show neurodegeneration but had early signs of neural apoptosis and selective reductions in receptors (dopamine, acetylcholine, and glutamate receptors) in the brain. In a third attempt, transgenic mice were created with full huntingtin complementary DNA with 89 CAG repeats. The phenotype of these mice more closely resembled human HD, with initial hyperactivity yielding to hypoactivity, subsequent akinesia, and death; neuropathological analysis showed selective neurodegeneration in the striatum and cortex, gliosis, and neuronal loss of about 20% (Reddy et al. 1999).

The critical pathogenic event in HD may be accelerated apoptosis. Apoptotic DNA fragments have been found in postmortem striatal tissue of HD patients (Butterworth et al. 1998). Mutant huntingtin is cleaved by caspase-3, an apoptotic enzyme, and this cleavage is enhanced by polyglutamate length (Martindale et al. 1998; Wellington et al. 1998). Mutant huntingtin is expressed abundantly by presynaptic cholinergic interneurons and cortical pyramidal cells that activate the striatal neurons that die (Fusco et al. 1999). This lends credence to the idea that excessive synaptic release of glutamate leads to excitotoxic striatal cell death (Sapp et al. 1999).

Potential Treatment

Thus far, only palliative treatment of symptoms exists for HD. A novel approach to therapy is to introduce trophic factors that may delay or retard excitotoxic damage of striatal neurons. In a nongenetic animal model for HD, in which rodents received intrastriatal injec-

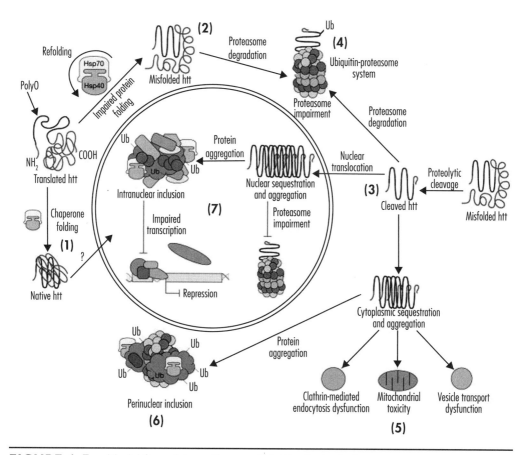

FIGURE 4–7. Model for cellular pathogenesis in Huntington's disease.

The molecular chaperones Hsp70 and Hsp40 promote the folding of newly synthesized huntingtin (htt) into a native structure. Wild-type htt is predominantly cytoplasmic and probably functions in vesicle transport, cytoskeletal anchoring, clathrin-mediated endocytosis, neuronal transport, or postsynaptic signaling. htt may be transported into the nucleus and have a role in transcriptional regulation (*1*). Chaperones can facilitate the recognition of abnormal proteins, promoting either their refolding or ubiquitination (Ub) and subsequent degradation by the 26S proteasome. The HD mutation induces conformational changes and is likely to cause the abnormal folding of htt, which, if not corrected by chaperones, leads to the accumulation of misfolded htt in the cytoplasm (*2*). Alternatively, mutant htt might also be proteolytically cleaved, giving rise to amino-terminal fragments that form sheet structures (*3*). Ultimately, toxicity might be elicited by mutant full-length htt or by cleaved N-terminal fragments, which may form soluble monomers, oligomers, or large insoluble aggregates. In the cytoplasm, mutant forms of htt may impair the ubiquitin-proteasome system (UPS), leading to the accumulation of more proteins that are misfolded (*4*). These toxic proteins might also impair normal vesicle transport and clathrin-mediated endocytosis. Also, the presence of mutant htt could activate proapoptotic proteins directly or indirectly by mitochondrial damage, leading to greater cellular toxicity and other deleterious effects (*5*). In an effort to protect itself, the cell accumulates toxic fragments into ubiquitinated cytoplasmic perinuclear aggregates (*6*). In addition, mutant htt can be translocated into the nucleus to form nuclear inclusions, which may disrupt transcription and the UPS (*7*).

Source. Reprinted by permission from Macmillan Publishers Ltd: Landles C, Bates GP: "Huntingtin and the Molecular Pathogenesis of Huntington's Disease" (Fourth in Molecular Medicine Review Series). *EMBO Report* 5:958–963, 2004. Copyright 2004, Macmillan Publishers, Ltd.

tion of excitatory amino acids, selective destruction of medium spiny neurons and motor and cognitive changes resulted, similar to what occurs in HD. When these animals received fibroblast grafts that secrete trophic factors, degeneration of striatal neurons was retarded, and motor and cognitive defects were prevented (Kordower et al. 1999). Small grafts induce widespread expression of catalase, a free radical scavenger, throughout the striatum. Neuroprotection is likely conferred by nerve growth factors' antioxidative properties or their effect on adenosine triphosphate (ATP) production. Simple infusion of trophic factors themselves was not effective.

Another potential therapy is the use of antioxidants (such as coenzyme Q10 and ubiquinone) that protect against glutamate toxicity and rescue mitochondrial metabolism and administration of creatine to buffer against energy depletion (Grunewald and Beal 1999). Others have proposed antiapoptosis agents, immunosuppressants, and fetal cell transplantation as possible therapeutic approaches for this fatal disease that as yet has no clear treatment.

PARKINSON'S DISEASE

PD is a progressive neurological disorder that is caused by the loss of dopaminergic neurons in the substantia nigra and nigrostriatal pathway of the midbrain. It was first described as "Shaking Palsy" in 1817 by James Parkinson because of the presence of a resting tremor and rigidity. The cardinal symptoms are poverty or slowness of movement (akinesia or bradykinesia), rigidity of the trunk and limb muscles, tremor or trembling that typically begins in the hands ("pill rolling"), and postural instability with impaired balance and coordination. Other common symptoms are a waxy facial expression, stooped posture, shuffling gait, and micrographia. The motor deficits arise from impairments in initiation, planning, and sequencing of voluntary movements. Some patients additionally experience difficulty in swallowing and chewing, speech impairments, and sleep disturbances. An associated dysfunction of the auto-nomic nervous system can cause urinary incontinence, constipation, sexual dysfunction, hypotension, and skin problems.

Many PD patients develop psychiatric syndromes, particularly depression, emotionality, and panic attacks, even in advance of the neurological signs. Treatment-emergent symptoms can include visual hallucinations, paranoid delusions, mania, and delirium. A sizable minority of patients develop cognitive slowing (bradyphrenia), and up to 40% of end-stage patients have dementia (Cedarbaum and Mc-Dowell 1987).

The onset is often subtle and gradual. Thereafter, the symptoms and their progression are quite variable, but PD frequently progresses to curtail walking, talking, and performing even simple tasks of daily living. There is no laboratory test for PD, which is diagnosed on the basis of the history and physical findings. The neuropathology includes a loss of pigmented (dopaminergic) neurons in the zona compacta of the substantia nigra and the presence of Lewy bodies in the remaining neurons. Noninvasive neuroimaging techniques can be used to examine the nigrostriatal pathophysiology (see Fischman 2005). Lewy bodies in other areas (cortex, amygdala, locus coeruleus, hypothalamus, dorsal medial nucleus of the vagus, and nucleus basalis of Meynert) may explain the nonmotor symptoms.

Epidemiological Studies

PD is a common condition, affecting about 1% of adults older than 60 years. Differences in case ascertainment and diagnostic criteria limit the ability to compare the incidence and prevalence of PD, but substantial variability is found between and within countries. The prevalence estimate is 133 in 100,000; the average age at onset is 63 years but may be increasing. The incidence of the disorder has been reported as 11 in 100,000 person-years (see Checkoway and Nelson 1999). PD may affect men at a slightly higher rate than women. Early-onset PD begins between ages 21 and 40 and accounts for 5%–10% of patients. The prevalence of PD increases with age, but it is not just an acceleration of normal aging; age is associated with a decline in striatal dopamine but not with changes in the caudate and putamen (van Dyck et al. 2002).

Secondary PD that is drug induced by dopamine antagonists (neuroleptics, antiemetics) or, less often, by calcium channel blockers is symmetric and resolves with drug discontinuation. PD can also be secondary to cerebrovascular disease that causes multiple lacunar strokes.

Family Studies

Most PD patients have no family history of PD, although a 2- to 14-fold increase in PD is seen in close relatives of affected individuals (Gasser et al. 1998). The greatest risk is found for the relatives of young probands; thus, 8.3% of the sibs of probands ages 35–44 were affected compared with 1.4% of the sibs of probands ages 65–74 years. Interestingly, PD is also increased in the relatives of probands with Alzheimer's disease, suggesting an etiological overlap between these disorders (Hofman et al. 1989). A strong familial nature for a syndrome is consistent with either shared genes or shared environments. Twin studies can be used to better disentangle these etiologies. Twin studies show that MZ and DZ twins of PD patients older than 60 have a similar concordance, consistent with the importance of environmental exposures, while for those with PD whose age at onset was 50 or younger, increased concordance in MZ twins was found (see Tanner et al. 1999). This suggests that, as in other diseases, there may be an early-onset form that has a greater genetic component. Some cases of PD can be attributed to specific gene mutations and toxic exposures, but the etiology of most cases is unknown. PD is a complex genetic disorder that probably results from the actions of multiple factors, including vulnerability genes, environmental exposures, aging, and gene-environment interactions.

Environmental Exposures

Research examining a role for environmental toxins in the etiology of PD was stimulated by

the finding that exposure to MPTP (1-methyl-4-phenyl-1,2,3,6-tetrahydropyridine), a toxic by-product made in the clandestine synthesis of a recreational drug, caused persistent PD in very young substance abusers (Langston et al. 1983) and in higher primates (Marsden and Jenner 1987). MPTP freely crosses the blood-brain barrier, where it is converted to a metabolite that is selectively taken up into dopaminergic neurons. The metabolite inhibits mitochondrial metabolism, leading to a decline in ATP and an accumulation of free radicals and oxidative damage. Investigation of the pathophysiology of MPTP yielded hypotheses about the etiology and pathophysiology of sporadic PD.

The risk for PD is also associated with other neurotoxins, including trace metals, cyanide, lacquer thinner, organic solvents, carbon monoxide, mercury, and carbon disulfide. In North America and Europe, early-onset PD appears to be associated with rural residence, perhaps reflecting exposure to pesticides, well water, or other toxins (Olanow and Tatton 1999). Preclinical parkinsonian symptoms are more common in regions of Israel where carbamates and organophosphates are detected (Herishanu et al. 1998). As reviewed by Kamel and Hoppin (2004), the accumulated data are compelling that pesticide exposure is associated with a significantly increased risk of PD, with risk estimates ranging from 1.6- to 7-fold (D.G. Le Couteur et al. 1999). The greatest evidence for association with a specific pesticide may be for paraquat (Liou et al. 1997), which produces selective degeneration of neurons (McCormack et al. 2002). Most studies focus on organopesticides, but other types of pesticides, including organochlorines, carbamates, fungicides, and fumigants, are known to be neurotoxic and may have similar effects. These toxins need not be selective for dopaminergic neurons because dopaminergic neurons may be comparatively more vulnerable than others in the brain. In sporadic PD, it may be that oxidant damage interferes with proteasomal cleavage of key gene products (synuclein), therefore leading to Lewy body formation (Jenner and Olanow 1998).

Infection may also increase the risk for PD, although these cases may be clinically and pathologically distinct from other PD (Gamboa et al. 1974). The great influenza pandemic of 1918 was linked to postencephalitic PD. Population studies also suggest that the risk for PD is increased by intrauterine influenza virus exposure, perhaps by the depletion of neurons in the developing substantia nigra (Mattock et al. 1988).

Cigarette smoking and tobacco use have an apparently protective effect against PD, according to numerous designs that showed lower relative risks for smokers than for non-smokers (reviewed in Checkoway and Nelson 1999). However, Allam et al. (2004) recently reviewed these studies and concluded that the apparently protective effect of cigarette smoking against PD actually resulted from reverse causation. Those individuals who developed PD were less likely to have strong smoking habits at younger ages, perhaps because of a prodromal condition. This line of research remains undetermined. Certainly, cigarette smoking would not be advanced as a protective strategy, in any case. Caffeine also may be protective against PD (G.W. Ross et al. 2000).

There are no consistent findings regarding PD and diet, despite expectations that vitamins A, C, and E would be protective given their antioxidant properties and that a high-fat diet would increase risk because of the potential for free radical generation (Checkoway and Nelson 1999). One study found an odds ratio of 9.0 for very high intake of animal fat (Logroscino et al. 1998).

Susceptibility Genes

Although strong familial patterns may also arise from shared exposures to toxins, several genes have been identified for patients with juvenile familial PD. These account for a small minority of cases but have illuminated pathology in the ubiquitin-proteasome system as the mechanism of neurodegeneration that may underlie PD in both familial and sporadic disease (reviewed by Samii et al. 2004). *PARK1* was the first gene linked to autosomal dominant PD. It codes for

α-synuclein protein, which is the major component of Lewy bodies. The gene may be involved in synaptic vesicle transport or uptake. In addition, elevation of this protein by a triplication of the normal gene (*PARK4*) was shown to precipitate early-onset PD in other families. The excessive or mutant α-synuclein protein may misfold or aggregate, causing it to be resistant to degradation by the ubiquitin-proteasome system (Figure 4–8). The most common gene defects may be in the *PARK2* gene, initially identified in recessive familial cases (Lucking et al. 2000). It codes for parkin, an enzyme (ubiquitin ligase) that is required for normal protein degradation. There are several parkin mutations, which may explain a half or more of the early-onset and juvenile-onset cases (see West et al. 2002), with other cases arising in parkin mutation heterozygotes. This defect leads to cell loss that typically is unaccompanied by Lewy bodies. Other mutations are described in the ubiquitin C-terminal hydrolase, which participates in the ubiquitin metabolism (Leroy et al. 1998); the DJ1 protein, which might be implicated in the response to oxidative stress (Bonifati et al. 2003); and *PINK1* (PTEN [phosphatase and tensin homologue deleted on chromosome 10]-induced kinase 1), which is a mitochondrial gene (Valente et al. 2004).

Molecular Mechanisms

Overall, the genetic findings provide strong evidence that the pathophysiology of PD involves a dysregulation of protein degradation by the ubiquitin-proteasome system. The ubiquitin-proteasome pathway affects many cellular processes and is a fundamental component of cell cycle regulation, although how it leads to cell death of dopaminergic neurons is still under investigation. Ubiquitin molecules are normally attached to damaged proteins as a signal for degradation.

Most cases do not involve gene defects in this pathway, suggesting that the damage is extrinsically determined. Such damage may arise from mitochondrial toxicity, oxidative stress, excitotoxicity, apoptosis, or inflammation (Gasser 2001). In some individuals, the ge-

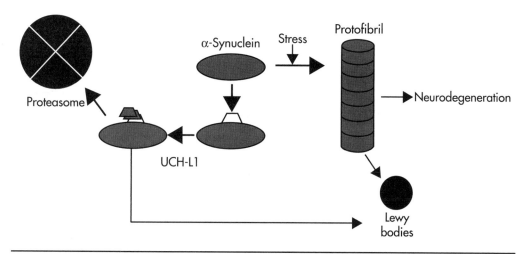

FIGURE 4–8.   Processing of α-synuclein, the major component of Lewy bodies, in Parkinson's disease.

The processing of α-synuclein by the ubiquitin-proteasome system can be potentially neurotoxic. In Parkinson's disease (PD), α-synuclein can oligomerize into protofibrils that in turn are potentially neurotoxic. The α-synuclein molecule can also be monoubiquitinated or polyubiquitinated; in either form, it can be processed by the proteasome and is involved in various mechanisms of pathogenesis of PD. UCH-L1 = ubiquitin carboxy-terminal hydrolase L1.

Source.   Adapted from Hasimoto M, Kawahara K, Bar-On P, et al.: "The Role of α-Synuclein Assembly and Metabolism in the Pathogenesis of Lewy Body Disease." *Journal of Molecular Neuroscience* 24(3):343–352, 2004. Used with permission.

netic susceptibility may be related to diminished detoxification of external agents by endogenous enzymes (Kuhn and Müller 1997; Langston 1998). Reports have linked PD to several metabolic enzymes. Cytochrome P450 (CYP) D6, a hepatic enzyme, and variants of CYPD6 weakly increase the risk for PD but may interact with glutathione S-transferase to elevate the risk for PD by 11- to 14-fold above that of the general population (Foley and Riederer 1999). An association between slow acetylation (N-acetyltransferase) and PD has been reported (Bandmann et al. 1997); slow acetylators may metabolize toxins more slowly, therefore potentiating their effect on vulnerable neurons. Also, in individuals with pesticide exposure, an association was found between PD and polymorphisms in a glutathione transferase locus (Menegon et al. 1998); the glutathione pathway plays a role in scavenging free radicals. Together, these observations suggest that many PD cases arise through a two-

hit gene-environment interaction pathway. In this model, risk entails both the genetic vulnerability and the toxic exposure, and neither factor is a sufficient cause of the disease.

WILSON'S DISEASE

In 1912, Wilson described a familial nervous disease associated with cirrhosis of the liver. Patients with this disorder (which is also known as hepatolenticular degeneration) may present with the triad of liver dysfunction, neuropsychiatric deterioration, and Kayser-Fleischer rings of the cornea. Renal impairment also may be present in patients with Wilson's disease (WD). The prevalence of WD is 1 in 30,000 (Schilsky 2002). Onset may be as early as age 4 or as late as the fifth decade.

WD occurs as a result of excessive copper accumulation and failure of copper excretion. Normally, copper is extracted from the portal circulation by hepatocytes and then either used for cellular metabolism, incorporated into ceruloplasmin, or excreted into bile. These last two pathways are impaired in WD. WD is diagnosed by measuring ceruloplasmin oxidase activity and hepatic copper content. A standard for disease diagnosis is the presence of more than 250 μg of copper per gram of liver (dry weight).

In WD, toxic amounts of copper accumulate first in the liver, where it leads to impaired protein synthesis, lipid peroxidation of membranes, DNA oxidative damage, and a reduced amount of cellular antioxidants. Mitochondria are especially vulnerable to this free radical damage and show early structural damage. Hepatocellular necrosis and apoptosis occur. Excess copper then spills out from damaged hepatocytes into the serum to infiltrate the brain, kidneys, and corneas. The basal ganglia are especially susceptible to the toxic effects of copper, possibly because the copper-containing enzyme dopamine β-hydroxylase is synthesized there (Ferenci 2004).

Neurological features in WD include spasticity, rigidity, dysarthria, dysphagia, apraxia, and a flapping tremor of the wrist and shoulder. Psychiatric manifestations are frequent and include personality changes, depressive episodes, cognitive dysfunction, and psychosis (Akil et al. 1991; Dening 1991). About one-third of the patients have psychiatric symptoms at the time of initial diagnosis (Ferenci 2004), and 10% of the patients present initially with only psychiatric symptoms (Akil et al. 1991). Although neuropsychiatric symptoms are nearly always accompanied by ocular Kayser-Fleischer rings (Schilsky 2002), they are not correlated with serum copper levels (Rathbun 1996) and hence may reflect active neurotoxicity rather than total copper load (Estrov et al. 2000). Interestingly, psychiatric symptoms are often exacerbated with chelation therapy of excess copper (Dening 1991; McDonald and Lake 1995). Magnetic resonance imaging shows loss of gray and white matter throughout the brain, including the caudate nucleus, brain stem, cerebrum, and cerebellum (Ferenci 2004).

Earlier onset of WD is more likely to be characterized by hepatic rather than neuropsychiatric signs (Cox et al. 1972). Nonetheless, many patients with signs of intellectual deterioration and movement disorder may present before age 10.

WD is progressive and fatal if untreated; death can occur from hemolytic crisis or liver failure. Treatment of WD involves removal of excess copper, either by using a chelating agent such as penicillamine (Walshe 1956) or trientene or by blocking intestinal copper absorption with zinc salts (Hoogenraad et al. 1979). Liver transplantation is also an effective treatment and cure for end-stage WD. Possible therapies in the future include liver cell transplantation and gene therapy with adenoviral vectors carrying the normal WD gene.

Genetics

WD is an autosomal recessive disorder. The *WD* locus (*WND*) was assigned to the long arm of chromosome 13 by close linkage with the red cell esterase D locus in a large Israeli-Arab kindred (Frydman et al. 1985). Bonne-Tamir et al. (1986) confirmed this linkage in two unrelated Druze kindreds and placed the *WND* locus distal to esterase D on chromosome 13. Haplotype analysis of 13q14.3 further defined the region surrounding the *WND* locus (G.R. Thomas et al. 1994). The identification of the WD gene, named *ATP7B*, was enabled by genetic study of Menkes' syndrome, which entails mutation in a related but different copper transporter (and which leads to copper deficiency rather than excess) (Daniel et al. 2004). Hence Petrukhin et al. (1994) reported the complete exon/intron structure of the WD gene, and individuals with WD were confirmed to have mutations at this locus. *ATP7B* has been cloned and found to encode a putative copper-transporting P-type ATPase (Figure 4–9) (Bull et al. 1993; Tanzi et al. 1993; Yamaguchi et al. 1993).

Identification and Diagnosis

More than 200 disease-specific mutations have been identified in WD (Schilsky 2002), including point mutations, deletions, insertions, and missense and splice site mutations. Most mutations occur either in transmembranous regions or at a site involved in ATP bind-

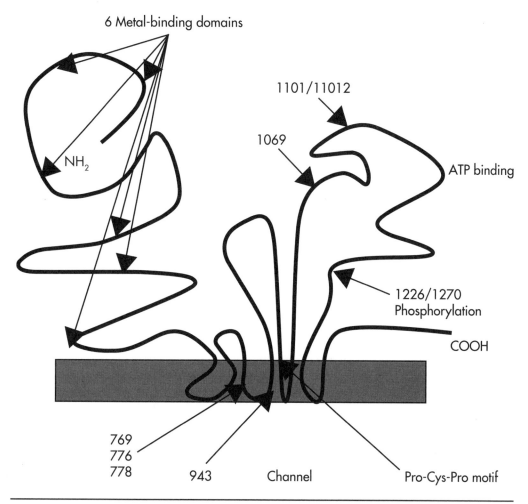

FIGURE 4–9.   P-type adenosine triphosphatase (ATPase) in Wilson's disease.

P-type adenosine triphosphatase (ATPase) is responsible for the binding and transport of copper. Note the six copper-binding domains, the adenosine triphosphate (ATP)–binding domain, the phosphorylation domain, and the channel domain. Pro-Cys-Pro = proline-cysteine-proline.

Source.   Reprinted from El-Youssef M: "Wilson Disease." *Mayo Clinic Proceedings* 78(9):1126–1136, 2003. Used with permission.

ing. The most frequent mutation (30% of patients of European descent) is a point mutation at position 1069, in which glutamine replaces histamine (H1069Q), which may be associated with later presentation and primarily neurological manifestation (Schiefermeier et al. 2000). The large number of mutations reduces the feasibility of a general screening test at this time. However, newer sequence analysis methodologies that screen the entire coding system of *ATP7B* may make such general screening plausible in the future. This will depend on differentiating disease-specific mutations from normal polymorphisms of the gene. At this time, haplotype analysis can be used for screening family members of patients with WD. At-risk siblings can have genetic and biochemical testing as toddlers; minimally toxic zinc therapy can begin as early as age 3 years to reduce copper absorption.

AUTISM

Autism is an uncommon neuropsychiatric disorder that is manifested by profound impairments in verbal and nonverbal communication and reciprocal social interrelationships and by interests and behaviors that are often repetitive and restrictive (American Psychiatric Association 2000). Onset of autism typically occurs before age 3 years, and the disorder persists throughout the life of the patient. Estimates of the population prevalence of autism are on the order of 5–10 per 10,000 (Bryson et al. 1988; Fombonne 1999). A consistently observed male-to-female ratio of 3–4:1 has been noted, with females often having more severe impairment, particularly in IQ (Volkmar et al. 1993).

FAMILY STUDIES

Beginning in the 1980s, family studies in which siblings of autistic probands were directly assessed showed rates of autism in the siblings of 2%–6% (Ritvo et al. 1989; Tsai et al. 1981). Another 20 subsequent studies continued to support these findings (Bailey et al. 1998). Szatmari (1999) pooled many such studies and estimated the risk to siblings as 2.2% (95% confidence interval [CI] = 1.1%–3.3%). Second- and third-degree relatives of autistic probands also have been assessed (DeLong and Dwyer 1988; Jorde et al. 1991; Pickles et al. 1995; Szatmari et al. 1995). These studies suggested an overall rate of autism of 0.2% in second-degree relatives and 0.1% in third-degree relatives. This dramatic decline in relative risk compared with that of first-degree relatives suggests a polygenic complex disorder. Family study data have been examined to determine whether a broader phenotype of pervasive developmental disorders (PDDs), of which autism is one, or other traits that occur in the relatives of autistic probands should be considered as phenotypes. On the whole, this research indicated that relatives of autistic probands can have a spectrum of behavioral traits, from isolated communication impairments and social difficulties to more severe disorders in the PDD spectrum (reviewed in Bailey et al. 1998). Although suggestive, this area of investigation has not been completely resolved, and it is clear that no evidence exists for "a behavioral or cognitive profile that is either universal or specific" (Bailey et al. 1998).

TWIN STUDIES

To determine whether the familial component of autism is genetic, several twin studies have been performed (Bailey et al. 1995; Folstein et and Rutter 1977; Ritvo et al. 1985; Steffenburg et al. 1989). These investigations, with a total of 108 twin pairs, reported a concordance rate of 36%–91% for MZ twins and 0%–24% for DZ twins. Only one group saw any concordance between DZ pairs (Ritvo et al. 1985). The observed nonconcordance in the DZ twins was probably secondary to the small sample number and low recurrence rate seen in siblings in family studies. These concordance rates yield heritability estimates in the range of 90%. This suggests that a substantial portion of the liability to autism is genetic in origin. These data also highlight the nonmendelian nature of its inheritance, implying multiple genes and epistatic gene interactions. Twin studies also support the inheritance of a broader phenotype. In an early study involving 21 twin pairs, concordance for cognitive and social abnormalities was 82% for MZ pairs and 10% for DZ pairs (Folstein and Rutter 1977). In a follow-up study that included the original group plus 28 new twin pairs, concordance for cognitive and social disorders was 92% for MZ pairs and again 10% for DZ pairs (Bailey et al. 1995). Imaging of MZ twins concordant or discordant for autism suggests a complex picture, with discordant twins showing cerebral white matter volumes similar to each other's yet different from those seen in nonautistic control subjects (Kates et al. 2004). Epidemiological data suggest that the process of twinning itself is not related to the high concordance rate (Hallmayer et al. 2002).

ADOPTION STUDIES

There are no known adoption studies for autistic disorder, although one study suggests that

PDD-like traits are more common in biological relatives of PDD probands than in nonbiological (including adoptive) relatives (Szatmari et al. 2000).

HIGH-RISK STUDIES

For several decades, clinicians have been describing the co-incidence of autism and various medical disorders. Depending on the stringency of the diagnostic criteria for autism and the comprehensiveness of the medical workup, this association is between 10% and 37% (Barton and Volkmar 1998; Gillberg and Coleman 1996; Rutter et al. 1994). Despite this variability in estimates and the ongoing debate on how they are derived, it is clear that the likelihood of a coexisting medical condition is related to a decreasing IQ (Ritvo et al. 1990; Steffenburg 1991). For example, one retrospective study that assessed 211 autistic subjects found that 24% of the subjects with an IQ greater than 50 had a broadly defined medical condition, whereas a full 40% of the individuals with an IQ less than 50 met the broad criteria for a medical condition (Barton and Volkmar 1998). Steffenburg (1991) used this association to propose potentially etiological subgroups of autism on the basis of the associated medical condition. These groupings included 1) pure hereditary autism, 2) other hereditary conditions (e.g., neurofibromatosis, tuberous sclerosis, fragile X syndrome), 3) other specific brain damage conditions (e.g., Möbius' syndrome, Rett's disorder), 4) nonspecific brain damage (e.g., epilepsy; hearing deficiencies; altered CSF, EEG, or CT scan results), and 5) unknown brain damage or genetic factors.

One well-documented disease association occurs with tuberous sclerosis. This condition is an autosomal dominant disorder involving the growth of hamartomas, which are abnormal benign lesions, in several organs, including the brain. The central nervous system (CNS) involvement is characterized by cortical and subependymal lesions, as well as seizures and mental retardation. Twenty-five percent of the patients with tuberous sclerosis also have au-

tism, and up to 40% have a disorder in the PDD spectrum (Smalley et al. 1998). Tuberous sclerosis has been reported to occur in 1%–2% of the patients with autism (Smalley 1992), and the rate is even higher in autistic individuals with a seizure disorder (Gillberg 1991). This co-occurrence between autism and tuberous sclerosis is much higher than would be predicted by prevalence rates of both of these rare disorders. Two genes have been identified— *TSC1* (Kandt et al. 1992) and *TSC2* (van Slegtenhorst et al. 1997)—whose gene products are known as hamartin and tuberin, respectively. The gene products of both genes are thought to be tumor suppressors (A. J. Green et al. 1994; van Slegtenhorst et al. 1997).

Smalley (1998) developed several hypotheses that may explain why genes thought to govern regulation of growth and differentiation could be associated with autism. First, and most favored, loss of tuberous sclerosis complex (TSC) protein function may lead to abnormal neural development in regions possibly related to autism. Second, TSC genes may actually be in close proximity, or linkage disequilibrium, to true autism genes. Finally, neuroanatomical and neuropsychological sequelae of tuberous sclerosis gene dysfunction, like seizures or tubers, may indirectly damage areas of the brain associated with autism. Further investigation of TSC gene products in neuronal function (Astrinidis et al. 2002; R. F. Lamb et al. 2000) may provide intriguing insights into one of a potential number of etiologies of autism.

MODE OF INHERITANCE

Several patterns of inheritance have been offered for autism, most deriving from particular clinical findings. The observation that the prevalence among girls is lower than among boys, yet female probands often have more autistic relatives, suggested a multifactorial hypothesis composed of genetic and nongenetic factors (Tsai et al. 1981). Likewise, the high male-to-female ratio and association with fragile X syndrome have suggested X-linked mechanisms, although enthusiasm for this theory has been tempered by the lack of linkage findings on the X chromosome (see following subsection, "Linkage Analysis"). Genomic imprinting also has been suggested as a mode of inheritance that attempts to solve the problem of unequal sex prevalence (Skuse 2000).

More formal attempts at understanding the mode of inheritance have had varied results. Ritvo et al. (1985) performed a classical segregation analysis on 46 multiple nuclear families (i.e., two or three autistic probands per family) and reported a segregation ratio close to that expected for an autosomal recessive mode of inheritance. They rejected both dominant and polygenic inheritance in these families. These data must be interpreted in light of the multiply affected ascertainment bias of the study. The same group produced different conclusions when they carried out a segregation analysis on all cases in a "well-defined" population (Jorde et al. 1991). Jorde et al. used a mixed model in 185 families and determined that the only inconsistent model was a single major locus model. Other analyses ruled out simple X-linked or imprinted X-linked segregation (Pickles et al. 2000). Pickles et al. (1995) used an analytic strategy that focused on the decrease in relative risk with degree of relatedness and estimated that three loci were most likely involved (range = 2–10). Together, these studies suggest that the interaction of multiple genes is more likely to cause autism than is a single major locus. The issues of selection resulting from low reproduction rates, phenotypic uncertainty, and genetic heterogeneity all complicate the elucidation of the mode of inheritance of autism. Attempts to determine clinical markers of heterogeneity have proven frustrating. One group found no obvious indicators of heterogeneity with estimations of clinical variability between and within MZ twin pairs (A. Le Couteur et al. 1996). A similar approach was used in 37 multiplex families, and again there was no concordance for IQ or specific autistic symptoms, although some repetitive and ritualistic behaviors seemed to show some intrafamily concordance (Spiker et al. 1994).

LINKAGE ANALYSIS

The last decade has seen the first attempts to identify susceptibility loci for autism. Multiple international multicenter genome scans have been published. Genetic linkage has been reported on the X chromosome and all but 5 of the 22 autosomes (Folstein and Rosen-Sheidley 2001; Wassink et al. 2005). Our brief review focuses on 7q and 2q, two genomic regions that have been most consistently observed between the various linkage studies. The first region is on the long arm of chromosome 7.

The International Molecular Genetic Study of Autism Consortium (IMGSAC) examined 87 European affected sibling pairs and observed a high score of 2.53 on 7q, with the score increasing to 3.55 in a subgroup of 56 of 66 families from the United Kingdom (International Molecular Genetic Study of Autism Consortium 1998). Subsequent analyses that used more markers and sibling pairs continued to support linkage to this region (International Molecular Genetic Study of Autism Consortium 2001a, 2001b). These analyses also suggest parent of origin and sex-limited effects on several chromosomes, including chromosome 7 (J. A. Lamb et al. 2005). The Collaborative Linkage Study of Autism, which included 75 multiplex families and 416 markers (Collaborative Linkage Study of Autism 2001), found maximum multipoint heterogeneity lod scores of 2.2 for a 7q marker, under a recessive model with 29% of the families being linked to this region. Another group focused on a segment of 7q in 76 families and found some evidence for linkage in this region (Ashley-Koch et al. 1999), a finding that remained when more families were genotyped (Shao et al. 2002b). An independent study of 110 families found no support for 7q until the authors genotyped additional markers in the area after adding 50 more families, resulting in a multipoint lod score of 2.13 (J. Liu et al. 2001). Increasing the number of families to 345 led to somewhat diminished support for 7q (Yonan et al. 2003). The same family set was used to link the 7q region to quantitative phenotypes involving repetitive behaviors and language in 152 families (Alarcon et al. 2002), although adding 235 additional families diminished this finding (Alarcon et al. 2005). These families also yielded evidence for a sex-limited effect in these linkage analyses, although not on chromosome 7 (Stone et al. 2004). Other genome scans provide minimal support for the 7q region (Auranen et al. 2000; Philippe et al. 1999), but some do not (Risch et al. 1999).

Chromosome arm 2q has also emerged as a potential location for an autism gene or genes. IMGSAC has found varying levels of support for linkage on 2q, from a multipoint maximum lod score of 0.65 in 99 families at 103 cM (International Molecular Genetic Study of Autism Consortium 1998), increasing to 1.6 at 111 cM and to 3.74 with a more telomeric marker (206 cM) and a broader phenotypic definition in a total of 152 families (International Molecular Genetic Study of Autism Consortium 2001b). Another group reported a multipoint heterogeneity lod score of 1.98 at 183 cM in 95 families (Buxbaum et al. 2001). A genome screen in 99 families showed a maximum lod score of 2.12 at 198 cM (Shao et al. 2002b), which increased to 2.86 in a subset of 45 families also segregating delays in phrase speech (Shao et al. 2002a).

From these studies, the region of 7q is clearly the most interesting. Other studies have focused linkage analyses on a region of common chromosomal abnormalities in autism and are discussed later in this chapter. The initial lack of consistent linkage findings on the X chromosome in some of the earliest genome scans mentioned earlier was of interest given the noted sex imbalance in prevalence. One older study in which 38 multiplex families were genotyped with 35 X chromosome markers showed no significant findings, with a single marker showing a maximum lod score of 1.24 (Hallmayer et al. 1996). More recently J. Liu et al. (2001) reported a finding on the X chromosome as their second highest (maximum lod score of 2.56), decreased to 1.78 when an additional 235 families were added (Yonan et al. 2003). A subsequent study of 99 families

again showed linkage to the X chromosome, although very distant from the previously discussed studies, with a multipoint score of 2.54 (Shao et al. 2002b), whereas a Finnish study observed a maximum score of 2.75 in 38 families at another point on the X chromosome (Auranen et al. 2002). Finally, 22 families were genotyped with X chromosome markers, and results showed modest support for linkage on the distal portion of the X chromosome.

In summary, these studies suggest evidence for autism susceptibility loci on 7q and 2q, even though several different samples with differing geographic origin and diagnostic classification were used. Positional cloning of candidate genes and higher-density marker scans will determine whether these remarkable findings hold true.

CHROMOSOMAL ABNORMALITIES

Chromosomal abnormalities have long been associated with autism. In a thorough review, Gillberg (1998) catalogs much of what has been described. On the basis of diagnostic criteria from DSM-III, DSM-III-R, DSM-IV (American Psychiatric Association 1980, 1987, 1994), and ICD-10 (World Health Organization 1992), some 49 individuals with autism have been reported to have abnormalities of 16 of 22 autosomes and both sex chromosomes. With less stringent criteria, only chromosomes 14 and 20 have not been associated with autism (Gillberg 1998). One survey found that 5% of autistic individuals had a major chromosomal abnormality (Ritvo et al. 1990). Anomalies occur most often in patients with mental retardation, with chromosome 15 abnormalities being particularly common and showing deletions and partial trisomy or tetrasomy in the 15q11–13 region. There appears to be some specificity to this region, as one study showed that 20 of 29 individuals selected for inverted duplications of chromosome 15 had "a high probability" of being autistic (Rineer et al. 1998). This is especially interesting in that deletions in this region are also implicated in Angelman syndrome, a behavioral syndrome that is characterized by prominent mental retardation, ataxic gait, and episodic smiling and laughing. In one survey of a population of 49,000 children, all 4 children diagnosed with Angelman syndrome also met the criteria for autism (Steffenburg et al. 1996). Interest in this region has spawned focused linkage studies, which have produced promising results (Bass et al. 1999; Cook et al. 1998), as well as successful efforts in physical mapping of the region (Maddox et al. 1999). Although it is still unclear what role chromosomal anomalies may play in autism, the strength of their association appears strong and thus will catalyze further investigation (Castermans et al. 2004).

CANDIDATE GENES

A recent review stated that at least 89 genes have been reported as candidate genes for autism (Wassink et al. 2005). Many genes are chosen on the basis of hypothesized pathways thought to be involved with autism or from observations in laboratory animal models of neurodevelopment (Bartlett et al. 2005). An example of this line of research stems from investigations that showed elevated blood serotonin levels in autistic individuals, when compared with control subjects (Abramson et al. 1989; Anderson et al. 1987). Serotonin levels were higher in autistic persons with autistic siblings, compared with autistic probands with no affected siblings, suggesting a relation between serotonin and a genetic diathesis for autism (Piven et al. 1991). The utility of serotonergic drugs in autism has rekindled interest in the serotonin system, particularly the serotonin transporter. A family-based study of 86 parent-proband trios showed significant linkage disequilibrium with a functional promoter polymorphism in the serotonin transporter gene (*SLC6A4*), the protein responsible for recycling synaptic serotonin and the target of many psychoactive medications (Cook et al. 1997). A dozen studies with similar design have been carried out, with ambiguous results rendering the role of this particular gene in autism still obscure.

A second strategy is an extension of the linkage studies described earlier, in which genes within regions of chromosomes linked to autism are further genotyped as polymorphic markers to assess association to that gene or are directly sequenced for disease or susceptibility variants. Some of these studies have not had positive results (Bacchelli et al. 2003; Bonora et al. 2002, 2005), although one gene, a mitochondrial aspartate/glutamate transporter located in the 2q interval, shows association with autism (Ramoz et al. 2004).

A third approach capitalizes on the rich catalog of cytogenetic abnormalities in autism, as described in the previous section. Examples include the neuroligin 3 and neuroligin 4 genes, which are found on the X chromosome and are involved with synaptogenesis. These genes lie in a region of the chromosome reported to be deleted in some autism patients (N.S. Thomas et al. 1999). Mutations in these genes have been described in carefully chosen autism families (Jamain et al. 2003; Laumonnier et al. 2004; Yan et al. 2005), although these mutations may be present in only a small subset of autism families (Gauthier et al. 2005; Vincent et al. 2004; Ylisaukko-oja et al. 2005). Another example involves the region of chromosome 15q11–13 that harbors several genes that may be interesting autism candidate genes (J.A. Lamb et al. 2000). A cluster of genes comprising the α_5, β_3, and γ_3 subunits of the γ-aminobutyric acid (GABA) receptor lies in the region. GABA is the chief inhibitory neurotransmitter in the CNS, and the GABA system is thought to be involved in seizure disorders. Mice deficient for the β_3 subunit show abnormal EEG findings, experience seizures, and engage in behavior reported to be similar to that in patients with Angelman syndrome (learning deficits, hyperactivity, poor motor coordination, and disturbed rest–activity patterns) (DeLorey et al. 1998). Cook et al. (1998) used a microsatellite marker located in the third intron of the human β_3 gene (*GABRB3*), as well as eight other markers in the region, to genotype 140 autistic families. The *GABRB3* marker was in significant linkage disequilibrium with autism, an observation confirmed by another group as well (Buxbaum et al. 2002). Linkage in this region was enhanced when phenotypic subtypes were used (Shao et al. 2003) but not with other subtypes (Ma et al. 2005a). Other groups have not replicated association to the region (Ma et al. 2005b; Maestrini et al. 1999).

In summary, despite extensive efforts to screen genes conjectured to be related to autism, very few have been unequivocally identified. Given the high genetic character of autism or "autisms," it is safe to conclude that genes that influence the phenotype will be identified. Efforts are being made to increase further the likelihood of identifying these genetic determinants. Such advances include developments in statistical genetics and refinements of the autism phenotype (Wassink et al. 2005). Laboratory innovations, such as use of whole genome association designs, use of microarray-based expression and DNA copy number analysis, screening of noncoding DNA based on comparative genomic data, and assessment of epigenetic modification, also may contribute to a better understanding of autism.

DEMENTIA

ALZHEIMER'S DISEASE

Alzheimer's disease is the most common cause of dementia, accounting for 50%–70% of all cases. It is a neurodegenerative disease that usually begins after age 65 years, although early-onset cases also occur. Alzheimer's disease is characterized by a progressive deterioration of mental abilities, particularly memory, language, abstract thought, and judgment. Psychiatric and behavioral disturbances are among its earliest symptoms, with overt neurological signs dominating the clinical picture as the illness progresses, including rigid limbs, frontal release findings, and seizures. The course leads inevitably to the loss of independent living and death over an average course of 8–10 years. The clinical picture, history, and laboratory studies permit a probable diagnosis of Alzheimer's disease, but the definitive diagnosis depends on postmortem studies.

The genetic discoveries in Alzheimer's disease have uncommonly complemented and extended what was known about the neuropathology of the disease. The pathognomonic neuropathology shows selective neuronal loss, with neurofibrillary tangles in the neurons and amyloid substance deposited in senile plaques and cerebral blood vessels. The neurofibrillary tangles consist of microtubule-associated tau proteins. These normally stabilize the microtubules of the neuronal cytoskeleton and are regulated by phosphorylation and dephosphorylation processes. In Alzheimer's disease, the microtubule-associated tau proteins become abnormally hyperphosphorylated and accumulate as paired helical filament tangles in degenerating neurons. The plaques are mainly built up by the deposition of β-amyloid protein, which is a proteolytic fragment of the larger precursor, β-amyloid precursor protein (β-APP).

Inflammation appears to be an important feature in many cases, perhaps initiated by immune reactions to β-amyloid plaques or tangles or reactions to the local vasculature or from systemic conditions. Alzheimer's disease and vascular dementia are not mutually exclusive, and pathological features of both disorders commonly coexist.

Epidemiological Studies

The prevalence estimates of Alzheimer's disease depend on the population sampled (community or nursing home residents), age, and diagnostic criteria (definition of "significant impairment"). Onset before age 65 distinguishes presenile (types 1, 3, 4) from senile (type 2) dementia, although the cutoff ages are indistinct. Presenile cases are more likely to be familial, to be rapidly progressive, and to show prominent temporal and parietal lobe features, including dysphasia or dyspraxia. Later-onset cases (type 2) have a more insidious course and generalized cognitive impairments.

About 3% of those ages 65–74 years and half of the population older than 85 have Alzheimer's disease. Alzheimer's disease rates approximately double every 5 years after age 40 years (Hendrie 1998); the prevalence is expected to swell as the average life span increases. Although age is the most important illness predictor, Alzheimer's disease pathology is not an expected feature of aging.

Geographic variations in the prevalence of Alzheimer's disease suggest the importance of environmental and lifestyle factors or variability in diagnosis and research methodology. Studies of migrant populations confirm the importance of environment and lifestyle. For example, the prevalence of Alzheimer's disease in Japan is 1.5%, whereas ethnic Japanese persons in Honolulu, Hawaii, have a prevalence of Alzheimer's disease of 5.4%, a rate comparable to that of white people in Hawaii (White et al. 1996).

Most Alzheimer's disease cases are sporadic, particularly the senile forms, and several demographic measures, lifestyle choices, environmental exposures, and medical conditions are associated with Alzheimer's disease risk. Even in the nonfamilial cases, it is expected that genetic susceptibility plays an important role. In particular, risk is associated with alleles of *APOE* (apolipoprotein E), which is a major component of very-low-density lipoproteins (VLDLs). The Alzheimer's disease risk for the ε4 homozygotes (*APOE*E4*) is especially elevated, although not all patients with Alzheimer's disease have *APOE*E4*, and many people with the ε4 allele remain free of disease. The *APOE*E4* allele is associated with an increased number of amyloid plaques, and it may interact with other susceptibility genes and environmental factors.

Females have a greater risk for Alzheimer's disease, even after accounting for their longer life span, with males showing a higher rate of vascular dementias. It was hypothesized that the risk for women could be due to menopause, and many long-term studies suggested that women who take estrogen-based hormone replacement therapy (HRT) have a lower risk of developing Alzheimer's disease. For example, the relative risk (RR) of Alzheimer's disease for HRT users versus nonusers was 0.46 (95% CI = 0.21–1.00) in the Baltimore Longitudinal Study (Kawas et al. 1997) and 0.24 (95% CI = 0.07–0.77) in the Italian Longitudinal Study on Aging (Baldereschi et al. 1998).

These associations remained significant after adjustment for age, education, age at menarche, age at menopause, smoking, alcohol use, body weight, and number of children. However, because HRT use was not random among these subjects, it is possible that women who are less likely to develop Alzheimer's disease for other reasons are just more likely to use HRT. Zandi et al. (2002) found no benefit of current HRT use except for those whose use exceeded 10 years. Recently, the Women's Health Initiative Memory Study surprised investigators by showing a doubling of the risk of all-cause dementia in women randomly assigned to receive Prempro, a specific form of combination hormone therapy, after age 64 years (Shumaker et al. 2003). This study was abruptly halted because the risks of HRT were found to "outweigh the benefits." Consequently, estrogen and progesterone combination therapy is not currently recommended for prevention of cognitive decline or dementia, and studies examining estrogen alone are being reexamined. There is new speculation that gonadotropins, rather than estrogen and progesterone, may play the key role in determining the risk for and progression of Alzheimer's disease. As recently reviewed (see Webber et al. 2005), women with Alzheimer's disease have higher levels of luteinizing hormone (LH) than do control subjects. Both LH and its receptor are expressed in brain regions that are susceptible to Alzheimer's disease pathology. Furthermore, because LH is mitogenic, it could dysregulate cell cycles as described in Alzheimer's disease neurons (see Casadesus et al. 2005).

A higher educational level is a protective factor (Launer et al. 1999), perhaps because of the increased synaptic and/or dendritic complexity attendant on learning demands. A well-controlled prospective study of at-risk individuals confirmed that low educational attainment was associated with a doubling of Alzheimer's disease incidence (Stern et al. 1994). The effect of education may be a result of higher socioeconomic status or linked to other factors that influence risk for Alzheimer's disease, such as lower stress or better diet. Determining whether education may directly mitigate the risk of developing Alzheimer's disease has implications for the prevention and treatment of Alzheimer's disease, such as using cognitive training to lower the risk for vulnerable individuals (Hendrie 1998).

Traumatic brain injury (TBI) has been related to Alzheimer's disease risk. A prospective study showed that TBI increased the incidence of Alzheimer's disease by fourfold over the next 5 years (RR = 4.1; 95% CI = 1.3–12.7), particularly in cases with *APOE*E4* (Mayeux et al. 1995; Tang et al. 1996). The association between TBI and Alzheimer's disease risk may be affected by the severity of the TBI (loss of consciousness or not) and by family history (Guo et al. 2000). One study suggested that TBI does not increase absolute risk but shortens the time to onset in those patients who will otherwise develop the disease (Nemetz et al. 1999). As reviewed by Jellinger (2004), some research findings support the plausibility of this association; *APOE* alleles are associated with prognosis following TBI, and neuropathological studies show that TBI can cause apolipoprotein B deposition and tau pathology.

Strong evidence supports a role for chronic inflammation in initiating and worsening Alzheimer's disease. Amyloid is a proinflammatory substance, and neuropathological examination shows that plaques are surrounded by signs of inflammation. Use of nonsteroidal anti-inflammatory drugs, such as ibuprofen, has shown protective effects (see Gasparini et al. 2005). Support for the inflammation hypothesis, reviewed by Finch (2005), includes C-reactive protein elevations, participation of activated brain microglia in amyloid plaque formation, and roles of the *APOE*E4* allele, which may exacerbate brain vascular abnormalities.

Cigarette smoking has been purported to have protective effects, but a pooled analysis of four prospective studies showed that it actually increased Alzheimer's disease risk, especially in men (Launer et al. 1999), and chronic nicotine exposure appears to enhance Alzheimer's disease pathology (Oddo et al. 2005). Oxidative stress may play a role in cellular damage, and antioxidants, such as vitamin E, are purported to slow the progression of Alzheimer's disease. In addition, low levels of vitamin B_{12} or folate may increase Alzheimer's disease risk, perhaps by increasing the amino acid homocysteine, which is also a cardiovascular disease risk factor that may cause inflammation. Aluminum exposure received a great deal of early attention as a risk factor, but this has not held up in controlled studies.

Hypertension also significantly elevates Alzheimer's disease risk, an effect that may be mediated by vascular injury and inflammation. In their review, Luchsinger and Mayeux (2004) highlighted the possible mechanisms linking cerebrovascular diseases with Alzheimer's disease. Diabetes and hyperinsulinemia are also likely to be important risk factors. Dysregulation of insulin or the insulin-like growth factor pathway, from either genetic mutations or metabolic derangements, could also mediate the disease risk (de la Monte and Wands 2005; Launer 2005).

Family and Twin Studies

Approximately a quarter of patients with Alzheimer's disease have another first-degree relative with Alzheimer's disease, and the familial nature of Alzheimer's disease has been established in case–control, family, and twin studies (reviewed in Richard and Amouyel 2001). The recurrence risks in family studies are small and variable: 0%–14.4% for parents and 3.8%–13.9% for siblings. The familial recurrences are more prominent in early-onset disease, although such cases may be just more easily ascertained, and both early- and late-onset cases frequently occur within a single family. Family studies are hindered by the late age at onset of Alzheimer's disease because vulnerable individuals often die from other conditions before the incidence age of Alzheimer's disease or may even develop dementia from another etiology.

Because family members have similar types of environmental exposures, twin studies are needed to determine whether familial factors are the result of shared genes. These studies consistently show higher concordance rates for MZ than for DZ twin pairs, ranging from 21% to 67% for MZ twin pairs and 8% to 50% for DZ twin pairs. For example, Raiha et al. (1996) showed pairwise concordance rates of 18.6% and 4.7% for MZ and DZ twins, respectively, with corresponding proband-wise concordance rates of 31.3% and 9.3%. These results show that heritability is a factor for at least some forms of Alzheimer's disease. Because of the late onset and strong environmental component to Alzheimer's disease risk, discordance among DZ twins may arise from different environmental influences or variation in incidence ages as well as from genetic differences. Variation in age at onset in MZ twins has been linked to events such as hysterectomy and infection (Nee and Lippa 1999).

Molecular Genetic Studies

Evidence has continued to accumulate that early- and later-onset forms differ in their underlying pathophysiology. The familial early-onset autosomal dominant forms, which explain less than 2% of Alzheimer's disease, are linked to mutations in three genes, as reviewed by Rubinsztein (1997): the *APP* gene on chromosome 21 (Goate et al. 1991), the presenilin 1 gene (*PSEN1*) on chromosome 14 (Sherrington et al. 1995), and the presenilin 2 gene (*PSEN2*) on chromosome 1 (Levy-Lehad et al. 1995; Rogaev et al. 1995).

The *APP* mutation on chromosome 21 causes "type 1" Alzheimer's disease. It explains about 15% of early-onset cases, and this is also the type of Alzheimer's disease that universally develops in individuals with Down syndrome, in whom the excess APP activity is due to a trisomy of the entire chromosome 21 rather than just the *APP* mutation. Another 18%–50% of the early-onset cases are from *PSEN1* mutations (type 3); this type has its onset during midlife, typically in the 40s, and progresses rapidly. Type 4 is caused by mutations in *PSEN2* and accounts for fewer than 1% of early-onset cases. It presents at ages 40–75 and follows a slowly deteriorating course that averages 11 years. Although

these three loci are uncommon causes of Alzheimer's disease, their identification has shed light on the biochemistry of amyloid formation and deposition in the human brain. Each of these mutations causes dysregulation of APP processing, leading to an increased production of β-amyloid peptide. This accumulation leads to misprocessing of the tau protein, which accumulates in amyloid plaques, explaining the typical neuropathology of Alzheimer's disease.

Most cases are late onset and sporadic (type 2), although clusters of late-onset cases in families exist. Except for the small percentage of patients with Alzheimer's disease who have mendelian inheritance patterns, the genetic component in most cases likely entails complex interactions between other genes and environmental exposures. APOE (chromosome 19) appears to play a role in all forms of Alzheimer's disease, both early-onset and late-onset familial and sporadic cases. *APOE* alleles act to modify the influence of other genotypes and exposures on the risk for Alzheimer's disease. Risk is increased by the ε4 allele and may be decreased by the ε2 allele. The most common allele (ε3) does not appear to influence risk. These effects are age-dependent and nonmendelian and vary between population samples, in keeping with the variability of genes and exposures.

Other purported susceptibility regions that could modulate the APOE effects include the APOE receptors. Of particular interest are the low-density lipoprotein (LDL) receptor–related protein and the VLDL receptor gene (Okuizumi et al. 1995) of the LDL receptor superfamily. Additional evidence shows associations between Alzheimer's disease and other genes, such as the α_1-antichymotrypsin gene (Kamboh et al. 1995), major histocompatibility genes, CYP genes (CYP2D6), and the gene encoding the nonamyloid component of senile plaques (*NACP*) (reviewed in Cruts et al. 1998).

The genetic and epidemiological research findings in Alzheimer's disease make an intriguing story that is gaining coherence as it progresses. These findings will almost certainly lead to advancements in the prevention, early detection, and treatment of Alzheimer's disease.

PRION DISEASES

Prions are proteinaceous infectious agents that cause a group of rare and fatal neurodegenerative disorders that were initially recognized as "transmissible spongiform encephalopathies." By the 1960s, it was recognized that the infectious agent was a protein because its infectivity was resistant to normal sterilization procedures and was susceptible to protein degradation (Alper et al. 1967). Stanley B. Prusiner (1982) subsequently discovered the prion protein, for which he received a Nobel Prize in 1997.

Prions are normal cellular membrane proteins that become infectious simply by changing shape, without a change in their nucleic acid sequence. When misfolded, they undergo a conformational change from an α-helix to a β-pleated sheet. These misfolded prions (PrPres) induce normal prion proteins (PrP) to change shape. The abnormal prion proteins can be transmitted from an exogenous source (consumed human flesh or beef, human endocrine injections, or dura mater transplants) or may derive from germline or somatic mutations in the *PRNP* gene. Although much has now been learned about prions, the mechanisms whereby a self-reproducing protein structure can cause infection remain intriguing and unknown.

The various prion diseases differ somewhat in their clinical profiles, but their presentation commonly includes impaired cognition, behavior changes, insomnia, and ataxia that progresses to include extrapyramidal and pyramidal symptoms, myoclonus, and akinetic mutism. Prion diseases have no effective treatments, but laboratory studies are conducted to verify that the symptoms have no treatable explanation. The definitive diagnosis is made by a brain biopsy. The neuropathology shows spongiform degeneration, with microglial activation, and a protease-resistant form of the host-derived prion protein.

Epidemiological Studies

Sporadic Creutzfeldt-Jakob disease.

The sporadic form of Creutzfeldt-Jakob disease (CJD) is the most common prion disease, accounting for approximately 60%–70% of all cases (see review of CJD variants by Gambetti et al. 2003). Its prevalence is 1 in 1 million. Sex ratios are nearly equal, although there may be an excess risk in men older than 60. Seventy-five percent of patients die within 6 months, although many die within a few weeks of the diagnosis (Knight 1998). CJD usually begins with a rapidly progressive dementia, although abnormal behavior or gait imbalance is the presenting symptom in about one-third of patients. The autopsy findings show gliosis, neuron loss, and spongiform change. Prion-containing amyloid deposits are identified by immunochemical staining.

Familial CJD.

The familial form of CJD shows autosomal dominant inheritance, but laboratory studies confirm that even these prion diseases are potentially transmissible. In affected families, about half of those with the mutant gene develop CJD. The clinical presentation of familial CJD varies, depending on the site of mutation within the *PRNP* gene. It can closely resemble the classic sporadic form of CJD or present a variant phenotype.

Gerstmann-Sträussler-Scheinker syndrome.

Gerstmann-Sträussler-Scheinker syndrome (GSS) is a rare familial autosomal dominant neurodegenerative disorder with an earlier age at onset than nonfamilial CJD. Its prevalence is estimated to be about 5 in 100 million (Belay 1999). Patients initially present with ataxia and later develop dementia; they also have dysarthria, ocular dysmetria, and hyporeflexia. Death ensues within 1–10 years. Neuropathological examination identifies neuronal vacuolation, astrocytic gliosis, and deposition of amyloid plaques. Although it is a familial condition, GSS can also be transmitted to subhuman primates and rodents via intracerebral inoculation as an infectious disease; infectivity is associated with the 27- to 30-kDa protein known as the *scrapie prion protein* (PrP^{Sc}). Antibodies to PrP^{Sc} react with the amyloid plaques seen in GSS.

Fatal familial insomnia. Fatal familial insomnia is extremely rare and has been identified in fewer than 20 families. As with other familial prion diseases, it has an autosomal dominant inheritance pattern. The mean age at onset in fatal familial insomnia is 49, and the disease lasts about a year. The course includes progressive insomnia, dementia, and motor findings of ataxia, dysphagia, dysarthria, tremor, and myoclonus. Autonomic abnormalities are common; psychiatric symptoms are also frequent and include panic attacks, phobias, and hallucinations. Late-appearing symptoms include primitive reflexes, breathing disorders, weight loss, mutism, and coma. Both slow-wave and rapid eye movement phases of sleep are lost, patients have enacted dream states, and the insomnia is near-total. Fatal familial insomnia involves nearly exclusive bilateral degeneration of the thalamus without spongiform changes or amyloid seen at postmortem examination. Despite its atypical presentation, the finding of abnormal prion protein on neuropathological examination confirmed that fatal familial insomnia is a prion disease (Medori et al. 1992).

Acquired Prion Diseases

Iatrogenic CJD depends on human-to-human transmission, typically via medical procedures. Its period of incubation depends on route of transmission: 12 years for peripheral hormone administration and 6 years for direct transplantation of brain tissue. Unlike other forms of CJD, the iatrogenic disease presents with ataxia and gait abnormalities, and only mild dementia is found in the late illness course (Belay 1999).

Other acquired prion diseases include kuru, now extinct, which was transmitted by cannibalism in New Guinea, and the recently defined new variant, or nvCJD. This variant is a new disease first identified in Great Britain that is thought to have derived from the infectious agent of bovine spongiform encephalopathy (BSE), more popularly known as "mad cow disease" (see Zeidler and Ironside 2000). The average age at onset in nvCJD is much younger,

at 27 years, than that of sporadic CJD. The duration of illness (14 months) is longer than in classic sporadic CJD. Common presenting symptoms are psychiatric, such as agitation, aggression, anxiety, depression, lability, and social withdrawal. Hallucinations, delusions, insomnia, and sensory distortions are not uncommon. Most patients do not show clear neurological signs until months after initial presentation. Many have had upgaze paresis, a symptom uncommon in sporadic CJD. Progressive dementia, ataxia, and myoclonus do occur, although later in the illness, and then in the context of delusions. Neuropathologically, nvCJD differs from the classic sporadic form: it has "daisy" or "florid" amyloid plaques surrounded by "petals" of spongiosis, which is also typical of sheep scrapie. It is of note that nvCJD can be detected in tonsils, appendix, spleen, and lymph nodes, as well as in the brain. Transmission across other mammalian species has previously been reported, with house cats (Pearson et al. 1991), ungulates (Kirkwood et al. 1990), and primates contracting spongiform encephalopathies after presumably eating contaminated food.

Molecular Studies

The inherited prion diseases are associated with autosomal mutations in the *PRNP* gene (Oesch et al. 1985), which encodes the prion protein. The human gene is located on chromosome 20 (see Glatzel et al. 2005). It has three exons, but its entire open reading frame is contained in only one exon. More than two dozen different amino acid–changing mutations have been identified in the coding region for these disorders. It is unclear what accounts for different types of prion activity, which have been described as strains that modify the course of illness. Some investigators hypothesize that an informational molecular component in addition to prion protein, perhaps a nucleic acid, accounts for different strains (Almond 1998).

Prion protein is expressed at its highest levels in the CNS and less so in the lymphoreticular system, heart, and skeleton. The normal protein is a copper-binding molecule, 33–35 kDa, which is localized to cell membranes in the CNS. Mice genetically engineered to have no prion protein have only subtle findings, other than being resistant to the development of prion diseases, which has complicated studies aimed at elucidating its normal biology (Weissmann and Flechsig 2003). The misfolded disease-associated prion protein PrP^{Sc} has a growing list of putative physiological roles, which include signal transduction, long-term memory, neuronal cell adhesion and neurite extension, and participation in cascades that resist cell death. Evidence suggests an ancient evolutionary past for prion-based inheritance because it is observed across phylogeny. Yet other research considers the possible role of prion proteins in modifying genomewide gene expression through epigenetic mechanisms (Shorter and Lindquist 2005). Prion diseases have illuminated a fascinating aspect of biology that is now being aggressively investigated.

SCHIZOPHRENIA

Schizophrenia comprises a group of serious psychiatric disorders that are characterized by "positive" (psychotic) symptoms, "negative" (deficit) symptoms, and cognitive impairment. Most patients are initially affected in young adulthood; 50% go on to experience some disability throughout their lives, and an additional 25% never recover and require lifelong care. The lifetime risk for schizophrenia is 0.9% (McGue and Gottesman 1991), and this risk is approximately equal for men and women, although women have a later mean onset by about 5 years and have a second and smaller postmenopausal peak of incidence (Häfner et al. 1993).

PATHOPHYSIOLOGY

Excessive subcortical transmission of dopamine has consistently been linked to the positive symptoms of schizophrenia (Abi-Dargham et al. 2000), whereas a deficit in dopamine activity in the prefrontal cortex is associated with negative symptoms. Hypofunction of both

excitatory N-methyl-D-aspartate (NMDA) glutamate (Heresco-Levy and Javitt 1998) and inhibitory GABA receptors is also believed to be involved in schizophrenia. Alterations of GABA neurotransmission in the dorsolateral prefrontal cortex may underlie the working memory deficits commonly seen in schizophrenic patients (D. A. Lewis et al. 2004).

In addition to neurotransmitter abnormalities, disruptions of synapses may underlie the clinical picture of schizophrenia. This theory is supported by postmortem studies in schizophrenia that reported increased packing of neuron cell bodies, with a decrease in the neuropil that composes the connections between neurons—specifically, dendritic branches and their spines, where synapses are concentrated (Glantz and Lewis 2000; Harrison 1999; Rosoklija et al. 2000). Postmortem studies also showed abnormal expression of a host of synaptic proteins and their corresponding mRNA (Harrison 1999). The idea of excessive synaptic pruning as the underlying mechanism for schizophrenia symptoms gains support from computer simulations of neuronal networks (McGlashan and Hoffman 2000). Reduction in neuropil also may explain the reduced brain volumes evident in schizophrenia (Harrison 1999).

The timing of pathophysiological processes in schizophrenia is not entirely clear. A common model of schizophrenia is that it results from abnormal prenatal neural development that remains latent until the affected region matures and is required to function optimally (Weinberger 1987). This model is consistent with the fact that schizophrenic patients have an excess of minor physical anomalies, which originate in utero, compared with control subjects (M. F. Green et al. 1994; Lohr and Flynn 1993). A neurodevelopmental model is also supported by the finding of subtle cognitive and motor abnormalities in the premorbid period during childhood (Done et al. 1994; Jones et al. 1994). Fish and colleagues (Fish 1977; Fish et al. 1992) coined the phrase *pandevelopmental retardation*, which refers to these premorbid subtle abnormalities found in multiple domains, including motor, sensory, cognitive, and cerebellar function, in children who go on to develop schizophrenia. Other studies confirm the presence of early and subtle abnormalities in at-risk children, such as compromised psychomotor performance and cognitive and motor dysfunction by age 10 years (Marcus et al. 1981). An innovative blinded review of home videotapes showed that raters could accurately identify which children would later develop schizophrenia by examining their motor skills (Walker et al. 1994). Other precursors of schizophrenia (albeit nonspecific) include delays in developmental milestones (e.g., walking and talking), more isolated play at ages 4 and 6 years, speech problems and clumsiness at ages 7 and 11 years, and poor school performance and social anxiety during the teen years (reviewed in Jones and Cannon 1998; Tarrant and Jones 1999). Global attentional dysfunction may be a biobehavioral marker for genetic liability to schizophrenia because attentional deficits exist in nearly half of all schizophrenic patients and in the offspring of parents with schizophrenia (Erlenmeyer-Kimling and Cornblatt 1978, 1992). Abnormal social behavior (e.g., trouble making friends, disciplinary problems, and unusual behavior in childhood and adolescence) may be another nonspecific indicator of risk for schizophrenia (Parnas et al. 1982a, 1982b).

However, evidence also indicates that patients are not "doomed from the womb" and that some postnatal exposures, including TBI and the use of drugs, such as cannabis, may increase the risk for schizophrenia (Arseneault et al. 2004; Malaspina et al. 2001). Dynamic changes in brain volumes over time in schizophrenic patients also provide support for the theory that progressive deteriorative processes occur in this putatively neurodevelopmental disorder. Cross-sectional imaging studies show increased ventricle size and reduced frontal and temporal lobe volumes in schizophrenic patients (Wright et al. 2000), abnormalities that are often evident by illness onset (Pantelis et al. 2003) and also present to some extent in those with increased genetic risk for illness

(Lawrie et al. 1999). However, volumetric changes may be an active process that continues beyond the onset of illness (Pantelis et al. 2003): for example, the superior temporal gyrus decreases in volume after onset of first psychosis (Kasai et al. 2003). These progressive reductions in brain volumes may be amenable to pharmacological intervention (Lieberman et al. 2005).

GENETICS AND MODE OF INHERITANCE

Evidence from family, twin, and adoption studies suggests that the liability to schizophrenia is at least in part inherited. First-degree relatives of schizophrenic probands have an increased risk of schizophrenia, with estimated risk rates of 6% for parents, 10% for siblings, and 13% and 46% for children with, respectively, one or two affected parents (McGue and Gottesman 1991). Identical twins have a concordance rate of 53%, whereas fraternal twins have a concordance rate of 15% (Kendler and Gardner 1997); the disparity in these rates suggests that 60%–90% of the liability to schizophrenia can be attributed to genes (Cannon et al. 1998; Jones and Cannon 1998). Interestingly, offspring of affected and unaffected (discordant) MZ twins have equal risk for schizophrenia (about 16%–18%), consistent with either incomplete penetrance or gene-environment interaction.

Adoption studies also support inheritance of schizophrenia liability (Heston 1966; Kety et al. 1994; Rosenthal et al. 1968) but cannot determine whether such effects are genetic or environmental (in utero) if mothers are the parent of comparison. When fathers are the parent in common (paternal half-siblings), however, the same increased risk in biological (vs. adopted) relatives holds (Kety 1988). Adoption studies also provide evidence for a gene-environment interaction, because adopted-away children of biological mothers with schizophrenia are even more likely to develop schizophrenia if they are raised in an adverse environment (Tienari 1991; Wahlberg et al. 1997).

Increased familial risk exists not only for schizophrenia but also for its spectrum disorders, such as schizotypal personality disorder (Battaglia and Torgersen 1996; Siever et al. 1993), and for features characteristic of schizophrenia (i.e., endophenotypes), including smooth-pursuit eye movement (Levy et al. 1994), neurological soft signs (Kinney et al. 1986), and gating impairments (Myles-Worsley et al. 1999).

Although schizophrenia is a genetic disorder, the nature of the genetic diathesis remains unclear. It is not simply a mendelian disorder (O'Donovan and Owen 1999). Most likely, schizophrenia results from epistasis, the interaction of multiple genes of small effect. A three-locus epistasis model can optimally account for the rapidly decreasing recurrence risk data for individuals with lowering degrees of relatedness to probands with schizophrenia (Risch 1990). As described, schizophrenia is likely etiologically heterogeneous, with various genetic, environmental, and interactive etiologies resulting in a common phenotype. Alleles that confer risk may be highly prevalent in the population, and illness may result from some constellation of disease genes when none or few may be sufficient by themselves.

Because the phenotype of schizophrenia is heterogeneous, some studies have focused on examining putative endophenotypes or intermediate phenotypes of schizophrenia genes. These lie on the pathway between genotype and disease and are usually measured differently (physiology, anatomy, neuropsychology). Endophenotypes are associated with illness, heritable, traitlike, and found also in family members without the disease. These may be easier to define than the diagnosis itself and may have a higher penetrance in humans. Also, endophenotypes can be studied in animal models to delineate pathophysiology. Promising candidate endophenotypes include aberrant smooth-pursuit eye movement (Crawford et al. 1998; O'Driscoll et al. 1998; R.G. Ross et al. 1998), N-acetylaspartate concentrations in the hippocampus (Callicott et al. 1998), abnormal hippocampal morphology (Csernansky et al. 1998), the P50 gating deficit (see "Chro-

mosome 15: α_7 Nicotinic Receptor" subsection later in this chapter), and abnormalities in working memory.

There is some evidence for anticipation in schizophrenia, which is the successive decrease in age at onset in newer generations of multiply affected pedigrees (Petronis and Kennedy 1995), as well as some evidence of increased trinucleotide repeat expansions, which account for anticipation in other illnesses such as Huntington's disease (Morris et al. 1995; O'Donovan et al. 1995). However, the location of these repeats and their relevance to schizophrenia etiology remain unknown (O'Donovan and Owen 1999).

The intriguing notion that schizophrenia can result from de novo genetic events in the paternal germ line was first suggested by Malaspina et al. (2001) to explain the strong relation of paternal age to the risk for schizophrenia. Since then, multiple studies in diverse populations have replicated the paternal age effect (Brown et al. 2002; Byrne et al. 2003; Dalman and Allebeck 2002; El-Saadi et al. 2004; Sipos et al. 2004; Zammit et al. 2003). In the Malaspina cohort, paternal age, overall, explained more than 25% of the risk for schizophrenia. Comparably, in Sweden, Sipos and Rasmussen (2004) estimated that 15% of the cases were attributable to paternal age greater than 30 years. The paternal age effect appears to be restricted to patients without a family history of psychosis (Byrne et al. 2003; Malaspina et al. 2002; Sipos et al. 2004). Sipos and colleagues found that paternal age was unrelated to the risk for familial cases, whereas the offspring of the oldest fathers showed a 5.5-fold increased risk for sporadic (nonfamilial) schizophrenia. The epidemiological evidence is convincing. There is a "dosage effect" of increasing paternal age on the relative risk for schizophrenia, and each cohort study has shown a tripling of risk for the offspring of the oldest fathers (>45–55 years). The studies have used prospective exposure data and validated psychiatric diagnoses, and they have together controlled for potential confounding factors, such as family history, maternal age, parental education and social ability, social class, birth order, birth weight, and birth complications. Furthermore, the studies showed specificity of late paternal age for the risk of schizophrenia compared with other psychiatric disorders, which is not the case for any other schizophrenia risk factor, including most of the susceptibility alleles (see the subsections later in this section). Furthermore, accumulating evidence suggests that sporadic (paternal age–related) schizophrenia may be a separate variant of the disease from familial cases (Malaspina et al. 1998, 2000a, 2000b, 2005).

Early linkage studies in schizophrenia were disappointing because of type I error, failures to replicate, small sample sizes, and the likelihood that each susceptibility gene has only a small effect. Two meta-analyses of linkage studies have supported 8p and 22q most strongly, among others, as regions associated with schizophrenia (Badner and Gershon 2002; C.M. Lewis et al. 2003). Candidate gene analysis focusing particularly on dopamine pathways also has provided a low yield for identifying schizophrenia genes. Of the many dopamine-related genes, evidence is strongest for the D_3 receptor, located on chromosome 3, which may confer some risk for schizophrenia (Kirov et al. 2005).

However, in the past few years, several putative susceptibility genes have been identified for schizophrenia, and they are listed here by chromosome number. Most of these genes code for proteins involved in excitatory glutamatergic pathways, and many influence synaptic function. With most of the genes identified thus far, specific mutant alleles or changes in the coding frame have not been identified as associated with increased schizophrenia risk. Overall, dysbindin and neuregulin have the greatest support as susceptibility genes, and good evidence supports disrupted-in-schizophrenia-1 (*DISC1*), *DAO/DAOA*, and regulator of G-protein signaling-4 (*RGS4*). Some of these regions and genes have been associated with bipolar disorder as well, including *DISC1*, neuregulin, and *DAOA* (Table 4–2) (Craddock et al. 2005).

Chromosome 1: *DISC1*

The major susceptibility gene for schizophrenia identified on chromosome 1 is *DISC1*. Its region—1q42—was initially identified as a potential locus for schizophrenia risk on the basis of an extended pedigree that had a balanced chromosomal translocation that involved this region (St. Clair et al. 1990). *DISC1* has shown linkage with schizophrenia in extended pedigrees (Ekelund et al. 2004) and has been associated with a broad phenotype that includes not only schizophrenia but also schizoaffective and bipolar disorders. The specific gene was identified as *DISC1* and was found in animal models to be associated with the putative endophenotype of electrophysiological abnormalities—specifically, reduced P300 (Blackwood et al. 2001). DISC1 protein is associated with the development and function of the hippocampus, particularly the growth of neuritis (Miyoshi et al. 2003), which is of interest as a leading model for schizophrenia pathophysiology as reduced neuropil and abnormal connectivity. *DISC1* also appears to be involved in cell migration, scaffolding and formation of the cytoskeleton, intracellular transport, mitochondrial function, and distribution of receptors in the membrane (Harrison and Weinberger 2005). The distribution of *DISC1* within the cell is altered in the orbitofrontal cortex in patients with psychosis (Sawamura et al. 2005). One allele has specifically been associated with hippocampal structure, neurochemistry, and function in both nonschizophrenic individuals and schizophrenic patients (Callicott et al. 2005).

RGS4

RGS4, located at 1q22, was targeted as a potential susceptibility gene because it had decreased gene expression in schizophrenia, as identified by postmortem microarray studies (Mirnics et al. 2001). Linkage was also established to this region in extended schizophrenia pedigrees, with a highly significant lod score of 6.50 (Brzustowicz et al. 2000). The expression of *RGS4* is regulated by dopaminergic activity, and itself modulates 5-HT$_{1A}$ activity. *RGS4* also

TABLE 4–2.   Schizophrenia susceptibility genes

Gene	Name	Gene locus
NRG1	Neuregulin-1	8p12–21
DTNBP1	Dysbindin	6p22
DAOA	D-Amino acid oxidase activator	12q24
G72	Interacts with DAOA	13q32–34
RGS4	Regulator of G-protein signaling-4	1q21–22
PRODH2	Proline dehydrogenase	22q11
COMT	Catechol O-methyltransferase	22q11
GRM3	Metabotropic glutamate receptor 3	7q21–22
DISC1	Disrupted-in-schizophrenia-1	1q42
PPP3CC	Calcineurin	8p21
Akt1	Protein kinase B	14q22–32
CHRNA7	α_7 Nicotinic receptor	15q13–14

interacts with an NRG1 receptor, ErbB3, whose expression is downregulated in schizophrenia.

Chromosome 6: Dysbindin or DTNBP1

The region of 6p22.3 was first identified as a region of interest in schizophrenia through extensive association mapping of illness with SNPs and haplotypes in extended German schizophrenia pedigrees (Straub et al. 2002). Association was also supported by studies of sibling pairs and parent-offspring trios (Kirov et al. 2004; Schwab et al. 2003) and other pedigrees (N.M. Williams et al. 2004), and significant associations have been found in more than 10 independent samples (Kirov et al. 2005). Specific risk alleles and haplotypes have not been identified, and susceptibility may be conferred by changes in message expression or processing. Reduced levels of dysbindin message have been found in the prefrontal cortex (Weickert et al. 2004), and dysbindin protein was reduced in glutamatergic terminals of the hippocampal formation (Talbot et al. 2004) in postmortem studies of schizophrenia. Mutant alleles are associated with differences in working and episodic memory in both patients and at-risk individuals (Harrison and Weinberger 2005). Dysbindin is part of the dystrophin-glycoprotein complex, which is located in postsynaptic densities, especially in the mossy fiber synaptic terminals in the hippocampus (and cerebellum). Dysbindin may regulate presynaptic proteins, such as SNAP25 and synapsin 1 (Numakawa et al. 2004) (which have differential neural expression in schizophrenia), and hence influence the presynaptic exocytotic release of glutamate.

Chromosome 8: NRG1

The association of the region of 8p21–22 with schizophrenia was first identified in a study in Iceland (Stefansson et al. 2002) and then replicated in diverse samples, including from Scotland, United Kingdom, Ireland, China, South Africa, and Portugal (Petryshen et al. 2005). Several potential schizophrenia genes are found in this region, including frizzled-3 and calcineurin A (Tosato et al. 2005), but the most promising candidate gene in the region is neuregulin. Neuregulin has been implicated in animal studies in a range of functions, including cell signaling, axon guidance, synaptogenesis, glial differentiation, myelination, and neurotransmission (Corfas et al. 2004; Michailov et al. 2004). Of interest, hypomorphic mice have increased ventricular volume, changes in α_7 nicotinic receptors, and failures of prepulse inhibition, all features that are characteristic of schizophrenia. Neuregulin also modifies expression of NMDA receptors, both through its own ErbB receptors and via actin. As with other putative susceptibility genes for schizophrenia, neuregulin also appears to be associated with bipolar disorder (with psychotic features) (E.K. Green et al. 2005).

Chromosomes 12 (*DAO*) and 13 (*DAOA*)

In French Canadian and Russian populations, novel susceptibility genes for schizophrenia were located on chromosome 13; one of these, identified as *G72*, was found to be primate-specific and to be expressed particularly in the caudate and amydala (Kirov et al. 2005). *G72* was localized to 13q33 (Addington et al. 2004), and polymorphisms of this gene have been associated with structural and functional abnormalities in both the prefrontal cortex and the hippocampus in patients with schizophrenia (Harrison and Weinberger 2005). *G72* was subsequently renamed *DAOA* because it was found to be an activator of *DAO* (D-amino acid oxidase), a susceptibility gene on chromosome 12. *DAO* oxidizes D-serine, a potent endogenous agonist of the NMDA glutamatergic receptor. Notably, *DAOA* has been associated in bipolar patients with persecutory delusions in particular (Schulze et al. 2005).

Chromosome 15: α_7 Nicotinic Receptor

Common in schizophrenia is a failure in sensory gating—namely, the failure to inhibit the P50 auditory evoked response to repeated stimuli, which appears to be inherited in an autosomal dominant fashion in schizophrenia pedigrees (Siegel et al. 1984). The endophenotype of this auditory evoked potential deficit has been linked to the α_7 subunit of the nicotinic acetylcholine receptor gene on 15q14 (Freedman et al. 1999).

Chromosome 22: *COMT*

The region of 22q11 has been of interest for several years because microdeletions in this region lead to a phenotype known as velo-cardiofacial syndrome, which frequently includes schizophrenia-like psychosis (about 24%) (Ivanov et al. 2003; K.C. Murphy et al. 1999). Linkage to this region has been found for schizophrenia (Badner and Gershon 2002; C.M. Lewis et al. 2003). Several genes within this region are part of the usual deletion zone and are plausible candidates for increasing schizophrenia susceptibility, including *COMT*, proline dehydrogenase (*PRODH*), and zinc finger, DHHC domain–containing protein 8 (*ZDHHC8*) (Kirov et al. 2005). Proline dehydrogenase mutations in mice are associated with abnormalities in sensorimotor gating analogous to schizophrenia (Gogos et al. 1999), as well as decreased levels of glutamate and GABA. Also, mutations are associated with hyperprolinemia, which has been found in schizophrenia. However, despite a finding of association of *PRODH* with schizophrenia in a Chinese sample (Li et al. 2004) and a microdeletion in this region in a schizophrenia pedigree (Jacquet et al. 2002), there have been several negative studies, and the association is not clear (Kirov et al. 2005). *ZDHHC8* codes for a transmembranous palmitoyl transferase and has been little studied (Kirov et al. 2005). In contrast, *COMT* has been extensively studied as a putative schizophrenia allele.

COMT (catechol O-methyltransferase) is a methylating enzyme that effectively inactivates dopamine and other catecholamines. It is largely responsible for dopamine clearance in the prefrontal cortex, which has a dearth of dopamine transporter in comparison to more subcortical brain regions. Alleles of interest vary at codon 148 of the brain-predominant membrane-bound form of COMT: the allele with valine at this position has higher activity and is associated with worse cognition (Egan et al. 2001; Malhotra et al. 2002).

The two alleles of interest are Val-*COMT* (valine) and Met-*COMT* (methionine), resulting from a substitution in a single base pair in the gene (codon 148). Val-*COMT* has higher enzyme activity and hence depletes more prefrontal dopamine; it is not surprising then that

Val-*COMT* is associated with worse cognition (Egan et al. 2001; Malhotra et al. 2002). However, no clear association of the valine allele alone with schizophrenia was found in a meta-analysis (Fan et al. 2005; Glatt et al. 2003). The association of specific haplotypes suggests that other codons in *COMT* or nearby genes may be responsible for the association (Kirov et al. 2005). However, among putative schizophrenia alleles, *COMT* alone has been implicated in a gene-environment interaction (Val-*COMT* × cannabis) in schizophrenia etiology (Caspi et al. 2005).

ENVIRONMENT

Several prenatal and early life environment factors contribute to schizophrenia in conjunction with genetic predisposition and family history. A 5%–8% excess of schizophrenia is seen among individuals born in the winter and early spring (Bembenek 2005), consistent with associations of maternal infections during pregnancy with schizophrenia risk (up to sevenfold), including rubella (Brown et al. 2001), influenza (Brown et al. 2004), and toxoplasmosis (Brown et al. 2005; Strous and Shoenfeld 2005). Postnatal infections (especially neonatal coxsackie B meningitis) are also associated with later schizophrenia (Rantakallio et al. 1997).

Other intrauterine and obstetrical risk factors besides infection associated with later schizophrenia include preeclampsia, low birth weight, hypoxic events (Canon et al. 2002), maternal cigarette smoking (O'Dwyer 1997; Sacker et al. 1995), Rh incompatibility (Hollister et al. 1996), maternal stress (Huttunen and Niskanen 1978; Van Os and Selten 1998), and exposure to famine or malnutrition early in gestation (e.g., the Dutch Hunger Winter of 1944–1945) (Dalman et al. 1999; Susser et al. 1996).

Other variables associated with schizophrenia risk include urban residence and upbringing (Pedersen and Mortensen 2001), immigration (Cantor-Graae et al. 2005), TBI (Malaspina et al. 1999), and use of drugs, particularly cannabis (Arseneault et al. 2004). Most exposures have small effects, with typical odds ratios or risk ratios of approximately 2. Questions of causation remain because premorbid or prodromal symptoms could increase risk of exposure (e.g., to head injury or drug use).

Immigration is associated with somewhat higher risk, compared with other exposures, because migration from poor countries to wealthy countries is associated with a 3- to 10-fold increase in schizophrenia risk, compared with both the host country and the country of origin (reviewed in Jones and Cannon 1998). This effect is greater for second-generation than for first-generation migrants, arguing against selective migration of at-risk individuals. It is not clear whether this finding reflects the effect of urbanization, stress, racism, or exposure to some new infectious or other environmental agent.

GENE-ENVIRONMENT INTERACTION

Increasingly, it is clear that gene-environment interactions must be considered for illness risk, with changes in gene expression as the likely mechanism (Quirion and Insel 2005). Data that support models of interaction between genetic vulnerability and the environment result from adoption studies. For adopted-away children of mothers with schizophrenia, adversity and poor family functioning in the adoptive home increase the risk for schizophrenia; however, no such effect is seen for adopted-away children of healthy mothers (Tienari 1991). In an Israeli study, children of mothers with schizophrenia had a higher risk of developing the illness themselves if raised in a kibbutz instead of a family home; again, this effect was not seen for children without genetic risk (Mirsky et al. 1985). Among the most exciting findings of gene-environment interaction for schizophrenia is the interaction of a specific allele of a susceptibility gene (i.e., Val-*COMT*) with an exposure (specifically, cannabis abuse) in increasing schizophrenia risk (Caspi et al. 2005).

RECOMMENDED READINGS

McGuffin P, Owen M, Gottesman I: Psychiatric Genetics and Genomics. Oxford, UK, Oxford University Press, 2002

Zorumski C, Rubin E: Psychopathology in the Genome and Neuroscience Era. Washington, DC, American Psychiatric Publishing, 2005

REFERENCES

Abi-Dargham A, Rodenhiser J, Printz D, et al: Increased baseline occupancy of D_2 receptors by dopamine in schizophrenia. Proc Natl Acad Sci U S A 97:8104–8109, 2000

Abramson RK, Wright HH, Carpenter R, et al: Elevated blood serotonin in autistic probands and their first-degree relatives. J Autism Dev Disord 19:397–407, 1989

Adams MD, Celniker SE, Holt RA, et al: The genome sequence of *Drosophila melanogaster*. Science 287:2185–2195, 2000

Addington AM, Gornick M, Sporn AL, et al: Polymorphisms in the 13q33.2 gene G70/G30 are associated with childhood-onset schizophrenia and psychosis not otherwise specified. Biol Psychiatry 10:976–980, 2004

Akil M, Schwartz JA, Dutchak D, et al: The psychiatric presentations of Wilson's disease [see comments]. J Neuropsychiatry Clin Neurosci 3:377–382, 1991

Alarcon M, Cantor RM, Liu J, et al: Evidence for a language quantitative trait locus on chromosome 7q in multiplex autism families. Am J Hum Genet 70:60–71, 2002

Alarcon M, Yonan AL, Gilliam TC, et al: Quantitative genome scan and Ordered-Subsets Analysis of autism endophenotypes support language QTLs. Mol Psychiatry 10:747–757, 2005

Alford RL, Ashizawa T, Jankovic J, et al: Molecular detection of new mutations, resolution of ambiguous results and complex genetic counseling issues in Huntington disease. Am J Med Genet 66:281–286, 1996

Allam MF, Campbell MJ, Del Castillo AS, et al: Parkinson's disease protects against smoking? Behav Neurol 15:65–71, 2004

Almond JW: Bovine spongiform encephalopathy and new variant Creutzfeldt-Jakob disease. Br Med Bull 54:749–759, 1998

Alper T, Cramp WA, Haig DA, et al: Does the agent of scrapie replicate without nucleic acid? Nature 214:764–766, 1967

Ambrose CM, Duyao MP, Barnes G, et al: Structure and expression of the Huntington's disease gene: evidence against simple inactivation due to an expanded CAG repeat. Somat Cell Mol Genet 20:27–38, 1994

American Psychiatric Association: Diagnostic and Statistical Manual of Mental Disorders, 3rd Edition. Washington, DC, American Psychiatric Association, 1980

American Psychiatric Association: Diagnostic and Statistical Manual of Mental Disorders, 3rd Edition, Revised. Washington, DC, American Psychiatric Association, 1987

American Psychiatric Association: Diagnostic and Statistical Manual of Mental Disorders, 4th Edition. Washington, DC, American Psychiatric Association, 1994

American Psychiatric Association: Diagnostic and Statistical Manual of Mental Disorders, 4th Edition, Text Revision. Washington, DC, American Psychiatric Association, 2000

Anderson GM, Freedman DX, Cohen DJ, et al: Whole blood serotonin in autistic and normal subjects. J Child Psychol Psychiatry 28:885–900, 1987

Andrews TC, Weeks RA, Turjanski N, et al: Huntington's disease progression: PET and clinical observations. Brain 122 (pt 12):2353–2363, 1999

Arseneault L, Cannon M, Witton J, et al: Causal association between cannabis and psychosis: examination of the evidence. Br J Psychiatry 184:110–117, 2004

Ashley-Koch A, Wolpert CM, Menold MM, et al: Genetic studies of autistic disorder and chromosome 7. Genomics 61:227–236, 1999

Astrinidis A, Cash TP, Hunter DS, et al: Tuberin, the tuberous sclerosis complex 2 tumor suppressor gene product, regulates Rho activation, cell adhesion and migration. Oncogene 21:8470–8476, 2002

Auranen M, Nieminen T, Majuri S, et al: Analysis of autism susceptibility gene loci on chromosomes 1p, 4p, 6q, 7q, 13q, 15q, 16p, 17q, 19q and 22q in Finnish multiplex families. Mol Psychiatry 5:320–322, 2000

Auranen M, Vanhala R, Varilo T, et al: A genome-wide screen for autism-spectrum disorders: evidence for a major susceptibility locus on chromosome 3q25–27. Am J Hum Genet 71:777–790, 2002

Bacchelli E, Blasi F, Biondolillo M, et al: Screening of nine candidate genes for autism on chromosome 2q reveals rare nonsynonymous variants in the cAMP-GEFII gene. Mol Psychiatry 8:916–924, 2003

Badner JA, Gershon ES: Meta-analysis of whole-genome linkage scans of bipolar disorder and schizophrenia. Mol Psychiatry 7:405–411, 2002

Bailey A, Le Couteur A, Gottesman I, et al: Autism as a strongly genetic disorder: evidence from a British twin study. Psychol Med 25:63–77, 1995

Bailey A, Palferman S, Heavey L, et al: Autism: the phenotype in relatives. J Autism Dev Disord 28:369–392, 1998

Baldereschi M, Di Carlo A, Lepore V, et al: Estrogen-replacement therapy and Alzheimer's disease in the Italian Longitudinal Study on Aging. Neurology 50:996–1002, 1998

Bandmann O, Vaughan J, Holmans P, et al: Association of slow acetylator genotype for N-acetyltransferase 2 with familial Parkinson's disease [see comments]. Lancet 350:1136–1139, 1997

Bartlett CW, Gharani N, Millonig JH, et al: Three autism candidate genes: a synthesis of human genetic analysis with other disciplines. Int J Dev Neurosci 23:221–234, 2005

Barton M, Volkmar F: How commonly are known medical conditions associated with autism? J Autism Dev Disord 28:273–278, 1998

Bass MP, Menold MM, Wolpert CM, et al: Genetic studies in autistic disorder and chromosome 15. Neurogenetics 2219–2226, 1999

Battaglia M, Torgersen S: Schizotypal disorder: at the crossroads of genetics and nosology. Acta Psychiatr Scand 94:303–310, 1996

Belay ED: Transmissible spongiform encephalopathies in humans. Annu Rev Microbiol 53:283–314, 1999

Bembenek A: Seasonality of birth in schizophrenia patients. Psychiatr Pol 39:259–270, 2005

Blackwood DH, Fordyce A, Walker MT, et al: Schizophrenia and affective disorders: cosegregation with a translocation at chromosome 1q42 that directly disrupts brain-expressed genes: clinical and P300 findings in a family. Am J Hum Genet 69:428–433, 2001

Boffelli D, Nobrega MA, Rubin EM: Comparative genomics at the vertebrate extremes. Nat Rev Genet 5:456–465, 2004

Bonifati V, Rizzu P, van Baren MJ, et al: Mutations in the DJ-1 gene associated with autosomal recessive early onset parkinsonism. Science 299:256–259, 2003

Bonne-Tamir B, Farrer LA, Frydman M, et al: Evidence for linkage between Wilson disease and esterase D in three kindreds: detection of linkage for an autosomal recessive disorder by the family study method. Genet Epidemiol 3:201–209, 1986

Bonora E, Bacchelli E, Levy ER, et al: Mutation screening and imprinting analysis of four candidate genes for autism in the 7q32 region. Mol Psychiatry 7:289–301, 2002

Bonora E, Lamb JA, Barnby G, et al: Mutation screening and association analysis of six candidate genes for autism on chromosome 7q. Eur J Hum Genet 13:198–207, 2005

Botstein D, White RL, Skolnick M, et al: Construction of a genetic linkage map using restriction fragment length polymorphisms. Am J Hum Genet 32:314–331, 1980

Brown AS, Cohen P, Harkavy-Friedman J, et al: A.E. Bennett Research Award: prenatal rubella, premorbid abnormalities, and adult schizophrenia. Biol Psychiatry 49:473–486, 2001

Brown AS, Schaefer CA, Wyatt RJ, et al: Paternal age and risk of schizophrenia in adult offspring. Am J Psychiatry 159:1528–1533, 2002

Brown AS, Begg MD, Gravenstein S, et al: Serologic evidence of prenatal influenza in the etiology of schizophrenia. Arch Gen Psychiatry 61:774–780, 2004

Brown AS, Schaefer CA, Quesenberry CP Jr, et al: Maternal exposure to toxoplasmosis and risk of schizophrenia in adult offspring. Am J Psychiatry 162:767–773, 2005

Bryson SE, Clark BS, Smith IM: First report of a Canadian epidemiological study of autistic syndromes. J Child Psychol Psychiatry 29:433–445, 1988

Brzustowicz LM, Hodgkinson KA, Chow EW, et al: Location of a major susceptibility locus for familial schizophrenia on chromosome 1q21-q22. Science 288:678–682, 2000

Bull PC, Thomas GR, Rommens M, et al: The Wilson disease gene is a putative copper transporting ATPase similar to the Menkes disease gene. Nat Genet 5:327–337, 1993

Butterworth NJ, Williams L, Bullock JY, et al: Trinucleotide (CAG) repeat length is positively correlated with the degree of DNA fragmentation in Huntington's disease striatum. Neuroscience 87:49–53, 1998

Buxbaum JD, Silverman JM, Smith CJ, et al: Evidence for a susceptibility gene for autism on chromosome 2 and for genetic heterogeneity. Am J Hum Genet 68:1514–1520, 2001

Buxbaum JD, Silverman JM, Smith CJ, et al: Association between a GABRB3 polymorphism and autism. Mol Psychiatry 7:311–316, 2002

Byrne M, Agerbo E, Ewald H, et al: Parental age and risk of schizophrenia: a case-control study. Arch Gen Psychiatry 60:673–678, 2003

Callicott JH, Egan MF, Bertolino A, et al: Hippocampal N-acetyl aspartate in unaffected siblings of patients with schizophrenia: a possible intermediate neurobiological phenotype. Biol Psychiatry 44:941–950, 1998

Callicott JH, Straub RE, Pezawas L, et al: Variation in DISC1 affects hippocampal structure and function and increases risk for schizophrenia. Proc Natl Acad Sci U S A 102:8627–8632, 2005

Cannon TD, Kaprio J, Lonnqvist J, et al: The genetic epidemiology of schizophrenia in a Finnish twin cohort: a population-based modeling study. Arch Gen Psychiatry 55:67–74, 1998

Canon M, Jones PB, Murray RM: Obstetric complications and schizophrenia. Am J Psychiatry 159:1080–1092, 2002

Cantor-Graae E, Zolkowska K, McNeil TF: Increased risk of psychotic disorder among immigrants in Malmo: a 3-year first-contact study. Psychol Med 35:1155–1163, 2005

Casadesus G, Atwood CS, Zhu X, et al: Evidence for the role of gonadotropin hormones in the development of Alzheimer disease. Cell Mol Life Sci 62:293–298, 2005

Caspi A, Moffitt TE, Cannon M, et al: Moderation of the effect of adolescent-onset cannabis use on adult psychosis by a functional polymorphism in the catechol-O-methyltransferase gene: longitudinal evidence of a gene x environment interaction. Biol Psychiatry 57:1117–1127, 2005

Castermans D, Wilquet V, Steyaert J, et al: Chromosomal anomalies in individuals with autism: a strategy towards the identification of genes involved in autism. Autism 8:141–161, 2004

Cedarbaum JM, McDowell FH: Sixteen-year follow-up of 100 patients begun on levodopa in 1968: emerging problems. Adv Neurol 45:469–472, 1987

C. elegans Sequencing Consortium: Genome sequence of the nematode C. elegans: a platform for investigating biology [published erratum appears in Science 283:35, 1999; 283:2103, 1999; 285:1493, 1999]. Science 282:2012–2018, 1998

Checkoway H, Nelson LM: Epidemiologic approaches to the study of Parkinson's disease etiology. Epidemiology 10:327–336, 1999

Chimpanzee Sequencing and Analysis Consortium: Initial sequence of the chimpanzee genome and comparison with the human genome. Nature 437:69–87, 2005

Collaborative Linkage Study of Autism: An autosomal genomic screen for autism. Am J Med Genet 105:609–615, 2001

Collins FS, Morgan M, Patrinos A: The Human Genome Project: lessons from large-scale biology. Science 300:286–290, 2003

Cook EH Jr, Courchesne R, Lord C, et al: Evidence of linkage between the serotonin transporter and autistic disorder. Mol Psychiatry 2:247–250, 1997

Cook EH Jr, Courchesne RY, Cox NJ, et al: Linkage-disequilibrium mapping of autistic disorder, with 15q11-13 markers. Am J Hum Genet 62:1077–1083, 1998

Corfas G, Roy K, Buxbaum JD: Neuregulin 1-erbB signaling and the molecular/cellular basis of schizophrenia. Nat Neurosci 7:575–580, 2004

Cox DW, Fraser FC, Sass-Kortsak A: A genetic study of Wilson's disease: evidence for heterogeneity. Am J Hum Genet 24:646–666, 1972

Craddock N, O'Donovan MC, Owen MJ: The genetics of schizophrenia and bipolar disorder: dissecting psychosis. J Med Genet 42:193–204, 2005

Crawford TJ, Sharma T, Puri BK, et al: Saccadic eye movements in families multiply affected with schizophrenia: the Maudsley Family Study. Am J Psychiatry 155:1703–1710, 1998

Cruts M, van Duijn CM, Backhovens H, et al: Estimation of the genetic contribution of presenilin-1 and -2 mutations in a population-based study of presenile Alzheimer disease. Hum Mol Genet 7:43–51, 1998

Csernansky JG, Joshi S, Wang L, et al: Hippocampal morphometry in schizophrenia by high dimensional brain mapping. Proc Natl Acad Sci U S A 95:11406–11411, 1998

Dalman C, Allebeck P: Paternal age and schizophrenia: further support for an association. Am J Psychiatry 159:1591–1592, 2002

Dalman C, Allebeck P, Cullberg J, et al: Obstetric complications and the risk of schizophrenia: a longitudinal study of a national birth cohort. Arch Gen Psychiatry 56:234–240, 1999

Daniel KG, Harbach RH, Guida WC, et al: Copper storage diseases: Menkes, Wilsons, and cancer. Front Biosci 9:2652–2662, 2004 de la Monte SM, Wands JR: Review of insulin and insulin-like growth factor expression, signaling, and malfunction in the central nervous system: relevance to Alzheimer's disease. J Alzheimers Dis 7:45–61, 2005

DeLong GR, Dwyer JT: Correlation of family history with specific autistic subgroups: Asperger's syndrome and bipolar affective disease. J Autism Dev Disord 18:593–600, 1988

DeLorey TM, Handforth A, Anagnostaras SG, et al: Mice lacking the beta$_3$ subunit of the GABA$_A$ receptor have the epilepsy phenotype and many of the behavioral characteristics of Angelman syndrome. J Neurosci 18:8505–8514, 1998

Dening TR: The neuropsychiatry of Wilson's disease: a review. Int J Psychiatry Med 21:135–148, 1991

Dermitzakis ET, Reymond A, Scamuffa N, et al: Evolutionary discrimination of mammalian conserved non-genic sequences (CNGs). Science 302:1033–1035, 2003

Done DJ, Crow TJ, Johnstone EC, et al: Childhood antecedents of schizophrenia and affective illness: social adjustment at ages 7 and 11. BMJ 309:699–703, 1994

Duyao MP, Auerbach AB, Ryan A, et al: Inactivation of the mouse Huntington's disease gene homolog Hdh. Science 269:407–410, 1995

Egan MF, Goldberg TE, Kolachana BS, et al: Effect of *COMT* Val 108/158 Met genotype on frontal lobe function and risk for schizophrenia. Proc Natl Acad Sci U S A 98:6917–6922, 2001

Ekelund J, Hennah W, Hiekkalinna T, et al: Replication of 1q42 linkage in Finnish schizophrenia pedigrees. Mol Psychiatry 9:1037–1041, 2004

El-Saadi O, Pedersen CB, McNeil TF, et al: Paternal and maternal age as risk factors for psychosis: findings from Denmark, Sweden and Australia. Schizophr Res 67:227–236, 2004

Erlenmeyer-Kimling L, Cornblatt B: Attentional measure in the study of children at high risk for schizophrenia. J Psychiatr Res 114:93–98, 1978

Erlenmeyer-Kimling L, Cornblatt BA: A summary of attentional findings in the New York High-Risk Project. J Psychiatr Res 26:405–426, 1992

Estrov Y, Scaglia F, Bodamer OA: Psychiatric symptoms of inherited metabolic disease. J Inherit Metab Dis 23:2–6, 2000

Fan JB, Zhang CS, Gu NF, et al: Catechol-O-methyltransferase gene Val/Met functional polymorphism and risk of schizophrenia: a large-scale association study plus meta-analysis. Biol Psychiatry 57:139–144, 2005

Ferenci P: Review article: diagnosis and current therapy of Wilson's disease. Aliment Pharmacol Ther 19:157–165, 2004

Finch CE: Developmental origins of aging in brain and blood vessels: an overview. Neurobiol Aging 26:281–291, 2005

Fischman AJ: Role of [^{18}F]-dopa-PET imaging in assessing movement disorders. Radiol Clin North Am 43:93–106, 2005

Fish B: Neurobiologic antecedents of schizophrenia in children: evidence for an inherited, congenital neurointegrative defect. Arch Gen Psychiatry 34:1297–1313, 1977

Fish B, Marcus J, Hans SL, et al: Infants at risk for schizophrenia: sequelae of a genetic neurointegrative defect: a review and replication analysis of pandysmaturation in the Jerusalem Infant Development Study. Arch Gen Psychiatry 49:221–235, 1992

Flint J, Valdar W, Shifman S, et al: Strategies for mapping and cloning quantitative trait genes in rodents. Nat Rev Genet 6:271–286, 2005

Foley P, Riederer P: Pathogenesis and preclinical course of Parkinson's disease. J Neural Transm Suppl 56:31–74, 1999

Folstein SE, Rosen-Sheidley B: Genetics of autism: complex aetiology for a heterogeneous disorder. Nat Rev Genet 2: 943–955, 2001

Folstein S, Rutter M: Infantile autism: a genetic study of 21 twin pairs. J Child Psychol Psychiatry 18:297–321, 1977

Folstein SE, Abbott MH, Chase GA, et al: The association of affective disorder with Huntington's disease in a case series and in families. Psychol Med 13:537–542, 1983

Fombonne E: The epidemiology of autism: a review. Psychol Med 29:769–786, 1999

Freedman R, Adler LE, Leonard S: Alternative phenotypes for the complex genetics of schizophrenia. Biol Psychiatry 45:551–558, 1999

Frydman M, Bonne-Tamir B, Farrer LA, et al: Assignment of the gene for Wilson disease to chromosome 13: linkage to esterase D locus. Proc Natl Acad Sci U S A 82:1819–1821, 1985

Fusco FR, Chen Q, Lamoreaux WJ, et al: Cellular localization of huntingtin in striatal and cortical neurons in rats: lack of correlation with neuronal vulnerability in Huntington's disease. J Neurosci 19:1189–1202, 1999

Gabriel SB, Schaffner SF, Nguyen H, et al: The structure of haplotype blocks in the human genome. Science 296:2225–2229, 2002

Gambetti P, Kong Q, Zou W, et al: Sporadic and familial CJD: classification and characterisation. Br Med Bull 66:213–239, 2003

Gamboa ET, Wolf A, Yahr MD, et al: Influenza virus antigen in postencephalitic parkinsonism brain: detection by immunofluorescence. Arch Neurol 31:228–232, 1974

Gasparini L, Ongini E, Wilcock D, et al: Activity of flurbiprofen and chemically related anti-inflammatory drugs in models of Alzheimer's disease. Brain Res Brain Res Rev 48:400–408, 2005

Gasser T: Genetics of Parkinson's disease. J Neurol 248:833–840, 2001

Gasser T, Muller-Myhsok B, Wszolek ZK, et al: A susceptibility locus for Parkinson's disease maps to chromosome 2p13. Nat Genet 18:262–265, 1998

Gauthier J, Bonnel A, St-Onge J, et al: *NLGN3/NLGN4* gene mutations are not responsible for autism in the Quebec population. Am J Med Genet B Neuropsychiatr Genet 132:74–75, 2005

Gillberg C: The treatment of epilepsy in autism. J Autism Dev Disord 21:61–77, 1991

Gillberg C: Chromosomal disorders and autism. J Autism Dev Disord 28:415–425, 1998

Gillberg C, Coleman M: Autism and medical disorders: a review of the literature. Dev Med Child Neurol 38:191–202, 1996

Giordani B, Berent S, Boivin MJ, et al: Longitudinal neuropsychological and genetic linkage analysis of persons at risk for Huntington's disease. Arch Neurol 52:59–64, 1995

Glantz LA, Lewis DA: Decreased dendritic spine density on prefrontal cortical pyramidal neurons in schizophrenia. Arch Gen Psychiatry 57:65–73, 2000

Glatt SJ, Faraone SV, Tsuang MT: Association between a functional catechol-O-methyltransferase gene polymorphism and schizophrenia: meta-analysis of case-control and family based studies. Am J Psychiatry 160:469–476, 2003

Glatzel M, Stoeck K, Seeger H, et al: Human prion diseases: molecular and clinical aspects. Arch Neurol 62:545–552, 2005

Goate A, Chartier-Harlin MC, Mullan M, et al: Segregation of a missense mutation in the amyloid precursor protein gene with familial Alzheimer's disease. Nature 349:704–706, 1991

Gogos JA, Santha M, Takacs Z, et al: The gene encoding proline dehydrogenase modulates sensorimotor gating in mice. Nat Genet 21:434–439, 1999

Green AJ, Johnson PH, Yates JR: The tuberous sclerosis gene on chromosome 9q34 acts as a growth suppressor. Hum Mol Genet 3:1833–1834, 1994

Green EK, Raybould R, Macgregor S, et al: Operation of the schizophrenia susceptibility gene, neuregulin 1, across traditional diagnostic boundaries to increase risk for bipolar disorder. Arch Gen Psychiatry 62:642–648, 2005

Green MF, Bracha HS, Satz P, et al: Preliminary evidence for an association between minor physical anomalies and second trimester neurodevelopment in schizophrenia. Psychiatry Res 53:119–127, 1994

Grunewald T, Beal MF: Bioenergetics in Huntington's disease. Ann N Y Acad Sci 893:203–213, 1999

Guo Z, Cupples LA, Kurz A, et al: Head injury and the risk of AD in the MIRAGE study. Neurology 54:1316–1323, 2000

Gusella JF, Wexler NS, Conneally PM, et al: A polymorphic DNA marker genetically linked to Huntington's disease. Nature 306:234–238, 1983

Gusella JF, MacDonald ME, Ambrose CM, et al: Molecular genetics of Huntington's disease. Arch Neurol 50:1157–1163, 1993

Häfner H, Maurer K, Löffler W, et al: The influence of age and sex on the onset and early course of schizophrenia. Br J Psychiatry 162:80–86, 1993

Hallmayer J, Hebert JM, Spiker D, et al: Autism and the X chromosome: multipoint sib-pair analysis. Arch Gen Psychiatry 53:985–989, 1996

Hallmayer J, Glasson EJ, Bower C, et al: On the twin risk in autism. Am J Hum Genet 71:941–946, 2002

Harper PS: New genes for old diseases: the molecular basis of myotonic dystrophy and Huntington's disease: the Lumleian Lecture 1995. J R Coll Physicians Lond 30:221–231, 1996

Harris GJ, Codori AM, Lewis RF, et al: Reduced basal ganglia blood flow and volume in presymptomatic, gene-tested persons at-risk for Huntington's disease. Brain 122 (pt 9):1667–1678, 1999

Harrison PJ: The neuropathology of schizophrenia: a critical review of the data and their interpretation. Brain 122 (pt 4):593–624, 1999

Harrison PJ, Weinberger DR: Schizophrenia genes, gene expression, and neuropathology: on the matter of their convergence. Mol Psychiatry 10:40–68, 2005

Hendrie HC: Epidemiology of dementia and Alzheimer's disease. Am J Geriatr Psychiatry 6:S3–S18, 1998

Hennekens CH, Buring JE: Epidemiology in Medicine. Boston, MA, Little, Brown, 1987

Heresco-Levy U, Javitt DC: The role of *N*-methyl-D-aspartate (NMDA) receptor-mediated neurotransmission in the pathophysiology and therapeutics of psychiatric syndromes. Eur Neuropsychopharmacol 8:141–152, 1998

Herishanu YO, Kordysh E, Goldsmith JR: A case-referent study of extrapyramidal signs (preparkinsonism) in rural communities of Israel. Can J Neurol Sci 25:127–133, 1998

Heston LL: Psychiatric disorders in foster home reared children of schizophrenic mothers. Br J Psychiatry 112:819–825, 1966

Hofman A, Collette HJ, Bartelds AI: Incidence and risk factors of Parkinson's disease in the Netherlands. Neuroepidemiology 8:296–299, 1989

Hollister JM, Laing P, Mednick SA: Rhesus incompatibility as a risk factor for schizophrenia in male adults. Arch Gen Psychiatry 53:19–24, 1996

Hoogenraad HU, Koevoet R, de Ruyter Korver EGWM: Oral zinc sulphate as long term treatment in Wilson's disease. Eur Neurol 18:205–211, 1979

Huntington Disease Collaborative Research Group: A novel gene containing a trinucleotide repeat that is expanded and unstable on Huntington disease chromosomes. Cell 72:971–983, 1993

Huttunen MO, Niskanen P: Prenatal loss of father and psychiatric disorders. Arch Gen Psychiatry 35:429–431, 1978

International HapMap Consortium: The International HapMap Project. Nature 426:789–796, 2003

International HapMap Consortium: A haplotype map of the human genome. Nature 437:1299–1320, 2005

International Human Genome Sequencing Consortium: Initial sequencing and analysis of the human genome. Nature 409:860–921, 2001

International Human Genome Sequencing Consortium: Finishing the euchromatic sequence of the human genome. Nature 431:931–945, 2004

International Molecular Genetic Study of Autism Consortium: Further characterization of the autism susceptibility locus AUTS1 on chromosome 7q. Hum Mol Genet 10:973–982, 2001a

International Molecular Genetic Study of Autism Consortium: A genomewide screen for autism: strong evidence for linkage to chromosomes 2q, 7q, and 16p. Am J Hum Genet 69:570–581, 2001b

International Molecular Genetic Study of Autism Consortium: A full genome screen for autism with evidence for linkage to a region on chromosome 7q. Hum Mol Genet 7:571–578, 1998

Ivanov D, Kirov G, Norton N, et al: Chromosome 22q11 deletions, velo-cardio-facial syndrome and early-onset psychosis: molecular genetic study. Br J Psychiatry 183:409–413, 2003

Jacquet H, Raux G, Thibaut F, et al: *PRODH* mutations and hyperprolinemia in a subset of schizophrenic patients. Hum Mol Genet 11:2243–2249, 2002

Jamain S, Quach H, Betancur C, et al: Mutations of the X-linked genes encoding neuroligins NLGN3 and NLGN4 are associated with autism. Nat Genet 34:27–29, 2003

Jellinger KA: Head injury and dementia. Curr Opin Neurol 17:719–723, 2004

Jenner P, Olanow CW: Understanding cell death in Parkinson's disease. Ann Neurol 44:S72–S84, 1998

Johnson GC, Esposito L, Barratt BJ, et al: Haplotype tagging for the identification of common disease genes. Nat Genet 29:233–237, 2001

Jones P, Cannon M: The new epidemiology of schizophrenia. Psychiatr Clin North Am 21:1–25, 1998

Jones P, Rodgers B, Murray R, et al: Child development risk factors for adult schizophrenia in the British 1946 birth cohort. Lancet 344:1398–1402, 1994

Jorde LB, Hasstedt SJ, Ritvo ER, et al: Complex segregation analysis of autism. Am J Hum Genet 49:932–938, 1991

Kamboh MI, Sanghera DK, Ferrell RE, et al: *APOE**4-associated Alzheimer's disease risk is modified by alpha 1-antichymotrypsin polymorphism [published erratum appears in Nat Genet 11:104, 1995]. Nat Genet 10:486–488, 1995

Kamel F, Hoppin JA: Association of pesticide exposure with neurologic dysfunction and disease. Environ Health Perspect 112:950–958, 2004

Kandt RS, Haines JL, Smith M, et al: Linkage of an important gene locus for tuberous sclerosis to a chromosome 16 marker for polycystic kidney disease. Nat Genet 2:37–41, 1992

Kasai K, Shenton ME, Salisbury DF, et al: Progressive decrease of left Heschl gyrus and planum temporale gray matter volume in first-episode schizophrenia: a longitudinal magnetic resonance imaging study. Arch Gen Psychiatry 60:766–775, 2003

Kates WR, Burnette C, Eliez S, et al: Neuroanatomic variation in monozygotic twin pairs discordant for the narrow phenotype for autism. Am J Psychiatry 161:539–546, 2004

Kawas C, Resnick S, Morrison A, et al: A prospective study of estrogen replacement therapy and the risk of developing Alzheimer's disease: the Baltimore Longitudinal Study of Aging [published erratum appears in Neurology 51:654, 1998]. Neurology 48:1517–1521, 1997

Kendler KS, Gardner CO: The risk for psychiatric disorders in relatives of schizophrenic and control probands: a comparison of three independent studies. Psychol Med 27:411–419, 1997

Kety SS: Schizophrenic illness in the families of schizophrenic adoptees: findings from the Danish national sample. Schizophr Bull 14:217–222, 1988

Kety SS, Wender PH, Jacobsen B, et al: Mental illness in the biological and adoptive relatives of schizophrenic adoptees: replication of the Copenhagen Study in the rest of Denmark. Arch Gen Psychiatry 51:442–455, 1994

Kidd KK: Genetic models for psychiatric disorders, in Genetic Research Strategies for Psychobiology and Psychiatry. Edited by Gershon ES, Matthysse S, Breakefield XO, et al. Pacific Grove, CA, Boxwood Press, 1981, pp 369–382

Kinney DK, Woods BT, Yurgelun-Todd D: Neurologic abnormalities in schizophrenic patients and their families; II: neurologic and psychiatric findings in relatives. Arch Gen Psychiatry 43:665–668, 1986

Kirkwood JK, Wells GA, Wilesmith JW, et al: Spongiform encephalopathy in an Arabian oryx (*Oryx leucoryx*) and a greater kudu (*Tragelaphus strepsiceros*) [see comments]. Vet Rec 127:418–420, 1990

Kirov G, Ivanov D, Williams NM, et al: Strong evidence for association between the dystrobrevin binding protein 1 gene (*DTNBP1*) and schizophrenia in 488 parent-offspring trios from Bulgaria. Biol Psychiatry 55:971–975, 2004

Kirov G, Donovan MC, Owen MJ: Finding schizophrenia genes. J Clin Invest 115:1440–1448, 2005

Klein RJ, Zeiss C, Chew EY, et al: Complement factor H polymorphism in age-related macular degeneration. Science 308:385–389, 2005

Knight R: Creutzfeldt-Jakob disease: clinical features, epidemiology and tests. Electrophoresis 19:1306–1310, 1998

Kordower JH, Isacson O, Emerich DF: Cellular delivery of trophic factors for the treatment of Huntington's disease: is neuroprotection possible? Exp Neurol 159:4–20, 1999

Kremer HPH, Goldberg YP, Andrew SE, et al: Worldwide study of the Huntington's disease mutation: the sensitivity and specificity of the repeated CAG sequences. N Engl J Med 330:1401–1406, 1994

Kuhn W, Müller T: [Therapy of Parkinson disease, 2: new therapy concepts for treating motor symptoms] (in German). Fortschr Neurol Psychiatr 65:375–385, 1997

Lamb JA, Moore J, Bailey A, et al: Autism: recent molecular genetic advances. Hum Mol Genet 9:861–868, 2000

Lamb JA, Barnby G, Bonora E, et al: Analysis of IMGSAC autism susceptibility loci: evidence for sex limited and parent of origin specific effects. J Med Genet 42:132–137, 2005

Lamb RF, Roy C, Diefenbach TJ, et al: The TSC1 tumour suppressor hamartin regulates cell adhesion through ERM proteins and the GTPase Rho. Nat Cell Biol 2:281–287, 2000

Landles C, Bates GP: Huntington and the molecular pathogenesis of Huntington's disease (Fourth in Molecular Medicine Review Series). EMBO Rep 5:958–963, 2004

Langlois S: Genomic imprinting: a new mechanism for disease. Pediatr Pathol 14:161–165, 1994

Langston JW: Epidemiology versus genetics in Parkinson's disease: progress in resolving an age-old debate. Ann Neurol 44 (3 suppl 1):S45–S52, 1998

Langston JW, Ballard P, Tetrud JW, et al: Chronic parkinsonism in humans due to a product of meperidine-analog synthesis. Science 219:979–980, 1983

Laumonnier F, Bonnet-Brilhault F, Gomot M, et al: X-linked mental retardation and autism are associated with a mutation in the NLGN4 gene, a member of the neuroligin family. Am J Hum Genet 74:552–557, 2004

Launer LJ: Diabetes and brain aging: epidemiologic evidence. Curr Diab Rep 5:59–63, 2005

Launer LJ, Andersen K, Dewey ME, et al: Rates and risk factors for dementia and Alzheimer's disease: results from EURODEM pooled analyses. EURODEM Incidence Research Group and Work Groups. European Studies of Dementia. Neurology 52:78–84, 1999

Lawrie SM, Whalley H, Kestelman JN, et al: Magnetic resonance imaging of brain in people at high risk of developing schizophrenia. Lancet 353(9146):30–33, 1999

Le Couteur A, Bailey A, Goode S, et al: A broader phenotype of autism: the clinical spectrum in twins. J Child Psychol Psychiatry 37:785–801, 1996

Le Couteur DG, McLean AJ, Taylor MC, et al: Pesticides and Parkinson's disease. Biomed Pharmacother 53:122–130, 1999

Leeflang EP, Zhang L, Tavare S, et al: Single sperm analysis of the trinucleotide repeats in the Huntington's disease gene: quantification of the mutation frequency spectrum. Hum Mol Genet 4:1519–1526, 1995

Leroy E, Boyer R, Auburger G, et al: The ubiquitin pathway in Parkinson's disease (letter). Nature 395:451–452, 1998

Levy DL, Holzman PS, Matthysse S, et al: Eye tracking and schizophrenia. Schizophr Bull 20:47–62, 1994

Levy-Lehad E, Lahad A, Wijsman EM, et al: Apolipoprotein E genotypes and age of onset in early onset familial Alzheimer's disease. Ann Neurol 38:678–680, 1995

Lewis CM, Levinson DF, Wise LH, et al: Genome scan meta-analysis of schizophrenia and bipolar disorder, part II: schizophrenia. Am J Hum Genet 73:34–48, 2003

Lewis DA, Volk DW, Hashimoto T: Selective alterations in prefrontal cortical GABA neurotransmission in schizophrenia: a novel target for the treatment of working memory dysfunction. Psychopharmacology 174:143–150, 2004

Li T, Ma X, Sham PC, et al: Evidence for association between novel polymorphisms in the *PRODH* gene and schizophrenia in a Chinese population. Am J Med Genet B Neuropsychiatr Genet 129:13–15, 2004

Lieberman JA, Tollefson GD, Charles C, et al: Antipsychotic drug effects on brain morphology in first-episode psychosis. HGDH Study Group. Arch Gen Psychiatry 62:361–370, 2005

Lindblad-Toh K, Wade CM, Mikkelsen TS, et al: Genome sequence, comparative analysis and haplotype structure of the domestic dog. Nature 438:803–819, 2005

Liou HH, Tsai MC, Chen CJ, et al: Environmental risk factors and Parkinson's disease: a case-control study in Taiwan. Neurology 48:1583–1588, 1997

Liu J, Nyholt DR, Magnussen P, et al: A genomewide screen for autism susceptibility loci. Am J Hum Genet 69:327–340, 2001

Logroscino G, Marder K, Graziano J, et al: Dietary iron, animal fats, and risk of Parkinson's disease. Mov Disord 13 (suppl 1):13–16, 1998

Lohr JB, Flynn K: Minor physical anomalies in schizophrenia and mood disorders. Schizophr Bull 19:551–556, 1993

Luchsinger JA, Mayeux R: Cardiovascular risk factors and Alzheimer's disease. Curr Atheroscler Rep 6:261–266, 2004

Lucking CB, Durr A, Bonifati V, et al: Association between early onset Parkinson's disease and mutations in the parkin gene. N Engl J Med 342:1560–1567, 2000

Ma DQ, Jaworski J, Menold MM, et al: Ordered-subset analysis of savant skills in autism for 15q11-q13. Am J Med Genet B Neuropsychiatr Genet 135:38–41, 2005a

Ma DQ, Whitehead PL, Menold MM, et al: Identification of significant association and gene-gene interaction of GABA receptor subunit genes in autism. Am J Hum Genet 77:377–388, 2005b

MacDonald ME, Barnes G, Srinidhi J, et al: Gametic but not somatic instability of CAG repeat length in Huntington's disease. J Med Genet 30:982–986, 1993

Maddox LO, Menold MM, Bass MP, et al: Autistic disorder and chromosome 15q11-q13: construction and analysis of a BAC/PAC contig. Genomics 62:325–331, 1999

Maestrini E, Lai C, Marlow A, et al: Serotonin transporter (*5-HTT*) and gamma-aminobutyric acid receptor subunit beta3 (*GABRB3*) gene polymorphisms are not associated with autism in the IMGSA families: the International Molecular Genetic Study of Autism Consortium. Am J Med Genet 88:492–496, 1999

Malaspina D, Friedman JH, Kaufmann C, et al: Psychobiological heterogeneity of familial and sporadic schizophrenia. Biol Psychiatry 43:489–496, 1998

Malaspina D, Sohler NL, Susser E: Interaction of genes and prenatal exposures in schizophrenia, in Prenatal Exposures in Schizophrenia. Edited by Susser E, Brown AS, Gorman JM. Washington, DC, American Psychiatric Press, 1999, pp 35–61

Malaspina D, Bruder G, Furman V, et al: Schizophrenia subgroups differing in dichotic listening laterality also differ in neurometabolism and symptomatology. J Neuropsychiatry Clin Neurosci 12:485–492, 2000a

Malaspina D, Goetz RR, Yale S, et al: Relation of familial schizophrenia to negative symptoms but not to the deficit syndrome. Am J Psychiatry 157:994–1003, 2000b

Malaspina D, Goetz RR, Friedman JH, et al: Traumatic brain injury and schizophrenia in members of schizophrenia and bipolar disorder pedigrees. Am J Psychiatry 158:440–446, 2001

Malaspina D, Brown A, Goetz D, et al: Schizophrenia risk and paternal age: a potential role for de novo mutations in schizophrenia vulnerability genes. CNS Spectr 7:26–29, 2002

Malaspina D, Reichenberg A, Weiser M, et al: Paternal age and intelligence: implications for age-related genomic changes in male germ cells. Psychiatr Genet15:117–125, 2005

Malhotra AK, Kestler LJ, Mazzanti C, et al: A functional polymorphism in the COMT gene and performance on a test of prefrontal cognition. Am J Psychiatry 159:652–654, 2002

Mangiarini L, Sathasivam K, Seller M, et al: Exon 1 of the HD gene with an expanded CAG repeat is sufficient to cause a progressive neurological phenotype in transgenic mice. Cell 87:493–506, 1996

Maraganore DM, de Andrade M, Lesnick TG, et al: High-resolution whole-genome association study of Parkinson disease. Am J Hum Genet 77:685–693, 2005

Marcus J, Auerbach J, Wilkinson L, et al: Infants at risk for schizophrenia: the Jerusalem Infant Development Study. Arch Gen Psychiatry 38:703–713, 1981

Margolis RL, Ross CA: Diagnosis of Huntington disease. Clin Chem 49:1726–1732, 2003

Mariappan SV, Silks LA III, Chen X, et al: Solution structures of the Huntington's disease DNA triplets, (CAG)n. J Biomol Struct Dyn 15:723–744, 1998

Marsden CD, Jenner PG: The significance of 1-methyl-4-phenyl-1,2,3,6-tetrahydropyridine. Ciba Found Symp 126:239–256, 1987

Martin ER, Lai EH, Gilbert JR, et al: SNPing away at complex diseases: analysis of single-nucleotide polymorphisms around APOE in Alzheimer disease. Am J Hum Genet 67:383–394, 2000

Martindale D, Hackam A, Wieczorek A, et al: Length of huntingtin and its polyglutamine tract influences localization and frequency of intracellular aggregates. Nat Genet 18:150–154, 1998

Mattock C, Marmot M, Stern G: Could Parkinson's disease follow intra-uterine influenza? A speculative hypothesis. J Neurol Neurosurg Psychiatry 51:753–756, 1988

Mayeux R, Ottman R, Maestre G, et al: Synergistic effects of traumatic head injury and apolipoprotein-epsilon 4 in patients with Alzheimer's disease [see comments]. Neurology 45:555–557, 1995

McCarthy MI, Kruglyak L, Lander ES: Sib-pair collection strategies for complex diseases. Genet Epidemiol 15:317–340, 1998

McCormack AL, Thiruchelvam M, Manning-Bog AB, et al: Environmental risk factors and Parkinson's disease: selective degeneration of nigral dopaminergic neurons caused by the herbicide paraquat. Neurobiol Dis 10:119–127, 2002

McDonald LV, Lake CR: Psychosis in an adolescent patient with Wilson's disease: effects of chelation therapy. Psychosom Med 57:202–204, 1995

McGlashan TH, Hoffman RE: Schizophrenia as a disorder of developmentally reduced synaptic connectivity. Arch Gen Psychiatry 57:637–648, 2000

McGue M, Gottesman II: The genetic epidemiology of schizophrenia and the design of linkage studies. Eur Arch Psychiatry Clin Neurosci 240:174–181, 1991

Medori R, Tritschler HJ, LeBlanc A, et al: Fatal familial insomnia, a prion disease with a mutation at codon 178 of the prion protein gene [see comments]. N Engl J Med 326:444–449, 1992

Menegon A, Board PG, Blackburn AC, et al: Parkinson's disease, pesticides, and glutathione transferase polymorphisms [see comments]. Lancet 352:1344–1346, 1998

Michailov GV, Sereda MW, Brinkmann BG, et al: Axonal neuregulin-1 regulates myelin sheath thickness. Science 304:700–703, 2004

Mirnics K, Middleton FA, Lewis DA, et al: Analysis of complex brain disorders with gene expression microarrays: schizophrenia as a disease of the synapse. Trends Neurosci 24:479–486, 2001

Mirsky AF, Silberman EK, Latz A, et al: Adult outcomes of high-risk children: differential effects of town and kibbutz rearing. Schizophr Bull 11:150–154, 1985

Miyoshi K, Honda A, Baba K, et al: Disrupted-In-Schizophrenia 1, a candidate gene for schizophrenia, participates in neurite outgrowth. Mol Psychiatry 8:685–694, 2003

Morris AG, Gaitonde E, McKenna PJ, et al: CAG repeat expansions and schizophrenia: association with disease in females and with early age-at-onset. Hum Mol Genet 4:1957–1961, 1995

Mouse Genome Sequencing Consortium: Initial sequencing and comparative analysis of the mouse genome. Nature 420:520–562, 2002

Murphy KC, Jones LA, Owen MJ: High rates of schizophrenia in adults with velo-cardio-facial syndrome. Arch Gen Psychiatry 56:940–945, 1999

Myers RH, Leavitt J, Farrer LA, et al: Homozygotes for Huntington's disease. Am J Hum Genet 45:614–618, 1989

Myles-Worsley M, Coon H, Tiobech J, et al: Genetic epidemiological study of schizophrenia in Palau, Micronesia: prevalence and familiality. Am J Med Genet 88:4–10, 1999

Nakamura Y, Leppert M, O'Connell P, et al: Variable number of tandem repeat (VNTR) markers for human gene mapping. Science 235:1616–1622, 1987

Nee LE, Lippa CF: Alzheimer's disease in 22 twin pairs—13-year follow-up: hormonal, infectious and traumatic factors. Dement Geriatr Cogn Disord 10:148–151, 1999

Nemetz PN, Leibson C, Naessens JM, et al: Traumatic brain injury and time to onset of Alzheimer's disease: a population-based study. Am J Epidemiol 149:32–40, 1999

Numakawa T, Yagasaki Y, Ishimoto T, et al: Evidence of novel neuronal functions of dysbindin, a susceptibility gene for schizophrenia. Hum Mol Genet 13:2699–2708, 2004

Oddo S, Caccamo A, Green KN, et al: Chronic nicotine administration exacerbates tau pathology in a transgenic model of Alzheimer's disease. Proc Natl Acad Sci U S A 102:3046–3051, 2005

O'Donovan MC, Owen MJ: Candidate-gene association studies of schizophrenia. Am J Hum Genet 65:587–592, 1999

O'Donovan MC, Guy C, Craddock N, et al: Expanded CAG repeats in schizophrenia and bipolar disorder. Nat Genet 10:380–381, 1995

O'Driscoll GA, Lenzenweger MF, Holzman PS: Antisaccades and smooth pursuit eye tracking and schizotypy. Arch Gen Psychiatry 55:837–843, 1998

O'Dwyer JM: Schizophrenia in people with intellectual disability: the role of pregnancy and birth complications. J Intellect Disabil Res 41 (pt 3):238–251, 1997

Oesch B, Westaway D, Walchli M, et al: A cellular gene encodes scrapie PrP 27–30 protein. Cell 40:735–746, 1985

Okuizumi K, Onodera O, Namba Y, et al: Genetic association of the very low density lipoprotein (VLDL) receptor gene with sporadic Alzheimer's disease. Nat Genet 11:207–209, 1995

Olanow CW, Tatton WG: Etiology and pathogenesis of Parkinson's disease. Annu Rev Neurosci 22:123–144, 1999

Ott J: Analysis of Human Genetic Linkage. Baltimore, MD, Johns Hopkins University Press, 1985

Pantelis C, Velakoulis D, McGorry PD, et al: Neuroanatomical abnormalities before and after onset of psychosis: a cross-sectional and longitudinal MRI comparison. Lancet 361:281–288, 2003

Parnas J, Schulsinger F, Schulsinger H, et al: Behavioral precursors of schizophrenia spectrum: a prospective study. Arch Gen Psychiatry 39:658–664, 1982a

Parnas J, Schulsinger F, Teasdale TW, et al: Perinatal complications and clinical outcome within the schizophrenia spectrum. Br J Psychiatry 140:416–420, 1982b

Pearson GR, Gruffydd-Jones TJ, Wyatt JM, et al: Feline spongiform encephalopathy (letter). Vet Rec 128:532, 1991

Pedersen CB, Mortensen PB: Family history, place and season of birth as risk factors for schizophrenia in Denmark: a replication and reanalysis. Br J Psychiatry 179:46–52, 2001

Petronis A, Kennedy JL: Unstable genes—unstable mind? Am J Psychiatry 152:164–172, 1995

Petrukhin K, Lutsenko S, Chernov I, et al: Characterization of the Wilson disease gene encoding a P-type copper transporting ATPase: genomic organization, alternative splicing, and structure/function predictions. Hum Mol Genet 3:1647–1656, 1994

Petryshen TL, Middleton FA, Kirby A, et al: Support for involvement of neuregulin 1 in schizophrenia pathophysiology. Mol Psychiatry 10:366–374, 328, 2005

Peyser CE, Folstein SE: Huntington's disease as a model for mood disorders: clues from neuropathology and neurochemistry. Mol Chem Neuropathol 12:99–119, 1990

Philippe A, Martinez M, Guilloud-Bataille M, et al: Genome-wide scan for autism susceptibility genes. Paris Autism Research International Sibpair Study. Hum Mol Genet 8:805–812, 1999

Pickles A, Bolton P, Macdonald H, et al: Latent-class analysis of recurrence risks for complex phenotypes with selection and measurement error: a twin and family history study of autism. Am J Hum Genet 57:717–726, 1995

Pickles A, Starr E, Kazak S, et al: Variable expression of the autism broader phenotype: findings from extended pedigrees. J Child Psychol Psychiatry 41:491–502, 2000

Piven J, Tsai GC, Nehme E, et al: Platelet serotonin, a possible marker for familial autism. J Autism Dev Disord 21:51–59, 1991

Prusiner SB: Novel proteinaceous infectious particles cause scrapie. Science 216:136–144, 1982

Quirion R, Insel TR: Psychiatry as a clinical neuroscience discipline. JAMA 294:2221–2224, 2005

Raiha I, Kaprio J, Koskenvuo M, et al: Dementia in twins. Lancet 347:1706, 1996

Ramoz N, Reichert JG, Smith CJ, et al: Linkage and association of the mitochondrial aspartate/glutamate carrier SLC25A12 gene with autism. Am J Psychiatry 161:662–669, 2004

Rantakallio P, Jones P, Moring J, et al: Association between central nervous system infections during childhood and adult onset schizophrenia and other psychoses: a 28-year follow-up. Int J Epidemiol 26:837–843, 1997

Rat Genome Sequencing Project Consortium: Genome sequence of the Brown Norway rat yields insights into mammalian evolution. Nature 428:493–521, 2004

Rathbun JK: Neuropsychological aspects of Wilson's disease. Int J Neurosci 85:221–229, 1996

Reddy PH, Charles V, Williams M, et al: Transgenic mice expressing mutated full-length HD cDNA: a paradigm for locomotor changes and selective neuronal loss in Huntington's disease. Philos Trans R Soc Lond B Biol Sci 354:1035–1045, 1999

Richard F, Amouyel P: Genetic susceptibility factors for Alzheimer's disease. Eur J Pharmacol 412:1–12, 2001

Richards RI, Sutherland GR: Dynamic mutations: a new class of mutations causing human disease. Cell 70:709–712, 1992

Ridley RM, Frith CD, Crow TJ, et al: Anticipation in Huntington's disease is inherited through the male line but may originate in the female. J Med Genet 25:589–595, 1988

Rineer S, Finucane B, Simon EW: Autistic symptoms among children and young adults with isodicentric chromosome 15. Am J Med Genet 81:428–433, 1998

Risch N: Linkage strategies for genetically complex traits, I: multilocus models. Am J Hum Genet 46:222–228, 1990

Risch N, Merikangas K: The future of genetic studies of complex human diseases. Science 273:1516–1517, 1996

Risch N, Spiker D, Lotspeich L, et al: A genomic screen of autism: evidence for a multilocus etiology. Am J Hum Genet 65:493–507, 1999

Ritvo ER, Spence MA, Freeman BJ, et al: Evidence for autosomal recessive inheritance in 46 families with multiple incidences of autism. Am J Psychiatry 142:187–192, 1985

Ritvo ER, Freeman BJ, Pingree C, et al: The UCLA–University of Utah epidemiologic survey of autism: prevalence. Am J Psychiatry 146:194–199, 1989

Ritvo ER, Mason-Brothers A, Freeman BJ, et al: The UCLA-University of Utah epidemiologic survey of autism: the etiologic role of rare diseases. Am J Psychiatry 147:1614–1621, 1990

Rogaev EI, Sherrington R, Rogaeva EA, et al: Familial Alzheimer's disease in kindreds with missense mutations in a gene on chromosome 1 related to the Alzheimer's disease type 3 gene. Nature 376:775–778, 1995

Rosenthal D, Wender PH, Kety SS, et al: Schizophrenics' offspring reared in adoptive homes. J Psychiatr Res 6:377–391, 1968

Rosoklija G, Toomayan G, Ellis SP, et al: Structural abnormalities of subicular dendrites in subjects with schizophrenia and mood disorders: preliminary findings. Arch Gen Psychiatry 57:349–356, 2000

Ross GW, Abbott RD, Petrovitch H, et al: Association of coffee and caffeine intake with the risk of Parkinson disease. JAMA 283:2674–2679, 2000

Ross RG, Olincy A, Harris JG, et al: Anticipatory saccades during smooth pursuit eye movements and familial transmission of schizophrenia. Biol Psychiatry 44:690–697, 1998

Rubinsztein DC: The genetics of Alzheimer's disease. Prog Neurobiol 52:447–454, 1997

Rutter M, Bailey A, Bolton P, et al: Autism and known medical conditions: myth and substance. J Child Psychol Psychiatry 35:311–322, 1994

Sacker A, Done DJ, Crow TJ, et al: Antecedents of schizophrenia and affective illness: obstetric complications. Br J Psychiatry 166:734–741, 1995

Samii A, Nutt JG, Ransom BR: Parkinson's disease. Lancet 363:1783–1793, 2004

Sapp E, Penney J, Young A, et al: Axonal transport of N-terminal huntingtin suggests early pathology of corticostriatal projections in Huntington disease. J Neuropathol Exp Neurol 58:165–173, 1999

Sawamura N, Sawamura-Yamamoto T, Ozeki Y, et al: A form of DISC1 enriched in nucleus: altered subcellular distribution in orbitofrontal cortex in psychosis and substance/alcohol abuse. Proc Natl Acad Sci U S A 102:1187–1192, 2005

Schiefermeier M, Kollegger H, Madl C, et al: The impact of apolipoprotein E genotypes on age at onset of symptoms and phenotypic expression in Wilson's disease. Brain 123 (pt 3):585–590, 2000

Schilsky ML: Diagnosis and treatment of Wilson's disease. Pediatr Transplant 6:15–19, 2002

Schulze TG, Ohlraun S, Czerski PM, et al: Genotype-phenotype studies in bipolar disorder showing association between the DAOA/G30 locus and persecutory delusions: a first step toward a molecular genetic classification of psychiatric phenotypes. Am J Psychiatry 162:2101–2108, 2005

Schwab SG, Knapp M, Mondabon S, et al: Support for association of schizophrenia with genetic variation in the 6p22.3 gene, dysbindin, in sib-pair families with linkage and in an additional sample of triad families. Am J Hum Genet 72:185–190, 2003

Shao Y, Raiford KL, Wolpert CM, et al: Phenotypic homogeneity provides increased support for linkage on chromosome 2 in autistic disorder. Am J Hum Genet 70:1058–1061, 2002a

Shao Y, Wolpert CM, Raiford KL, et al: Genomic screen and follow-up analysis for autistic disorder. Am J Med Genet 114:99–105, 2002b

Shao Y, Cuccaro ML, Hauser ER, et al: Fine mapping of autistic disorder to chromosome 15q11-q13 by use of phenotypic subtypes. Am J Hum Genet 72:539–548, 2003

Sherrington R, Rogaev EI, Liang Y, et al: Cloning of a gene bearing missense mutations in early onset familial Alzheimer's disease. Nature 375:754–760, 1995

Shorter J, Lindquist S: Prions as adaptive conduits of memory and inheritance. Nat Rev Genet 6:435–450, 2005

Shumaker SA, Legault C, Rapp SR, et al: WHIMS Investigators. Estrogen plus progestin and the incidence of dementia and mild cognitive impairment in postmenopausal women: the Women's Health Initiative Memory Study: a randomized controlled trial. JAMA 289:2651–2662, 2003

Siegel C, Waldo M, Mizner G, et al: Deficits in sensory gating in schizophrenic patients and their relatives: evidence obtained with auditory evoked responses. Arch Gen Psychiatry 41:607–612, 1984

Siever LJ, Kalus OF, Keefe RS: The boundaries of schizophrenia. Psychiatr Clin North Am 16:217–244, 1993

Sipos A, Rasmussen F, Harrison G, et al: Paternal age and schizophrenia: a population based cohort study. BMJ 329:1070, 2004

Skuse DH: Imprinting, the X-chromosome, and the male brain: explaining sex differences in the liability to autism. Pediatr Res 47:9–16, 2000

Smalley SL: Autism and tuberous sclerosis. J Autism Dev Disord 28:407–414, 1998

Smalley SL, Tanguay PE, Smith M, et al: Autism and tuberous sclerosis. J Autism Dev Disord 22:339–355, 1992

Spiker D, Lotspeich L, Kraemer HC, et al: Genetics of autism: characteristics of affected and unaffected children from 37 multiplex families. Am J Med Genet 54:27–35, 1994

St. Clair D, Blackwood D, Muir W, et al: Association within a family of a balanced autosomal translocation with major mental illness. Lancet 336:13–16, 1990

Stefansson H, Sigurdsson E, Steinthorsdottir V, et al: Neuregulin 1 and susceptibility to schizophrenia. Am J Hum Genet 71:877–892, 2002

Steffenburg S: Neuropsychiatric assessment of children with autism: a population-based study. Dev Med Child Neurol 33:495–511, 1991

Steffenburg S, Gillberg C, Hellgren L, et al: A twin study of autism in Denmark, Finland, Iceland, Norway and Sweden. J Child Psychol Psychiatry 30:405–416, 1989

Steffenburg S, Gillberg CL, Steffenburg U, et al: Autism in Angelman syndrome: a population-based study. Pediatr Neurol 14:131–136, 1996

Stern Y, Gurland B, Tatemichi TK, et al: Influence of education and occupation on the incidence of Alzheimer's disease [see comments]. JAMA 271:1004–1010, 1994

Stone JL, Merriman B, Cantor RM, et al: Evidence for sex-specific risk alleles in autism spectrum disorder. Am J Hum Genet 75:1117–1123, 2004

Straub RE, Jiang Y, MacLean CJ, et al: Genetic variation in the 6p22.3 gene *DTNBP1*, the human ortholog of the mouse dysbindin gene, is associated with schizophrenia. Am J Hum Genet 71:337–348, 2002

Strous RD, Shoenfeld Y: Revisiting old ghosts: prenatal viral exposure and schizophrenia. Isr Med Assoc J 7:43–45, 2005

Susser E, Neugebauer R, Hoek HW, et al: Schizophrenia after prenatal famine: further evidence [see comments]. Arch Gen Psychiatry 53:25–31, 1996

Szatmari P: Heterogeneity and the genetics of autism. J Psychiatry Neurosci 24:159–165, 1999

Szatmari P, Archer L, Fisman S, et al: Asperger's syndrome and autism: differences in behavior, cognition, and adaptive functioning. J Am Acad Child Adolesc Psychiatry 34:1662–1671, 1995

Szatmari P, MacLean JE, Jones MB, et al: The familial aggregation of the lesser variant in biological and nonbiological relatives of PDD probands: a family history study. J Child Psychol Psychiatry 41:579–586, 2000

Talbot K, Eidem WL, Tinsley CL, et al: Dysbindin-1 is reduced in intrinsic, glutamatergic terminals of the hippocampal formation in schizophrenia. J Clin Invest 113:1353–1363, 2004

Tang MX, Maestre G, Tsai WY, et al: Effect of age, ethnicity, and head injury on the association between APOE genotypes and Alzheimer's disease. Ann NY Acad Sci 802:6–15, 1996

Tanner CM, Ottman R, Goldman SM, et al: Parkinson disease in twins: an etiologic study. JAMA 281:341–346, 1999

Tanzi RE, Petrukhin K, Chernov I, et al: The Wilson disease gene is a copper transporting ATPase with homology to the Menkes disease gene. Nat Genet 5:344–350, 1993

Tarrant CJ, Jones PB: Precursors to schizophrenia: do biological markers have specificity? [see comments]. Can J Psychiatry 44:335–349, 1999

Telenius H, Kremer HPH, Theilmann J, et al: Molecular analysis of juvenile Huntington's disease: the major influence on (CAG)n repeat length is the sex of the affected parent. Hum Mol Genet 2:1535–1540, 1993

Thomas GR, Bull PC, Roberts EA, et al: Haplotype studies in Wilson disease. Am J Hum Genet 54:71–78, 1994

Thomas NS, Sharp AJ, Browne CE, et al: Xp deletions associated with autism in three females. Hum Genet 104:43–48, 1999

Tienari P: Interaction between genetic vulnerability and family environment: the Finnish adoptive family study of schizophrenia. Acta Psychiatr Scand 84:460–465, 1991

Tosato S, Dazzan P, Collier D: Association between the neuregulin 1 gene and schizophrenia: a systematic review. Schizophr Bull 31:613–617, 2005

Tsai L, Stewart MA, August G: Implication of sex differences in the familial transmission of infantile autism. J Autism Dev Disord 11:165–173, 1981

Valente EM, Abou-Sleiman PM, Caputo V, et al: Hereditary early onset Parkinson's disease caused by mutations in PINK1. Science 304:1158–1160, 2004

van Dyck CH, Seibyl JP, Malison RT, et al: Age-related decline in dopamine transporters: analysis of striatal subregions, nonlinear effects, and hemispheric asymmetries. Am J Geriatr Psychiatry 10:36–43, 2002

Van Os J, Selten JP: Prenatal exposure to maternal stress and subsequent schizophrenia: the May 1940 invasion of The Netherlands [see comments]. Br J Psychiatry 172:324–326, 1998

van Slegtenhorst M, de Hoogt R, Hermans C, et al: Identification of the tuberous sclerosis gene *TSC1* on chromosome 9q34. Science 277:805–808, 1997

Venter JC, Adams MD, Myers EW, et al: The sequence of the human genome. Science 291:1304–1351, 2001

Vincent JB, Kolozsvari D, Roberts WS, et al: Mutation screening of X-chromosomal neuroligin genes: no mutations in 196 autism probands. Am J Med Genet B Neuropsychiatr Genet 129:82–84, 2004

Volkmar FR, Szatmari P, Sparrow SS: Sex differences in pervasive developmental disorders. J Autism Dev Disord 23:579–591, 1993

Wahlberg KE, Wynne LC, Oja H, et al: Gene-environment interaction in vulnerability to schizophrenia: findings from the Finnish Adoptive Family Study of Schizophrenia. Am J Psychiatry 154:355–362, 1997

Walker EF, Savoie T, Davis D: Neuromotor precursors of schizophrenia. Schizophr Bull 20:441–451, 1994

Walshe JM: Penicillamine: a new oral therapy for Wilson's disease. Am J Med 21:487–495, 1956

Wang DG, Fan JB, Siao CJ, et al: Large-scale identification, mapping, and genotyping of single-nucleotide polymorphisms in the human genome. Science 280:1077–1082, 1998

Wassink TH, Brzustowicz LM, Bartlett CW, et al: The search for autism disease genes. Ment Retard Dev Disabil Res Rev 10:272–283, 2005

Webber KM, Casadesus G, Marlatt MW, et al: Estrogen bows to a new master: the role of gonadotropins in Alzheimer pathogenesis. Ann N Y Acad Sci 1052:201–209, 2005

Weickert CS, Straub RE, McClintock BW, et al: Human dysbindin (*DTNBP1*) gene expression in normal brain and in schizophrenic prefrontal cortex and midbrain. Arch Gen Psychiatry 61:544–555, 2004

Weinberger DR: Implications of normal brain development for the pathogenesis of schizophrenia. Arch Gen Psychiatry 44:660–669, 1987

Weissmann C, Flechsig E: PrP knock-out and PrP transgenic mice in prion research. Br Med Bull 66:43–60, 2003

Wellington CL, Ellerby LM, Hackam AS, et al: Caspase cleavage of gene products associated with triplet expansion disorders generates truncated fragments containing the polyglutamine tract. J Biol Chem 273:9158–9167, 1998

West A, Periquet M, Lincoln S, et al: Complex relationship between Parkin mutations and Parkinson disease. Am J Med Genet 114:584–591, 2002

Wexler NS, Young AB, Tanzi R, et al: Homozygotes for Huntington's disease. Nature 3326:194–197, 1987

Wexler NS, Lorimer J, Porter J, et al: Venezuelan kindreds reveal that genetic and environmental factors modulate Huntington's disease age of onset. Project US-VCR. Proc Natl Acad Sci U S A 101:3498–3503, 2004

White L, Petrovitch H, Ross GW, et al: Prevalence of dementia in older Japanese-American men in Hawaii: the Honolulu-Asia Aging Study [see comments]. JAMA 276:955–960, 1996

Williams NM, Preece A, Morris DW, et al: Identification in 2 independent samples of a novel schizophrenia risk haplotype of the dystrobrevin binding protein (DTNBP1). Arch Gen Psychiatry 61:336–344, 2004

World Health Organization: The ICD-10 Classification of Mental and Behavioural Disorders. Geneva, Switzerland, World Health Organization, 1992

Wright IC, Rabe-Hesketh S, Woodruff PW, et al: Meta-analysis of regional brain volumes in schizophrenia. Am J Psychiatry 157:16–25, 2000

Yamaguchi Y, Heiny ME, Gitlin JD: Isolation and characterization of a human liver cDNA as a candidate gene Wilson disease. Biochem Biophys Res Commun 197:271–277, 1993

Yan J, Oliveira G, Coutinho A, et al: Analysis of the neuroligin 3 and 4 genes in autism and other neuropsychiatric patients. Mol Psychiatry 10:329–332, 2005

Ylisaukko-oja T, Rehnstrom K, Auranen M, et al: Analysis of four neuroligin genes as candidates for autism. Eur J Hum Genet 13:1285–1292, 2005

Yonan AL, Alarcon M, Cheng R, et al: A genome-wide screen of 345 families for autism-susceptibility loci. Am J Hum Genet 73:886–897, 2003

Zammit S, Allebeck P, Dalman C, et al: Paternal age and risk for schizophrenia. Br J Psychiatry 183:405–408, 2003

Zandi PP, Carlson MC, Plassman BL, et al; Cache County Memory Study Investigators: Hormone replacement therapy and incidence of Alzheimer disease in older women: the Cache County Study. JAMA 288:2123–2129, 2002

Zeidler M, Ironside JW: The new variant of Creutzfeldt-Jakob disease. Rev Sci Tech 19:98–120, 2000

5

NEUROPSYCHIATRIC ASPECTS OF DELIRIUM

Paula T. Trzepacz, M.D.
David J. Meagher, M.D., M.R.C.Psych.

Delirium is a commonly occurring neuropsychiatric syndrome primarily, but not exclusively, characterized by impairment in cognition, which causes a "confusional state." Delirium is an altered state of consciousness between normal alertness and awakeness and stupor or coma. Delirium may have a rapid, forceful onset with many symptoms, or it may be preceded by a subacute "subclinical" delirium with gradual changes over the course of a few days, such as alterations in sleep pattern or aspects of cognition. Emergence from coma usually involves a period of delirium before normal consciousness is achieved, except in drug-induced comatose states (Ely and Dittus 2004; McNicoll et al. 2003).

Because delirium has a wide variety of underlying etiologies—identification of which is part of clinical management—it is considered a syndrome. It may, however, represent dysfunction of a final common neural pathway that leads to its characteristic symptoms. Its broad constellation of symptoms includes not only the diffuse cognitive deficits implicit for its diagnosis but also delusions, perceptual disturbances, affective lability, language abnormalities, disordered thought processes, sleep-wake cycle disturbance, and psychomotor changes. Table 5–1 presents details of symptoms of delirium that affect nearly every neuropsychiatric domain, including characteristic features that help differentiate delirium from other psychiatric disorders.

Unlike symptoms of most other psychiatric disorders, those of delirium typically fluctuate in intensity over a 24-hour period, where relatively lucid or quiescent periods often occur. Daily Delirium Rating Scale (DRS) ratings of postoperative patients showed patterns where symptoms diminished but reappeared consistent with either serial short episodes or diminution to subclinical levels (Rudberg et al. 1997).

Delirium can occur at any age, and the less mature neural pathways of children may put

---

TABLE 5–1.   Signs and symptoms of delirium

Diffuse cognitive deficits

Attention

Orientation (time, place, person)

Memory (short- and long-term; verbal and visual)

Visuoconstructional ability

Executive functions

Temporal course

Acute or abrupt onset

Fluctuating severity of symptoms over 24-hour period

Usually reversible

Subclinical syndrome may precede and/or follow the episode

Psychosis

Perceptual disturbances (especially visual), including illusions, hallucinations, metamorphosias

Delusions (usually paranoid and poorly formed)

Thought disorder (tangentiality, circumstantiality, loose associations)

Sleep-wake disturbance

Fragmented throughout 24-hour period

Reversal of normal cycle

Sleeplessness

Psychomotor behavior

Hyperactive

Hypoactive

Mixed

Language impairment

Word-finding difficulty/dysnomia/paraphasia

Dysgraphia

Altered semantic content

Severe forms can mimic expressive or receptive aphasia

Altered or labile affect

Any mood can occur, usually incongruent to context

Anger or increased irritability common

Hypoactive delirium often mislabeled as depression

Lability (rapid shifts) common

Unrelated to mood preceding delirium

---

them at high risk. Although delirium in children is vastly understudied, descriptions indicate that symptoms are essentially identical to those in adults (Platt et al. 1994b; Prugh et al. 1980; Turkel et al. 2003, 2006).

Delirium is the accepted term to denote acute disturbances of global cognitive function, encompassing a unitary syndrome with multiple possible different etiologies, as defined in both DSM-IV/DSM-IV-TR and ICD-10 research classification systems (American Psychiatric Association 1994, 2000; World Health Organization 1992). Unfortunately, multiple synonyms, based on the etiology or setting in which delirium is encountered, persist both in the literature and between disciplines in clinical practice. Examples include *acute confusional state, intensive care unit (ICU) psychosis, hepatic encephalopathy, toxic psychosis, acute brain failure*, and *posttraumatic amnesia*. The term *reversible cognitive deficit* is used in geriatric literature but is poorly defined and not synonymous with delirium; it could instead represent subclinical delirium or cognitive impairment related to many other causes (e.g., pain, poor sleep, medication adverse events). Recent research shows that DSM-IV-TR delirium occurs after traumatic brain injury (Sherer et al. 2005), despite misnomers and poor recognition by nonpsychiatrists. Consistent and proper use of the term *delirium* will greatly enhance medical communication, diagnosis, and research.

DIAGNOSIS

DIAGNOSTIC CRITERIA SYSTEMS

Diagnostic criteria for delirium first appeared in DSM-III (American Psychiatric Association 1980). Symptom rating scales for delirium began to appear around the time of DSM-III.

DSM-IV (as well as its text revision, DSM-IV-TR) (see Table 5–2) has five categories of delirium; the criteria are the same for each category except the one for etiology. The categories are delirium due to 1) a general medical condition, 2) substance intoxication, 3) substance withdrawal, or 4) multiple etiologies, and 5) delirium not otherwise specified. This notation of etiology in DSM-IV is reminiscent of the first DSM.

DSM-III through DSM-IV-TR include the major criterion that describes altered state of consciousness, considered as either inattention or "clouding of consciousness." The elements of consciousness that are altered are not specified, nor is it clear how "clouding" differs from "level" of consciousness. Attentional disturbance distinguishes delirium from dementia, for which the first criterion is memory impairment. Attentional disturbances in delirium range from general, nonspecific reduction in alertness (typically associated with nicotinic, cholinergic, histaminergic, or adrenergic actions) to decreased selective focusing or sustaining of attention (which may be related to muscarinic cholinergic dysfunction). The contribution of attentional deficits to the altered awareness that occurs in delirium is insufficient by itself to account for other prominent symptoms—formal thought disorder, language and sleep-wake cycle disturbances, and other cognitive-perceptual deficits.

The characteristic features of the temporal course of delirium—acute onset and fluctuation of symptoms—have constituted a separate criterion in DSM-III, DSM-III-R (American Psychiatric Association 1987), and DSM-IV. Temporal features assist in distinguishing delirium from most types of dementia.

TABLE 5–2.   DSM-IV-TR criteria for diagnosis of delirium due to a general medical condition

A.   Disturbance of consciousness (i.e., reduced clarity of awareness of the environment) with reduced ability to focus, sustain, or shift attention.

B.   A change in cognition (such as memory deficit, disorientation, language disturbance) or the development of a perceptual disturbance that is not better accounted for by a preexisting, established, or evolving dementia.

C.   The disturbance develops over a short period of time (usually hours to days) and tends to fluctuate during the course of the day.

D.   There is evidence from the history, physical examination, or laboratory findings that the disturbance is caused by the direct physiological consequences of a general medical condition.

Source.   Reprinted from the *Diagnostic and Statistical Manual of Mental Disorders*, 4th Edition, Text Revision. Washington, DC, American Psychiatric Association, 2000. Copyright 2000, American Psychiatric Association. Used with permission.

Dysexecutive symptoms (impairment of prefrontal executive cognition) are not mentioned in any DSM edition, despite the importance of prefrontal involvement in delirium (Trzepacz 1994a). Psychosis has not received much attention except in DSM-II (American Psychiatric Association 1968), despite the occurrence of delusions in about one-third of patients and hallucinations in slightly more (Meagher 2005; Morita et al. 2004; Webster and Holroyd 2000). Characteristic features of delusions (which are usually paranoid and poorly formed) and hallucinations (often visual) have not been specified in DSM criteria, despite their usefulness to the clinician.

The World Health Organization's ICD-10 (1992) research diagnostic criteria for delirium are similar to DSM-IV-TR criteria but diverge from them in that cognitive dysfunction is manifested by both memory impairment and disorientation, and also by a disturbance in sleep.

Lesser diagnostic emphasis on disorganized thinking in DSM-IV accounts for its greater sensitivity and inclusivity (but lower specificity) in comparison to the other systems.

PRODROMAL SYMPTOMS

Although delirium is usually characterized by an acute onset replete with many symptoms, it may be subclinical. Matsushima et al. (1997) prospectively studied 10 cardiac care unit patients who met DSM-III-R criteria for delirium and 10 nondelirious control subjects and found prodromal changes of background slowing on electroencephalography (EEG) (theta/alpha ratio) and sleep disturbance associated with changing consciousness. Duppils and Wikblad (2004) studied elderly hip surgery patients and found that delirium was preceded by prodromal symptoms in 62%, including disorientation, calls for assistance, and anxiety 2 days before full delirium. De Jonghe et al. (2005) studied delirium symptoms daily with the Delirium Rating Scale—Revised-98 (DRS-R98) in elderly patients undergoing hip surgery. Disorientation, short- and long-term memory disturbance, and inattention occurred during 3 days

before emergence of full delirium, whereas sleep-wake cycle disturbance, hallucinations, and thought process disorder occurred 1 day before, suggesting that cognitive impairments precede sleep-wake and psychotic symptoms. Kaneko et al. (1999) found a close correlation between development of postoperative delirium and decreased nocturnal and excessive daytime sleep. Fann et al. (2005) prospectively followed patients undergoing stem cell transplantation and found both psychobehavioral and cognitive disturbances predated onset of full delirium by 4 days. The best brief tool to assess for prodromal symptoms with a high degree of predictability has not been determined. Nonspecific symptoms such as anxiety or calls for assistance may be less useful than cognitive and sleep-wake items.

SUBSYNDROMAL DELIRIUM

Subsyndromal delirium symptoms in elderly persons may be associated with poorer prognosis, approaching that of the full syndrome. Cole et al. (2003b) prospectively studied subsyndromal delirium in 164 elderly medical patients with one or more of four symptoms—clouding of consciousness, inattention, disorientation, and perceptual disturbances. More symptoms predicted worse prognosis, as evidenced by longer inpatient stays, poorer cognitive and functional status, and greater subsequent mortality at 12-month follow-up. Bourdel-Marchasson et al. (2004) found that subsyndromal delirium (equivalently to full syndromal delirium) predicted postdischarge need for institutional care among elderly patients admitted to medical facilities. Marcantonio et al. (2002) found that reduced independent-living status in elderly postoperative hip surgery patients with subsyndromal delirium was similar to that of patients with mild delirium when both groups were assessed at 6-month follow-up. Moreover, in postacute skilled nursing facilities mortality rates were lower for subsyndromal delirium (18%) than for full delirium (25%) but significantly higher than rates for nondelirious patients (5%) (Marcantonio et al. 2005). Research is lacking in children and nongeriatric adults in whom frailty, diminished cognitive reserve, and dementia are not confounding issues.

MISDIAGNOSIS

Delirium frequently goes undetected in clinical practice. Between one-third and two-thirds of cases are missed across a range of therapeutic settings and by various specialists, including psychiatrists and neurologists (Johnson et al. 1992). Nonrecognition results in poorer outcomes, including increased mortality (Kakuma et al. 2003; Rockwood et al. 1994). Altered mental status was noted in only 16% of elderly emergency department patients with delirium (Hustey et al. 2003).

Misdiagnosis of delirium is more likely in patients who are older; who have sensory impairments, preexisting dementia, or a hypoactive presentation; and who are referred from surgical or intensive care settings (S.C. Armstrong et al. 1997; Inouye et al. 2001). Delirium is commonly misdiagnosed as depression by nonpsychiatrists (Farrell and Ganzini 1995; Nicholas and Lindsey 1995; Trzepacz et al. 1985). ICU populations have delirium prevalence rates ranging from 40% to 87% (Ely et al. 2001b), but delirium is unfortunately understudied and neglected, either because it is "expected" to happen during severe illness or because medical resources are preferentially dedicated to managing the more immediate "life-threatening" problems.

The stereotyped image of delirium as an agitated psychotic state misrepresents most of the patients, who may not have psychotic symptoms or may have a hypoactive presentation (Meagher and Trzepacz 2000). Detection can be improved by assessing cognitive function, improving awareness of the varied presentations of delirium, and routinely using a screening tool (O'Keeffe et al. 2005; Rockwood et al. 1994).

DIFFERENTIAL DIAGNOSIS

Because delirium encompasses so many domains of higher cortical functions, its differ-

ential diagnosis is broad, and it can be mistaken for dementia, depression, primary or secondary psychosis, anxiety and somatoform disorders, and, particularly in children, behavioral disturbance (Table 5–3). Accurate diagnosis requires close attention to symptoms, temporal onset, and results of tests (e.g., cognitive and laboratory measures, EEG, and chart review including medication lists and anesthesia records). Given that delirium can be the presentation for serious medical illness, any patient experiencing a sudden deterioration in cognitive function should be assessed for possible delirium. Urinary tract infections in nursing home patients commonly present as delirium. Delirium occurs commonly in stroke patients (Caeiro et al. 2004a; Ferro et al. 2002) and is frequently the first indication of cerebrovascular accident (L.A. Wahlund and Bjorlin 1999).

Delirium Versus Dementia

The most difficult differential diagnosis for delirium is dementia, the other cause of generalized cognitive impairment. Lewy body dementia has a more aggressive temporal course than Alzheimer's disease and mimics delirium, with fluctuation of symptom severity, visual hallucinations, attentional impairment, alteration of consciousness, and delusions (Robinson 2002). Dementia is a potent predisposing factor for the development of delirium and is often comorbid with delirium in elderly patients.

Despite this substantial overlap, delirium and dementia can be reliably distinguished by a combination of careful history-taking for onset of characteristic symptoms and clinical investigation. Abrupt onset and fluctuating course are highly characteristic of delirium. In addition, attention is markedly disturbed in delirium but relatively intact in uncomplicated dementia, in which memory impairment is instead the cardinal feature. Dementia patients often awaken at night, mistaking it as daytime, whereas disruption of the sleep-wake cycle, including fragmentation throughout 24 hours or even sleeplessness, is more characteristic in patients with delirium.

TABLE 5–3. Differential diagnosis of delirium

	Delirium	Dementia	Depression	Schizophrenia
Onset	Acute	Insidious[a]	Variable	Variable
Course	Fluctuating	Often progressive	Diurnal variation	Variable
Reversibility	Usually[b]	Not usually	Usually but can be recurrent	No, but has exacerbations
Level of consciousness	Impaired	Unimpaired until late stages	Generally unimpaired	Unimpaired (perplexity in acute stage)
Attention and memory	Inattention is primary with poor memory	Poor memory without marked inattention	Mild attention problems, inconsistent pattern, memory intact	Poor attention, inconsistent pattern, memory intact
Hallucinations	Usually visual; can be auditory, tactile, gustatory, olfactory	Can be visual or auditory	Usually auditory	Usually auditory
Delusions	Fleeting, fragmented, usually persecutory	Paranoid, often fixed	Complex and mood congruent	Frequent, complex, systematized, often paranoid

[a]Except for large strokes, which can be abrupt, and Lewy body dementia, which can be subacute.
[b]Can be chronic (as in paraneoplastic syndrome, central nervous system adverse effects of medications, or severe brain damage).

Only a few studies have investigated differences in symptom profile between patients with delirium and patients with dementia (O'Keeffe 1994; Trzepacz and Dew 1995). Trzepacz et al. (2002) used the DRS-R98 and noted significant differences (after Bonferroni correction) between delirium and dementia groups (who had been blindly evaluated) for sleep-wake cycle disturbances, thought process abnormalities, motor agitation, attention, and visuospatial ability, which were more impaired in delirium, but no differences for delusions, affective lability, language, motor retardation, orientation, and short- or long-term memory. Careful assessment can distinguish groups of patients with these two disorders, but more work is needed to clarify differentiating features between delirium and dementia that can be applied to individual cases in clinical practice.

Even more challenging is distinguishing delirium from comorbid delirium-dementia. Most studies find few differences between groups (Cole et al. 2002b; Liptzin et al. 1993; Trzepacz et al. 1998; Voyer et al. 2006). Thus, it appears that when delirium and dementia are comorbid, delirium phenomenology generally overshadows that of the dementia, but when delirium and dementia are assessed as individual conditions, more symptoms can distinguish them, at least by mean scores. These research findings are consistent with the clinical rule of thumb for preventing misattribution of delirium to dementia, namely that "altered cognition reflects delirium until proven otherwise."

Most tools used for delirium assessment have not been validated for their ability to distinguish delirium from dementia, although three have been—the DRS (Trzepacz and Dew 1995), DRS-R98 (Trzepacz et al. 2001, 2002), and Cognitive Test for Delirium (CTD; Hart et al. 1996). Although abnormalities of the EEG are common to both delirium and dementia, diffuse slowing occurs more frequently (81% vs. 33%) in delirium and favors its diagnosis. In contrast, electroencephalographic slowing occurs later in the course of most degenerative dementias, although slowing occurs sooner with viral and prion dementias. The percentage of theta activity on quantitative EEGs allows differentiation of delirium from dementia (Jacobson and Jerrier 2000).

Delirium Versus Mood Disorders

Hypoactive delirium is frequently mistaken for depression (Nicholas and Lindsey 1995). Farrell and Ganzini (1995) found that more than half of delirious patients referred to a consultation-liaison service for "depression" had thoughts of death, and almost one-quarter had suicidal thoughts. Although some symptoms of major depression occur in delirium (e.g., psychomotor slowing, sleep disturbances, irritability), in major depression, symptom onset tends to be less acute, and mood disturbances tend to be more sustained and typically dominate the clinical picture.

The distinction of delirium from depression is particularly important because in addition to delayed treatment, use of antidepressants can aggravate delirium. The more widespread and profound cognitive changes of delirium, along with the etiological backdrop and differing clinical course, usually enable a firm distinction, and EEG can be diagnostic.

Delirium Versus Psychotic Disorders

Abnormalities of thought process and content and misperceptions can occur in both delirium and schizophrenia, but they differ. Delusions in delirium are rarely as fixed or stereotyped as in schizophrenia, and first-rank symptoms are uncommon (Cutting 1987). Delusions are usually persecutory, and sometimes grandiose or somatic, and fragmented because they incorporate aspects of the environment that are poorly comprehended. Paranoid concerns about immediate well-being or perceived danger in the environment are common themes. Unlike in schizophrenia, hallucinations in delirium are more often visual and, on occasion, olfactory, tactile, or gustatory. Tactile hallucinations (including formications) often suggest a hyperdopaminergic or hypocholinergic state. Illusions are common in delirium, while depersonalization, derealization, and delusional misidentification are less common.

Level of consciousness, attention, and memory are generally unimpaired in schizophrenia. Careful physical examination, coupled with EEG and/or a delirium-specific instrument, distinguishes delirium or allows diagnosis of superimposed delirium in medically ill schizophrenic patients.

EPIDEMIOLOGY

INCIDENCE AND PREVALENCE

Delirium occurs at any age. It is understudied in children and adolescents. Most epidemiological studies focus on the elderly, who are at higher risk to develop delirium due to medical burden, frailty, central nervous system (CNS) degeneration, and changes in the brain with aging. Decreased cholinergic activity, often referred to as "reduced brain reserve," underlies many of these factors. CNS disorders (e.g., stroke, hypertensive and diabetic vessel changes, tumor, dementia) further increase vulnerability to delirium.

During the next three decades, the population of those age 60 and older will increase by 159% in less developed countries and by 59% in more developed countries (Jackson 1999). One would expect delirium rates to increase in parallel to the dementia prevalence rates.

Turkel et al. (2003) evaluated children and adolescents (ages 6 months to 19 years) with DSM-IV delirium and found DRS scores comparable to those for adults, with the only difference being fewer delusions and hallucinations in the younger children (mean age = 8 years). Turkel et al. (2006) compared the frequency of delirium symptoms between children and adults across many studies and, despite differences in methodologies and incidences, found delirium phenomenology essentially the same. In preverbal children or noncommunicative adults, clinicians must rely more on inference and observation of changed or unusual behaviors. Hallucinations in delirious children can be misattributed to imaginary friends (Prugh et al. 1980). When the diagnosis is uncertain, EEG shows generalized slowing that normalizes as delirium resolves in children, as in adults (Okamura et al. 2005).

Fann (2000) reviewed prospective studies and found an incidence range from 3% to 42% and a prevalence range from 5% to 44% in hospitalized patients. Up to 60% of nursing home patients older than age 65 (Sandberg et al. 1998), 10%–15% of elderly persons upon hospitalization, and another 10%–40% during hospitalization have delirium. A clinical rule of thumb is that approximately a fifth of general hospital patients have delirium sometime during hospitalization, increasing to 80%–90% in medical ICU and terminal cancer patients (Ely et al. 2001a; Lawlor et al. 2000a).

MORBIDITY AND MORTALITY

Delirium is associated with high rates of morbidity and mortality. It is not known whether the increased mortality rate is 1) solely attributable to the physiological perturbations resulting from the underlying medical causes of delirium, 2) attributable to indirect effects on the body related to perturbations of neuronal (or neuronal-endocrine-immunological) function during delirium, 3) attributable to damaging effects on the brain from neurochemical abnormalities associated with delirium (e.g., dysfunctional cellular metabolism or glutamatergic surges), or 4) related to consequences of delirious patients not fully cooperating with their medical care and rehabilitative programs during hospitalization. Furthermore, their behaviors can directly reduce the effectiveness of procedures meant to treat their medical problems (e.g., removing tubes and intravenous lines, climbing out of bed), as well as result in a higher incidence of serious complications (e.g., falls, infections due to hypostasis, bedsores), which adds to morbidity and possibly to further physiological injury and mortality.

The interpretation of studies of mortality risk associated with delirium is complicated by methodological inconsistencies and shortcomings. Some studies do not compare delirium with control groups, most do not address the effects of treatment, many include comorbid dementia, many do not control for differences in severity or type of medical comorbidity, most do not address effects of advanced age as a separate risk factor, and specific delirium rating instruments are rarely used.

Given these caveats, mortality rates during index hospitalization for a delirium episode range from 4% to 65% (Cameron et al. 1987; Gustafson et al. 1988). When delirium present on admission was excluded, the index mortality rate for incident cases was as low as about 1.5% (Inouye et al. 1999). Some studies found significantly elevated mortality rates for delirium compared with control subjects (Cameron et al. 1987; Jitapunkul et al. 1992; Pompeii et al. 1994; Rabins and Folstein 1982; van Hemert et al. 1994), whereas other studies did not (Forman et al. 1995; George et al. 1997; Gustafson et al. 1988; Inouye et al. 1998, 1999; Kishi et al. 1995). Many studies of longer-term follow-up of delirium mortality rates (more than 3 months after discharge) did find worse mortality rates in delirium groups. Excessive mortality in some reports was attributed to greater age (Gustafson et al. 1988; Huang et al. 1998; Kishi et al. 1995; Trzepacz et al. 1985; Weddington 1982), more serious medical problems (Cole and Primeau 1993; Jitapunkul et al. 1992; Magaziner et al. 1989; Trzepacz et al. 1985), and dementia (Cole and Primeau 1993; Gustafson et al. 1988) as well as severity of delirium symptoms (Marcantonio et al. 2002). Conversely, Curyto et al. (2001) found an increased mortality of 75% at 3 years for delirious compared with control (51%) elderly patients despite no differences in prehospital levels of depression, global cognitive performance, physical functioning, or medical comorbidity. Frail elderly individuals living in nursing facilities studied for 3 months during and after an acute medical hospitalization had high mortality rates of 18% in the hospital and 46% at 3 months that were associated with severe and persistent delirium (Kelly et al. 2001). Leslie et al. (2005) found that hospitalized elderly patients with delirium had a 62% increased risk of mortality at 1-year follow-up

and lost an average of 13% of a year of life compared with nondelirious control subjects.

Inouye et al. (1998) found that delirium significantly increased mortality risk, even after controlling for age, sex, dementia, activities of daily living (ADL) level, and Acute Physiology and Chronic Health Evaluation II (APACHE II; Knaus et al. 1985) scores. Ely et al. (2004a) reported that delirium in medical ICU patients was independently associated with a greater than 300% increased likelihood of dying at 6 months ($P = 0.008$), even after correcting for numerous covariates including coma and use of psychoactive medications. McCusker et al. (2002) found delirium a significant predictor of 12-month mortality for older inpatients, even after adjusting for age, sex, marital status, living location, comorbidity, acute physiological severity, illness severity, dementia, and hospital service. Pitkälä and colleagues (2005) found delirium predicted mortality and institutionalization in an elderly population at both 1- and 2-year follow-up, even when level of frailty was accounted for.

Better outcomes, including reduced mortality, result when delirium is actively identified and treated. In emergency departments, 30 delirious and 77 nondelirious elderly patients who had been discharged to their homes were assessed at 6-month follow-up intervals until 18 months (Kakuma et al. 2003). After adjusting for age, sex, functional level, cognitive status, comorbidity, and number of medications, delirium was significantly associated with increased mortality. Those whose delirium was not detected by the emergency department staff had the highest mortality over 6 months compared with those whose delirium was detected; no mortality difference was seen between the patients whose delirium was detected and the nondelirious patients, emphasizing the importance of detection.

Even though the mechanism is not understood, delirium is associated with an increased risk for mortality, extending well beyond the index hospitalization, that might be reduced by aggressive treatment of both the delirium and its comorbid medical problems, except possibly in the frailest elderly patients.

LENGTH OF STAY

Most, but not all, studies have found significantly increased length of stay (LOS) associated with delirium. A meta-analysis of eight studies (Cole and Primeau 1993) supports both numerical and statistical differences between delirium patient and control groups' LOS. Delirium duration was associated with LOS in both the medical ICU and the hospital ($P \leq 0.0001$) and was the strongest predictor of LOS, even after Ely et al. (2001a) adjusted for illness severity, age, gender, and days of opiate and narcotic use. McCusker et al. (2003b) studied elderly medical inpatients and found significantly longer LOS for incident, but not prevalent, delirium. The Academy of Psychosomatic Medicine Task Force on Mental Disorders in General Medical Practice (Saravay and Strain 1994) reviewed outcomes of delirium and reported that comorbid delirium increased LOS 100% in general medical patients (R.I. Thomas et al. 1988), 114% in elderly patients (Schor et al. 1992), 67% in stroke patients (Cushman et al. 1998), 300% in critical care patients (Kishi et al. 1995), 27% in cardiac surgery patients, and 200%–250% in hip surgery patients (Berggren et al. 1987). They noted that delirium contributes to increased LOS via medical and behavioral mechanisms, including decreased motivation to participate in treatment and rehabilitation, medication refusal, disruptive behavior, incontinence and urinary tract infections, falls and fractures, and decubitus. Saravay et al. (2004) prospectively assessed chronology of cognitive and behavioral symptoms in hospitalized patients and found that delirium and dementia contribute to increased LOS via their consequences, such as falls, pulled intravenous lines, incontinence, restraints, and decreased cooperation.

REDUCED INDEPENDENCE

Decreased independent living status and increased rate of institutionalization in the elderly during follow-up after a delirium episode were found in many studies (Cole and Primeau 1993; George et al. 1997; Inouye et al. 1998; Pitkälä et al. 2005), as were reduction in ambulation and/or ADL level at follow-up (Francis and Kapoor 1992; Gustafson et al. 1988; Inouye et al. 1998; Minagawa et al. 1996; Murray et al. 1993). Pitkälä et al. (2005) identified delirium as an independent predictor of loss of independence and mortality at 2-year follow-up in a study of frail elderly patients older than 70 years. Elderly femoral neck fracture patients who had delirium on admission or postoperatively were more dependent in their ADL both at discharge and 4 months later (B. Olofsson et al. 2005). Even subsyndromal delirium is reported to increase index admission LOS and reduce postdischarge functional level and mortality after adjusting for age, sex, marital status, previous living arrangement, comorbidity, dementia status, and clinical or physiological severity of illness (Cole et al. 2003b; Marcantonio et al. 2005).

COST OF CARE

Delirium results in greater costs of care. Franco et al. (2001) found higher professional consultation, technical, and routine nursing care costs in delirious patients older than 50 years who were undergoing elective surgery. Milbrandt et al. (2004) found 39% increased cost associated with having at least one delirium episode in 183 mechanically ventilated medical ICU patients, even though analysis controlled for multiple confounds such as age, comorbidity of illness, degree of organ dysfunction, and nosocomial infection. Median ICU costs per patient were 60% greater and total hospital costs were 65% higher in delirious patients. Fick et al. (2005) studied health care costs from administrative records of a managed care organization for 76,000 community-dwelling elderly patients and found that costs were twice as high for patients with delirium and especially increased for patients with delirium superimposed on dementia compared with those with either condition alone. The elevated health care costs were related to cerebrovascular disease, urinary tract infections, pneumonia, and dehydration and resulted in greater facility costs and more emergency department and nursing home visits.

DISTRESS AND PSYCHOLOGICAL SEQUELAE

Delirium is frequently a distressing experience for patients and their caregivers. Delirium-recovered patients may be uncomfortable discussing their delirium episodes—even to the extent of denial—because of fear that they may be "senile" or "mad" (Schofield 1997). When Breitbart et al. (2002a) used the Delirium Experience Questionnaire to rate 101 cancer patients with a resolved delirium episode, their spouses, and their nurses, 43% recalled their episode, and recall depended on delirium severity. Mean distress levels were high for patients at 3.2 points (scored 0–4) and nurses at 3.1, but were highest for spouses at 3.8. However, among delirious patients who did not recall the episode ($n = 47$), the mean distress level was only 1.5. Fann et al. (2005) found that in patients undergoing hematopoietic stem cell transplantation, level of affective distress was closely linked to delirium severity. In nondemented elderly patients with delirium, O'Keeffe (2005) found that more than half were able to recall psychotic symptoms and that many continued to be distressed by their recollections 6 months later. Thus, delirium can have a great psychological effect on patients and those who care for them, yet it is often overlooked in the treatment care plan.

REVERSIBILITY OF A DELIRIUM EPISODE

Delirium traditionally has been distinguished from dementia by its potential for reversal and its transient neurobiological state. Bedford's (1957) study of delirium found that only 5% of the patients were still "confused" at 6-month follow-up. Elderly patients may not have full resolution of symptoms at hospital discharge. Levkoff et al. (1992) found that only 4% of the elderly patients with delirium had complete

resolution of symptoms at discharge, 20.8% at 6 weeks, and 17.7% at 6 months, but they did not exclude comorbid dementia patients. McCusker et al. (2003a) found that 12 months after diagnosis of delirium in elderly medical inpatients, inattention, disorientation, and poor memory were the most persistent individual symptoms both in those with and in those without concomitant dementia (see next section, "Persistent Cognitive Deficits").

One explanation for persisting impairments may be incomplete treatment or recurring course of delirium (Meagher 2001a). The ever-increasing financial pressures to shorten hospital stays have resulted in many patients being discharged from the hospital before delirium has resolved, even though families and nursing homes are not resourced to manage delirium to its resolution. Kiely et al. (2004) studied 2,158 patients from seven Boston-area skilled nursing facilities and found that 16% had a full-blown delirium. They warned of the adverse effect of delirium persisting in subacute care settings. Marcantonio et al. (2005) assessed 1,248 elderly patients soon after admission to postacute facilities and found that 15% had delirium and another 51% had subsyndromal delirium.

PERSISTENT COGNITIVE DEFICITS

In the elderly, the term *persistent cognitive impairment* in the weeks or months following a delirium episode during a medical-surgical hospitalization is used, but its neuropsychological pattern and etiology are not clear and are highly confounded by difficult-to-measure comorbid pathophysiologies. Possible causes of persistent cognitive difficulties in patients who have experienced delirium are shown in Figure 5–1.

The increased diagnosis of dementia in patients who had an episode of delirium suggests a preexisting dementia heralded by the delirium. Kolbeinsson and Jonsson (1993) found that delirium was complicated by dementia at follow-up in 70% of patients. Rahkonen et al. (2000) found that when the index episode of delirium resolved, a new diagnosis of dementia was made in 27% of 51 prospectively studied

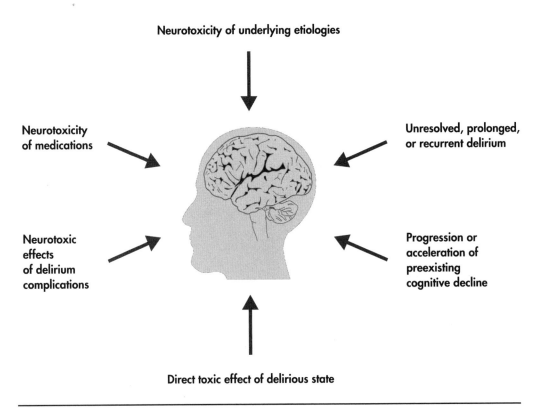

Neurotoxicity of underlying etiologies

Neurotoxicity of medications

Unresolved, prolonged, or recurrent delirium

Neurotoxic effects of delirium complications

Progression or acceleration of preexisting cognitive decline

Direct toxic effect of delirious state

FIGURE 5–1. Possible reasons for persistent cognitive impairment in patients after an episode of delirium.

community-dwelling elderly individuals, and at 2-year follow-up, a total of 55% had a new diagnosis of dementia. Rockwood et al. (1999) reported an 18% annual incidence of dementia in patients with delirium—a more than three times higher risk than in nondelirious patients when the confounding effects of comorbid illness severity and age were adjusted for.

Persistent cognitive deficits appear to indicate a previously undiagnosed dementia that progresses after delirium resolution. In 252 community-dwelling older people, 64% had a new diagnosis of dementia (Sternberg et al. 2000). Koponen et al.'s (1994) 5-year longitudinal study of delirium in the elderly attributed persistence and progression of symptoms more to the underlying dementia than to the previous delirium episode. Similarly, in a cross-sectional study of consecutive psychogeriatric admissions, the only factor significantly linked to incomplete symptom resolution in

delirium was the presence of preexisting cognitive impairment (Camus et al. 2000). Kasahara et al. (1996) compared delirium and dementia in young (35–45 years) and aged (older than 60 years) alcoholic patients and found similar frequency of delirium but no cases of dementia in the younger group, compared with 62% of the aged group. Therefore, younger adults with delirium either have better brain recovery than elders do or are at less risk for degenerative and vascular dementias that can be misattributed to delirium persistence.

RISK FACTORS FOR DELIRIUM

Risk factors are external or intrinsic variables that increase the likelihood of experiencing delirium and should not be confused with causes of delirium. Delirium is particularly common during hospitalization when there is a confluence of both predisposing factors—that is, vulnerabilities related to the individual, including genetics—and precipitating factors related to external stressors, medications, illness, surgery, and so on. Patient-related, illness-related, procedure-related, pharmacological, and environmental factors have been identified as risk factors for delirium, as illustrated in Figure 5–2. Risk factors identified for the elderly are not the same as those for ICU patients or children. More research is needed to identify setting-specific and age-specific risk factors that are highly predictive and possibly modifiable as preventive strategies.

Stress-vulnerability models for the occurrence of delirium have been long recognized. Henry and Mann (1965) described "delirium readiness." More recent models of causation describe cumulative interactions between predisposing (vulnerability) factors and precipitating insults (Inouye and Charpentier 1996; O'Keeffe and Lavan 1996). Baseline risk is a more potent predictor of the likelihood of delirium: if baseline vulnerability is low, then patients are very resistant to the development of delirium despite exposure to significant precipitating factors, whereas if baseline vulnerability is high, then delirium is likely even in response to minor precipitants. Tsutsui et al. (1996), for example, found that in patients older than 80 years, delirium occurred in 52% after emergency surgery and in 20% after elective procedures, whereas no case of delirium was noted in patients younger than 50 undergoing either elective or emergency procedures. It is generally believed that the aged brain is more vulnerable to delirium, in part related to structural and degenerative changes as well as altered neurochemical flexibility. Children are also considered to be at higher risk for delirium, possibly related to developmental immaturity of brain structure and chemistry.

Although the value of reducing risk factors appears self-evident, many risk factors may simply be markers of general morbidity, and therefore studies documenting preventive effects are important. Some risk factors are proxies for actual causes—in the elderly, a bladder catheter may increase risk for delirium because of infection risk or may indicate an infection that is an etiology.

Some risk factors are potentially modifiable and thus are targets for preventive or prompter interventions. Medication exposure is probably the most readily modifiable risk factor for delirium, being implicated as a cause in 20%–40% of cases of delirium. Marcantonio et al. (2001) reported that proactive geriatric consultation with a protocol advising on 10 aspects of care reduced both incidence and severity of delirium in an elderly hip fracture population. In contrast, systematic detection of and multidisciplinary care for delirium produced minimal improvement in outcome of older medical inpatients, many with comorbid dementia (Cole et al. 2002a).

AGE

The aged brain is more vulnerable to delirium, in part related to structural and degenerative changes and reduced neurochemical flexibility. However, children are also considered at higher risk for delirium, possibly because of ongoing microstructural and neurochemical brain development. For example, pruning of synaptic bulbs and maturation of the cholinergic system continue into mid-adolescence, particularly in layer III of the prefrontal cortex. This layer is an associative area that interconnects with other brain association regions and is important for executive cognitive functions; this layer develops slowly throughout childhood, is especially affected by Alzheimer's neuropathological changes in the elderly, and is highly cholinergic. Perhaps immaturity or degeneration of this prefrontal cholinergic layer is relevant to vulnerability for delirium. Advanced age is also associated with a higher frequency of other risk factors such as cognitive impairment and vulnerability to drug toxicity. The elderly have diminished renal and hepatic function as well as reduced water-to-fat content ratio. Moreover, the effects of drugs are mitigated less by counterregulatory homeostatic mechanisms (Turnheim 2003).

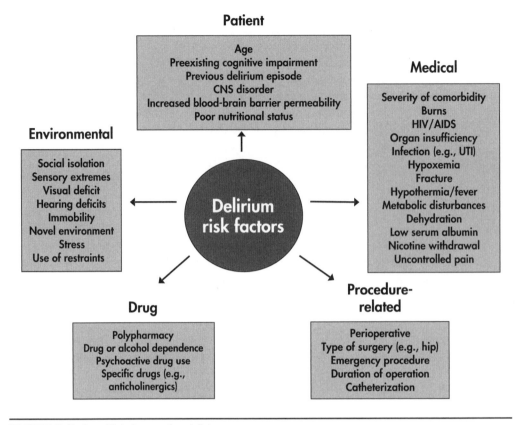

FIGURE 5–2.   Risk factors for delirium.

AIDS = acquired immunodeficiency syndrome; CNS = central nervous system; HIV = human immunodeficiency virus; UTI = urinary tract infection.

PREEXISTING COGNITIVE IMPAIRMENT

Up to two-thirds of the cases of delirium occur superimposed on preexisting cognitive impairment (L. A. Wahlund and Bjorlin 1999). Delirium is 2–3.5 times more common in patients with dementia than in control subjects without dementia (Erkinjuntti et al. 1986; Jitapunkul et al. 1992). Delirium risk appears to be greater in Alzheimer's disease of late onset and in vascular dementia than in other dementias, perhaps reflecting the relatively widespread neuronal disturbance associated with these conditions (Robertsson et al. 1998). Marcantonio et al. (2005) found that nondelirious elderly patients admitted to postacute facilities had virtually no preexisting dementia compared with those who had become delirious.

MEDICATIONS

Polypharmacy and drug intoxication or withdrawal may be the most common causes of delirium, but drug use is also a risk factor (Gaudreau et al. 2005b; Hales et al. 1988; Inouye and Charpentier 1996; Kagansky et al. 2004; Trzepacz et al. 1985). Benzodiazepines, opiates, and drugs with anticholinergic activity have a particular association with delirium (T. M. Brown 2000; Marcantonio et al. 1994). In hospitalized cancer patients, delirium risk is increased at cumulative daily doses of greater than 90 mg of morphine equivalents, greater than 15 mg of dexamethasone equivalents, and greater than 2 mg of lorazepam equivalents (Gaudreau et al. 2005a). In elderly hip fracture patients, midazolam use was significantly related to delirium incidence (Santos et al.

2005). L. Han et al. (2001) studied older patients with preexisting delirium and found that exposure to anticholinergic medications worsened delirium. Many drugs (and their metabolites) can unexpectedly contribute to delirium as a result of unrecognized anticholinergic effects. Ten of the 25 most commonly prescribed drugs for the elderly had sufficient in vitro anticholinergic activity identified by radioreceptor assay to cause memory and attention impairment in elderly subjects without delirium (Tune et al. 1992). White et al. (2005) identified altered drug metabolism as a possible factor in delirium. Spectrophotometry identified reduced plasma esterase activity (including acetylcholinesterase and butyrylcholinesterase) in elderly patients with delirium compared with nondelirious control subjects and also found that mortality was associated with low plasma esterase activity at admission. It is therefore important to minimize drug exposure, especially when elderly patients are facing high-risk periods such as the perioperative phase.

NEUROLOGICAL INSULTS

Delirium can be an important presenting feature of cerebrovascular disease. L. A. Wahlund and Bjorlin (1999) found that stroke without other neurological signs accounted for 14% of all cases of delirium, and Ferro et al. (2002) found that delirium can complicate the course of acute stroke in up to 48% of patients. Caeiro et al. (2004b) found that delirium was more common after hemorrhagic rather than ischemic stroke and that anticholinergic medications were a particular risk factor. Delirium was more common after hemispheric than brain stem or cerebellar stroke—in particular, after right middle cerebral artery lesions—and after intracerebral rather than subarachnoid hemorrhage or cerebral infarct (Caeiro et al. 2004a). Delirium incidence was 16% in 68 consecutive cases of acute subarachnoid hemorrhage and was associated with admission computed tomography scan evidence of intraventricular bleeding, hydrocephalus, and basofrontal hematomas, suggesting damage to

networks subserving attention, declarative memory, and emotional expression (Caeiro et al. 2005).

PAIN CONTROL MEDICATIONS

Delirium has a relationship to both overuse of pain control medications and undertreatment of acute pain. Delirium was nine times more likely in older patients undergoing hip surgery deemed to have undertreated pain (Morrison et al. 2003), and delirium was associated with higher scores of bodily pain perioperatively (Duppils and Wikblad 2004). Similarly, Adunsky et al. (2002) found lower use of analgesia in patients developing delirium. Fann et al. (2005) found that a rise in pain severity predated delirium severity by 3 days. B. Gagnon et al. (2001) identified alterations in the circadian pattern that the experience of pain typically follows as indicated by greater use of analgesia for breakthrough pain in delirious patients. Use of meperidine may be associated with an elevated risk of delirium (Adunsky et al. 2002; Morrison et al. 2003). An open-label switch from morphine to fentanyl in delirious cancer patients was associated with reduced delirium and pain severity and an escalation of opioid doses (Morita et al. 2005). Patient-controlled analgesia is associated with less overall opiate use, reduced delirium incidence (Tokita et al. 2001), and shorter duration of delirium when it occurs (Mann et al. 2000). Therefore, careful attention to pain medicine use is important.

NUTRITIONAL FACTORS

Thiamine deficiency is an underappreciated cause of and/or risk factor for delirium in pediatric intensive care and oncology patients (Seear et al. 1992) and nonalcoholic elderly patients (O'Keeffe et al. 1994). Thiamine is a cofactor necessary for adequate functioning of cholinergic neurons.

Low serum albumin is an important risk factor at any age and may signify poor nutrition, chronic disease, or liver or renal insufficiency. Hypoalbuminemia results in a greater bioavailability of many drugs that are transported in the bloodstream by albumin, and this is associated with an increased risk of side effects, including delirium (Dickson 1991; Trzepacz and Francis 1990). This increased biological drug activity occurs within the therapeutic range and is not recognized because increased levels of free drug are not reported separately in assays. Serum albumin was identified by discriminant analysis, along with Trail Making Test Part B and EEG dominant posterior rhythm, to sensitively distinguish delirious from nondelirious liver transplant candidates (Trzepacz et al. 1988b). Low serum albumin, along with advanced age, cognitive impairment, bone metastases, and a hematological malignancy, was predictive of delirium in oncology patients (Ljubisljevic and Kelly 2003).

PERIOPERATIVE FACTORS

Postoperative delirium (excluding emergence from anesthesia) appears most frequently at day 3. Van der Mast and Fekkes (2000) proposed that surgery induces immune activation and a physical stress response. This comprises of increased limbic-hypothalamic-pituitary-adrenocortical axis activity, low triiodothyronine syndrome, and altered blood-brain barrier permeability. Increased blood-brain barrier permeability is a risk factor for delirium, as occurs in uremia. A large multicenter study (International Study of Post-Operative Cognitive Dysfunction) found age, duration of anesthesia, lower education level, second operation, postoperative infection, and respiratory complications to be predictors of postoperative cognitive impairment (Moller et al. 1998). Other work has identified type of surgery (e.g., cardiothoracic), duration of operation, intraoperative complications, and emergency nature of procedure as perioperative factors associated with an elevated risk of delirium (Agnoletti et al. 2005; Bucerius et al. 2004). In postcardiotomy surgery, urgency of operation, intraoperative factors, and cerebrovascular disease were independent predictors of delirium (Bucerius et al. 2004).

Pratico and colleagues (2005) have proposed a model by which anesthetics acting on central cholinergic systems may cause postoperative delirium, but in a review of 20 randomized controlled trials that examined the role of anesthetic choice in postoperative cognitive dysfunction, Wu et al. (2004) found no evidence that general anesthetics were associated with a greater risk than regional anesthetics.

GENETIC FACTORS

Several studies have addressed the influence of genetic factors in delirium vulnerability. To date, these have focused mostly on alcohol withdrawal delirium and suggest positive associations between the risk of delirium tremens and polymorphisms of genes for neuropeptide Y (Koehnke et al. 2002), a glutamatergic kainate receptor subunit (Preuss et al. 2003, 2006), a cannabinoid receptor (Schmidt et al. 2002), and brain-derived neurotrophic factor (BDNF) (Matsushita et al. 2004). Conversely, studies of genes for norepinephrine transporter (Samochowiec et al. 2002), dopamine β-hydroxylase (Köhnke et al. 2006), glutamate transporter (Sander et al. 2000), metabotropic glutamate receptors (Preuss et al. 2002), BDNF (Matsushita et al. 2004), and N-methyl-D-aspartate receptor subunits (Rujescu et al. 2005; Tadic et al. 2005) have not identified significant associations with delirium propensity. Studies of the dopamine transporter gene have been both positive (Gorwood et al. 2003; Wernicke et al. 2002) and negative (Köhnke et al. 2005).

A few studies addressed the role of genetic factors in the expression of delirium symptoms as well as treatment response to antipsychotics in delirium. These studies suggested that visual hallucinations during alcohol withdrawal delirium are more frequent in subjects with the A9 allele of the dopamine transporter gene (Limosin et al. 2004), cholecystokinin A receptor (Okubo et al. 2002) and promoter gene (Okubo et al. 2000) polymorphisms, catechol-O-methyltransferase (COMT) polymorphisms (A. Nakamura et al. 2001), and NRH:quinone oxidoreductase 2 polymorphisms (an enzyme involved in alcohol metabolism) (Okubo et al. 2003). J.Y. Kim et al. (2005) did not find any relation between dopamine transporter gene polymorphisms and responsiveness to risperidone or haloperidol in medical-surgical patients. Pomara et al. (2004) studied the relation between the apolipoprotein E (APOE) genotype and sensitivity to anticholinergic medication exposure (trihexyphenidyl hydrochloride) in cognitively intact elderly individuals and found that subjects with the *APOE*E4* allele experienced significantly greater cognitive impairment. On a similar note, van Munster et al. (2005) studied the *APOE* genotype in a small sample of elderly general hospital patients and were unable to find an association with delirium risk.

ETIOLOGIES OF DELIRIUM

Delirium has a wide variety of etiologies alone or in combination. Figure 5–3 is a part of the Delirium Etiology Checklist (Paula Trzepacz, personal communication, 2006), a standardized tool used to determine etiologies within 13 categories; the etiologies can then be rated for degree of likelihood on the basis of overall clinical evaluation of a patient (scoresheet not shown). These categories include primary CNS disorders, systemic disturbances that affect cerebral function, and drug or toxin exposure (including intoxication and withdrawal). Often multiple etiologies occur serially in addition to concurrently and may prolong the delirium episode. We hypothesize that delirium severity is a function of an individual's baseline delirium vulnerability, such as age or genetics, interacting with multiple overlapping or serial etiologies, as illustrated in Figure 5–4.

Between two and six possible causes are typically identified (Breitbart et al. 1996; Francis et al. 1990; Meagher et al. 1996; O'Keeffe 1999; Trzepacz et al. 1985), with a single etiology identified in 50% or fewer of the cases (Camus et al. 2000; Morita et al. 2001; O'Keeffe 1999; S.M. Olofsson et al. 1996; Ramirez-Bermudez et al. 2006). It is important that clinicians consider further investigation after one likely cause is determined. Multiple-etiology delirium is more frequent in the elderly and those with terminal illness. For example, delirium in cancer patients can be due to the direct

effect of the primary tumor or an indirect effect of metastases, metabolic problems (organ failure or electrolyte disturbance), chemotherapy, radiation and other treatments, infections, vascular complications, nutritional deficits, and paraneoplastic syndromes.

Some causes occur more frequently in particular populations. Drugs and polypharmacy commonly cause or contribute to delirium, especially in elderly patients (T.M. Brown 2000). Drug-related causes are more commonly reported in psychiatric populations. Delirium in children and adolescents involves the same categories of etiologies as in adults, although specific causes may differ. Delirium related to illicit drugs is more common in younger populations, whereas that due to prescribed drugs and polypharmacy is more common in older populations. Cerebral hypoxia is common at age extremes, with chronic obstructive airway disease, myocardial infarction, and stroke common in older patients and hypoxia due to foreign body inhalation, drowning, or asthma more frequent in younger patients. Poisonings are also more common in children than in adults, whereas children and the elderly both have high rates of delirium related to head trauma—bicycle accidents in children and falls in the elderly.

Once the diagnosis of delirium is made, a careful and thorough, although prioritized, search for causes must be conducted. Ameliorations of specific underlying causes are important in resolving delirium, although this should not preclude treatment of the delirium itself, which can reduce symptoms even before underlying medical causes are rectified (Breitbart et al. 1996).

DELIRIUM DETECTION, SCREENING, AND ASSESSMENT

Given the high rates of missed diagnosis, there is a great need for brief screening tools that enable prompt recognition of delirium with high sensitivity even if specificity is lower. Screening tools can provide a provisional diag-

Drug Intoxication
1❑ Alcohol   3❑ Opiate   5❑ Hallucinogenic   6❑ Prescribed drug _____
2❑ Sedative-hypnotic   4❑ Psychostimulant   7❑ Other _____
                                                                8❑ OTC _____

Drug Withdrawal
1❑ Alcohol   3❑ Prescribed drug _____
2❑ Sedative-hypnotic   4❑ Other drug _____

Metabolic/Endocrine Disturbance
1❑ Volume depletion   6❑ Uremia   12❑ Hypoalbuminemia   21❑ Hypomagnesiemia
2❑ Volume overload   7❑ Anemia   13❑ Hyperalbuminemia   22❑ Hypermagnesiemia
3❑ Acidosis   8❑ Avitaminosis _____   14❑ Bilirubinemia   23❑ Hypophosphatemia
4❑ Alkalosis   9❑ Hypervitaminosis _____   15❑ Hypocalcemia   24❑ Hypothyroidism
5❑ Hypoxia   10❑ Hypoglycemia   16❑ Hypercalcemia   25❑ Hyperthyroidism
                       11❑ Hyperglycemia   17❑ Hypokalemia   26❑ Hypoparathyroidism
                                           18❑ Hyperkalemia   27❑ Hyperparathyroidism
                                           19❑ Hyponatremia   28❑ Cushing's syndrome
30❑ Other_____   20❑ Hypernatremia   29❑ Addison's disease

❑ Traumatic Brain Injury

❑ Seizures

Intracranial Infection
1❑ Meningitis   3❑ Abscess   5❑ HIV
2❑ Encephalitis   4❑ Neurosyphilis   6❑ Other _____

Systemic Infection
1❑ Bacteremia   3❑ Fungal   5❑ Viral   7❑ Urinary
2❑ Sepsis   4❑ Protozoal   6❑ Respiratory   8❑ Other _____

Intracranial Neoplasm
1❑ Primary   2❑ Metastasis   3❑ Meningeal carcinomatosis
Histology _____   Site _____

Extracranial Neoplasm
Site of primary lesion _____   ❑ Paraneoplastic syndrome

Cerebrovascular Disorder
1❑ Transient ischemic attack   3❑ Stroke   6❑ Intraparenchymal hemorrhage
2❑ Subarachnoid hemorrhage   4❑ Subdural hemorrhage 7❑ Cerebral vasculitis
                                5❑ Cerebral edema   8❑ Other _____

Organ Insufficiency
1❑ Cardiac   3❑ Hepatic   5❑ Pancreatic
2❑ Pulmonary   4❑ Renal   6❑ Other _____

Other CNS
1❑ Parkinson's disease   3❑ Multiple sclerosis   5❑ Hydrocephalus
2❑ Huntington's disease   4❑ Wilson's disease   6❑ Other _____

Other Systemic
1❑ Heatstroke   3❑ Radiation   5❑ Immunosuppressed   7❑ Fractures
2❑ Hypothermia   4❑ Postoperative state   6❑ Other_____
© Trzepacz 1999

FIGURE 5–3.   Delirium Etiology Checklist worksheet.

Contact author for copy of complete checklist (PTT@lilly.com).

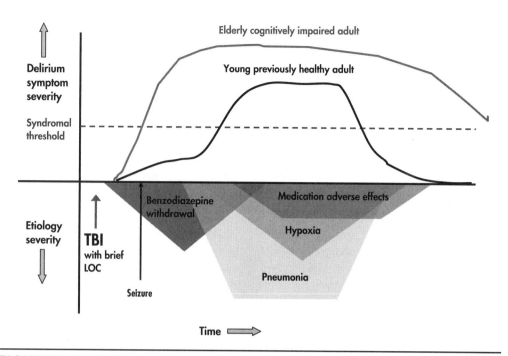

FIGURE 5–4. Delirium severity as a function of an individual's baseline delirium vulnerability interacting with multiple overlapping or serial etiologies.

TBI = traumatic brain injury; LOC = loss of consciousness.

nosis but often have poor differential diagnostic capability.

Screening tools for delirium need to be convenient for use in day-to-day practice as well as suitable for use by nonpsychiatric physicians and nurses. The Confusion Assessment Method (CAM) is probably the most widely used delirium screening tool in general hospitals (Inouye et al. 1990). It is based on DSM-III-R criteria and requires the presence of three of four cardinal symptoms of delirium. It is intended for use by nonpsychiatric clinicians in hospital settings and is useful for case finding, although nurses' ratings were much less sensitive than those done by physicians (1.00 vs. 0.13) when compared with an independent physician's DSM-III-R diagnosis (Rolfson et al. 1999). It has not been well studied for its ability to distinguish delirium from dementia, depression, or other psychiatric disorders. Cole et al. (2003a) assessed the sensitivity and specificity of the full CAM in patients with DSM-III-R–diagnosed delirium, dementia, or comor-

bid delirium-dementia. When these investigators used a cutoff of 6 of 11 items present, they found 95% sensitivity and 83% specificity in delirium-only cases and 98% sensitivity and 76% specificity in comorbid cases; however, when they used fewer items, such as a minimum cutoff of 3 symptoms, the specificities were greatly reduced, to 60% for delirium and 47% for comorbid delirium-dementia.

Because delirium is primarily a cognitive disorder, bedside assessment of cognition is critical to proper diagnosis. All cognitive domains are affected—orientation, attention, short- and long-term memory, visuoconstructional ability, and executive functions (the latter are poorly studied in delirium)—even though attentional deficits are most specifically emphasized in DSM. Pattern and timing of deficits assist in differential diagnosis from dementias and amnestic disorders.

Use of bedside screening tests such as the Mini-Mental State Examination (MMSE) allows documentation of the presence of a cognitive disorder, although the MMSE alone is insufficient to distinguish delirium from dementia (Rolfson et al. 1999; Trzepacz et al. 1988a). The MMSE is easy for many people (ceiling effect) and has a limited breadth of items, particularly for prefrontal executive and right hemisphere functions.

Trail Making Test Part B along with reduced serum albumin and EEG dominant posterior rhythm distinguished delirious from nondelirious liver transplant candidates with 97% sensitivity and 83% specificity (Trzepacz et al. 1988a). Fann et al. (2002) found that patients who developed delirium after stem cell transplantation had lower Trail Making Test Part B scores pretransplant. The Trail Making Test Part B may be a useful test to screen for delirium risk or monitor delirium, although the patient needs to be able to write.

The Clock Drawing Test assesses constructional praxis, visuospatial ability, executive function, and verbal and semantic memory. Fisher and Flowerdew (1995) found that the Clock Drawing Test was superior to the MMSE for predicting risk of postoperative delirium in older patients. Manos (1997) found the Clock Drawing Test to be a useful screen for cognitive impairment in medically ill patients, even though it did not discriminate between delirium and dementia. K.Y. Kim et al. (2003) used the Clock Drawing Test and MMSE to plot treatment response to quetiapine in delirium and found that scores on both tests improved as delirium resolved over a 4-week period. However, Rolfson et al. (1999) found that neither the Clock Drawing Test nor the MMSE was a sensitive marker of delirium in elderly cardiac surgery patients. The Clock Drawing Test detects overall cognitive impairment in elderly medical inpatients but lacks specificity for either the severity or the presence of delirium (Adamis et al. 2005); however, it correlated reasonably with the DRS ($r=-0.60$) and MMSE ($r=0.70$).

COGNITIVE ASSESSMENT

The CTD (Hart et al. 1996) is a bedside cognitive test designed specifically for delirious patients, who are often unable to speak or write in a medical setting. The CTD correlates highly with the MMSE ($r=0.82$) in delirium patients and was performable in 42% of the ICU patients in whom the MMSE was not. It has two equivalent forms that correlate highly ($r=0.90$), which allows for repeated measurements. However, it correlates less well with symptom rating scales for delirium that include noncognitive symptoms—for example, the Medical College of Virginia Nurses Rating Scale for Delirium (Hart et al. 1996) ($r=-0.02$) or the DRS-R98 (Trzepacz et al. 2001) ($r=-0.62$). The CTD has many nonverbal (nondominant hemisphere) items and includes abstraction questions. R.E. Kennedy et al. (2003) tested the CTD in 65 traumatic brain injury patients in a neurorehabilitation hospital and found 72% sensitivity and 70% specificity compared with DSM-IV diagnoses of delirium.

It has been theorized that prefrontal and right hemisphere circuits are especially important in delirium neuropathophysiology (Trzepacz 1994a, 1999b, 2000). Two studies found that just a few cognitive tests (e.g., similarities and Digit Span Forward) were able to discriminate delirious from nondelirious medical patients. One assessed only right hemisphere functions—visual attention span forward and recognition memory for pictures (Hart et al. 1997)—and the other assessed prefrontal functions (Bettin et al. 1998).

DELIRIUM ASSESSMENT INSTRUMENTS

Diagnostic criteria are important in diagnosing delirium, and cognitive tests are useful to document cognitive impairment. Rating the severity of the broad range of delirium symptoms, however, requires other methods. The choice of instrument is dictated by many factors, as listed in Table 5–4. Unfortunately, the increase in the number of instruments developed for delirium assessment has not been matched by an equivalent body of research to support their use by confirming suitability for use in different populations with well-designed psychometric studies. More than 10 instruments have

TABLE 5–4. Factors relevant to choice of delirium assessment instrument

Purpose of the assessment

Screening

Diagnosis

Severity

Serial measurement of profile

Range of symptoms measured

Assessor

Nurse

Physician

Trained researcher

Ease of use

Time available

Need for training

Population to be studied and location

Ability to cooperate with procedure

Validity in different populations

Psychometric properties of the instrument

Reliability

Internal consistency

Validity

been proposed to assess symptoms of delirium for screening, diagnosis, or symptom severity rating (Trzepacz 1994b). However, only a few of these have been used broadly (see descriptions below). Three instruments operationalized DSM-III criteria: the Saskatoon Delirium Checklist (Miller et al. 1988), the Organic Brain Syndrome Scale (Berggren et al. 1987), and the Delirium Assessment Scale (O'Keeffe 1994). In these, DSM-III–derived items are rated along a continuum of mild, moderate, and severe. None has been well described or validated. The Delirium Assessment Scale could not distinguish delirium from dementia patients. A more recently developed severity scale, the Confusional State Evaluation (Robertsson 1999), assessed 22 items, but 12 were

determined a priori to be "key symptoms." It was not validated against control groups, and dementia patients were included in the delirium group.

The most commonly used delirium assessment tool by nurses is the NEECHAM Confusion Scale (Neelon et al. 1986). It is scored from 0 to 30 with cutoffs for levels of confusion severity and was originally validated in elderly acute medical and nursing home settings without a control group. Interrater reliability was 0.96, correlation with the MMSE was 0.81, and correlation with nurses' subjective ratings was 0.46. It has three sections—information processing, behavior, and physiological measurement. Internal consistency was between 0.73 and 0.82 (Cronbach α) in 73 elderly hip surgery patients, and factor analysis detected three factors (Johansson et al. 2002). The psychometric qualities of the NEECHAM scale also have been assessed in elderly ICU patients, indicating internal consistency (0.81) and concordance with DSM-III-R criteria (0.68) (Csokasy 1999). It has been translated into Swedish, Norwegian, Dutch, and Japanese.

The DRS (Trzepacz et al. 1988a) is a 10-item scale assessing a breadth of delirium features and can function both to clarify diagnosis and to assess symptom severity because of its hierarchical nature (Trzepacz 1999a; van der Mast 1994). It has been translated into Italian, French, Spanish, Korean, Japanese, Mandarin Chinese, Dutch, Swedish, German, Portuguese, and a language of India for international use. It is generally used by those who have some psychiatric training. The DRS has high interrater reliability and validity even compared with other psychiatric patient groups, and it distinguishes delirium from dementia. It has been modified by some researchers to a 7- or 8-item subscale for repeated measures. In one study (Treloar and MacDonald 1997), the DRS and CAM diagnosed delirium with a high level of agreement ($r = 0.81$). It has been used to assess delirium in children and adolescents (Turkel et al. 2003).

The Memorial Delirium Assessment Scale (MDAS) is a 10-item severity rating scale for use after a diagnosis of delirium has been made (Breitbart et al. 1997). It was intended for repeated ratings within a 24-hour period, as occurs in treatment studies. It does not include items for temporal onset and fluctuation of symptoms, which are characteristic symptoms that help to distinguish delirium from dementia. The MDAS correlated highly with the DRS ($r=0.88$) and the MMSE ($r=-0.91$). The Japanese version of the MDAS was validated in 37 elderly patients with delirium, dementia, mood disorder, or schizophrenia and was found to distinguish among them ($P<0.0001$), with a mean score of 18 in the delirium group (Matsuoka et al. 2001). It correlated reasonably well with the DRS Japanese version ($r=-0.74$) and the Clinician's Global Rating of Delirium ($r=0.67$) and less well with the MMSE ($r=0.54$). The Italian version of the MDAS (Grassi et al. 2001) correlated well with the DRS Italian version in a study of 105 consecutive cancer patients (66 had delirium). When the CAM was used as the diagnostic standard, the MDAS had a high specificity (94%) but low sensitivity (68%), whereas the DRS with a cutoff of 10 had high sensitivity (95%) and low specificity (68%) and with a cutoff of 12 had a sensitivity of 80% and a specificity of 76%. In this same study, the MMSE had 96% sensitivity but only 38% specificity. Factor analysis showed a three-factor structure for the DRS and a two-factor structure for the MDAS. Lawlor et al. (2000b) used the MDAS in cancer patients with DSM-IV– diagnosed delirium and found two factors: Cronbach $\alpha=0.78$ and a correlation ($r=0.55$) with the MMSE.

The DRS-R98 is a substantially revised version of the DRS that addresses the shortcomings of the DRS (Trzepacz et al. 2001). It allows for repeated measurements and includes separate or new items for language, thought processes, motor agitation, motor retardation, and five cognitive domains. The DRS-R98 has 16 items, with 3 diagnostic items separable from the 13-item severity subscale for serial measurements. Anchored severity descriptions for a broad range of symptoms known to occur

in delirium use standard phenomenological definitions, without a priori assumptions about which symptoms occur more frequently. The total scale is used for the initial evaluation of delirium to so as allow discrimination from other disorders. The DRS-R98 total score ($P<0.001$) distinguished delirium from dementia, schizophrenia, depression, and other medical conditions during blind ratings, with sensitivities ranging from 91% to 100% and specificities from 85% to 100%, depending on the cutoff score chosen. It has high internal consistency (Cronbach $\alpha=0.90$), correlates well with the DRS ($r=0.83$) and the CTD ($r=-0.62$), and has high interrater reliability (intraclass correlation coefficient $=0.99$). In a review of delirium assessment tools, Timmers and colleagues (2005) concluded that the DRS-R98 was the best overall of currently available delirium rating tools largely because of its range of symptoms and suitability for use by physicians and research assistants. Translations exist or are in progress for Spanish, Portuguese, Japanese, Korean, Greek, Danish, Dutch, German, French, Lithuanian, Norwegian, Italian, and modern and traditional Chinese versions. Japanese, Korean, Chinese, Dutch, Portuguese, and Spanish (Spain and Colombia) versions have been validated and published (De Rooij 2005a; Fonseca et al. 2005; Kishi et al. 2001). A Palm Pilot version has been used for clinical research (Hill et al. 2002).

On the basis of issues such as instrument design, purpose, available translations, and breadth of use, a few of the available instruments are recommended (Table 5–5). They can be used together or separately depending on the clinical or research need. For example, a screening tool can be used for case detection, followed by a more thorough assessment for meeting DSM or ICD criteria and symptom severity.

ELECTROENCEPHALOGRAPHY

In the 1940s, Engel and Romano (1944, 1959; Romano and Engel 1944) began a series of classic papers that described the relationship of delirium, as measured by cognitive impair-

TABLE 5–5.   **Recommended delirium assessment instruments[a]**

Instrument	Type	Rater
Confusion Assessment Method (Inouye et al. 1990)	4-item diagnostic screener	Nonpsychiatric clinician
Confusion Assessment Method for ICU (Ely et al. 2001b)	4-item diagnostic screener anchored by objective tests	ICU nurses
Delirium Rating Scale[b] (Trzepacz et al. 1988a)	10-item severity/ diagnostic scale	Psychiatrically trained clinician
Memorial Delirium Assessment Scale (Breitbart et al. 1997)	10-item severity scale	Clinician
Delirium Rating Scale—Revised-98 (Trzepacz et al. 2001)	16-item scale (severity and diagnostic subscales)	Psychiatrically trained clinician
Cognitive Test for Delirium (Hart et al. 1996)	5 cognitive domains as bedside test	Trained technician or clinician

Note.   ICU = intensive care unit.
[a]See text for descriptions.
[b]Has been used in children.

ment, to electroencephalographic slowing. In their seminal work, they showed an association between abnormal electrical activity of the brain and the psychiatric symptoms of delirium; the reversibility of both conditions; the ubiquity of electroencephalographic changes for different underlying disease states; and an improvement in electroencephalography background rhythm that paralleled clinical improvement. The thalamus drives the normal awake, resting alpha rhythm, and cholinergic activity is necessary such that anticholinergic agents cause slowing of the dominant posterior rhythm. Abnormalities in evoked potentials support a role for the thalamus in delirium (Trzepacz et al. 1989).

Working with burn patients, Andreasen et al. (1977) showed that the time course of electroencephalographic slowing could precede or lag behind overt clinical symptoms of delirium, although sensitive delirium symptom ratings were not used. Although generalized slowing is the typical EEG pattern for both hypoactive and hyperactive presentations of delirium and for most etiologies of delirium, delirium tremens is associated with predominantly low-

voltage fast activity (Kennard et al. 1945), making it an important exception. An animal model for delirium that used atropine found similar electroencephalographic slowing in rats as in humans that was associated over time with worsened cognitive function (maze performance) (Leavitt et al. 1994; Trzepacz et al. 1992).

EEG characteristics in delirium include slowing or dropout of the dominant posterior rhythm, diffuse theta or delta waves (i.e., slowing), poor organization of background rhythm, and loss of reactivity on EEG to eye opening and closing (Jacobson and Jerrier 2000). Similarly, quantitative EEG (QEEG) in delirium shows parallel findings affecting slowing of power bands' mean frequency (see Figure 5–5) as compared with nondelirious control subjects.

Table 5–6 describes different EEG patterns that can be seen clinically in delirium. Although diffuse slowing is the most common presentation, false-negative results occur when a person's characteristic dominant posterior rhythm does not slow sufficiently to drop from the alpha to the theta range, thereby being read

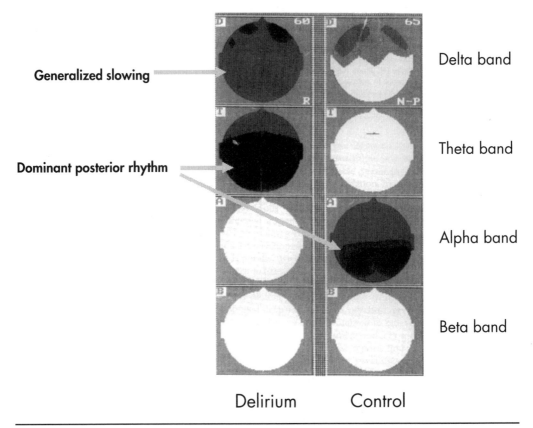

Generalized slowing

Dominant posterior rhythm

Delta band

Theta band

Alpha band

Beta band

Delirium   Control

FIGURE 5–5.   Quantitative electroencephalography (QEEG) brain map in delirium.
Relative power in each of four frequency bands (higher power in darker color).

Source.   Reprinted from Jacobson S, Jerrier H: "EEG in Delirium." *Seminars in Clinical Neuropsychiatry* 5:86–92, copyright 2000, with permission from Elsevier.

as normal despite the presence of abnormal slowing for that individual. (Generally, a change of more than 1 Hz from an individual's baseline is considered abnormal.) Comparison with prior baseline EEGs is often helpful to document that slowing has in fact occurred. Less commonly, but nonetheless important, an EEG may detect focal problems, such as ictal and subictal states or a previously unsuspected tumor that presents with prominent confusion. These include toxic ictal psychosis, nonconvulsive status, and complex partial status epilepticus (Drake and Coffey 1983; Trzepacz 1994a) or focal lesions (Jacobson and Jerrier 2000). New-onset complex partial seizures are underappreciated in the elderly, related to ischemic damage (Sundaram and Dostrow

1995). Jacobson and Jerrier (2000) warned that it can be difficult to distinguish delirium from drowsiness and light sleep unless the technologist includes standard alerting procedures during the EEG. In most cases, EEGs are not needed to make a clinical diagnosis of delirium, instead being used when seizures are suspected or differential diagnosis is difficult, such as in schizophrenic patients with medical illness.

More recent advances in electroencephalographic technologies have expanded our knowledge. Koponen et al. (1989b) used spectral analysis of delirious elderly patients (about 75% of whom also had dementia) and found significant reductions in alpha percentage, increased theta and delta activity, and slowing of

TABLE 5–6.   Electroencephalographic patterns in patients with delirium

Electroencephalographic finding	Comment	Causes
Diffuse slowing	Most typical delirium pattern	Many causes, including anticholinergicity, posttraumatic brain injury, hepatic encephalopathy, hypoxia
Low-voltage fast activity	Typical of delirium tremens	Alcohol withdrawal; benzodiazepine intoxication
Spikes/polyspikes, frontocentral	Toxic ictal pattern (nonconvulsive)	Hypnosedative drug withdrawal; tricyclic and phenothiazine intoxication
Left/bilateral slowing or delta bursts; frontal intermittent rhythmic delta	Acute confusional migraine	Usually in adolescents
Epileptiform activity, frontotemporal or generalized	Status with prolonged confusional states	Nonconvulsive status and complex partial status epilepticus

the peak and mean frequencies. All of these findings are consistent with electroencephalographic slowing. The study also found a correlation between the severity of cognitive decline and the length of the patient's hospital stay and the degree of electroencephalographic slowing. Jacobson et al. (1993a) could use QEEG to distinguish delirious from nondelirious individuals with the relative power of the alpha frequency band and could distinguish delirious from demented patients according to theta activity and the relative power of the delta band. Serial EEGs of delirious patients showed associations between the relative power of the alpha band and cognitive ability, whereas in demented patients, the absolute power of the delta band was associated with cognitive changes (Jacobson et al. 1993b). QEEG could replace conventional EEG for delirium assessment in the future (Jacobson and Jerrier 2000).

Evoked potentials also may be abnormal in delirium, suggesting thalamic or subcortical involvement in the production of symptoms. Metabolic causes of delirium precipitate abnormalities in visual, auditory, and somatosensory evoked potentials (Kullmann et al. 1995; Trzepacz et al. 1989), whereas somatosensory

evoked potentials are abnormal in patients whose delirium is due to posttraumatic brain injury, suggesting damage to the medial lemniscus. In general, normalization of evoked potentials parallels clinical improvement, although evoked potentials are not routinely recorded for clinical purposes.

EEGs and evoked potentials in children with delirium show patterns similar to those in adults, with diffuse slowing on EEG and increased latencies of evoked potentials (J.A. Katz et al. 1988; Okamura et al. 2005; Prugh et al. 1980; Ruijs et al. 1993, 1994). The degree of slowing on EEGs and evoked potentials recorded serially over time in children and adolescents correlates with the severity of delirium and with recovery from delirium (Foley et al. 1981; Montgomery et al. 1991; Onofrj et al. 1991).

PHENOMENOLOGY OF DELIRIUM

Wolff and Curran's (1935) classic descriptive report of 106 consecutive "dysergastic reaction" patients is still consistent with modern-day notions of delirium symptoms. Inconsistent terminology, unclear definitions of symptoms, and underuse of standardized symptom assessment tools have hampered subsequent efforts to describe delirium phenomenology more carefully or to compare symptom incidences across studies and etiological populations (Meagher and Trzepacz 1998). Most studies are cross-sectional, so we lack an understanding of how various symptoms change over the course of an episode.

More recent longitudinal research including daily delirium ratings has focused on total scale scores and not the occurrence of individual symptoms and their pattern over time. Rudberg et al. (1997) used the DRS and DSM-III-R criteria to rate daily 432 medical-surgical patients 65 years or older at a university hospital. They found a 15% incidence of delirium ($n = 63$), in 69% of whom the delirium lasted for only a day. Mean DRS scores on day 1 were significantly higher (i.e., worse) in those whose delirium occurred for multiple days than in those whose delirium lasted 1 day, suggesting a relation between severity and duration in delirium episodes. Marcantonio et al. (2003) studied delirium symptom progression measured with nursing staff ratings of minimum data set symptoms over the first week after admission to postacute facilities. They noted that all six symptoms measured (distractibility, altered perception, disorganized speech, restlessness, lethargy, and mental fluctuation) persisted in two-thirds of patients, with symptoms worsening in 12%. Fann et al. (2005) prospectively studied patients undergoing hematopoietic stem cell transplantation with thrice-weekly assessments with the DRS and MDAS from pretransplantation to day 30 posttransplant. They found that neuropsychiatric features (psychomotor changes, sleep-wake cycle disturbance, and psychotic symptoms) dominated in the early phases but that cognitive impairment peaked a week into delirium and dominated thereafter.

Despite across-study inconsistencies (see Table 5–7) for symptom frequencies, certain symptoms occur more often than do others, consistent with the proposal that delirium has core symptoms irrespective of etiology (Trzepacz 1999b, 2000). The most recent data used the DRS-R98 to assess more symptoms with greater consistency than in prior studies. Only one study reported symptoms in children (Turkel et al. 2006) that differed significantly from those in adults: less frequent delusions, more fluctuation of symptoms, greater sleep-wake cycle disturbance, more affective lability, and more agitation. However, none of those adult studies used the DRS-R98, and generally symptom collection was neither well standardized nor comprehensive. In contrast, Turkel and colleagues' (2006) data in children showed frequencies more consistent with the adult DRS-R98 studies.

Figure 5–6 illustrates how multiple etiologies for delirium may "funnel" into a final common neural pathway (Trzepacz 1999b, 2000) so that the phenomenological expression becomes similar despite a breadth of different physiologies. This implies, as well, that certain brain circuits and neurotransmitter systems are more affected (Trzepacz 1994a, 1999b, 2000).

CORE SYMPTOMS

Candidates for "core" symptoms include attentional deficits, memory impairment, disorientation, sleep-wake cycle disturbance, thought process abnormalities, language disturbances, and motor alterations (see "Motor Subtypes" section below), whereas "associated" or noncore symptoms would include perceptual disturbances (illusions, hallucinations), delusions, and affective changes (Trzepacz 1999b). Analysis of DRS-R98 blinded ratings supports this separation of so-called core from associated symptoms on the basis of their relative prevalence (Trzepacz et al. 2001). The occurrence of the less frequent associated symptoms might suggest involvement of particular etiologies and their specific pathophysiologies or individual differences in brain circuitry and vulnerability.

The severity of symptoms in delirium typically fluctuates in intensity over any 24-hour period, unlike that in most other psychiatric

TABLE 5–7. Studies of delirium phenomenology

	Frequency (%) in children	Frequencies (%) from adult studies that used various classifications	Frequencies (%) from studies that used DRS-R98
Disorientation	77	43, 70, 78, 80, 88, 94, 96, 100	76, 96
Attentional deficits	100	17, 62, 100, 100, 100	97, 100
Sustained attention		89	
Shifting attention		87	
Clouded consciousness	93	58, 65, 65, 87, 91, 100	
Memory impairment (unspecified)	52	64, 90, 95, 100	
Short-term memory			88, 92
Long-term memory			89, 96
Visuospatial impairment			87, 96
Language abnormalities		41, 47, 62, 76, 93	57, 67
Disorganized thinking/thought process abnormalities		57, 64, 76, 95	54, 79
Incoherence		77	
Sleep-wake cycle disturbance	98	25, 49, 77, 95, 96	92, 97
Perceptual disturbance/hallucinations	43	24, 35, 35, 41, 45, 46, 71	50, 63
Delusions		18, 19, 25, 37, 38, 45, 68	21, 31
Affective lability/emotional disturbance	79	43, 63, 97, 97	53, 54
Apathy	68	86	
Anxiety	61	55	
Irritability	86		
Psychomotor changes (general)		38, 53, 55, 83, 88, 92, 93	
Motor agitation	69	59	62, 79
Motor retardation		71	29, 62

Note. DRS-R98 = Delirium Rating Scale—Revised-98.

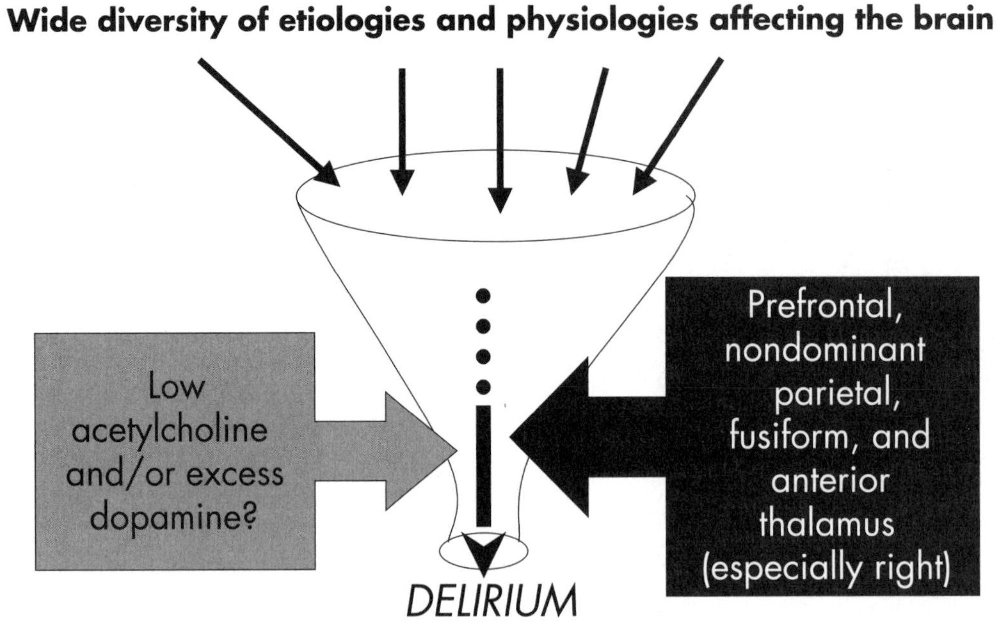

Wide diversity of etiologies and physiologies affecting the brain

FIGURE 5–6. Delirium final common pathway.

disorders. Symptom fluctuation is thus an important indicator of delirium and is emphasized in diagnostic classifications (American Psychiatric Association 1994, 2000; World Health Organization 1992). During this characteristic waxing and waning of symptoms, relatively lucid or quiescent periods pose challenges for accurate diagnosis and severity ratings. Some lucid periods may restore enough capacity for patients to communicate their management choices (Bostwick and Masterson 1998). The underlying reason for this fluctuation in symptom severity is not understood—it may relate to shifts between hypoactive and hyperactive periods or fragmentations of the sleep-wake cycle, including daytime rapid eye movement (REM) sleep and circadian disturbances.

Historically, delirium has been viewed by some neurologists primarily as a disturbance of attention; less importance has been attributed to its other cognitive deficits and behavioral symptoms. Attentional disturbance is the cardinal symptom required for diagnosis of delirium yet is unlikely to explain the breadth of delirium symptoms. The nondominant poste-

rior parietal and prefrontal cortices, as well as the brain stem and anteromedial thalamus, play roles in subserving attention, but other brain regions are likely to be involved in other symptoms of delirium. Distractibility, inattention, and poor environmental awareness can be evident during interview and on formal testing. Attentional impairment was found in 100% of delirium patients in a blinded assessment with the DRS-R98 (Trzepacz et al. 2001). O'Keeffe and Gosney (1997) found that attentional deficits discriminated delirium patients from either patients with dementia or elderly inpatients without psychiatric disorders when they used sensitive tests such as Digit Span Backward and the Digit Cancellation Test.

Memory impairment occurs often in delirium, affecting both short- and long-term memory, although most reports have not distinguished between types of memory impairment. In delirium due to posttraumatic brain injury, procedural and declarative memory are impaired, and procedural memory improves first (Ewert et al. 1985). Patients are usually amnestic for some or all of their delirium episodes, although recent studies have highlighted

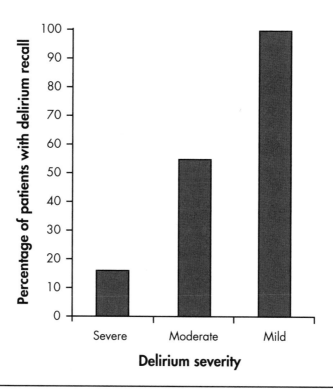

FIGURE 5–7. Ability to recall an episode of delirium worsens with more severe delirium symptoms.

Source. Reprinted from Breitbart W, Gibson C, Tremblay A: "The Delirium Experience: Delirium Recall and Delirium-Related Distress in Hospitalized Patients With Cancer, Their Spouses/Caregivers, and Their Nurses." *Psychosomatics* 43:183–194, 2002. Copyright 2002 American Psychiatric Publishing, Inc. Used with permission.

that many patients can recall some of the often distressing experiences of delirium. Breitbart et al. (2002a) found that about half of their patients with resolved delirium were amnestic for their episode and that more severe amnesia was associated with greater severity of delirium on the MDAS, suggesting a defect in new learning during delirium (see Figure 5–7). Similarly, O'Keeffe (2005) found that about half of elderly nondemented delirious patients recalled their delirium, many of whom continued to be disturbed by their recollections 6 months later. Trzepacz et al. (2001) found a high correlation between the DRS-R98 short- and long-term memory items ($r=0.51$, $P=0.01$) in delirious patients, with attention correlating with short-term memory ($r=0.44$, $P=0.03$) but not with long-term memory. This outcome is consistent with adequate attention

being a prerequisite for information to enter short-term (working) memory, followed by storage of selected data from working memory into long-term memory.

Disturbances of the sleep-wake cycle are especially common in patients with delirium. The DRS-R98 identified sleep-wake cycle disturbances in 92%–97% of delirious patients (Meagher et al. 2007; Trzepacz et al. 2001). Sleep disturbances range from napping and nocturnal disruptions to a more severe disintegration of the normal circadian cycle. The role of sleep disturbances in early or prodromal phases of delirium is uncertain; some have suggested that sleep disturbances may be a central feature of delirium evolution, possibly related to disturbed melatonin secretion (Charlton and Kavanau 2002; Shigeta et al. 2001). However, Harrell and Othmer (1987), in a study of postcardiotomy delirium, found that sleep disturbance mirrored reductions in MMSE scores but did not predate them. Similarly, de Jonghe et al. (2005) found that the prodromal phase of delirium was characterized principally by cognitive disturbances rather than behavioral or sleep disturbances. A retrospective study measured treatment response—2 or more consecutive nights of undisturbed sleep was equated with delirium resolution (Dautzenberg et al. 2004).

Visuospatial disturbances have not been studied in detail in delirium, but Clock Drawing Test deficits and wandering behaviors indicate difficulties. Accuracy of both the overall shapes and the details of drawings is impaired, suggesting dysfunction of bilateral posterior parietal lobes and prefrontal cortex. Meagher et al. (2007) found disturbances of visuospatial function in 87% of delirious patients and noted that these were moderate or severe in 64%.

Language disturbances in delirium include dysnomia, paraphasias, impaired comprehension, dysgraphia, and word-finding difficulties. In extreme cases, language resembles a fluent dysphasia. Incoherent speech or speech disturbance is reported commonly. Dysgraphia was once believed to be specific to delirium (Chedru and Geschwind 1972), but comparison of writing samples from patients with other psychiatric disorders found that dysgraphia was not specific to delirium (Patten and Lamarre 1989); rather, abnormal semantic content of language was more differentiating in delirium. The language item on the DRS-R98 did not distinguish delirium and dementia patients, but the CTD comprehension item, which incorporates language and executive function, did (Trzepacz et al. 2002).

Disorganized thinking was found in 95% of delirious patients in one study (Rockwood 1993) and was noted by Cutting (1987) to be different from schizophrenic thought processes. However, very little work has been done to characterize thought process disorder in patients with delirium, which clinically ranges from tangentiality and circumstantiality to loose associations. On the DRS-R98, 21% of delirium patients had tangentiality or circumstantiality, whereas 58% had loose associations (Trzepacz et al. 2001). Greater severity of thought process disturbances can distinguish delirium when it occurs with concomitant dementia (Laurila et al. 2004), and thought disorder is significantly worse in delirium than in dementia (Trzepacz et al. 2002). Besides thought process abnormality, other indications of psychosis include abnormal thought content and perceptual disturbances, although these occur less often than do core symptoms (Trzepacz et al. 2001).

ASSOCIATED SYMPTOMS

Psychotic symptoms occur in both agitated and quiet presentations and are important determinants of the delirium experience for patients and their caregivers (Breitbart et al. 2002a). A retrospective study of 227 consecutively evaluated delirium patients found that 25.6% had delusions, 27% had visual hallucinations, 12.4% had auditory hallucinations, and 2.7% had tactile hallucinations (Webster and Holroyd 2000). O'Keeffe (2005) prospectively studied 105 elderly nondemented patients with delirium and found that 70% had delusions or misperceptions or both during delirium. Cutting (1987) noted that delusional content tended to involve delusional misidentification, imminent misadventure to others, or bizarre happenings in the patient's environment. Although psychotic symptoms are commonly equated with hyperactive presentations, recent reports emphasized their occurrence in quieter presentations (Breitbart et al. 2002a; Meagher 2005).

The type of perceptual disturbance and delusion distinguishes delirium from schizophrenia (Cutting 1987). Clinically, the occurrence of visual (as well as tactile, olfactory, and gustatory) hallucinations heightens the likelihood of an identifiable medical problem or drug toxicity, although primary psychiatric disorders do occasionally present with visual misperceptions. Visual hallucinations range from patterns or shapes to complex and vivid animations, which may vary according to which part of the brain is being affected (Trzepacz 1994a). Simple forms or colors suggest dysfunction closer to the primary visual cortex, whereas more complex ones implicate the temporal or fusiform regions, with peduncular hallucinations causing movielike hallucinations. Persecutory delusions that are poorly formed (not systematized) are the most common type in delirium, but other types can occur (e.g., somatic or grandiose).

Affective lability that involves unpredictable mood changes within minutes is characteristic of delirium. Mood alterations can take many forms (e.g., anxiety, fear, anger, dysphoria, elation, euphoria, apathy), with rapid changes from one type to another without obvious relation to the context (i.e., incongruent) and outside of self-control. In a study of patients referred by a consultation-liaison psychiatrist for suspected mood disorder who actually had delirium, 24% experienced suicidal thoughts, 52% had frequent thoughts of death, and 32% believed that there was no point in taking medications (Farrell and Ganzini 1995). These findings highlight the importance of careful monitoring of mental state in delirious patients. Affective lability occurred less often than did core symptoms (Meagher et al. 2007; Trzepacz et al. 2001).

MOTOR SUBTYPES

Disturbances of motor behavior are almost invariable in delirium (Camus et al. 2000; Gupta et al. 2005; Meagher 2005) and have been considered as candidates for inclusion among its core symptoms. The varying motor presentations of delirium have been described since ancient times, when two patterns were distinguished—"phrenitis" and "lethargicus" (Lipowski 1990). Contemporary medicine recognizes three patterns: excited ("hyperactive"), lethargic ("hypoactive"), and "mixed." Often motor disturbances are characterized more as psychomotor behaviors (including hyperalertness, wandering, uncooperativeness or hypersomnolence, disinterest, and unawareness) that encompass nonmotor symptoms that may or may not have any specificity for delirium.

These motor variants are important not only because of their effect on delirium detection and management but also because of their relation to prognosis and differences in underlying etiology and pathophysiology. Delusions, hallucinations, mood lability, speech incoherence, and sleep disturbances may be somewhat more frequent in hyperactive patients (Meagher and Trzepacz 2000; Ross et al. 1991) but also occur in hypoactive patients. Neurologists have differentiated delirium such that disorientation with reduced motor activity has been called "acute confusion," whereas hyperactive disoriented patients were labeled "delirious" (Mesulam 1985; Mori and Yamadori 1987). In a study of infarctions of the right middle cerebral artery, Mori and Yamadori (1987) found that acute confusional states are disturbances of attention, resulting from frontostriatal damage, whereas acute agitated deliria are disturbances of emotion and affect resulting from injury to the middle temporal gyrus. However, these distinctions are not supported by data or neural circuitry (Trzepacz 1994a). Temporal-limbic information is linked to prefrontal cortex via the basotemporal-limbic pathways and the thalamo-frontal-striatal circuits. Evidence suggests delirium likely relates to both frontal and temporal-limbic dysfunction.

Motor subtypes have similar degrees of overall cognitive impairment and electroencephalographic slowing, which are objective and diagnostic aspects of delirium (Koponen et al. 1989b; Ross et al. 1991). Studies suggest that these motorically defined subtypes differ in relation to the frequency of nonmotor symptoms (Gupta et al. 2005; Meagher et al. 2000; Sandberg et al. 1999), etiology (Gupta et al. 2005; Meagher et al. 1998; Morita et al. 2001; Ross et al. 1991), pathophysiology (Balan et al. 2003), detection rates (Inouye 1994), treatment experience (Breitbart et al. 2002b; Meagher et al. 1996; Uchiyama et al. 1996), and duration of episode.

However, methodological inconsistencies and variability of findings across studies make the interpretation of these findings difficult (Meagher and Trzepacz 2000; Meagher et al.

2008). In particular, the definitions of motor subtypes vary considerably and include symptoms that do not directly relate to motor disturbance and have uncertain value in subtyping (e.g., affective changes, aggressive behavior, alterations in verbal output). Moreover, waxing and waning of symptom severity and sleep-wake cycle abnormalities complicate our understanding of motor subtypes, as does reliance on subjective and retrospective reports of behavior over 24-hour periods. Wide variation is seen among reports of relative frequencies of motor subtypes, even when alcohol withdrawal cases are excluded. In a prospective study of delirious patients, Meagher et al. (2008) found a remarkably low level of concordance (34%) among four different methods of defining psychomotor subtypes.

Balan et al. (2003) showed that levels of the melatonin metabolite 6-SMT correlated closely with motor presentation during the delirium episode but normalized thereafter, with highest levels in hypoactive patients, followed by mixed motor presentation, and with lowest levels in those with hyperactivity. These findings echo those noted in studies of melatonin function and psychomotor profile in mood disorders (B. Wahlund et al. 1998). Melatonin is involved in regulation of the sleep-wake circadian cycle at the hypothalamus and has recognized hypnotic effects. It is also involved in regulation of immune response and aging, and its secretion is increased by immobilization and decreased during the daytime by light exposure. Balan et al. (2003) hypothesized that disruption of melatonin secretion is key to the emergence of delirium and that the interaction of certain extrinsic factors (e.g., abnormal light exposure in medical ICU settings) may interact with intrinsic factors to shape motor profile according to whether secretion is increased (relative hypoactivity) or decreased (relative hyperactivity).

Delirium due to drug-related causes is most commonly hyperactive, whereas delirium due to metabolic disturbances, including hypoxia, is more frequently hypoactive in presentation (Meagher et al. 1998; Morita et al. 2001; O'Keeffe and Lavan 1999; S.M. Olofsson et al. 1996;

Ross et al. 1991). Patients with a hyperactive subtype may have better outcomes after an episode of delirium, with shorter LOS, lower mortality rates, and a higher rate of full recovery (Kobayashi et al. 1992; Liptzin and Levkoff 1992; S.M. Olofsson et al. 1996). However, these differences may reflect variations in underlying causes, recognition rates, or treatment practices. Underdetection and misdiagnosis are especially common in hypoactive patients. In fact, Meagher et al. (1996) found that use of psychotropic medication and supportive environmental ward strategies were related to level of hyperactivity rather than to degree of cognitive disturbance. S.M. Olofsson et al. (1996) reported better outcome in patients with hyperactive delirium but noted that they received less haloperidol than did nonhyperactive patients. O'Keeffe and Lavan (1999) reported greater use of neuroleptics and shorter hospital stays in hyperactive patients but attributed this to less severe illness at the onset of delirium and a lower incidence of hospital-acquired infections and bedsores in those who were hyperactive. Even when actively screened for earlier detection or more active investigation, hypoactive patients still may have a poorer outcome (O'Keeffe and Lavan 1999). Other work has found similar outcomes in the different motor groups (Camus et al. 2000). All work focused on implication of motor presentations of delirium may need reevaluation when motor activity monitoring redefines these categories objectively.

Treatment studies have not been designed specifically to assess response or effectiveness for different motor subtypes. In clinical practice, it is often presumed that neuroleptic agents are useful in delirium solely for sedative or antipsychotic purposes and thus more effective for hyperactive patients. However, a prospective study found comparable efficacy for haloperidol in treating both hypo- and hyperactive delirious medical patients (Platt et al. 1994a), whereas another study (Breitbart et al. 2002b) found that hypoactive symptoms were somewhat less responsive to olanzapine in an uncontrolled open trial; however, structural brain lesions may have been confounds.

Uchiyama et al. (1996) found better response rates to mianserin in delirium with hyperactive motor presentation compared with hypoactive motor profile, attributed to its sedating effects. Overall, the relation between motor subtype and treatment and outcome remains unclear and confounded by methodological issues.

TREATMENT OF DELIRIUM

Delirium is an example par excellence of a disorder requiring a multifaceted biopsychosocial approach to assessment and treatment. After the diagnosis of delirium is made, the process of identifying and reversing suspected causes begins. Rapid treatment is important because of the high morbidity and mortality rates associated with delirium. Treatments include medication, environmental manipulation, and patient and family psychosocial support (American Psychiatric Association 1999). However, no drug has a U.S. Food and Drug Administration (FDA) indication for the treatment of delirium. Randomized double-blind, placebo-controlled, adequately powered efficacy trials are lacking. The American Psychiatric Association (1999) "Practice Guidelines for the Treatment of Patients With Delirium" note the need for such research, and this is ever more pertinent given the escalating range of therapeutic options available in delirium, including atypical antipsychotics, procholinergic agents, and melatonergic compounds. Most prospective drug studies use open-label designs (Table 5–8); more is published about atypical antipsychotics than about conventional neuroleptics in these studies. Whether any neuroleptic agent adequately targets all core symptoms of delirium has not been shown. Cholinergic agents hold more promise in chronic prophylactic dosing, although shorter-acting agents such as physostigmine, which offer faster onset of action in acute settings, have not been tried for non-drug-induced delirium.

PREVENTION STRATEGIES

Preoperative patient education and preparation were helpful in reducing delirium symptom rates (Chatham 1978; Owens and Hutelmyer 1982; Schindler et al. 1989; M. A. Williams et al. 1985). However, studies that used caregiver education and environmental or risk factor interventions had mixed results, with two not finding any significant effect on delirium rate (Nagley 1986; Wanich et al. 1992) and one (Rockwood et al. 1994) finding modest gains in delirium diagnosis (3%–9%) through special internal medicine house staff education efforts. In contrast, Inouye et al. (1999) studied the effect on delirium of preventive measures that minimized six of the risk factors identified in their previous work with hospitalized elderly patients. They used standardized protocols in a prospective study of 852 elderly medical inpatients to address cognitive impairment, sleep deprivation, immobility, visual impairment, hearing impairment, and dehydration, which resulted in significant reductions in the number (62 vs. 90) and duration (105 vs. 161 days) of delirium episodes relative to control subjects. Effects of adherence to the delirium risk protocol were subsequently reported for 422 elderly patients during implementation (Inouye et al. 2003): adherence ranged from 10% for the sleep protocol to 86% for orientation. Higher levels of adherence by staff resulted in lower delirium rates up to a maximum of an 89% reduction, even after the investigators controlled for confounding variables such as medical comorbidity, functional status, and illness severity. At 6-month follow-up of 705 survivors from this intervention study of six risk factors, no differences were seen between groups for any of 10 outcome measures except for less frequent incontinence in the intervention group (Bogardus et al. 2003), suggesting that the intervention's effect was essentially during the index hospitalization, without longer-lasting benefits. When a subset of patients at high risk for delirium at baseline were compared, however, patients who received the intervention had significantly better self-rated health and functional status at follow-up.

Marcantonio et al. (2001) found that proactive geriatric consultation in patients undergoing hip surgery was associated with sig-

TABLE 5–8.   Prospective studies of drug treatment in delirium

Study	Agent	Population	Design	Purpose	Measure[a]	Diagnosis
Conventional antipsychotics						
Breitbart et al. 1996	Haloperidol vs. chlorpromazine vs. lorazepam	30 AIDS inpatients	Double-blind, randomized	Efficacy	DRS	DSM-III-R
K.J. Kalisvaart et al. 2005	Haloperidol vs. placebo	430 elderly hip surgery inpatients	Double-blind, randomized	Prophylaxis (acute)	DRS-R98	DSM-IV
Kaneko et al. 1999	Intravenous haloperidol vs. intravenous placebo	78 gastrointestinal postoperative inpatients	Randomized, not blinded	Prophylaxis (acute) and rescue	Clinical assessment	DSM-III-R
Atypical antipsychotics						
Horikawa et al. 2003	Risperidone	10 consultation-liaison referrals	Open label	Efficacy	DRS	DSM-IV
Mittal et al. 2004	Risperidone	10 medical-surgical admissions	Open label	Efficacy	DRS	DSM-IV
Parellada et al. 2004	Risperidone	64 medical inpatients	Open label	Efficacy	DRS	DSM-IV
Toda et al. 2005	Risperidone	10 elderly inpatients	Open label	Efficacy	DRS	DSM-IV
C. S. Han and Kim 2004	Risperidone vs. haloperidol	28 consultation-liaison referrals	Double-blind, randomized	Efficacy	MDAS	DSM-III-R
J. Y. Kim et al. 2005	Haloperidol vs. risperidone	42 medical-surgical patients	Open label, not randomized	Efficacy	DRS-R98	DSM-IV
Sipahimalani and Masand 1998	Olanzapine vs. haloperidol	22 consultation-liaison referrals	Open label, not randomized	Efficacy	DRS	Not specified
K. S. Kim et al. 2001	Olanzapine	20 medical-surgical patients	Open label	Efficacy	DRS	DSM-IV
Breitbart et al. 2002b	Olanzapine	79 cancer inpatients	Open label	Efficacy	MDAS	DSM-IV

TABLE 5–8. Prospective studies of drug treatment in delirium (continued)

Study	Agent	Population	Design	Purpose	Measure[a]	Diagnosis
Hill et al. 2002	Olanzapine vs. risperidone vs. haloperidol	50 general hospital patients	Open label, not randomized	Efficacy	DRS-R98	DSM-IV
Skrobik et al. 2004	Olanzapine vs. haloperidol	103 ICU patients	Randomized, not blinded	Efficacy	Delirium Index	ICU delirium screening checklist
Straker et al. 2006	Aripiprazole	14 general hospital patients	Open label	Efficacy	DRS-R98	DSM-IV
K. Y. Kim et al. 2003	Quetiapine	12 geriatric medical patients	Open label	Efficacy	DRS	DSM-IV
Sasaki et al. 2003	Quetiapine	12 patients	Open label	Efficacy	DRS	DSM-IV
Pae et al. 2004	Quetiapine	22 inpatients	Open label	Efficacy	DRS-R98	DSM-IV
Lee et al. 2005	Amisulpride vs. quetiapine	40 patients	Open label, randomized	Efficacy	DRS-R98	DSM-IV
Procholinergic						
Diaz et al. 2001	Citicoline vs. placebo	81 elderly nondemented hip surgery patients	Randomized	Prophylaxis (acute)	CAM AMT	DSM-III-R
Liptzin et al. 2005	Donepezil vs. placebo	80 elderly elective hip surgery patients	Double-blind, randomized	Prophylaxis (acute)	DSI	DSM-IV
Moretti et al. 2004	Rivastigmine vs. Cardioaspirin	230 elderly vascular dementia outpatients	Case–control, not randomized	Prophylaxis (chronic)	CAM Index at 2 years	DSM-IV
Other						
J. Nakamura et al. 1994	Mianserin vs. haloperidol vs. oxypertine	23 general hospital inpatients	Not specified	Efficacy	DRS	Not specified
J. Nakamura et al. 1995	Mianserin vs. haloperidol	65 consultation-liaison referrals	Open label, not randomized	Efficacy	DRS	DSM-III-R

TABLE 5–8.   **Prospective studies of drug treatment in delirium (continued)**

Study	Agent	Population	Design	Purpose	Measure[a]	Diagnosis
Other (continued)						
Uchiyama et al. 1996	Mianserin	62 psychogeriatric inpatients	Open label	Efficacy	DRS	DSM-IV
J. Nakamura et al. 1997a	Mianserin vs. haloperidol	66 consultation-liaison referrals	Open label, not randomized	Efficacy	DRS	DSM-IV
J. Nakamura et al. 1997b	Mianserin suppositories	16 consultation-liaison patients	Open label	Efficacy	DRS	DSM-IV
Bayindir et al. 2000	Ondansetron	35 postcardiotomy patients	Open label	Efficacy	4-point clinical scale	Not specified
B. Gagnon et al. 2005	Methylphenidate	14 cancer patients	Open label	Efficacy	MMSE	DSM-IV

[a]Primary outcome measure.

Note.   AMT = Abbreviated Mental Test; CAM = Confusion Assessment Method; DRS = Delirium Rating Scale; DRS-R98 = Delirium Rating Scale—Revised-98; DSI = Delirium Symptom Inventory; ICU = intensive care unit; MDAS = Memorial Delirium Assessment Scale; MMSE = Mini-Mental State Examination.

nificantly reduced incidence and severity of delirium in the intervention group who had received a mean of 10 recommendations regarding risk factor prevention and active treatment of emergent delirium. Interestingly, more than three-quarters of these recommendations were adhered to, but with relatively less adherence to suggestions regarding analgesia, nutritional inadequacies, and correction of sensory impairments. Young and George (2003) studied the effect of introducing consensus guidelines for delirium management in general hospital settings and found that management processes improved only when the intervention was reinforced by regular teaching sessions, but these effects did not reach statistical significance.

Milisen et al. (2001) compared delirium rates in two cohorts of elderly hip surgery patients (each $n = 60$)—each before and after implementing an intervention composed of nurse education, cognitive screening, consultation by a nurse or physician geriatric/delirium specialist, and a scheduled pain protocol. They found no effect on delirium incidence but, rather, a shorter delirium duration (median = 1 vs. 4 days) and lower delirium severity score in the intervention group as measured by a modified (not validated) CAM. Marcantonio et al. (2001) used a different study design and randomly assigned 62 elderly hip fracture patients to either a perioperative geriatric consultation or usual care. Daily ratings on the MMSE, Delirium Symptom Inventory, CAM, and MDAS indicated a lower delirium rate (32% vs. 50%) and fewer severe delirium cases (12% vs. 29%) in the consultative group. LOS was not affected, and the effect of consultation was greatest in those patients without preexisting dementia or poor ADL, in contrast to the subgroup analysis of Bogardus et al. (2003), in which most benefit accrued at follow-up for high-risk patients.

PHARMACOLOGICAL PROPHYLAXIS

Cholinergic agents have engendered the most interest, consistent with the cholinergic deficiency hypothesis for delirium. Perioperative piracetam use during anesthesia was reviewed across eight studies, mostly from the 1970s, and was believed to have a positive effect on reducing postoperative delirium symptoms (Gallinat et al. 1999). Citicoline, 1.2 mg/day, given 1 day before and on each of 4 days after surgery, was assessed for acute prophylaxis of delirium in a randomized, placebo-controlled trial of 81 nondemented hip surgery patients (Diaz et al. 2001). Although no significant difference was found between groups on the Abbreviated Mental Test or the CAM, the placebo group had numerically more delirium cases (17.4% vs. 11.7%). In a retrospective review of delirium incidence in hospitalized elderly medical patients who received various treatments over an 18-month period, Dautzenberg et al. (2004) found a lower incidence of delirium in patients who had received chronic rivastigmine treatment. A double-blind, randomized, placebo-controlled trial of donepezil given 2 weeks before and after elective orthopedic surgery in an elderly population did not find a group difference, a result that was attributed to low delirium incidence and underpowering of the study in this cognitively intact low-risk cohort (Liptzin et al. 2005). In a 24-month prophylaxis study comparing rivastigmine with Cardioaspirin in elderly patients with vascular dementia, Moretti et al. (2004) found reduced occurrence of delirium (40% vs. 62%), shorter episode duration (4 vs. 7.5 days), and lower use of benzodiazepines and antipsychotics in the cholinesterase inhibitor group, supporting a role for cholinergic deficiency in delirium in these at-risk patients.

Kaneko et al. (1999) compared postoperative prophylaxis with 5 mg/day of intravenous haloperidol with intravenous saline in a randomized but not blinded trial of gastrointestinal surgery patients and found that the incidence of delirium was only 10.5% in the active drug group compared with 32.5% in the saline group ($P<0.05$). Rescue with haloperidol and flunitrazepam was allowed, however, in both groups as soon as delirium symptoms appeared, but mean doses were not reported. K. J. Kalisvaart et al. (2005) studied 430 elderly hip surgery patients in a randomized, double-blind, acute prophylaxis study in which either haloperidol or placebo was given up to 3 days before and 3 days after surgery. Although they found a nonsignificant lower numerical difference only for delirium incidence (23% vs. 32%) with the use of haloperidol, significant differences were found for shorter delirium duration (4.4 vs. 12 days), lower DRS-R98 scores (13.6 vs. 18.2), and shorter LOS (12 vs. 23.8 days) in the active treatment group. This was the first double-blind, randomized, placebo-controlled trial of use of a neuroleptic agent for delirium, but dosing was lower than in an efficacy design.

Adjusting the types of routinely used medications can reduce iatrogenic delirium. Maldonado et al. (2004) reported an interim data analysis showing significantly reduced delirium incidence (DSM-IV and DRS) when a novel α_2-adrenergic receptor agonist—dexmedetomidine (5%)—was administered for postoperative sedation, compared with propofol (54%) or fentanyl/midazolam (46%), in patients who had cardiac valve surgery. Improved pain control after hepatectomy surgery in elderly patients using patient-controlled epidural anesthesia with bupivacaine and fentanyl ($n = 14$) compared with continuous epidural mepivacaine ($n = 16$) was associated with lower incidences of moderate and severe delirium (36% vs. 75% and 14% vs. 50%, respectively), and antipsychotic drug use was also lower in that group (Tokita et al. 2001). Similarly, an open-label switch from morphine to fentanyl in delirious cancer patients resulted in decreased MDAS and pain scores in 13 of 20 patients on day 3, although 4 received neuroleptic rescue doses (Morita et al. 2005). Ely and Dittus (2004) encourage individual titration of sedating agents to avoid iatrogenic delirium and unresponsive states in ICU patients.

NONPHARMACOLOGICAL TREATMENT OF A DELIRIUM EPISODE

The principles of good ward management of delirious patients include ensuring the safety of the patient and his or her immediate surroundings (including sitters), achieving optimal levels of environmental stimulation, and minimizing the effects of any sensory impediments. The complications of delirium can be minimized by careful attention to the potential for falls and avoidance of prolonged hypostasis. The use of orienting techniques (e.g., calendars, night-lights, and reorientation by staff) and familiarizing the patient with the environment (e.g., with photographs of family members) are sometimes comforting, although it is important to remember that environmental manipulations alone do not reverse delirium (American Psychiatric Association 1999; S.D. Anderson 1995). It also has been suggested that diurnal cues from natural lighting reduce sensory deprivation and incidence of delirium (L.M. Wilson 1972), although sensory deprivation alone is insufficient to cause delirium (Francis 1993). Unfortunately, the routine implementation of nursing interventions occurs primarily in response to hyperactivity and behavioral management challenges rather than to the core cognitive disturbances of delirium (Meagher et al. 1996).

An alternative approach is home-based care ("hospital in the home"), which results in reduced incidence and duration of delirium and substantially reduced rehabilitation costs in elderly patients undergoing physical rehabilitation (Caplan et al. 2005). The "flying delirium team" uses a nurse-led coordinated approach to multidisciplinary care (psychiatry, geriatrics, and neurology) of hospitalized patients with delirium (Lemey et al. 2005). The "Delirium Room" (Flaherty et al. 2003) is a specialized four-bed unit for management and mobilization of disturbed elderly patients without the use of restraints (use being a well-recognized risk factor for delirium [McCusker et al. 2001]) that involves comprehensive delirium-oriented treatment to minimize risk and aggravating factors and medication use with daily multidisciplinary reviews of progress. Preliminary investigation suggests that exposure to delirium risk factors and mortality rates are reduced in this model of care. McCaffrey and Locsin (2004) found a lower incidence of delirium in elderly postoperative patients provided with passive ("easy listening") music therapy via a bedside compact disc player, with a calming effect on the ward atmosphere.

Supportive interaction with relatives and caregivers is fundamental to good management of delirium. During implementation of a psychoeducational intervention for family caregivers of terminally ill cancer patients, P. Gagnon et al. (2002) found that few caregivers were aware of the risk of delirium or that it could be treated. The intervention was associated with significant improvements in caregiver confidence. Lundstrom et al. (2005) found reduced delirium duration and mortality in patients receiving care on a ward where staff had received training in delirium assessment and treatment and where improved caregiver-patient interaction was emphasized. Although relatives can play an integral role in efforts to support and reorient delirious patients, they can add to the burden if they are ill-informed, critical, or anxious, whereby medical staff members respond to their distress by inappropriately medicating patients. Recovered delirium patients reported that simple but firm communication, reality orientation, a visible clock, and the presence of a relative contributed to a heightened sense of control (Schofield 1997). Clarification of the cause and meaning of symptoms combined with recognition of treatment goals can allow better management of what is a distressing experience for both patient and loved ones (Breitbart et al. 2002a; Meagher 2001b).

PHARMACOLOGICAL TREATMENT OF DELIRIUM

Current delirium pharmacotherapies are borrowed from the treatment of primary psychiatric disorders. Pharmacological treatment with a neuroleptic agent (dopamine D_2 antagonist) is the clinical standard of delirium treatment, although other agents have been tried and are described in this section (see Table 5–8). Doses need to be modified for elderly patients; however, Hally and Cooney (2005) found that these modifications were frequently over-

looked for both haloperidol (62%) and lorazepam (47%) prescribing.

Benzodiazepines

Benzodiazepines are generally reserved for delirium due to ethanol or sedative-hypnotic withdrawal, for which they are first-line agents (Mayo-Smith et al. 2004). Lorazepam or clonazepam (the latter for alprazolam withdrawal) is often used. However, Klijn and van der Mast (2005) warned about overlooking other causes of delirium when patients have alcohol withdrawal, and contend that haloperidol should be the first-choice treatment in these patients as well.

Some clinicians use lorazepam as an adjunctive medication with haloperidol in the most severe cases of delirium or when extra assistance with sleep is needed. Benzodiazepine monotherapy is generally not effective for non-substance-related delirium and may exacerbate the delirium, as shown in Breitbart and colleagues' (1996) controlled blinded study. None of the survey respondents from the American Geriatrics Society would use lorazepam alone to treat severe delirium in elderly postoperative patients (Carnes et al. 2003). Anticholinergic toxicity–induced delirium and agitation were controlled and reversed with physostigmine (87% and 96%, respectively), whereas benzodiazepines controlled agitation in 24% and were ineffective in treating delirium in a retrospective report of 52 consecutive toxicology consultations (Burns et al. 2000). Additionally, patients who received physostigmine had a lower incidence of complications (7% vs. 46%) and a shorter time to recovery (median = 12 vs. 24 hours) compared with patients who received benzodiazepines. Pandharipande et al. (2006) found a significant deliriogenic effect, in medical ICU patients, only for benzodiazepines when compared with other commonly used medications (propofol, morphine, and fentanyl), even though higher doses of all of these agents were used in delirious than in nondelirious ICU patients. A survey of ICU physicians found that 66% of the respondents treated delirium with haloperidol, 12% used lorazepam, and fewer than 5% used atypical anti-

psychotics. More than 55% administered haloperidol and lorazepam at daily doses of 10 mg or
less, but some used more than 50 mg/day of either medication (Ely et al. 2004b).

Cholinergic Enhancer Drugs

The cholinergic deficiency hypothesis of delirium suggests that treatment with a cholinergic
enhancer drug—generally acetylcholinesterase
inhibitors—could be therapeutic. Physostigmine reverses anticholinergic delirium (Stern
1983), but its side effects (seizures) and short
half-life make it unsuitable for routine clinical
treatment of delirium. Tacrine also was shown
to reverse central anticholinergic syndrome
(Mendelson 1977), but it has not been studied
formally. Three case reports found that donepezil improved delirium in postoperative state,
comorbid Lewy body dementia, and comorbid
alcohol dementia (Burke et al. 1999; Wengel
et al. 1998, 1999). Physostigmine administered in the emergency department to patients
suspected of having muscarinic toxicity
resulted in reversal of delirium in 22 of 39
patients, including several in whom the cause
could not be determined (Schneir et al. 2003);
only 1 of the 39 patients had an adverse event
(brief seizure). C. J. Kalisvaart et al. (2004)
reported that three cases of prolonged delirium that was unresponsive to haloperidol or
atypical antipsychotics rapidly resolved when
treatment was switched to rivastigmine. (See
also "Pharmacological Prophylaxis" subsection
earlier in this chapter.)

Neuroleptics

Haloperidol is the neuroleptic most often chosen for the treatment of delirium. It can be
administered orally, intramuscularly, or intravenously (Adams 1984, 1988; Dudley et al.
1979; Gelfand et al. 1992; Moulaert 1989;
Sanders and Stern 1993; Tesar et al. 1985),
although the intravenous route has not been
approved by the FDA. Intravenously administered haloperidol is twice as potent as that
taken orally (Gelfand et al. 1992). Bolus intravenous doses usually range from 0.5 to 20 mg,
although larger doses are sometimes given. In

severe, refractory cases, continuous intravenous infusions of 15–25 mg/hour (up to 1,000
mg/day) can be given (Fernandez et al. 1988;
J.L. Levenson 1995; Riker et al. 1994; Stern
1994). The specific brain effects of haloperidol
in alleviating delirium are not known, but
positron emission tomography scans show
reduced glucose utilization in the limbic cortex, thalamus, caudate, and frontal and anterior cingulate cortices (Bartlett et al. 1994).
These regions are important for behavior and
cognition and have been implicated in the neuropathogenesis of delirium. Milbrandt et al.
(2005) found in nearly 1,000 ICU patients
that use of haloperidol was associated with
reduced mortality.

Clinical use of haloperidol traditionally has
been considered to be relatively safe in the seriously medically ill and does not cause as much
hypotension as droperidol (Gelfand et al.
1992; Moulaert 1989; Tesar et al. 1985). Haloperidol does not antagonize dopamine-
induced increases in renal blood flow (D.H.
Armstrong et al. 1986). Even when haloperidol
is given intravenously at high doses in delirium,
extrapyramidal symptoms (EPS) are usually
not a problem except in more sensitive patients
(e.g., those with human immunodeficiency virus (HIV) infection or Lewy body dementia)
(Fernandez et al. 1989; McKeith et al. 1992;
Swenson et al. 1989). In a case series, five ICU
patients receiving 250–500 mg/day of continuous or intermittent intravenous haloperidol
had self-limited withdrawal dyskinesia following high-dose haloperidol (Riker et al. 1997).
Intravenous lorazepam is sometimes combined
with intravenous haloperidol in critically ill patients to lessen EPS and increase sedation.

Cases of prolonged QTc interval on electrocardiogram (ECG) and torsades de pointes ta-
chyarrhythmia (multifocal ventricular tachycardia) have been increasingly recognized and
attributed to intravenously administered haloperidol (Hatta et al. 2001; Huyse 1988; Kriwisky et al. 1990; Metzger and Friedman 1993;
O'Brien et al. 1999; Perrault et al. 2000; Wilt
et al. 1993; Zee-Cheng et al. 1985). The American Psychiatric Association (1999) "Practice

Guidelines for the Treatment of Patients With Delirium" recommend that QTc prolongation greater than 450 ms or greater than 25% over a previous ECG may warrant telemetry, cardiology consultation, dose reduction, or discontinuation. They also recommend monitoring serum magnesium and potassium in critically ill delirious patients whose QTc is 450 ms or greater, because of the common use of concomitant drugs and/or electrolyte disturbances that also can prolong the QTc interval.

Empirical evidence for neuroleptic benefits in treating delirium is substantial, but efficacy trials are mostly open label. Itil and Fink (1966) found that chlorpromazine reversed anticholinergic delirium. In a double-blind, randomized, controlled design, Breitbart et al. (1996) found that delirium in acquired immunodeficiency syndrome (AIDS) patients significantly improved with haloperidol or chlorpromazine, but not with lorazepam, but DRS and MMSE scores still did not return to normal. In addition, both hypoactive and hyperactive subtypes responded to treatment with haloperidol or chlorpromazine, and improvement was noted within hours of treatment, even before the underlying medical causes were addressed (Platt et al. 1994a).

Haloperidol use in pediatric patients with delirium is not well documented, despite its use in adult delirium and in other childhood psychiatric disorders (Teicher and Glod 1990). Its efficacy in children for delusions, hallucinations, thought disorder, aggressivity, stereotypies, hyperactivity, social withdrawal, and learning disability (Teicher and Glod 1990) suggests that it may have a potentially beneficial role in pediatric delirium. Clinical experience with haloperidol in pediatric delirium supports its beneficial effects, although no controlled studies have been done. A retrospective report of 30 children (mean age 7 ± 1.0 years, range 8 months to 18 years) with burn injuries supports the use of haloperidol for agitation, disorientation, hallucinations, delusions, and insomnia (R.L. Brown et al. 1996). The mean haloperidol dose was 0.47 ± 0.002 mg/kg, with a mean maximum dose in

24 hours of 0.46 mg/kg, administered intravenously, orally, and intramuscularly. Mean efficacy, as scored on a 0- to 3-point scale (3 = excellent), was 2.3 ± 0.21, but the drug was not efficacious in 17% of cases (four of five of these failures were via the oral route). EPS were not observed, and one episode of hypotension occurred with the intravenous route.

Droperidol has been used to treat acute agitation and confusion from a variety of causes, including mania and delirium (Hooper and Minter 1983; Resnick and Burton 1984; H. Thomas et al. 1992), and was superior to placebo (van Leeuwen et al. 1977). Compared with haloperidol, droperidol is more sedating, has a faster onset of action, can be used only parenterally in the United States, and is very hypotensive because of its potent α-adrenergic antagonism (Moulaert 1989). It is not recommended for use in delirium, however, because of serious cardiac safety concerns resulting from significant prolongation of the QTc interval in a dose-related manner (Lawrence and Nasraway 1997; Lischke et al. 1994; Reilly et al. 2000).

Atypical Antipsychotic Agents

Atypical antipsychotic agents differ from haloperidol and other conventional neuroleptics in a variety of neurotransmitter activities, especially serotonin. In addition to presynaptic serotonin type 2 (5-HT_2) receptor antagonism, it is hypothesized that loose binding at the dopamine D_2 receptor may define atypicality (Kapur and Seeman 2001). Some atypical antipsychotics are being used routinely to treat delirium, and literature on their use is accumulating. Hally and Cooney (2005) surveyed prescribing practices for delirium among general hospital medical staff and noted that risperidone was the second most frequently prescribed antipsychotic agent (38%) after haloperidol. In several patients who had a poor response to haloperidol, delirium improved after treatment was switched to an atypical antipsychotic agent (Al-Samarrai et al. 2003; Leso and Schwartz 2002; Passik and Cooper 1999). Haloperidol is avoided in posttraumatic brain injury delirium because dopamine blockade is thought to be deleterious to cognitive recovery; two traumatic brain injury patients with delirium given low-dose olanzapine showed remarkable improvement within a short time (Ovchinsky et al. 2002), suggesting a possible role for atypical antipsychotics in this population.

Because atypical antipsychotics differ in their chemical structures and are not a pharmacological class per se, they may differ in how they affect delirium. Receptor activities and adverse event profiles differ among the atypical agents, and their associated EPS, QTc prolongation, and effects on cognition are particularly relevant to any use in delirium. Ziprasidone was implicated in causing QTc prolongation in a patient with delirium (Leso and Schwartz 2002) and was temporally related to runs of torsades de pointes and QTc prolongation during rechallenge in a patient with delirium (Heinrich et al. 2006). In some case reports, risperidone, quetiapine, and olanzapine were implicated in causing delirium (Chen and Cardasis 1996; Karki and Masood 2003; Ravona-Springer et al. 1998; Samuels and Fang 2004; Sim et al. 2000).

A few reports included more than one atypical agent or compared conventional agents with atypical agents. Al-Samarrai et al. (2003) reported two cases of delirium that did not respond to either haloperidol or risperidone but settled soon after initiation of quetiapine. Three elderly patients with postoperative delirium responded quickly to olanzapine up to 10 mg/day and tolerated it well, despite not responding to or having excessive sedation from either haloperidol or risperidone (Khouzam and Gazula 2001). Hill et al. (2002) compared DRS-R98 daily ratings from 50 consecutive delirium cases treated with haloperidol, olanzapine, or risperidone and found a significant main effect of drug and time at 3 days, with olanzapine being more effective in reducing delirium severity than either haloperidol or risperidone. Skrobik et al. (2004) found similar efficacy for haloperidol and olanzapine in ICU patients, with more EPS in the haloperidol group, but standardized delirium ratings were not used and investigators were not blinded to

drug. J.Y. Kim et al. (2005) used the DRS-R98 to compare haloperidol and risperidone in an open-label nonrandomized trial and found equivalent efficacy. Blinded, randomized comparator studies are clearly needed to determine whether therapeutic differences exist.

Clozapine—the first atypical antipsychotic—is clinically distinct from the others and is not recommended for delirium treatment. It is very sedating, has significant anticholinergic side effects, causes sinus tachycardia, lowers seizure threshold, and is associated with causing agranulocytosis. Clozapine treatments ($n = 391$) resulted in about an 8% incidence of delirium episodes among 315 psychiatric inpatients, and in 7 of 33 episodes it was the only drug used (Gaertner et al. 1989). The incidence and risk factors for delirium were evaluated in 139 psychiatric patients with a mean age of 41 years who were given an average daily dose of 282 ± 203 mg/day for 18.9 ± 16.4 days (Centorrino et al. 2003). Delirium was diagnosed in 10.1%, and 71.4% of those cases were moderate to severe; cotreatment with other centrally active antimuscarinic drugs, poor clinical outcome, older age, and longer hospitalization (by 17.5 days) were associated with delirium in these patients. Cholinergic agents can reverse clozapine-induced delirium (Schuster et al. 1977).

Risperidone in doses up to 5 mg/day has been reported to reduce delirium severity as measured by the DRS in an open-label case series (Sipahimalani and Masand 1997) and several prospective open trials (Horikawa et al. 2003; Mittal et al. 2004; Parellada et al. 2004; Toda et al. 2005). Double-blind, placebo-controlled studies (I.R. Katz et al. 1999) have reported that risperidone has dose-related EPS beginning at about 2 mg/day. The combination of risperidone and the selective serotonin reuptake inhibitor paroxetine was reported to induce delirium as part of serotonin syndrome in two elderly patients (ages 78 and 86 years) (Karki and Masood 2003). Liu et al. (2004), in a retrospective analysis, found that risperidone had efficacy similar to that of haloperidol in treating hyperactive symptoms of delirium, but patients receiving risperidone required much less anticholinergic medication for EPS.

Eleven patients with delirium taking olanzapine showed similar response on the DRS to 11 patients with delirium taking haloperidol in an open-label, nonrandomized case series, although 5 haloperidol-treated patients had EPS or excessive sedation compared with none in the olanzapine-treated group (Sipahimalani and Masand 1998). Breitbart et al. (2002b) found resolution of delirium according to the MDAS with olanzapine treatment in 79% of patients by day 3 with overall good tolerability but less responsiveness in older patients with brain damage as a result of metastases or dementia. K. S. Kim et al. (2001) found decreased DRS scores in 20 patients with delirium (mean age = 46 years) taking olanzapine, which was well tolerated without EPS. Olanzapine has a favorable EPS profile and does not appear to have a clinically significant effect on the QTc interval at therapeutic doses in schizophrenic patients (Czekalla et al. 2001). Olanzapine increases acetylcholine release measured by in vivo microdialysis in both rat prefrontal cortex (Meltzer et al. 1999) and hippocampus (Schirazi et al. 2000), consistent with procholinergic activity. J. S. Kennedy et al. (2001) theorized that presynaptic blockade by olanzapine at 5-HT_3, 5-HT_6, and muscarinic type 2 (M_2) receptors may account for this increased acetylcholine release (see discussion of ondansetron in "Agents With Serotonergic Actions" subsection later in this chapter).

Open-label studies of patients with delirium treated with quetiapine with flexible dosing suggested that it was well tolerated and associated with symptom reduction on the DRS (K. Y. Kim et al. 2003; Sasaki et al. 2003) or DRS-R98 (Pae et al. 2004). Lee et al. (2005) compared amisulpride (mean dose = 156 mg/day) with quetiapine (mean dose = 113 mg/day) in an open-label, randomized study of delirium and found similar reductions in DRS-R98 scores, and both drugs were well tolerated.

Aripiprazole, an atypical antipsychotic with prodopaminergic effects related to partial agonism, was reported to be efficacious in an open-label trial in which the DRS-R98 was used and to have a low rate of adverse events (Straker et al. 2006).

Atypical agents in intramuscular formulations are therapeutic options being tried by clinicians whose medically ill patients cannot take oral medications. However, recent concerns about a possible increased risk of cerebrovascular events in elderly patients with dementia receiving chronic oral atypical antipsychotics (Brodaty et al. 2003; I. R. Katz et al. 1999) suggest a need for greater caution in their use, particularly in view of the high rate of concomitant dementia in patients with delirium. The risk of adverse cerebrovascular events is comparable for risperidone, quetiapine, and olanzapine, but the risk is elevated when they are used in patients with dementia compared with other indications (Layton et al. 2005). Other work suggests that stroke is no higher in elderly patients receiving atypical antipsychotics compared with typical antipsychotics (Herrmann et al. 2004) and that medication choice should be guided by a careful consideration of the overall risk-benefit ratio (L. S. Schneider et al. 2005).

Psychostimulants

Psychostimulants can worsen delirium—probably via increased dopaminergic activity—and their use when a depressed mood is present is contentious (J. A. Levenson 1992; P. B. Rosenberg et al. 1991). Morita et al. (2000) reported improvement of hypoactive delirium in a terminally ill cancer patient due to disseminated intravascular coagulation and multiorgan failure when methylphenidate, 10–20 mg/day, was administered, which raised the arousal level within 1 day and improved MDAS and DRS scores. They attributed the improvement to amelioration of an overstimulated γ-aminobutyric acid (GABA) system. In an open-label study, B. Gagnon et al. (2005) administered 20–30 mg of methylphenidate to 14 patients with advanced metastatic cancer and hypoactive delirium; median MMSE scores improved at 1-hour postdose. Cases with psychosis were excluded.

Anticonvulsant Agents

Anticonvulsant agents such as valproic acid may have a role in some cases of delirium, and they are first-line treatments when ictal states are the cause of delirium (Bourgeois et al. 2005; A. Schneider 2005).

Agents With Serotonergic Actions

Agents with serotonergic actions may be of therapeutic value in delirium. L-Tryptophan administered thrice daily was associated with improved MMSE scores and reduced tranquilizer requirement in an uncontrolled study of 32 patients with substance-related delirium (Hebenstreit et al. 1989). Mianserin, a serotonergic tetracyclic antidepressant, has been used in Japan for delirium in elderly medical and postsurgical cohorts, administered either orally or as a suppository. Several open-label studies found reductions in the DRS scores similar to those seen with haloperidol (J. Nakamura et al. 1995, 1997a, 1997b; Uchiyama et al. 1996). Its efficacy was theorized to be related to effects on reducing agitation and improving sleep or to its weak D_2 receptor antagonism in conjunction with blockade of postsynaptic $5\text{-}HT_2$, presynaptic α-adrenergic, and H_1 and H_2 histaminic receptor blockade.

A single 8-mg intravenous dose of ondansetron, a $5\text{-}HT_3$ antagonist, was reported to reduce agitation in patients with delirium when a 4-point rating scale was applied prospectively in 35 postcardiotomy patients (mean age = 51 years) (Bayindir et al. 2000). Blockade of presynaptic $5\text{-}HT_3$ and $5\text{-}HT_6$ receptors increases release of acetylcholine, possibly the mechanism for ondansetron's apparent beneficial effects.

POSTDELIRIUM MANAGEMENT

Treatment of delirium should continue until symptoms have fully resolved, but the role of continued treatment thereafter is uncertain. Alexopoulos et al. (2004) surveyed 52 experts on the treatment of older adults and found consensus that treatment of delirium should be continued for at least a week after response before tapering and discontinuation are attempted. However, many patients experiencing delirium are discharged before full resolution of symptoms, and, unfortunately, continued monitoring and management are often not part of postdischarge planning. Problems with attention and orientation are especially persistent (McCusker et al. 2003a). Further episodes may be prevented by addressing risk factors such as medication exposure and sensory impairments. There has been little study of the psychological aftermath of delirium, but recent work suggests that approximately 50% of patients can recall the episode (Breitbart et al. 2002a; O'Keeffe 2005). Depression and posttraumatic stress disorder have been described, but most dismiss the episode once it has passed, often despite lingering concerns that the episode heralds a first step toward loss of mental faculties and independence (Schofield 1997). Other patients experience silent delirium and are ashamed or afraid to admit to symptoms. Explicit recognition and discussion of the meaning of delirium can facilitate adjustment but also can allow more detailed discussion of how best to minimize future risk. A follow-up visit can facilitate postdelirium adjustment by clarifying the transient nature of delirium symptoms in contrast to dementia (Easton and MacKenzie 1988) and by providing any ongoing medication adjustments.

NEUROPATHOPHYSIOLOGY OF DELIRIUM

Delirium is considered to result from a generalized disturbance of higher cerebral cortical processes, as reflected by diffuse slowing on the EEG and a breadth of neuropsychiatric symptoms (cognition, perception, sleep, motor, language, and thought). It is not accompanied by primary motor or sensory deficits except when related to a specific etiology (e.g., asterixis), although progressive loss of control of motor functions occurs as severity increases (e.g., difficulty with hygiene and self-feeding; incontinence) (Engel and Romano 1959). Thus, not all brain regions are equally affected in delirium. Certain regions, circuits, and neurochemistry may be integral in the neuropathogenesis of delirium (Trzepacz 1994a, 1999b, 2000). Henon et al. (1999) found that laterality of lesion location and not metabolic factors accounted for the differences in delirium incidence for superficial cortical lesions.

Even though delirium has many different etiologies, each with its own physiological effects on the body, its constellation of symptoms is largely stereotyped, with many considered "core" symptoms (Meagher et al. 2007; Trzepacz et al. 2001). Somehow this diversity of physiological perturbations translates into a common clinical expression that may well relate to dysfunction of certain neural circuits (as well as neurotransmitters)—that is, a final common neural pathway (Trzepacz 1999b, 2000). An analogy of a funnel (see Figure 5–6) can be used to represent this common neural circuitry.

NEUROANATOMICAL CONSIDERATIONS

Studies support certain neural pathways being involved in delirium. Specifically, bilateral or right prefrontal cortex, superficial right posterior parietal cortex, basal ganglia, either right or left fusiform cortex (ventromesial temporoparietal) and lingual gyrus, and right anterior thalamus appear to be particularly associated with delirium (Trzepacz 2000). In addition, the pathways linking them (thalamic-frontal-subcortical and temporolimbic-frontal/subcortical) are likely involved. This hypothesis is largely based on structural neuroimaging reports of associated lesions (Table 5–9), only a few of which are consecutive and prospective in design, and a limited number of functional neuroimaging studies.

Lateralization to more right-sided circuitry involvement in delirium is supported by evidence besides lesion studies. The right prefrontal cortex cognitively processes novel situations, in contrast to the left (which processes familiar situations), and this may account for delirium patients' difficulties with comprehending new environments (E.L. Goldberg 1998). The right posterior parietal cortex subserves sustained attention and attention to the environment (Posner and Boies 1971), and both are often impaired in delirium. Bipolar patients had the highest incidence of delirium (35.5%) among 199 psychiatric inpatients (Ritchie et al. 1996), and because right-sided anterior and subcortical pathways have been implicated in mania (Blumberg et al. 1999), this suggests a predisposition to delirium possibly based on neuroanatomy. Bell's mania is a severe form of mania that causes pseudodelirium. Visual attention and visual memory tests—assessing nondominant hemisphere cognitive functions—distinguished delirious from nondelirious patients (Hart et al. 1997). Dopamine neurotransmission is lateralized such that activity is normally higher in the left prefrontal cortex (Glick et al. 1982), and this difference may become more extreme if right-sided pathways are affected in delirium.

Lesions of the right posterior parietal cortex may be present with severe delirium that overshadows sensory deficits (Boiten and Lodder 1989; Koponen et al. 1989a; Mesulam et al. 1979; Price and Mesulam 1985). Infarctions distributed in the right middle cerebral artery produce fewer localizing neurological signs when they are accompanied by agitated delirium (Schmidley and Messing 1984). Lesions of the fusiform region may be associated with an acute, agitated delirium accompanied by visual impairment (Horenstein et al. 1967; Medina et al. 1974, 1977). Despite their posterior location, lesions in this basal temporal region also may affect functions of the prefrontal cortex via temporal-limbic-frontal pathways.

The thalamus is uniquely positioned to filter, integrate, and regulate information among the brain stem, cortex, and subcortex. Abnormal EEG results and somatosensory evoked potential slowing are consistent with thalamic dysfunction in delirium (see subsection "Electroencephalography" earlier in this chapter). The anterior, medial, and dorsal thalamic nuclei have important interconnections with prefrontal, subcortical, and limbic areas that are involved in cognitive and behavioral functions.

TABLE 5–9.   Lesions associated with delirium in structural neuroimaging studies

Study	Lesions associated with delirium
Mesulam et al. 1979; Price and Mesulam 1985	CVA in R posterior parietal, R prefrontal, ventromedial temporal, or occipital cortex
Horenstein et al. 1967	CVAs in fusiform and calcarine cortices
Medina et al. 1977	L or bilateral mesial temporal-occipital CVA
Medina et al. 1974	L hippocampal or fusiform CVA
Vaphiades et al. 1996	R mesial occipital, parahippocampal, and hippocampal (with visual hallucinations)
Nighoghossian et al. 1992	R subcortical CVA (with frontal deactivation)
Bogousslavsky et al. 1988	R anterior thalamus CVA on preexisting L caudate lesion (with ↓ frontal perfusion on SPECT)
Figiel et al. 1989; Martin et al. 1992	Lesions in caudate nucleus (in depressed patients treated with ECT or medications)
Figiel et al. 1991	Parkinson's disease patients (depressed and treated with ECT or medications)
Koponen et al. 1989a	R prefrontal or posterior parietal cortex CVA (many with comorbid dementia)
Dunne et al. 1986	R temporoparietal CVA
Mullaly et al. 1982	R temporal or parietal CVA
Boiten and Lodder 1989	R inferior parietal lobule CVA
Friedman 1985; Santamaria et al. 1984	R anteromedial thalamus CVA
Henon et al. 1999	R superficial CVA (prospective sample)
Caeiro et al. 2004b	CVAs in R MCA hemispheric, thalamus, and caudate

Note.   CVA = cerebrovascular accident (stroke); ECT = electroconvulsive therapy; MCA = middle cerebral artery; R = right; L = left; SPECT = single-photon emission computed tomography.

Source.   Adapted from Trzepacz PT: "Is There a Final Common Neural Pathway in Delirium? Focus on Acetylcholine and Dopamine." *Seminars in Clinical Neuropsychiatry* 5:132–148, copyright 2000, with permission from Elsevier.

Because the thalamus is extensively and reciprocally interconnected with all areas of cerebral cortex, a relatively small thalamic lesion can cause delirium. The thalamus is rich in GABAergic interneurons and glutamatergic neurons (Sherman and Kock 1990) and receives cholinergic, noradrenergic, and serotonergic afferents from brain stem nuclei. Muscarinic influences at the thalamus affect baseline electroencephalographic rhythm. Strokes in the right paramedian and anteromedial thalamus (Bogousslavsky et al. 1988; Friedman 1985; Santamaria et al. 1984) can cause delirium. Gaudreau and Gagnon (2004) have proposed a model of delirium in which both "positive" symptoms (psychosis) and "negative" symptoms (inattention) can be caused by thalamic sensory overload caused by excessive dopaminergic or glutamatergic activity and/or reduced cholinergic or GABAergic activity.

Basal ganglia lesions are also associated with delirium. Preexisting lesions of the caudate nucleus (Figiel et al. 1989; Martin et al. 1992) and Parkinson's disease (Figiel et al. 1991) increase the risk of delirium during electroconvulsive therapy and with the use of tricyclic antidepressants. From a study of delirium incidence among 175 consecutive dementia patients, Robertsson et al. (1998) concluded that subcortical damage increased delirium risk and that patients with vascular dementia were more at risk than were those with early Alzheimer's or frontotemporal dementia.

A retrospective study of 661 stroke patients found 33% to be acutely confused on presentation (Dunne et al. 1986). The 19 patients diagnosed as having delirium almost exclusively had right-sided temporoparietal cortex lesions, although another 26 patients with similar lesions were not classified as having delirium because they lacked "clouded consciousness," and thus the frequency of delirium associated with such lesions was likely underdiagnosed. A retrospective study of 309 neurology consultations found 60 patients with acute confusional state; those with focal lesions had mostly right temporal or parietal locations (Mullaly et al. 1982).

A few prospective studies of stroke location and delirium incidence have been done. Ramirez-Bermudez et al. (2006) surveyed 202 neurological emergencies and found that delirium (incidence = 15%) was associated with lesions in the frontal and temporal lobes, but did not report laterality for individual cases. When DSM-IV criteria and a DRS score of 10 or more points were used to define cases, 202 consecutive stroke patients had a 25% incidence of delirium (Henon et al. 1999). Right-sided superficial cortical lesions were more associated with delirium than were left-sided lesions ($P = 0.009$), whereas deep lesions did not show laterality. Computed tomography scans for 69 consecutively admitted delirious (DSM-III diagnosis) elderly patients, many of whom had comorbid dementia, were compared with scans for 31 age-matched control subjects with other neurological disorders (Koponen et al. 1989a). Delirious patients had more generalized atrophy and focal changes—in particular, right hemisphere lesions in the parieto-occipital association area. On the basis of DSM-III-R criteria, 48% of 155 consecutive stroke patients were acutely confused (Gustafson et al. 1991). Among these, more patients with left-sided lesions were confused (58%) than those with right-sided lesions (38%), although the study was not designed to assess effects of laterality. Caeiro et al. (2004b) used the DRS to assess delirium prospectively in 218 consecutive acute stroke patients and a control group of 50 acute coronary syndrome patients; they found a higher incidence of delirium in the stroke patients (13% vs. 2%). Hemispheric strokes were more associated with delirium than were brain stem or cerebellar strokes, and the most common lesions were large right middle cerebral artery infarcts, and independent predictors included neglect (a nondominant cerebral dysfunction) and increased odds ratios for thalamus (1.3), caudate (6.7), and middle cerebral artery (2.4) lesion locations. Thus, many patients with strokes can become delirious through a variety of chemical or structural mechanisms—for example, glutamatergic surges and cholinergic deficiency—

but most evidence supports laterality for cortical and thalamic lesions.

Findings from single-photon emission computed tomography and positron emission tomography scans also support the relevance of the prefrontal cortex and subcortical regions in patients with delirium (Trzepacz 1994a). These tests usually show reduced flow or metabolism in the frontal cortex and either increased or decreased flow in subcortical regions. Yokota and colleagues (2003) used xenon-enhanced computed tomography and found widespread reduction in regional cerebral blood flow (cerebral cortex, thalamus, basal ganglia) in delirious patients that returned to normal when delirium improved. Reishies et al. (2005) found altered cognition following electroconvulsive therapy that was associated with increased slow-wave activity that was most pronounced in the anterior cingulate cortex, a region important for higher cognitive functions such as error processing, working memory, verbal fluency, selective attention, and long-term memory. Dysfunction in both cortical and subcortical regions in delirium is also supported by EEG slowing and slowing of evoked potentials (see subsection "Electroencephalography" earlier in this chapter).

NEUROTRANSMISSION

A final common neural pathway for delirium would be composed of both neuroanatomical and neurochemical dimensions. The preponderance of evidence in the literature supports a low cholinergic/excess dopaminergic state for this proposed final common neural pathway (Trzepacz 1996, 2000). Although other neurotransmitter systems are known to be involved for certain etiologies (e.g., hepatic insufficiency or alcohol withdrawal delirium), the activity of cholinergic and dopaminergic pathways can be regulated and affected by other neurotransmitters, including serotonergic, opiatergic, GABAergic, noradrenergic, and glutamatergic systems; altered metabolic states; physiological changes of inflammatory and stress responses; and glial activity. Thus,

many factors can interact with the final common pathway to culminate in delirium.

Neurotransmission may be altered in many ways, including through widespread effects on oxidative metabolism. Glucose and oxygen are both critical for brain function, and their delivery is dependent on properly functioning cardiovascular and pulmonary systems. Pathways for the metabolism of glucose and production of adenosine triphosphate involve oxygen and vitamins (cofactors for enzymes) as well as substrates related to neurotransmission (e.g., amino acids and acetyl coenzyme A), so the citric acid cycle is very important for general brain metabolism and production of neurotransmitters. Seaman et al. (2006) retrospectively found that measures of oxidative stress (hemoglobin, hematocrit, and pulse oximetry) and presence of pneumonia or sepsis were worse in patients who developed delirium in an ICU than in those who did not, even though no differences in overall medical morbidity were identified with APACHE II scores. During severe illness, surgery, and trauma, ratios of plasma amino acids may affect synthesis in the brain of neurotransmitters that are associated with immune activation and adaptive metabolic changes that redirect energy consumption (van der Mast and Fekkes 2000).

Alterations in the blood-brain barrier, such as during uremia, allow penetration of molecules and drugs that would not ordinarily enter the CNS and thereby produce unwanted effects on function of the brain regions and pathways. Vascular endothelial cells and perivascular cells at the interface between peripheral blood and brain parenchyma are proposed to be involved in transmission of inflammation from periphery to brain such that signals are transmitted via activation of those parenchymal microglia, according to postmortem human brain tissue studies (Uchikado et al. 2004). This is a suggested mechanism whereby systemic inflammatory responses are relayed to the brain despite an intact blood-brain barrier and may cause delirium through release of cytokines that alter neurotransmission without overt structural damage to the brain.

Whereas some etiologies of delirium alter neurotransmission via general metabolism, others may antagonize or interfere with specific receptors and neurotransmitters. Evidence indicates both specific and widespread effects on neurotransmission in delirium. In addition to changes in major neurotransmitter systems, neurotoxic metabolites, such as quinolinic acid from tryptophan metabolism (Basile et al. 1995), and false transmitters, such as octopamine in patients with liver failure, can alter neurotransmission and also have been implicated in the neuropathogenesis of delirium. Because glia regulate neurotransmitter amounts in the synapse, glial dysfunction also may be involved.

A wide variety of medications and their metabolites have anticholinergic activity and cause delirium. Some act postsynaptically; others act presynaptically; and still others, such as norfentanyl and normeperidine, have anticholinergic metabolites (Coffman and Dilsaver 1988). Tune et al. (1992) studied and measured the anticholinergic activity of many medications in "atropine equivalents." They identified significant anticholinergic effects in many medications usually not recognized as being anticholinergic (e.g., digoxin, nifedipine, cimetidine, and codeine). However, the assay used did not discriminate among the five muscarinic receptor subtypes, activity at which can result in opposite effects in the brain depending on location in the synapse; for example, blockade of presynaptic M_2 receptors results in an increased release of acetylcholine. Delirium induced by anticholinergic drugs is associated with generalized electroencephalographic slowing and is reversed by treatment with physostigmine or neuroleptics (Itil and Fink 1966; Stern 1983). Centrally active anticholinergic agents can cause electroencephalographic slowing and reduced verbal memory (Sloan et al. 1992).

A rat model of delirium in which a range of atropine doses was used showed similar features as human delirium: cognitive impairment, electroencephalographic slowing and increased amplitude, and hyperactivity during objective motor monitoring (Leavitt et al. 1994; Trzepacz et al. 1992) (see Figure 5–8). A different rat model in which lower atropine doses were used showed cognitive impairment, but because EEGs were not recorded, intoxication, but not delirium per se, was found (O'Hare et al. 1997).

In addition, several medical conditions have anticholinergic effects, including thiamine deficiency, hypoxia, and hypoglycemia, all of which may reduce acetylcholine by affecting the oxidative metabolism of glucose and the production of acetyl coenzyme A, the rate-limiting step for acetylcholine synthesis (Trzepacz 1994a, 1996). Consistent with these findings, glucose has been shown to enhance memory performance via a CNS muscarinic mechanism (Kopf and Baratti 1994). Parietal cortex levels of choline are reduced in chronic hepatic encephalopathy, as measured by magnetic resonance imaging (MRI) spectroscopy (Kreis et al. 1991).

Serum levels of anticholinergic activity are elevated in patients with postoperative delirium and correlate with severity of cognitive impairment (Tune et al. 1981), improving with resolution of the delirium (Mach et al. 1995). Post–electroconvulsive therapy delirium is also associated with higher serum anticholinergic levels (Mondimore et al. 1983). Higher serum anticholinergic activity levels were associated with reduced self-care ability among nursing home patients (Rovner et al. 1988). A double-blind intervention study in a nursing home showed that reduction of anticholinergic drugs improved cognitive status in those who had had elevated serum anticholinergic levels (Tollefson et al. 1991). This assay also detects substances circulating in peripheral blood that reflect inflammation and are not specific to the cholinergic system but may still have relevance to delirium.

Age-associated changes in cholinergic function also increase delirium propensity. Alzheimer's and vascular dementias reduce cholinergic activity and are associated with increased risk for delirium. Lewy body dementia mimics delirium with its fluctuating symptom severity,

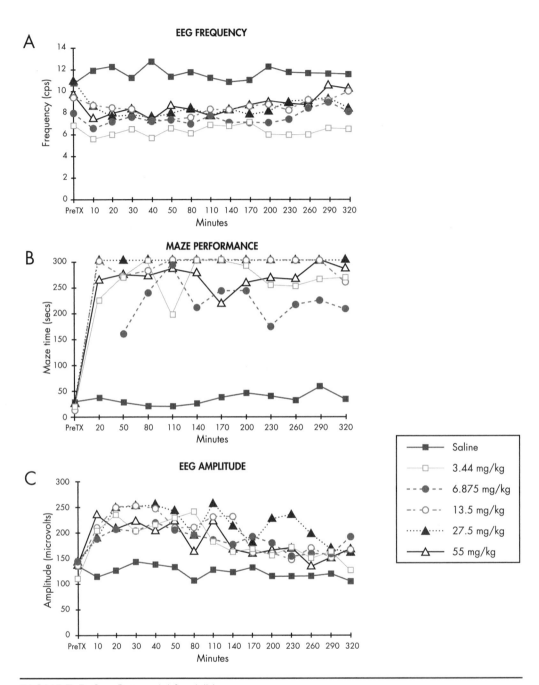

FIGURE 5–8.   Rat model for delirium.

Panel A. Electroencephalographic (EEG) frequency for saline control group and atropine dose groups at all times. *Panel B*. Maze performance for saline control group and atropine dose groups at all times. *Panel C*. EEG amplitude for saline control group and atropine dose groups at all times. PreTX = baseline; cps = cycles per second.

Source.   Reprinted from Leavitt M, Trzepacz PT, Ciongoli K: "Rat Model of Delirium: Atropine Dose-Response Relationships." *Journal of Neuropsychiatry and Clinical Neurosciences* 6:279–284, 1994. Copyright 1994, American Psychiatric Press, Inc. Used with permission.

confusion, hallucinations (especially visual), delusions, and electroencephalographic slowing and is associated with significant loss of cholinergic nucleus basalis neurons (Robinson 2002). Its delirium symptoms respond to donepezil (Kaufer et al. 1998). Use of cholinergic agents has been associated with reduced delirium incidence or improvement in delirium (see subsection "Pharmacological Treatment of Delirium" earlier in this chapter) (Dautzenberg et al. 2004; Diaz et al. 2001; Moretti et al. 2004), including in vascular dementia patients.

Stroke and traumatic brain injury are associated with decreased cholinergic activity—especially in the thalamus, amygdala, frontal cortex, hippocampus, and basal forebrain (Yamamoto et al. 1988)—and with increased vulnerability to antimuscarinic drugs (Dixon et al. 1994). The low cholinergic state seems to correlate temporally with delirium following the acute event (see Figure 5–9). Thus, broad support exists for an anticholinergic mechanism from diverse mechanisms of delirium: metabolic, neurochemical, and structural.

Cholinergic toxicity from organophosphate insecticides, nerve poisons, and tacrine (Trzepacz et al. 1996) also can cause delirium, although this is not as well described as anticholinergic delirium. Perhaps delirium results from extreme imbalances of cholinergic neurotransmitter activity levels.

Dopamine activity may be increased as a result of reduced cholinergic activity, conceptualized as an imbalance of the activities of dopamine and acetylcholine relative to each other. Hypoxia is associated with increased release of dopamine while decreasing the release of acetylcholine (Broderick and Gibson 1989). In striatum, D_2 receptor stimulation reduces acetylcholine release, whereas D_1 stimulation increases it (Ikarashi et al. 1997). Phasic dopamine release is associated with salience attribution to external stimuli, and it mediates working memory in the prefrontal cortex, which is essential for problem solving and decision making (Kienast and Heinz 2006). Both of these functions are important for a delirious

patient trying to interact with the environment. D_1 receptors are highly involved in the modulation of working memory and their activation follows an inverted U-shaped curve, so that too little or too much D_1 agonism disrupts performance.

Delirium can occur from intoxication with dopaminergic drugs, including levodopa, dopamine, and bupropion (Ames et al. 1992), and from cocaine binges (Wetli et al. 1996). Patients with alcohol withdrawal delirium are more likely to have the A9 allele of the dopamine transporter gene compared with matched control subjects without delirium (Sander et al. 1997), suggesting a role for dopamine in delirium propensity, although subsequent reports were inconsistent (Köhnke et al. 2005). Delirium from opiates may be mediated by increased dopamine and glutamate activity in addition to decreased acetylcholine (Gibson et al. 1975). Excess dopamine levels occur during hepatic encephalopathy, presumably as a result of increased levels of tyrosine and phenylalanine in cerebrospinal fluid (Knell et al. 1974) or changes in dopamine regulation by altered serotonin activity. Dopamine agonists (active at D_1 and D_2 receptors) have been shown to cause electroencephalographic slowing and behavioral arousal in rats (Ongini et al. 1985), findings similar to those seen in rats treated with atropine (Leavitt et al. 1994; Trzepacz et al. 1992). A rat model for delirium that used apomorphine (a direct D_1 and D_2 agonist) in a choice reaction task showed reversal of performance deficits by administration of haloperidol and aniracetam, a cholinomimetic, but not by administration of tacrine, which worsened deficits (K. Nakamura et al. 1998). The investigators concluded that cognitive deficits were mediated by a D_2 mechanism, but because EEGs were not recorded, it is not clear if this could be a delirium animal model.

Little is known about which dopamine receptor subtypes are involved in the neuropathogenesis of delirium, although those related to the mesolimbic and mesofrontal dopaminergic pathways are probably involved. Antidopaminergic agents, particularly neuro-

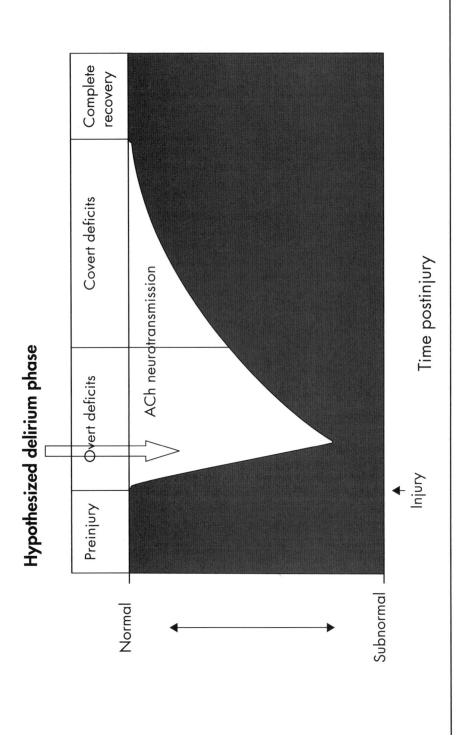

FIGURE 5–9.   Cholinergic hypofunction after traumatic brain injury.

ACh = acetylcholine.

Source.   Reprinted from Dixon CE, Hamm RJ, Taft WC, et al.: "Increased Anticholinergic Sensitivity Following Closed Skull Impact and Controlled Cortical Impact Traumatic Brain Injury in the Rat." *Journal of Neurotrauma* 11:275–287, 1994. Copyright 1994. Used with permission.

leptics, can be successfully used to treat delirium, including that arising from anticholinergic causes (Itil and Fink 1966; Platt et al. 1994a). Traditional neuroleptics that are effective in treating delirium are not subtype specific; haloperidol predominantly affects D_2 receptors, although it also affects D_1, D_3, and D_4 receptors (Piercey et al. 1995). Use of selective dopamine antagonists might shed light on the mechanism underlying delirium. For example, differential effects on D_1, D_2, and D_3 receptors might underlie different motor presentations during an individual delirium episode (Trzepacz 2000). Polymorphisms in genes related to dopamine receptors (e.g., through mutations, single-nucleotide polymorphisms, and variable number tandem repeats) may mediate more subtle differences in dopamine receptor function and open the door to better understanding of delirium occurrence and risk as well as treatment through genetic studies (Wong et al. 2000).

Norepinephrine is well known for its importance in cognition, especially with regard to attention, working memory, and executive functioning. J. Nakamura et al. (1997a) described decreased concentration of plasma-free 3-methoxy-4-hydroxy-phenylglycol (MHPG), a norepinephrine metabolite, in association with improvement on the DRS in response to treatment, reaching levels for nondelirious control subjects, but no difference in plasma-free homovanillic acid. This suggests that delirium is a hyperadrenergic state, even though plasma levels may not reflect CNS levels. Norepinephrine modulates and attenuates the effect of dopamine's disruption of normal gating; that is, suppression of irrelevant information at the nucleus accumbens. Low doses of dopamine can enhance gating, whereas higher doses disrupt it; this may be related to distractibility in delirium (Swerdlow et al. 2006).

Both increased and decreased GABA have been implicated in causing delirium. Increased GABAergic activity, in addition to reduced glutamate and increased serotonin activity, is one of several putative mechanisms implicated in hepatic encephalopathy (Mousseau and But-

terworth 1994). Increased GABA activity may result from elevated ammonia levels, which increase levels of glutamate and glutamine, which are then converted into GABA (B. Anderson 1984; Schafer and Jones 1982). Consistent with this hypothesis is the improvement observed in some patients with hepatic encephalopathy who are taking flumazenil, which blocks $GABA_A$-benzodiazepine receptors. Glutamine levels have been shown to be elevated in hepatic encephalopathy, as measured by MRI spectroscopy, although the chemical relations among glutamine, GABA, and glutamate confound the meaning of this measurement (Kreis et al. 1991). Reduced GABA activity occurs in delirium during withdrawal from ethanol and from sedative-hypnotic drugs. Decreased GABA activity is also implicated in the mechanism of antibiotic delirium caused by penicillins, cephalosporins, and quinolones (Akaike et al. 1991; Mathers 1987).

Both low and excessive levels of serotonin are associated with delirium (van der Mast and Fekkes 2000). Serotonin activity may be increased in patients with hepatic encephalopathy—related to increased tryptophan uptake in the brain (Mousseau and Butterworth 1994; van der Mast and Fekkes 2000)—as well as in sepsis (Mizock et al. 1990) and serotonergic syndromes (R. J. Goldberg and Huk 1992). The precursor of serotonin, tryptophan, is also implicated in delirium. Increases in free tryptophan levels in plasma correlate with reductions in cerebral blood flow on xenon-enhanced computed tomography scans in patients with subclinical hepatic encephalopathy (Rodriguez et al. 1987), and L-5-hydroxytryptophan induces delirium (Irwin et al. 1986). In contrast, tryptophan is decreased in patients with postcardiotomy delirium (van der Mast et al. 1994). Serotonin regulates dopamine activity in some brain regions, including the striatum and limbic system (Meltzer 1993), which may explain why neuroleptics are useful in treating serotonergic deliria.

Histamine may play a role in delirium through its effects on arousal and hypothalamic regulation of sleep-wake circadian rhythms. H_1 agonists and H_3 antagonists increase wakefulness (Monti 1993), whereas antihistamines (H_1 antagonists) reduce arousal and are associated with REM sleep (Marzanatti et al. 1989) and delirium (Tejera et al. 1994). H_1 antagonists increase catechols and serotonin levels and have anticholinergic properties (Jones et al. 1986), possibly mediating delirium. H_2 antagonists also cause delirium, possibly related to their anticholinergic properties (Picotte-Prillmayer et al. 1995), although they do not affect brain sleep centers.

Glutamate release is increased during hypoxia, and glutamatergic receptors may be activated by quinolone antibiotics (P.D. Williams and Helton 1991). Activation of glutamatergic receptors is a possible mechanism for quinolones causing delirium. Dopamine and glutamate are both neurotransmitters at the thalamus, a region potentially important in the neuropathogenesis of delirium.

Disruption of normal biological rhythms is well recognized in delirium, particularly in relation to sleep-wake cycles and other circadian cycles. Melatonin receptors exist at the suprachiasmatic nucleus of the hypothalamus. Several studies have suggested a possible relation between these disruptions and altered melatonin metabolism; tryptophan is the precursor for both melatonin and serotonin. Shigeta et al. (2001) compared melatonin secretion patterns of nondelirious and delirious patients with and without complications after major abdominal surgery. In the patients with delirium, reduced melatonin levels were not associated with complications, and markedly elevated melatonin levels resulted in complications (infection, shock, cardiac failure). Similarly, K. Olofsson et al. (2004) advocated a trial of melatonin as a treatment for delirium on the basis of observed disruption of the circadian rhythm of melatonin secretion in ICU patients. Balan et al. (2003) found high levels of melatonin metabolites in the urine in delirium, especially in patients with hypoactive delirium. Lewis and Barnett (2004) proposed that administration of melatonin in delirium may restore tryptophan levels by reducing its breakdown and thereby treat not only hypoactive but also hyperactive forms by blunting activity of an alternative metabolic pathway for tryptophan that produces an abnormal metabolite that is believed to produce excitatory symptoms.

CYTOKINES AND INFLAMMATORY RESPONSE

Cytokines have been implicated as causes of inflammatory or infection-induced delirium, and they also may have a role in sleep (Moldofsky et al. 1986). They are polypeptide hormones secreted in the CNS by glia and macrophages, whose normally low extracellular levels are increased during stress, rapid growth, inflammation, tumor, trauma, and infection (Hopkins and Rothwell 1995; Stefano et al. 1994). Although cytokines are not yet identified as neurotransmitters per se, they may influence the activities of catecholamines, indoleamines, GABA, and acetylcholine (Hopkins and Rothwell 1995) and can cause increased release and turnover of dopamine and norepinephrine (Stefano et al. 1994) and reduction of acetylcholine levels (Willard et al. 1999), thereby causing delirium. Cytokines acting as neurotoxins, as in HIV dementia, is another mechanism for causing brain dysfunction (Lipton and Gendelman 1995), although Broadhurst and Wilson (2001) have highlighted that inhibition of growth factor–mediated neuroprotective effects may be a significant mechanism by which cytokines enhance neurodegeneration, especially in a compromised CNS.

The use of interleukins in cancer patients is commonly associated with delirium (S. Rosenberg et al. 1989). Interleukin-1 (IL-1) is an endogenous pyrogen, high doses of IL-2 cause delirium, IL-6 levels predict lesion size in stroke, and tumor necrosis factor α is a cytotoxic cytokine, whereas insulinlike growth factor–1 (IGF-1) is neuroprotective and inhibits cytotoxic cytokines (K. Wilson et al. 2005). K. Wilson et al. (2005) found that low premorbid IGF-1 levels predicted delirium incidence in a prospective study. De Rooij (2005b) found increased levels of IL-6, IL-8, and C-reactive protein in hospitalized elderly patients with delirium. Conversely, somatostatin and IGF-1 have been shown to improve cognitive function in preclinical and clinical studies of cognitively impaired subjects (Craft et al. 1999; Saatman et al. 1997) and may therefore have a role in prevention and treatment of delirium. Further work on the protective role of IGF-1 in patients at risk for delirium is needed.

CONCLUSION

Delirium is a common neuropsychiatric disorder affecting cognition, thinking, perception, sleep, language, and other behaviors. It is associated with increased mortality following an episode, the attribution of which to delirium itself or underlying medical problems is unclear. It affects persons of any age, although elderly patients may be particularly vulnerable, especially if they have dementia. Research in nongeriatric adults and children is sorely needed lest we risk error in applying data from elderly to younger persons. Clinical assessment of delirium can be aided through the use of diagnostic criteria and rating scales, as well as knowledge of which populations are at risk. Research could greatly benefit from consensus on using certain valid, specific, and sensitive instruments across studies. Underdetection and misdiagnosis are rampant, begging for valid, concise screening and monitoring tools.

Certain symptoms of delirium may represent "core" symptoms, whereas others may be associated symptoms that occur under various conditions, possibly more related to etiology or idiopathic features. Core symptoms may reflect dysfunction of certain brain regions and neurotransmitter systems that constitute a "final common neural pathway" that is responsible for the presentation of the syndrome of delirium. Regions implicated include prefrontal cortex, thalamus, basal ganglia, right temporoparietal cortex, and fusiform and lingual gyri. Diverse physiologies related to the wide variety of etiologies may funnel into a common neurofunctional expression for delirium via elevated brain dopaminergic and reduced cholinergic activity or a relative imbalance between

these. Other neurochemical candidates include serotonin, melatonin, norepinephrine, GABA, glutamate, and cytokines, although these may interact to regulate or alter activity of acetylcholine and dopamine in key circuitry.

The clinical standard of treatment involves a dopamine antagonist medication—usually haloperidol—although, theoretically, procholinergic drugs should help. Drug treatment studies for delirium, particularly double-blind studies, are few, and no placebo-controlled, appropriately powered efficacy trials have been done. Newer agents deserve more study as well. It is important to initiate treatment even before medical causes have been rectified and for both hypoactive and hyperactive psychomotor presentations because target symptoms are probably cognition, thought, sleep, and language. That delirium is common yet inadequately detected; associated with increased morbidity, mortality, and length of hospitalization; and potentially caused by virtually anything from a textbook of medicine has been well substantiated. The travesty is the lack of a specific efficacious and well-tolerated treatment as substantiated by a regulatory approval in any country. Clearly, delirium needs to become a top priority for regulatory agencies and national research funding institutions.

RECOMMENDED READINGS

Breitbart W, Gibson C, Tremblay A: The delirium experience: delirium recall and delirium-related distress in hospitalized patients with cancer, their spouses/caregivers, and their nurses. Psychosomatics 43:183–194, 2002

Engel GL, Romano J: Delirium, a syndrome of cerebral insufficiency. J Chronic Dis 9:260–277, 1959

Kalisvaart KJ, de Jonghe JFM, Bogaards MJ, et al: Haloperidol prophylaxis for elderly hip surgery patients at risk for delirium: a randomized, placebo-controlled study. J Am Geriatr Soc 53:1658–1666, 2005

Marcantonio ER, Flacker JM, Wright RJ, et al: Reducing delirium after hip fracture: a randomized trial. J Am Geriatr Soc 49:516–522, 2001

Meagher D: Delirium: optimizing management. BMJ 322:144–149, 2001

Trzepacz PT: Is there a final common neural pathway in delirium? Focus on acetylcholine and dopamine. Semin Clin Neuropsychiatry 5:132–148, 2000

REFERENCES

Adamis D, Morrison C, Treloar A, et al: The performance of the Clock Drawing Test in elderly medical inpatients: does it have utility in the identification of delirium? J Geriatr Psychiatry Neurol 18:129–133, 2005

Adams F: Neuropsychiatric evaluation and treatment of delirium in the critically ill cancer patient. Cancer Bull 36:156–160, 1984

Adams F: Emergency intravenous sedation of the delirious medically ill patient. J Clin Psychiatry 49(suppl):22–26, 1988

Adunsky A, Levy R, Mizrahi E, et al: Exposure to opioid analgesia in cognitively impaired and delirious elderly hip fracture patients. Arch Gerontol Geriatr 35:245–251, 2002

Agnoletti V, Ansaloni L, Catena F, et al: Postoperative delirium after elective and emergency surgery: analysis and checking of risk factors: a study protocol. BMC Surg 5:12, 2005

Akaike N, Shirasaki T, Yakushiji T: Quinolone and fenbufen interact with GABA-A receptors in dissociated hippocampal cells of rats. J Neurophysiol 66:497–504, 1991

Alexopoulos GS, Streim J, Carpenter D, et al: Using antipsychotic agents in older patients. Expert Consensus Panel for Using Antipsychotic Drugs in Older Patients. J Clin Psychiatry 65 (suppl 2):5–99, 2004

Al-Samarrai S, Dunn J, Newmark T, et al: Quetiapine for treatment-resistant delirium. Psychosomatics 44:350–351, 2003

American Psychiatric Association: Diagnostic and Statistical Manual of Mental Disorders, 2nd Edition. Washington, DC, American Psychiatric Association, 1968

American Psychiatric Association: Diagnostic and Statistical Manual of Mental Disorders, 3rd Edition. Washington, DC, American Psychiatric Association, 1980

American Psychiatric Association: Diagnostic and Statistical Manual of Mental Disorders, 3rd Edition, Revised. Washington, DC, American Psychiatric Association, 1987

American Psychiatric Association: Diagnostic and Statistical Manual of Mental Disorders, 4th Edition. Washington, DC, American Psychiatric Association, 1994

American Psychiatric Association: Practice guidelines for the treatment of patients with delirium. Am J Psychiatry 156(suppl):1–20, 1999

American Psychiatric Association: Diagnostic and Statistical Manual of Mental Disorders, 4th Edition, Text Revision. Washington, DC, American Psychiatric Association, 2000

Ames D, Wirshing WC, Szuba MP: Organic mental disorders associated with bupropion in three patients. J Clin Psychiatry 53:53–55, 1992

Anderson B: A proposed theory for the encephalopathies of Reye's syndrome and hepatic encephalopathy. Med Hypotheses 15:415–420, 1984

Anderson SD: Treatment of elderly patients with delirium. Can Med Assoc J 152:323–324, 1995

Andreasen NJC, Hartford CE, Knott JR, et al: EEG changes associated with burn delirium. Dis Nerv Syst 38:27–31, 1977

Armstrong DH, Dasts JF, Reilly TE, et al: Effect of haloperidol on dopamine-induced increase in renal blood flow. Drug Intell Clin Pharm 20:543–546, 1986

Armstrong SC, Cozza KL, Watanabe KS: The misdiagnosis of delirium. Psychosomatics 38:433–439, 1997

Balan S, Leibovitz A, Zila SO, et al: The relation between the clinical subtypes of delirium and the urinary level of 6-SMT. J Neuropsychiatry Clin Neurosci 15:363–366, 2003

Bartlett EJ, Brodie JD, Simkowitz P, et al: Effects of haloperidol challenge on regional cerebral glucose utilization in normal human subjects. Am J Psychiatry 151:681–686, 1994

Basile AS, Saito K, Li Y, et al: The relationship between plasma and brain quinolinic acid levels and the severity of hepatic encephalopathy in animal models of fulminant hepatic failure. J Neurochem 64:2607–2614, 1995

Bayindir O, Akpinar B, Can E, et al: The use of the 5-HT$_3$ antagonist ondansetron for the treatment of post-cardiotomy delirium. J Cardiothorac Vasc Anesth 14:288–292, 2000

Bedford PD: General medical aspects of confusional states in elderly people. BMJ 2:185–188, 1957

Berggren D, Gustafson Y, Eriksson B, et al: Postoperative confusion following anesthesia in elderly patients treated for femoral neck fractures. Anesth Analg 66:497–504, 1987

Bettin KM, Maletta GJ, Dysken MW, et al: Measuring delirium severity in older general hospital inpatients without dementia: the Delirium Severity Scale. Am J Geriatr Psychiatry 6:296–307, 1998

Blumberg HP, Stern E, Ricketts S, et al: Rostral orbitofrontal prefrontal cortex dysfunction in the manic state of bipolar disorder. Am J Psychiatry 156:1986–1988, 1999

Bogardus ST Jr, Desai MM, Williams CS, et al: The effects of a targeted multicomponent delirium intervention on postdischarge outcomes for hospitalized older adults. Am J Med 114:383–390, 2003

Bogousslavsky J, Ferranzzini M, Regli F, et al: Manic delirium and frontal-like syndrome with paramedian infarction of the right thalamus. J Neurol Neurosurg Psychiatry 51:116–119, 1988

Boiten J, Lodder J: An unusual sequela of a frequently occurring neurologic disorder: delirium caused by brain infarct. Ned Tijdschr Geneeskd 133:617–620, 1989

Bostwick JM, Masterson BJ: Psychopharmacological treatment of delirium to restore mental capacity. Psychosomatics 39:112–117, 1998

Bourdel-Marchasson I, Vincent S, Germain C, et al: Delirium symptoms and low dietary intake in older inpatients are independent predictors of institutionalization: a 1-year prospective population-based study. J Gerontol A Biol Sci Med Sci 59:350–354, 2004

Bourgeois JA, Koike AK, Simmons JE, et al: Adjunctive valproic acid for delirium and/or agitation on a consultation-liaison service: a report of six cases. J Neuropsychiatry Clin Neurosci 17:232–238, 2005

Breitbart W, Marotta R, Platt MM, et al: A double-blind trial of haloperidol, chlorpromazine, and lorazepam in the treatment of delirium in hospitalized AIDS patients. Am J Psychiatry 153:231–237, 1996

Breitbart W, Rosenfeld B, Roth A, et al: The Memorial Delirium Assessment Scale. J Pain Symptom Manage 13:128–137, 1997

Breitbart W, Gibson C, Tremblay A: The delirium experience: delirium recall and delirium-related distress in hospitalized patients with cancer, their spouses/caregivers, and their nurses. Psychosomatics 43:183–194, 2002a

Breitbart W, Tremblay A, Gibson C: An open trial of olanzapine for the treatment of delirium in hospitalized cancer patients. Psychosomatics 43:175–182, 2002b

Broadhurst C, Wilson K: Immunology of delirium: new opportunities for treatment and research. Br J Psychiatry 179:288–289, 2001

Brodaty H, Ames D, Snowdon J, et al: A randomized placebo-controlled trial of risperidone for the treatment of aggression, agitation, and psychosis of dementia. J Clin Psychiatry 64:134–143, 2003

Broderick PA, Gibson GE: Dopamine and serotonin in rat striatum during in vivo hypoxic-hypoxia. Metab Brain Dis 4:143–153, 1989

Brown RL, Henke A, Greenhalgh DG, et al: The use of haloperidol in the agitated, critically ill pediatric patient with burns. J Burn Care Rehabil 17:34–38, 1996

Brown TM: Drug-induced delirium. Semin Clin Neuropsychiatry 5:113–125, 2000

Bucerius J, Gummert JF, Borger MA, et al: Predictors of delirium after cardiac surgery delirium: effect of beating-heart (off-pump) surgery. J Thorac Cardiovasc Surg 127:57–64, 2004

Burke WJ, Roccaforte WH, Wengel SP: Treating visual hallucinations with donepezil. Am J Psychiatry 156:1117–1118, 1999

Burns MJ, Linden CH, Graudins A, et al: A comparison of physostigmine and benzodiazepines for the treatment of anticholinergic poisoning. Ann Emerg Med 35:374–381, 2000

Caeiro L, Ferro JM, Albuquerque R, et al: Delirium in the first days of acute stroke. J Neurol 251:171–178, 2004a

Caeiro L, Ferro JM, Claro MI, et al: Delirium in acute stroke: a preliminary study of the role of anticholinergic medications. Eur J Neurol 11:699–704, 2004b

Caeiro L, Menger C, Ferro JM, et al: Delirium in acute subarachnoid haemorrhage. Cerebrovasc Dis 19:31–38, 2005

Cameron DJ, Thomas RI, Mulvihill M, et al: Delirium: a test of DSM-III criteria on medical inpatients. J Am Geriatr Soc 35:1007–1010, 1987

Camus V, Gonthier R, Dubos G, et al: Etiologic and outcome profiles in hypoactive and hyperactive subtypes of delirium. J Geriatr Psychiatry Neurol 13:38–42, 2000

Caplan GA, Coconis J, Board N, et al: Does home treatment affect delirium? A randomised controlled trial of rehabilitation of elderly and care at home or usual treatment (The REACH-OUT trial). Age Ageing 35:53–60, 2005

Carnes M, Howell T, Rosenberg M, et al: Physicians vary in approaches to the clinical assessment of delirium. J Am Geriatr Soc 51:234–239, 2003

Centorrino F, Albert MJ, Drago-Ferrante G, et al: Delirium during clozapine treatment: incidence and associated risk factors. Pharmacopsychiatry 36:156–160, 2003

Charlton BG, Kavanau JL: Delirium and psychotic symptoms: an integrative model. Med Hypotheses 58:24–27, 2002

Chatham MA: The effect of family involvement on patients' manifestations of postcardiotomy psychosis. Heart Lung 7:995–999, 1978

Chedru F, Geschwind N: Writing disturbances in acute confusional states. Neuropsychologia 10:343–353, 1972

Chen B, Cardasis W: Delirium induced by lithium and risperidone combination. Am J Psychiatry 153:1233–1234, 1996

Coffman JA, Dilsaver SC: Cholinergic mechanisms in delirium. Am J Psychiatry 145:382–383, 1988

Cole MG, Primeau FJ: Prognosis of delirium in elderly hospital patients. Can Med Assoc J 149:41–46, 1993

Cole MG, McCusker J, Bellavance F, et al: Systematic detection and multidisciplinary care of delirium in older medical inpatients: a randomized trial. Can Med Assoc J 167:753–759, 2002a

Cole M[G], McCusker J, Dendukuri N, et al: Symptoms of delirium among elderly medical inpatients with or without dementia. J Neuropsychiatry Clin Neurosci 14:167–175, 2002b

Cole MG, Dendukuri N, McCusker J, et al: An empirical study of different diagnostic criteria for delirium among elderly medical inpatients. J Neuropsychiatry Clin Neurosci 15:200–207, 2003a

Cole M[G], McCusker J, Dendukuri N, et al: The prognostic significance of subsyndromal delirium in elderly medical inpatients. J Am Geriatr Soc 51:754–760, 2003b

Craft S, Asthana MD, Newcomer JW, et al: Enhancement of memory in Alzheimer's disease with insulin and somatostain, but not glucose. Arch Gen Psychiatry 56:1135–1140, 1999

Csokasy J: Assessment of acute confusion: use of the NEECHAM confusion scale. Appl Nurs Res 12:51–55, 1999

Curyto KJ, Johnson J, TenHave T, et al: Survival of hospitalized elderly patients with delirium: a prospective study. Am J Geriatr Psychiatry 9:141–147, 2001

Cushman LA: Secondary neuropsychiatric complications in stroke: implications for acute care. Arch Phys Med Rehabil 69:877–879, 1998

Cutting J: The phenomenology of acute organic psychosis: comparison with acute schizophrenia. Br J Psychiatry 151:324–332, 1987

Czekalla J, Beasley CM Jr, Dellva MA, et al: Analysis of the QTc interval during olanzapine treatment of patients with schizophrenia and related psychoses. J Clin Psychiatry 62:191–198, 2001

Dautzenberg PL, Mulder LJ, Olde Rikkert MG, et al: Delirium in elderly hospitalized patients: protective effects of chronic rivastigmine usage. Int J Geriatr Psychiatry 19:641–644, 2004

de Jonghe JFM, Kalisvaart KJ, Eikelenboom P, et al: Early symptoms in the prodromal phase of delirium in elderly hip-surgery patients. Int Psychogeriatr 17 (suppl 2):148, 2005

De Rooij S: Delirium subtype identification and the validation of the Delirium Rating Scale—Revised-98 (Dutch version) in hospitalised elderly patients. Int Psychogeriatr 17 (suppl 2):262, 2005a

De Rooij S: Raised levels of interleukin-6, interleukin-8, and C-reactive protein in hospitalised elderly patients with delirium. Int Psychogeriatr 17 (suppl 2):146–157, 2005b

Diaz V, Rodriguez J, Barrientos P, et al: Use of procholinergics in the prevention of postoperative delirium in hip fracture surgery in the elderly: a randomized controlled trial. Rev Neurol 33:716–719, 2001

Dickson LR: Hypoalbuminemia in delirium. Psychosomatics 32:317–323, 1991

Dixon CE, Hamm RJ, Taft WC, et al: Increased anticholinergic sensitivity following closed skull impact and controlled cortical impact traumatic brain injury in the rat. J Neurotrauma 11:275–287, 1994

Drake ME, Coffey CE: Complex partial status epilepticus simulating psychogenic unresponsiveness. Am J Psychiatry 140:800–801, 1983

Dudley DL, Rowlett DB, Loebel PJ: Emergency use of intravenous haloperidol. Gen Hosp Psychiatry 1:240–246, 1979

Dunne JW, Leedman PJ, Edis RH: Inobvious stroke: a cause of delirium and dementia. Aust N Z J Med 16:771–778, 1986

Duppils GS, Wikblad K: Delirium: behavioural changes before and during the prodromal phase. J Clin Nurs 13:609–616, 2004

Easton C, MacKenzie F: Sensory-perceptual alterations: delirium in the intensive care unit. Heart Lung 17:229–237, 1988

Ely EW, Dittus RS: Pharmacological treatment of delirium in the intensive care unit. JAMA 292:168, 2004

Ely EW, Gautam S, Margolin R, et al: The impact of delirium in the intensive care unit on hospital length of stay. Intensive Care Med 27:1892–1900, 2001a

Ely EW, Gordan S, Francis J, et al: Evaluation of delirium in critically ill patients: validation of the Confusion Assessment Method for the intensive care unit (CAM-ICU). Crit Care Med 29:1370–1379, 2001b

Ely EW, Shintani A, Truman B, et al: Delirium as a predictor of mortality in mechanically ventilated patients in the intensive care unit. JAMA 291:1753–1762, 2004a

Ely EW, Stephens RK, Jackson JC, et al: Current opinions regarding the importance, diagnosis, and management of delirium in the intensive care unit: a survey of 912 healthcare professionals. Crit Care Med 32:106–112, 2004b

Engel GL, Romano J: Delirium, II: reversibility of electroencephalogram with experimental procedures. Arch Neurol Psychiatry 51:378–392, 1944

Engel GL, Romano J: Delirium, a syndrome of cerebral insufficiency. J Chronic Dis 9:260–277, 1959

Erkinjuntti T, Wikstrom J, Parlo J, et al: Dementia among medical inpatients: evaluation of 2000 consecutive admissions. Arch Intern Med 146:1923–1926, 1986

Ewert J, Levin HS, Watson MG, et al: Procedural memory during posttraumatic amnesia in survivors of severe closed head injury: implications for rehabilitation. Arch Neurol 46:911–916, 1985

Fann JR: The epidemiology of delirium: a review of studies and methodological issues. Semin Clin Neuropsychiatry 5:86–92, 2000

Fann JR, Roth-Roemer S, Burington BE, et al: Delirium in patients undergoing hematopoietic stem cell transplantation. Cancer 95:1971–1981, 2002

Fann JR, Alfano CM, Burington BE, et al: Clinical presentation of delirium in patients undergoing hematopoietic stem cell transplantation. Cancer 103:810–820, 2005

Farrell KR, Ganzini L: Misdiagnosing delirium as depression in medically ill elderly patients. Arch Intern Med 155:2459–2464, 1995

Fernandez F, Holmes VF, Adams F, et al: Treatment of severe, refractory agitation with a haloperidol drip. J Clin Psychiatry 49:239–241, 1988

Fernandez F, Levy JK, Mansell PWA: Management of delirium in terminally ill AIDS patients. Int J Psychiatry Med 19:165–172, 1989

Ferro JM, Caeiro L, Verdelho A: Delirium in acute stroke. Curr Opin Neurol 15:51–55, 2002

Fick DM, Kolanowski AM, Waller JL, et al: Delirium superimposed on dementia in a community-dwelling managed care population: a three-year retrospective study of occurrence, costs and utilization. J Gerontol Med Sci 60A:748–753, 2005

Figiel GS, Krishman KR, Breitner JC, et al: Radiologic correlates of antidepressant-induced delirium: the possible significance of basal ganglia lesions. J Neuropsychiatry Clin Neurosci 1:188–190, 1989

Figiel GS, Hassen MA, Zorumski C, et al: ECT-induced delirium in depressed patients with Parkinson's disease. J Neuropsychiatry Clin Neurosci 3:405–411, 1991

Fisher BW, Flowerdew G: A simple model for predicting postoperative delirium in older patients undergoing elective orthopedic surgery. J Am Geriatr Soc 43:175–178, 1995

Flaherty JH, Tariq SH, Raghavan S, et al: A model for managing delirious older inpatients. J Am Geriatr Soc 51:1031–1035, 2003

Foley CM, Polinsky MS, Gruskin AB, et al: Encephalopathy in infants and children with chronic renal disease. Arch Neurol 38:656–658, 1981

Fonseca F, Bulbena A, Navarrete R, et al: Spanish version of the Delirium Rating Scale—Revised-98: reliability and validity. Psychosom Res 59:147–151, 2005

Forman LJ, Cavalieri TA, Galski T, et al: Occurrence and impact of suspected delirium in hospitalized elderly patients. J Am Osteopath Assoc 95:588–591, 1995

Francis J: Sensory and environmental factors in delirium. Paper presented at Delirium: Current Advancements in Diagnosis, Treatment and Research, Geriatric Research, Education, and Clinical Center (GRECC), Veterans Administration Medical Center, Minneapolis, MN, September 13–14, 1993

Francis J, Kapoor WN: Prognosis after hospital discharge of older medical patients with delirium. J Am Geriatr Soc 40:601–606, 1992

Francis J, Martin D, Kapoor WN: A prospective study of delirium in hospitalized elderly. JAMA 263:1097–1101, 1990

Franco K, Litaker D, Locala J, et al: The cost of delirium in the surgical patient. Psychosomatics 42:68–73, 2001

Friedman JH: Syndrome of diffuse encephalopathy due to nondominant thalamic infarction. Neurology 35:1524–1526, 1985

Gaertner HJ, Fischer E, Hoss J: Side effects of clozapine. Psychopharmacology 99:S97–S100, 1989

Gagnon B, Lawlor PG, Mancini IL, et al: The impact of delirium on the circadian distribution of breakthrough analgesia in advanced cancer patients. J Pain Symptom Manage 22:826–833, 2001

Gagnon B, Low G, Schreier G: Methylphenidate hydrochloride improves cognitive function in patients with advanced cancer and hypoactive delirium: a prospective clinical study. J Psychiatry Neurosci 30:100–107, 2005

Gagnon P, Charbonneau C, Allard P, et al: Delirium in advanced cancer; a psychoeducational intervention for family caregivers. J Palliat Care 18:253–261, 2002

Gallinat J, Moller HJ, Hegerl U: Piracetam in anesthesia for prevention of postoperative delirium. Anasthesiol Intensivmed Notfallmed Schmerzther 34:520–527, 1999

Gaudreau JD, Gagnon P: Psychotogenic drugs and delirium pathogenesis: the central role of the thalamus. Med Hypotheses 64:471–475, 2004

Gaudreau JD, Gagnon P, Harel F, et al: Fast, systematic, and continuous delirium assessment in hospitalized patients: the Nursing Delirium Screening Scale. J Pain Symptom Manage 29:368–375, 2005a

Gaudreau JD, Gagnon P, Harel F, et al: Psychoactive medications and risk of delirium in hospitalized cancer patients. J Clin Oncol 23:6712–6728, 2005b

Gelfand SB, Indelicato J, Benjamin J: Using intravenous haloperidol to control delirium (abstract). Hosp Community Psychiatry 43:215, 1992

George J, Bleasdale S, Singleton SJ: Causes and prognosis of delirium in elderly patients admitted to a district general hospital. Age Ageing 26:423–427, 1997

Gibson GE, Jope R, Blass JP: Decreased synthesis of acetylcholine accompanying impaired oxidation of pyruvate in rat brain slices. Biochem J 26:17–23, 1975

Glick SD, Ross DA, Hough LB: Lateral asymmetry of neurotransmitters in human brain. Brain Res 234:53–63, 1982

Goldberg EL: Lateralization of frontal lobe functions and cognitive novelty. J Neuropsychiatry Clin Neurosci 6:371–378, 1998

Goldberg RJ, Huk M: Serotonergic syndrome from trazodone and buspirone (letter). Psychosomatics 33:235–236, 1992

Gorwood P, Limosin F, Batel P, et al: The A9 allele of the dopamine transporter gene is associated with delirium tremens and alcohol-withdrawal seizure. Biol Psychiatry 53:85–92, 2003

Grassi L, Caraceni A, Beltrami E, et al: Assessing delirium in cancer patients: the Italian versions of the Delirium Rating Scale and the Memorial Delirium Assessment Scale. J Pain Symptom Manage 21:59–68, 2001

Gupta AK, Saravay SM, Trzepacz PT, et al: Delirium motoric subtypes (abstract). Psychosomatics 46:158, 2005

Gustafson Y, Berggren D, Brahnstrom B, et al: Acute confusional states in elderly patients treated for femoral neck fracture. J Am Geriatr Soc 36:525–530, 1988

Gustafson Y, Olsson T, Eriksson S, et al: Acute confusional state (delirium) in stroke patients. Cerebrovasc Dis 1:257–264, 1991

Hales RE, Polly S, Orman D: An evaluation of patients who received an organic mental disorder diagnosis on a psychiatric consultation-liaison service. Gen Hosp Psychiatry 11:88–94, 1988

Hally O, Cooney C: Delirium in the hospitalized elderly: an audit of NCHD prescribing practice. Ir J Psychol Med 22:133–136, 2005

Han CS, Kim YK: A double-blind trial of risperidone and haloperidol for the treatment of delirium. Psychosomatics 45:297–301, 2004

Han L, McCusker J, Cole M, et al: Use of medications with anticholinergic effect predicts clinical severity of delirium symptoms in older medical inpatients. Arch Intern Med 161:1099–1105, 2001

Harrell R, Othmer E: Postcardiotomy confusion and sleep loss. J Clin Psychiatry 48:445–446, 1987

Hart RP, Levenson JL, Sessler CN, et al: Validation of a cognitive test for delirium in medical ICU patients. Psychosomatics 37:533–546, 1996

Hart RP, Best AM, Sessler CN, et al: Abbreviated Cognitive Test for Delirium. J Psychosom Res 43:417–423, 1997

Hatta K, Takahashi T, Nakamura H, et al: The association between intravenous haloperidol and prolonged QT interval. J Clin Psychopharmacol 21:257–261, 2001

Hebenstreit GF, Fellerer K, Twerdy B, et al: L-Tryptophan in pre-delirium and delirium conditions. Infusionstherapie 16:92–96, 1989

Heinrich TW, Biblo LA, Schneider J: Torsades de pointes associated with ziprasidone. Psychosomatics 47:264–268, 2006

Henon H, Lebert F, Durieu I, et al: Confusional state in stroke: relation to preexisting dementia, patient characteristics and outcome. Stroke 30:773–779, 1999

Henry WD, Mann AM: Diagnosis and treatment of delirium. Can Med Assoc J 93:1156–1166, 1965

Herrmann N, Mamdani M, Lanctot KL: Atypical antipsychotics and risk of cerebrovascular accidents. Am J Psychiatry 161:1113–1115, 2004

Hill EH, Blumenfield M, Orlowski B: A modification of the Trzepacz Delirium Rating Scale—Revised-98 for use on the Palm Pilot, and a presentation of data of symptom monitoring using haloperidol, olanzapine, and risperidone in the treatment of delirious hospitalized patients (abstract). Psychosomatics 43:158, 2002

Hooper JF, Minter G: Droperidol in the management of psychiatric emergencies. J Clin Psychopharmacol 3:262–263, 1983

Hopkins SJ, Rothwell NJ: Cytokines and the nervous system, I: expression and recognition. Trends Neurosci 18:83–88, 1995

Horenstein S, Chamberlin W, Conomy J: Infarction of the fusiform and calcarine regions: agitated delirium and hemianopia, in Translations of the American Neurological Association 1967, Vol 92. Edited by Yahr MD. New York, Springer, 1967, pp 85–89

Horikawa N, Yamazaki T, Miyamoto K, et al: Treatment for delirium with risperidone: results of a prospective open trial with 10 patients. Gen Hosp Psychiatry 25:289–292, 2003

Huang S-C, Tsai S-J, Chan C-H, et al: Characteristics and outcome of delirium in psychiatric inpatients. Psychiatry Clin Neurosci 52:47–50, 1998

Hustey FM, Meldon SW, Smith MD, et al: The effect of mental status screening on the care of elderly emergency department patients. Ann Emerg Med 41:678–684, 2003

Huyse F: Haloperidol and cardiac arrest. Lancet 2:568–569, 1988

Ikarashi Y, Takahashi A, Ishimaru H, et al: Regulation of dopamine D1 and D2 receptors on striatal acetylcholine release in rats. Brain Res Bull 43:107–115, 1997

Inouye SK: The dilemma of delirium: clinical and research controversies regarding diagnosis and evaluation of delirium in hospitalized elderly medical patients. Am J Med 7:278–288, 1994

Inouye SK, Charpentier PA: Precipitating factors for delirium in hospitalized elderly patients: predictive model and interrelationships with baseline vulnerability. JAMA 275:852–857, 1996

Inouye SK, van Dyke CH, Alessi CA, et al: Clarifying confusion: the Confusion Assessment Method. Ann Intern Med 113:941–948, 1990

Inouye SK, Rushing JT, Foreman MD, et al: Does delirium contribute to poor hospital outcome? J Gen Intern Med 13:234–242, 1998

Inouye SK, Bogardus ST, Charpentier PA, et al: A multicomponent intervention to prevent delirium in hospitalized older patients. N Engl J Med 340:669–676, 1999

Inouye SK, Foreman MD, Mion LC, et al: Nurses' recognition of delirium and its symptoms: comparison of nurse and researcher ratings. Arch Intern Med 161:2467–2473, 2001

Inouye SK, Bogardus ST Jr, Williams CS, et al: The role of adherence on the effectiveness of nonpharmacologic interventions: evidence from the delirium prevention trial. Arch Intern Med 163:958–964, 2003

Irwin M, Fuentenebro F, Marder SR, et al: L-5-Hydroxytryptophan-induced delirium. Biol Psychiatry 21:673–676, 1986

Itil T, Fink M: Anticholinergic drug-induced delirium: experimental modification, quantitative EEG, and behavioral correlations. J Nerv Ment Dis 143:492–507, 1966

Jackson SA: The epidemiology of aging, in Principles of Geriatric Medicine and Gerontology. Edited by Hazzard WR, Blass JP, Ettinger WH, et al. New York, McGraw-Hill, 1999, pp 203–226

Jacobson S, Jerrier S: EEG in delirium. Semin Clin Neuropsychiatry 5:86–92, 2000

Jacobson SA, Leuchter AF, Walter DO: Conventional and quantitative EEG diagnosis of delirium among the elderly. J Neurol Neurosurg Psychiatry 56:153–158, 1993a

Jacobson SA, Leuchter AF, Walter DO, et al: Serial quantitative EEG among elderly subjects with delirium. Biol Psychiatry 34:135–140, 1993b

Jitapunkul S, Pillay I, Ebrahim S: Delirium in newly admitted elderly patients: a prospective study. Q J Med 83:307–314, 1992

Johansson IS, Hamrin EK, Larsson G: Psychometric testing of the NEECHAM Confusion Scale among patients with hip fracture. Res Nurs Health 25:203–211, 2002

Johnson JC, Kerse NM, Gottlieb G, et al: Prospective versus retrospective methods of identifying patients with delirium. J Am Geriatr Soc 40:316–319, 1992

Jones J, Dougherty J, Cannon L: Diphenhydramine-induced toxic psychosis. Am J Emerg Med 4:369–371, 1986

Kagansky N, Rimon E, Naor S, et al: Low incidence of delirium in very old patients after surgery for hip fractures. Am J Geriatr Psychiatry 12:306–314, 2004

Kakuma R, du Fort GG, Arsenault L, et al: Delirium in older emergency department patients discharged home: effect on survival. J Am Geriatr Soc 51:443–450, 2003

Kalisvaart CJ, Boelaarts L, de Jonghe JF, et al: [Successful treatment of three elderly patients suffering from prolonged delirium using the cholinesterase inhibitor rivastigmine] (in Dutch). Ned Tijdschr Geneeskd 148:1501–1504, 2004

Kalisvaart KJ, de Jonghe JF, Bogaards MJ, et al: Haloperidol prophylaxis for elderly hip-surgery patients at risk for delirium: a randomized placebo-controlled study. J Am Geriatr Soc 53:1658–1666, 2005

Kaneko T, Cai J, Ishikura T, et al: Prophylactic consecutive administration of haloperidol can reduce the occurrence of postoperative delirium in gastrointestinal surgery. Yonago Acta Med 42:179–184, 1999

Kapur S, Seeman P: Does fast dissociation from the dopamine d(2) receptor explain the action of atypical antipsychotics? A new hypothesis. Am J Psychiatry 158:360–369, 2001

Karki SD, Masood GR: Combination risperidone and SSRI-induced serotonin syndrome. Ann Pharmacother 37:388–391, 2003

Kasahara H, Karasawa A, Ariyasu T, et al: Alcohol dementia and alcohol delirium in aged alcoholics. Psychiatry Clin Neurosci 50:115–123, 1996

Katz IR, Jeste DV, Mintzer JE, et al: Comparison of risperidone and placebo for psychosis and behavioral disturbances associated with dementia: a randomized double-blind trial. J Clin Psychiatry 60:107–115, 1999

Katz JA, Mahoney DH, Fernbach DJ: Human leukocyte alpha-interferon induced transient neurotoxicity in children. Invest New Drugs 6:115–120, 1988

Kaufer DI, Catt KE, Lopez OL, et al: Dementia with Lewy bodies: response of delirium-like features to donepezil. Neurology 51:1512–1513, 1998

Kelly KG, Zisselman M, Cutillo-Schmitter T, et al: Severity and course of delirium in medically hospitalized nursing facility residents. Am J Geriatr Psychiatry 9:72–77, 2001

Kennard MA, Bueding E, Wortis WB: Some biochemical and electroencephalographic changes in delirium tremens. Q J Stud Alcohol 6:4–14, 1945

Kennedy JS, Zagar A, Bymaster F, et al: The central cholinergic system profile of olanzapine compared with placebo in Alzheimer's disease. Int J Geriatr Psychiatry 16:S24–S32, 2001

Kennedy RE, Nakase-Thompson R, Nick TG, et al: Use of the Cognitive Test for Delirium in patients with traumatic brain injury. Psychosomatics 44:283–289, 2003

Khouzam HR, Gazula K: Clinical experience of olanzapine during the course of post operative delirium associated with psychosis in geriatric patients: a report of three cases. International Journal of Psychiatry in Clinical Practice 5:63–68, 2001

Kiely DK, Bergmann MA, Jones RN, et al: Characteristics associated with delirium persistence among newly admitted post-acute facility patients. J Gerontol A Biol Sci Med Sci 59:344–349, 2004

Kienast T, Heinz A: Dopamine and the diseased brain. CNS Neurol Disord Drug Targets 5:109–131, 2006

Kim JY, Jung IK, Han C, et al: Antipsychotics and dopamine transporter gene polymorphisms in delirium patients. Psychiatry Clin Neurosci 59:183–188, 2005

Kim KS, Pae CU, Chae JH, et al: An open pilot trial of olanzapine for delirium in the Korean population. Psychiatry Clin Neurosci 55:515–519, 2001

Kim KY, Bader GM, Kotlyar V, et al: Treatment of delirium in older adults with quetiapine. J Geriatr Psychiatry Neurol 16:29–31, 2003

Kishi Y, Iwasaki Y, Takezawa K, et al: Delirium in critical care unit patients admitted through an emergency room. Gen Hosp Psychiatry 17:371–379, 1995

Kishi Y, Hosaka T, Yoshikawa E, et al: Delirium Rating Scale—Revised (DRS-R-98), Japanese version. Seishin Igaku 43:1365–1371, 2001

Klijn IA, van der Mast RC: Pharmacotherapy of alcohol withdrawal delirium in patients admitted to a general hospital (comment). Arch Intern Med 165:346, 2005

Knaus WA, Draper EA, Wagner DP, et al: APACHE II: a severity of disease classification system. Crit Care Med 13:818–829, 1985

Knell AJ, Davidson AR, Williams R, et al: Dopamine and serotonin metabolism in hepatic encephalopathy. BMJ 1:549–551, 1974

Kobayashi K, Takeuchi O, Suzuki M, et al: A retrospective study on delirium type. Jpn J Psychiatry Neurol 46:911–917, 1992

Koehnke MD, Schick S, Lutz U, et al: Severity of alcohol withdrawal symptoms and the T1128C polymorphism of the neuropeptide Y gene. J Neural Transm 109:1423–1429, 2002

Köhnke MD, Batra A, Kolb W, et al: Association of the dopamine transporter gene with alcoholism. Alcohol Alcohol 40:339–342, 2005

Köhnke MD, Kolb W, Kohnke AM, et al: *DBH (*) 444G/A* polymorphism of the dopamine beta hydroxylase gene is associated with alcoholism but not with severe alcohol withdrawal symptoms. J Neural Transm 113:869–876, 2006

Kolbeinsson H, Jonsson A: Delirium and dementia in acute medical admissions of elderly patients in Iceland. Acta Psychiatr Scand 87:123–127, 1993

Kopf SR, Baratti CM: Memory-improving actions of glucose: involvement of a central cholinergic muscarinic mechanism. Behav Neural Biol 62:237–243, 1994

Koponen H, Hurri L, Stenback U, et al: Computed tomography findings in delirium. J Nerv Ment Dis 177:226–231, 1989a

Koponen H, Partanen J, Paakkonen A, et al: EEG spectral analysis in delirium. J Neurol Neurosurg Psychiatry 52:980–985, 1989b

Koponen H, Sirvio J, Lepola U, et al: A long-term follow-up study of cerebrospinal fluid acetylcholinesterase in delirium. Eur Arch Psychiatry Clin Neurosci 243:347–351, 1994

Kreis R, Farrow N, Ross BN: Localized NMR spectroscopy in patients with chronic hepatic encephalopathy: analysis of changes in cerebral glutamine, choline, and inositols. NMR Biomed 4:109–116, 1991

Kriwisky M, Perry GY, Tarchitsky, et al: Haloperidol-induced torsades de pointes. Chest 98:482–484, 1990

Kullmann F, Hollerbach S, Holstege A, et al: Subclinical hepatic encephalopathy: the diagnostic value of evoked potentials. J Hepatol 22:101–110, 1995

Laurila JV, Pitkala KH, Strandberg TE, et al: Delirium among patients with and without dementia: does the diagnosis according to the DSM-IV differ from the previous classifications? Int J Geriatr Psychiatry 19:271–277, 2004

Lawlor PG, Gagnon B, Mancini IL, et al: Occurrence, causes and outcome of delirium in patients with advanced cancer. Arch Intern Med 160:786–794, 2000a

Lawlor PG, Nekolaichuk C, Gagnon B, et al: Clinical utility, factor analysis, and further validation of the Memorial Delirium Assessment Scale in patients with advanced cancer: assessing delirium in advanced cancer. Cancer 88:2859–2867, 2000b

Lawrence KR, Nasraway SA: Conduction disturbances associated with administration of butyrophenone antipsychotics in the critically ill: a review of the literature. Pharmacotherapy 17:531–537, 1997

Layton D, Harris S, Wilton LV, et al: Comparison of incidence rates of cerebrovascular accidents and transient ischaemic attacks in observational cohort studies of patients prescribed risperidone, quetiapine or olanzapine in general practice in England including patients with dementia. J Psychopharmacol 19:473–482, 2005

Leavitt M, Trzepacz PT, Ciongoli K: Rat model of delirium: atropine dose-response relationships. J Neuropsychiatry Clin Neurosci 6:279–284, 1994

Lee KU, Won WY, Lee HK, et al: Amisulpride versus quetiapine for the treatment of delirium: a randomized, open prospective study. Int Clin Psychopharmacol 20:311–314, 2005

Lemey L, Vranken C, Simoens K, et al: The "flying delirium room": towards an adequate approach of acute delirium in a general hospital. Int Psychogeriatr 17 (suppl 2):260, 2005

Leslie DL, Zhang Y, Holford TR, et al: Premature death associated with delirium at 1-year follow-up. Arch Intern Med 165:1657–1662, 2005

Leso L, Schwartz TL: Ziprasidone treatment of delirium. Psychosomatics 43:61–62, 2002

Levenson JA: Should psychostimulants be used to treat delirious patients with depressed mood? (letter). J Clin Psychiatry 53:69, 1992

Levenson JL: High-dose intravenous haloperidol for agitated delirium following lung transplantation. Psychosomatics 36:66–68, 1995

Levkoff SE, Evans DA, Liptzin B, et al: Delirium: the occurrence and persistence of symptoms among elderly hospitalized patients. Arch Intern Med 152:334–340, 1992

Lewis MC, Barnett SR: Postoperative delirium: the tryptophan dysregulation model. Med Hypotheses 63:402–406, 2004

Limosin F, Loze JY, Boni C, et al: The A9 allele of the dopamine transporter gene increases the risk of visual hallucinations during alcohol withdrawal in alcohol-dependent women. Neurosci Lett 362:91–94, 2004

Lipowski ZJ: Delirium: Acute Confusional States. New York, Oxford University Press, 1990

Lipton SA, Gendelman HE: Dementia associated with the acquired immunodeficiency syndrome. N Engl J Med 332:934–940, 1995

Liptzin B, Levkoff SE: An empirical study of delirium subtypes. Br J Psychiatry 161:843–845, 1992

Liptzin B, Levkoff SE, Gottlieb GL, et al: Delirium: background papers for DSM-IV. J Neuropsychiatry Clin Neurosci 5:154–160, 1993

Liptzin B, Laki A, Garb JL, et al: Donepezil in the prevention and treatment of post-surgical delirium. Am J Geriatr Psychiatry 13:1100–1106, 2005

Lischke V, Behne M, Doelken P, et al: Droperidol causes a dose-dependent prolongation of the QT interval. Anesth Analg 79:983–986, 1994

Liu CY, Juang YY, Liang HY, et al: Efficacy of risperidone in treating the hyperactive symptoms of delirium. Int Clin Psychopharmacol 19:165–168, 2004

Ljubisljevic V, Kelly B: Risk factors for development of delirium among oncology patients. Gen Hosp Psychiatry 25:345–352, 2003

Lundstrom M, Edlund A, Karlsson S, et al: A multifactorial intervention program reduces the duration of delirium, length of hospitalization, and mortality in delirious patients. J Am Geriatr Soc 53:622–628, 2005

Mach J, Dysken M, Kuskowski M, et al: Serum anticholinergic activity in hospitalized older persons with delirium: a preliminary study. J Am Geriatr Soc 43:491–495, 1995

Magaziner J, Simonsick EM, Kashner M, et al: Survival experience of aged hip fracture patients. Am J Public Health 79:274–278, 1989

Maldonado JR, van der Starre P, Wysong A, et al: Dexmedetomide: can it reduce the incidence of ICU delirium in postcardiotomy patients? Proceedings of 50th annual meeting of the Academy of Psychosomatic Medicine. Psychosomatics 45:145–175, 2004

Mann C, Pouzeratte Y, Boccara G, et al: Comparison of intravenous or epidural patient-controlled analgesia in the elderly after major abdominal surgery. Anesthesiology 92:433–441, 2000

Manos PJ: The utility of the ten-point clock test as a screen for cognitive impairment in general hospital patients. Gen Hosp Psychiatry 19:439–444, 1997

Marcantonio ER, Juarez G, Goldman L, et al: The relationship of postoperative delirium with psychoactive medications. JAMA 272:1518–1522, 1994

Marcantonio ER, Flacker JM, Wright RJ, et al: Reducing delirium after hip fracture: a randomized trial. J Am Geriatr Soc 49:516–22, 2001

Marcantonio E[R], Ta T, Duthie E, et al: Delirium severity and psychomotor types: their relationship with outcomes after hip fracture repair. J Am Geriatr Soc 50:850–857, 2002

Marcantonio ER, Simon SE, Bergmann MA, et al: Delirium symptoms in post-acute care: prevalent, persistent, and associated with poor functional recovery. J Am Geriatr Soc 51:4–9, 2003

Marcantonio ER, Kiely DK, Simon SE, et al: Outcomes of older people admitted to postacute facilities with delirium. J Am Geriatr Soc 53:963–969, 2005

Martin M, Figiel G, Mattingly G, et al: ECT-induced interictal delirium in patients with a history of a CVA. J Geriatr Psychiatry Neurol 5:149–155, 1992

Marzanatti M, Monopoli A, Trampus M, et al: Effects of nonsedating histamine H-1 antagonists on EEG activity and behavior in the cat. Pharmacol Biochem Behav 32:861–866, 1989

Mathers DA: The GABA-A receptor: new insights from single channel recording. Synapse 1:96–101, 1987

Matsuoka Y, Miyake Y, Arakaki H, et al: Clinical utility and validation of the Japanese version of the Memorial Delirium Assessment Scale in a psychogeriatric inpatient setting. Gen Hosp Psychiatry 23:36–40, 2001

Matsushima E, Nakajima K, Moriya H, et al: A psychophysiological study of the development of delirium in coronary care units. Biol Psychiatry 41:1211–1217, 1997

Matsushita S, Kimura M, Miyakawa T, et al: Association study of brain-derived neurotrophic factor gene polymorphism and alcoholism. Alcohol Clin Exp Res 28:1609–1612, 2004

Mayo-Smith MF, Beecher LH, Fischer TL, et al: Management of alcohol withdrawal delirium: an evidence-based practice guideline. Working Group on the Management of Alcohol Withdrawal Delirium, Practice Guidelines Committee, American Society of Addiction Medicine. Arch Intern Med 164:1405–1412, 2004

McCaffrey R, Locsin R: The effect of music listening on acute confusion and delirium in elders undergoing elective hip and knee surgery. J Clin Nurs 13:91–96, 2004

McCusker J, Cole M, Abrahamowicz M, et al: Environmental risk factors for delirium in hospitalized older people. J Am Geriatr Soc 49:1327–1334, 2001

McCusker J, Cole M, Abrahamowicz M, et al: Delirium predicts 12-month mortality. Arch Intern Med 162:457–463, 2002

McCusker J, Cole MG, Dendukuri N, et al: The course of delirium in older medical inpatients: a prospective study. J Gen Intern Med 18:696–704, 2003a

McCusker J, Cole MG, Dendukuri N, et al: Does delirium increase hospital stay? J Am Geriatr Soc 51:1539–1546, 2003b

McKeith I, Fairbairn A, Perry R, et al: Neuroleptic sensitivity in patients with senile dementia of Lewy body type. BMJ 305:673–678, 1992

McNicoll L, Pisani MA, Zhang Y, et al: Delirium in the intensive care unit: occurrence and clinical course in older patients. J Am Geriatr Soc 51:591–598, 2003

Meagher D: Delirium episode as a sign of undetected dementia among community dwelling elderly subjects. J Neurol Neurosurg Psychiatry 70:821, 2001a

Meagher D: Delirium: optimising management. BMJ 7279:144–149, 2001b

Meagher D[J]: Clearing the confusion: psychopathology, cognition, and motoric profile in 100 consecutive cases of delirium. Int Psychogeriatr 17 (suppl 2):120–121, 2005

Meagher DJ, Trzepacz PT: Delirium phenomenology illuminates pathophysiology, management and course. J Geriatr Psychiatry Neurol 11:150–157, 1998

Meagher DJ, Trzepacz PT: Motoric subtypes of delirium. Semin Clin Neuropsychiatry 5:76–86, 2000

Meagher DJ, O'Hanlon D, O'Mahony E, et al: Use of environmental strategies and psychotropic medication in the management of delirium. Br J Psychiatry 168:512–515, 1996

Meagher DJ, O'Hanlon D, O'Mahoney E, et al: Relationship between etiology and phenomenological profile in delirium. J Geriatr Psychiatry Neurol 11:146–149, 1998

Meagher DJ, O'Hanlon D, O'Mahony E, et al: Relationship between symptoms and motoric subtype of delirium. J Neuropsychiatry Clin Neurosci 12:51–56, 2000

Meagher DJ, Moran M, Raju B, et al: Phenomenology of 100 consecutive adult cases of delirium. Br J Psychiatry 190:135–141, 2007

Meagher DJ, Moran M, Raju B, et al: Motor symptoms in 100 patients with delirium versus control subjects: comparison of subtyping methods. Psychosomatics 49:300–308, 2008

Medina JL, Rubino FA, Ross E: Agitated delirium caused by infarctions of the hippocampal formation and fusiform and lingual gyri. Neurology 24:1181–1183, 1974

Medina JL, Sudhansu C, Rubino FA: Syndrome of agitated delirium and visual impairment: a manifestation of medial temporo-occipital infarction. J Neurol Neurosurg Psychiatry 40:861–864, 1977

Meltzer HY: Serotonin-dopamine interactions and atypical antipsychotic drugs. Psychiatr Ann 23:193–200, 1993

Meltzer HY, O'Laughlin IA, Dai J, et al: Atypical antipsychotic drugs but not typical increased extracellular acetylcholine levels in rat medial prefrontal cortex in the absence of acetylcholinesterase inhibition (abstract). Abstr Soc Neurosci 25:452, 1999

Mendelson G: Pheniramine aminosalicylate overdosage: reversal of delirium and choreiform movements with tacrine treatment. Arch Neurol 34:313, 1977

Mesulam M-M: Attention, confusional states, and neglect, in Principles of Behavioral Neurology. Edited by Mesulam M-M. Philadelphia, PA, FA Davis, 1985, pp 125–168

Mesulam M-M, Waxman SG, Geschwind N, et al: Acute confusional states with right middle cerebral artery infarction. J Neurol Neurosurg Psychiatry 39:84–89, 1979

Metzger E, Friedman R: Prolongation of the corrected QT and torsades de pointes cardiac arrhythmia associated with intravenous haloperidol in the medically ill. J Clin Psychopharmacol 13:128–132, 1993

Milbrandt EB, Deppen S, Harrison PL, et al: Costs associated with delirium in mechanically ventilated patients. Crit Care Med 32:955–962, 2004

Milbrandt EB, Kersten A, Kong L, et al: Haloperidol use is associated with lower hospital mortality in mechanically ventilated patients. Crit Care Med 33:226–229, 2005

Milisen K, Foreman MD, Abraham IL, et al: A nurse-led interdisciplinary intervention program for delirium in elderly hip-fracture patients. J Am Geriatr Soc 49:523–532, 2001

Miller PS, Richardson JS, Jyu CA, et al: Association of low serum anticholinergic levels and cognitive impairment in elderly presurgical patients. Am J Psychiatry 145:342–345, 1988

Minagawa H, Uchitomi Y, Yamawaki S, et al: Psychiatric morbidity in terminally ill cancer patients: a prospective study. Cancer 78:1131–1137, 1996

Mittal D, Jimerson NA, Neely EP, et al: Risperidone in the treatment of delirium: results from a prospective open-label trial. J Clin Psychiatry 65:662–667, 2004

Mizock BA, Sabelli HC, Dubin A, et al: Septic encephalopathy: evidence for altered phenylalanine metabolism and comparison with hepatic encephalopathy. Arch Intern Med 150:443–449, 1990

Moldofsky H, Lue FA, Eisen J, et al: The relationship of interleukin-1 and immune functions to sleep in humans. Psychosom Med 48:309–318, 1986

Moller JT, Cluitmans P, Rasmussen LS, et al: Long-term postoperative cognitive dysfunction in the elderly ISPOCD1 study. ISPOCD investigators. International Study of Post-Operative Cognitive Dysfunction. Lancet 351:857–861, 1998

Mondimore FM, Damlouji N, Folstein MF, et al: Post-ECT confusional states associated with elevated serum anticholinergic levels. Am J Psychiatry 140:930–931, 1983

Montgomery EA, Fenton GW, McClelland RJ, et al: Psychobiology of minor head injury. Psychosom Med 21:375–384, 1991

Monti JM: Involvement of histamine in the control of the waking state. Life Sci 53:1331–1338, 1993

Moretti R, Torre P, Antonello RM, et al: Cholinesterase inhibition as a possible therapy for delirium in vascular dementia: a controlled, open 24-month study of 246 patients. Am J Alzheimers Dis Other Demen 19:333–339, 2004

Mori E, Yamadori A: Acute confusional state and acute agitated delirium. Arch Neurol 44:1139–1143, 1987

Morita T, Otani H, Tsunoda J, et al: Successful palliation of hypoactive delirium due to multiorgan failure by oral methylphenidate. Support Care Cancer 8:134–137, 2000

Morita T, Tei Y, Tsunoda J, et al: Underlying pathologies and their associations with clinical features in terminal delirium of cancer patients. J Pain Symptom Manage 22:997–1006, 2001

Morita T, Hirai K, Sakaguchi Y, et al: Family perceived distress about delirium-related symptoms of terminally ill cancer patients. Psychosomatics 45:107–113, 2004

Morita T, Takigawa C, Onishi H, et al: Opioid rotation from morphine to fentanyl in delirious cancer patients: an open-label trial. J Pain Symptom Manage 30:96–103, 2005

Morrison RS, Magaziner J, Gilbert M, et al: Relationship between pain and opioid analgesics on the development of delirium following hip fracture. J Gerontol A Biol Sci Med Sci 58:76–81, 2003

Moulaert P: Treatment of acute nonspecific delirium with IV haloperidol in surgical intensive care patients. Acta Anaesthesiol Belg 40:183–186, 1989

Mousseau DD, Butterworth RF: Current theories on the pathogenesis of hepatic encephalopathy. Proc Soc Exp Biol Med 206:329–344, 1994

Mullally W, Huff K, Ronthal M, et al: Frequency of acute confusional states with lesions of the right hemisphere (abstract). Ann Neurol 12:113, 1982

Murray AM, Levkoff SE, Wetle TT, et al: Acute delirium and functional decline in the hospitalized elderly patient. J Gerontol 48:M181–M186, 1993

Nagley SJ: Predicting and preventing confusion in your patients. J Gerontol Nurs 12:27–31, 1986

Nakamura A, Inada T, Kitao Y, et al: Association between catechol-O-methyltransferase (COMT) polymorphism and severe alcoholic withdrawal symptoms in male Japanese alcoholics. Addict Biol 6:233–238, 2001

Nakamura J, Uchimura N, Yamada S, et al: Effects of mianserin hydrochloride on delirium: comparison with the effects of oxypertine and haloperidol. Nihon Shinkei Seishin Yakurigaku Zasshi 14:269–277, 1994

Nakamura J, Uchimura N, Yamada S, et al: The effect of mianserin hydrochloride on delirium. Hum Psychopharmacol 10:289–297, 1995

Nakamura J, Uchimura N, Yamada S, et al: Does plasma free-3-methoxy-4-hydroxyphenyl(ethylene)glycol increase the delirious state? A comparison of the effects of mianserin and haloperidol on delirium. Int Clin Psychopharmacol 12:147–152, 1997a

Nakamura J, Uchimura N, Yamada S, et al: Mianserin suppositories in the treatment of postoperative delirium. Hum Psychopharmacol 12:595–599, 1997b

Nakamura K, Kurasawa M, Tanaka Y: Apomorphine-induced hypoattention in rat and reversal of the choice performance impairment by aniracetam. Eur J Pharmacol 342:127–138, 1998

Neelon VJ, Champagne MT, Carlson JR, et al: The NEECHAM scale: construction, validation, and clinical testing. Nurs Res 45:324–330, 1986

Nicholas LM, Lindsey BA: Delirium presenting with symptoms of depression. Psychosomatics 36:471–479, 1995

Nighoghossian N, Trouillas P, Vighetto A, et al: Spatial delirium following a right subcortical infarct with frontal deactivation. J Neurol Neurosurg Psychiatry 55:334–335, 1992

O'Brien JM, Rockwood RP, Suh KI: Haloperidol-induced torsades de pointes. Ann Pharmacother 33:1046–1050, 1999

O'Hare E, Weldon DT, Bettin K, et al: Serum anticholinergic activity and behavior following atropine sulfate administration in the rat. Pharmacol Biochem Behav 56:151–154, 1997

Okamura A, Nakano T, Fukumoto Y, et al: Delirious behaviour in children with influenza: its clinical features and EEG findings. Brain Dev 27:271–274, 2005

O'Keeffe ST: Rating the severity of delirium: the Delirium Assessment Scale. Int J Geriatr Psychiatry 9:551–556, 1994

O'Keeffe ST: Clinical subtypes of delirium in the elderly. Dement Geriatr Cogn Disord 10:380–385, 1999

O'Keeffe S[T]: The experience of delirium in older people. Int Psychogeriatr 17 (suppl 2):120, 2005

O'Keeffe ST, Gosney MA: Assessing attentiveness in older hospitalized patients: global assessment vs. test of attention. J Am Geriatr Soc 45:470–473, 1997

O'Keeffe ST, Lavan JN: Predicting delirium in elderly patients: development and validation of a risk-stratification model. Age Ageing 25:317–321, 1996

O'Keeffe ST, Lavan JN: Clinical significance of delirium subtypes in older people. Age Ageing 28:115–119, 1999

O'Keeffe ST, Tormey WP, Glasgow R, et al: Thiamine deficiency in hospitalized elderly patients. Gerontology 40:18–24, 1994

O'Keeffe ST, Mulkerrin EC, Nayeem K, et al: Use of serial Mini-Mental State Examinations to diagnose and monitor delirium in elderly hospital patients. J Am Geriatr Soc 53:867–870, 2005

Okubo T, Harada S, Higuchi S, et al: Genetic polymorphism of the CCK gene in patients with alcohol withdrawal symptoms. Alcohol Clin Exp Res 24 (4 suppl):2–4, 2000

Okubo T, Harada S, Higuchi S, et al: Investigation of quantitative loci in the CCKAR gene with susceptibility to alcoholism. Alcohol Clin Exp Res 26 (8 suppl):2–5, 2002

Okubo T, Harada S, Higuchi S, et al: Association analyses between polymorphisms of the phase II detoxification enzymes (GSTM1, NQO1, NQO2) and alcohol withdrawal symptoms. Alcohol Clin Exp Res 27 (8 suppl):68S–71S, 2003

Olofsson B, Lundström M, Borssén B, et al: Delirium is associated with poor rehabilitation outcome in elderly patients treated for femoral neck fractures. Scand J Caring Sci 19:119–127, 2005

Olofsson K, Alling C, Lundberg D, et al: Abolished circadian rhythm of melatonin secretion in sedated and artificially ventilated intensive care patients. Acta Anaesthesiol Scand 48:679–684, 2004

Olofsson SM, Weitzner MA, Valentine AD, et al: A retrospective study of the psychiatric management and outcome of delirium in the cancer patient. Support Care Cancer 4:351–357, 1996

Ongini E, Caporali MG, Massotti M: Stimulation of dopamine D-1 receptors by SKF 38393 induces EEG desynchronization and behavioral arousal. Life Sci 37:2327–2333, 1985

Onofrj M, Curatola L, Malatesta G, et al: Reduction of P3 latency during outcome from post-traumatic amnesia. Acta Neurol Scand 83:273–279, 1991

Ovchinsky N, Pitchumoni S, Skotzko CE: Use of olanzapine for the treatment of delirium following traumatic brain injury. Psychosomatics 43:147–148, 2002

Owens JF, Hutelmyer CM: The effect of postoperative intervention on delirium in cardiac surgical patients. Nurs Res 31:60–62, 1982

Pae CU, Lee SJ, Lee CU, et al: A pilot trial of quetiapine for the treatment of patients with delirium. Hum Psychopharmacol 19:125–127, 2004

Pandharipande P, Shintani A, Peterson J, et al: Lorazepam is an independent risk factor for transitioning to delirium in intensive care unit patients. Anesthesiology 104:21–26, 2006

Parellada E, Baeza I, de Pablo J, et al: Risperidone in the treatment of patients with delirium. J Clin Psychiatry 65:348–353, 2004

Passik SD, Cooper M: Complicated delirium in a cancer patient successfully treated with olanzapine. J Pain Symptom Manage 17:219–223, 1999

Patten SB, Lamarre CJ: Dysgraphia (letter). Can J Psychiatry 34:746, 1989

Perrault LP, Denault AY, Carrier M, et al: Torsades de pointes secondary to intravenous haloperidol after coronary artery bypass graft surgery. Can J Anesth 47:251–254, 2000

Picotte-Prillmayer D, DiMaggio JR, Baile WF: H-2 blocker delirium. Psychosomatics 36:74–77, 1995

Piercey MF, Camacho-Ochoa M, Smith MW: Functional roles for dopamine-receptor subtypes. Clin Neuropharmacol 18:S34–S42, 1995

Pitkälä KH, Laurila JV, Strandberg TE, et al: Prognostic significance of delirium in frail older people. Dement Geriatr Cogn Disord 19:158–163, 2005

Platt MM, Breitbart W, Smith M, et al: Efficacy of neuroleptics for hypoactive delirium. J Neuropsychiatry Clin Neurosci 6:66–67, 1994a

Platt MM, Trautman P, Frager G, et al: Pediatric delirium: research update. Paper presented at the annual meeting of the Academy of Psychosomatic Medicine, Phoenix, AZ, November 1994b

Pomara N, Willoughby LM, Wesnes K, et al: Increased anticholinergic challenge-induced memory impairment associated with the APOE-epsilon4 allele in the elderly: a controlled pilot study. Neuropsychopharmacology 29:403–409, 2004

Pompeii P, Foreman M, Rudberg MA, et al: Delirium in hospitalized older persons: outcomes and predictors. J Am Geriatr Soc 42:809–815, 1994

Posner ML, Boies SJ: Components of attention. Psychol Rev 78:391–408, 1971

Pratico C, Quattrone D, Lucanto T, et al: Drugs of anesthesia acting on central cholinergic system may cause post-operative cognitive dysfunction and delirium. Med Hypotheses 65:972–982, 2005

Preuss UW, Koller G, Bahlmann M, et al: No association between metabotropic glutamate receptors 7 and 8 (mGlur7 and mGlur8) gene polymorphisms and withdrawal seizures and delirium tremens in alcohol-dependent individuals. Alcohol Alcohol 37:174–178, 2002

Preuss UW, Koller G, Zill P, et al: Alcoholism-related phenotypes and genetic variants of the CB1 receptor. Eur Arch Psychiatry Clin Neurosci 253:275–280, 2003

Preuss UW, Zill P, Koller G, et al: Ionotropic glutamate receptor gene *GRIK3 SER310ALA* functional polymorphism is related to delirium tremens in alcoholics. Pharmacogenomics J 6:34–41, 2006

Price BH, Mesulam M: Psychiatric manifestations of right hemisphere infarctions. J Nerv Ment Dis 173:610–614, 1985

Prugh DG, Wagonfeld S, Metcalf D, et al: A clinical study of delirium in children and adolescents. Psychosom Med 42:177–195, 1980

Rabins PV, Folstein MF: Delirium and dementia: diagnostic criteria and fatality rates. Br J Psychiatry 140:149–153, 1982

Rahkonen T, Luukkainen-Markkula R, Paanila S, et al: Delirium as a sign of undetected dementia among community dwelling elderly subjects: a 2 year follow up study. J Neurol Neurosurg Psychiatry 69:519–521, 2000

Ramirez-Bermudez J, Lopez-Gomez M, Sosa Ana L, et al: Frequency of delirium in a neurological emergency room. J Neuropsychiatry Clin Neurosci 18:108–112, 2006

Ravona-Springer R, Dohlberg OT, Hirschman S, et al: Delirium in elderly patients treated with risperidone: a report of three cases. J Clin Psychopharmacol 18:171–172, 1998

Reilly JG, Ayis AS, Ferrier IN, et al: QTc-interval abnormalities and psychotropic drug therapy in psychiatric patients. Lancet 355:1048–1052, 2000

Reishies FM, Neuhaus AH, Hansen ML, et al: Electrophysiological and neuropsychological analysis of a delirious state: the role of the anterior cingulate gyrus. Psychiatry Res 138:171–181, 2005

Resnick M, Burton BT: Droperidol versus haloperidol in the initial management of acutely agitated patients. J Clin Psychiatry 45:298–299, 1984

Riker RR, Fraser GL, Cox PM: Continuous infusion of haloperidol controls agitation in critically ill patients. Crit Care Med 22:433–440, 1994

Riker RR, Fraser GL, Richen P: Movement disorders associated with withdrawal from high-dose intravenous haloperidol therapy in delirious ICU patients. Chest 111:1778–1781, 1997

Ritchie J, Steiner W, Abrahamowicz M: Incidence of and risk factors for delirium among psychiatric patients. Psychiatr Serv 47:727–730, 1996

Robertsson B: Assessment scales in delirium. Dement Geriatr Cogn Disord 10:368–379, 1999

Robertsson B, Blennow K, Gottfries CG, et al: Delirium in dementia. Int J Geriatr Psychiatry 13:49–56, 1998

Robinson MJ: Probable Lewy body dementia presenting as "delirium." Psychosomatics 43:84–86, 2002

Rockwood K: The occurrence and duration of symptoms in elderly patients with delirium. J Gerontol 48:M162–M166, 1993

Rockwood K, Cosway S, Stolee P, et al: Increasing the recognition of delirium in elderly patients. J Am Geriatr Soc 42:252–256, 1994

Rockwood K, Cosway S, Carver D, et al: The risk of dementia and death after delirium. Age Ageing 28:551–556, 1999

Rodriguez G, Testa R, Celle G, et al: Reduction of cerebral blood flow in subclinical hepatic encephalopathy and its correlation with plasma-free tryptophan. J Cereb Blood Flow Metab 7:768–772, 1987

Rolfson DB, McElhaney JE, Jhangri GS, et al: Validity of the Confusion Assessment Method in detecting postoperative delirium in the elderly. Int Psychogeriatr 11:431–438, 1999

Romano J, Engel GL: Delirium, I: electroencephalographic data. Arch Neurol Psychiatry 51:356–377, 1944

Rosenberg PB, Ahmed I, Hurwitz S: Methylphenidate in depressed medically ill patients. J Clin Psychiatry 52:263–267, 1991

Rosenberg S, Loetz M, Yang J: Experience with the use of high-dose interleukin-2 in the treatment of 652 cancer patients. Ann Surg 210:474–484, 1989

Ross CA, Peyser CE, Shapiro I, et al: Delirium: phenomenologic and etiologic subtypes. Int Psychogeriatr 3:135–147, 1991

Rothwell NJ, Hopkins SJ: Cytokines and the nervous system, II: actions and mechanisms of action. Trends Neurosci 18:130–136, 1995

Rovner BW, David A, Lucas-Blaustein MJ, et al: Self-care capacity and anticholinergic drug levels in nursing home patients. Am J Psychiatry 145:107–109, 1988

Rudberg MA, Pompei P, Foreman MD, et al: The natural history of delirium in older hospitalized patients: a syndrome of heterogeneity. Age Ageing 26:169–174, 1997

Ruijs MB, Keyser A, Gabreels FJ, et al: Somatosensory evoked potentials and cognitive sequelae in children with closed head injury. Neuropediatrics 24:307–312, 1993

Ruijs MB, Gabreels FJ, Thijssen HM: The utility of electroencephalography and cerebral CT in children with mild and moderately severe closed head injuries. Neuropediatrics 25:73–77, 1994

Rujescu D, Soyka M, Dahmen N, et al: GRIN1 locus may modify the susceptibility to seizures during alcohol withdrawal. Am J Med Genet B Neuropsychiatr Genet 133:85–87, 2005

Saatman KE, Contreras PC, Smith DH, et al: Insulin-like growth factor-1 improves both neurological motor and cognitive outcome following experimental brain injury. Exp Neurol 147:418–427, 1997

Samochowiec J, Kucharska-Mazur J, Kaminski R, et al: Norepinephrine transporter gene polymorphism is not associated with susceptibility to alcohol dependence. Psychiatry Res 111:229–233, 2002

Samuels S, Fang M: Olanzapine may cause delirium in geriatric patients. J Clin Psychiatry 65:582–583, 2004

Sandberg O, Gustafson Y, Brannstrom B, et al: Prevalence of dementia, delirium and psychiatric symptoms in various care settings for the elderly. Scand J Soc Med 26:56–62, 1998

Sandberg O, Gustafson Y, Brannstrom B, et al: Clinical profile of delirium in older patients. J Am Geriatr Soc 47:1300–1306, 1999

Sander T, Harms H, Podschus J, et al: Alleleic association of a dopamine transporter gene polymorphism in alcohol dependence with withdrawal seizures or delirium. Biol Psychiatry 41:299–304, 1997

Sander T, Ostapowicz A, Samochowiec J, et al: Genetic variation of the glutamate transporter *EAAT2* gene and vulnerability to alcohol dependence. Psychiatr Genet 10:103–107, 2000

Sanders KM, Stern TA: Management of delirium associated with use of the intra-aortic balloon pump. Am J Crit Care 2:371–377, 1993

Santamaria J, Blesa R, Tolosa ES: Confusional syndrome in thalamic stroke. Neurology 34:1618–1619, 1984

Santos FS, Wahlund LO, Varli F, et al: Incidence, clinical features and subtypes of delirium in elderly patients treated for hip fractures. Dement Geriatr Cogn Disord 20:231–237, 2005

Saravay SM, Strain JJ: APM Task Force on Funding Implications of Consultation-Liaison Outcome Studies. Psychosomatics 35:227–232, 1994

Saravay SM, Kaplowitz M, Kurek J, et al: How do delirium and dementia increase length of stay of elderly general medical inpatients. Psychosomatics 45:235–242, 2004

Sasaki Y, Matsuyama T, Inoue S, et al: A prospective, open-label, flexible-dose study of quetiapine in the treatment of delirium. J Clin Psychiatry 64:1316–1321, 2003

Schafer DF, Jones EA: Hepatic encephalopathy and the gamma-aminobutyric acid neurotransmitter system. Lancet 1:18–20, 1982

Schindler BA, Shook J, Schwartz GM: Beneficial effects of psychiatric intervention on recovery after coronary artery bypass graft surgery. Gen Hosp Psychiatry 11:358–364, 1989

Schirazi S, Rodriguez D, Nomikos GG: Effects of typical and atypical antipsychotic drugs on acetylcholine release in the hippocampus. Abstr Soc Neurosci 26:2144, 2000

Schmidley JW, Messing RO: Agitated confusional states with right hemisphere infarctions. Stroke 5:883–885, 1984

Schmidt LG, Samochowiec J, Finckh U, et al: Association of a CB1 cannabinoid receptor gene (*CNR1*) polymorphism with severe alcohol dependence. Drug Alcohol Depend 65:221–224, 2002

Schneider A: Use of intravenous valproate (Depacon) in the treatment of delirium: a case series. Neurobiol Aging 25 (suppl 2):S302–S303, 2005

Schneider LS, Dagerman KS, Insel P: Risk of death with atypical antipsychotic drug treatment for dementia: meta-analysis of randomized placebo-controlled trials. JAMA 294:1934–1943, 2005

Schneir AB, Offerman SR, Ly BT, et al: Complications of diagnostic physostigmine administration to emergency department patients. Ann Emerg Med 42:14–19, 2003

Schofield I: A small exploratory study of the reaction of older people to an episode of delirium. J Adv Nurs 25:942–952, 1997

Schor JD, Levkoff SE, Lipsitz LA, et al: Risk factors for delirium in hospitalized elderly. JAMA 267:827–831, 1992

Schuster P, Gabriel E, Kufferle B, et al: Reversal by physostigmine of clozapine-induced delirium. Clin Toxicol 10:437–441, 1977

Seaman JS, Schillerstrom J, Carroll D, et al: Impaired oxidative metabolism precipitates delirium: a study of 101 ICU patients. Psychosomatics 47:56–61, 2006

Seear M, Lockitch G, Jacobson B, et al: Thiamine, riboflavin and pyridoxine deficiency in a population of critically ill children. J Pediatr 121:533–538, 1992

Sherer M, Nakas-Thompson R, Yablon SA, et al: Multidimensional assessment of acute confusion after traumatic brain injury. Arch Phys Med Rehabil 86:896–904, 2005

Sherman SM, Kock C: Thalamus, in The Synaptic Organization of the Brain, 3rd Edition. Edited by Shepherd GM. New York, Oxford University Press, 1990, pp 246–278

Shigeta H, Yasui A, Nimura Y, et al: Postoperative delirium and melatonin levels in elderly patients. Am J Surg 182:449–454, 2001

Sim FH, Brunet DG, Conacher GN: Quetiapine associated with acute mental status changes (letter). Can J Psychiatry 3:299, 2000

Sipahimalani A, Masand PS: Use of risperidone in delirium: case reports. Ann Clin Psychiatry 9:105–107, 1997

Sipahimalani A, Masand PS: Olanzapine in the treatment of delirium. Psychosomatics 39:422–430, 1998

Skrobik YK, Bergeron N, Dumont M, et al: Olanzapine vs haloperidol: treating delirium in a critical care setting. Intensive Care Med 30:444–449, 2004

Sloan EP, Fenton GW, Standage KP: Anticholinergic drug effects on quantitative EEG, visual evoked potentials, and verbal memory. Biol Psychiatry 31:600–606, 1992

Stefano GB, Bilfinger TV, Fricchione GL: The immune-neuro-link and the macrophage: postcardiotomy delirium, HIV-associated dementia and psychiatry. Prog Neurobiol 42:475–488, 1994

Stern TA: Continuous infusion of physostigmine in anticholinergic delirium: a case report. J Clin Psychiatry 44:463–464, 1983

Stern TA: Continuous infusion of haloperidol in agitated critically ill patients. Crit Care Med 22:378–379, 1994

Sternberg SA, Wolfson C, Baumgarten M: Undetected dementia in community-dwelling older people: the Canadian Study of Health and Aging. J Am Geriatr Soc 48:1430–1434, 2000

Straker DA, Shapiro PA, Muskin PR: Aripiprazole in the treatment of delirium. Psychosomatics 47:385–391, 2006

Sundaram M, Dostrow V: Epilepsy in the elderly. Neurologist 1:232–239, 1995

Swenson JR, Erman M, Labelle J, et al: Extrapyramidal reactions: neuropsychiatric mimics in patients with AIDS. Gen Hosp Psychiatry 11:248–253, 1989

Swerdlow NR, Bongiovanni MJ, Tochen L, et al: Separable noradrenergic and dopaminergic regulation of prepulse inhibition in rats: implications for predictive validity and Tourette syndrome. Psychopharmacology 186:246–254, 2006

Tadic A, Dahmen N, Szegedi A, et al: Polymorphisms in the NMDA subunit 2B are not associated with alcohol dependence and alcohol withdrawal-induced seizures and delirium tremens. Eur Arch Psychiatry Clin Neurosci 255:129–135, 2005

Teicher MH, Glod CA: Neuroleptic drugs: indications and guidelines for their rational use in children and adolescents. J Child Adolesc Psychopharmacol 1:33–56, 1990

Tejera CA, Saravay SM, Goldman E, et al: Diphenhydramine-induced delirium in elderly hospitalized patients with mild dementia. Psychosomatics 35:399–402, 1994

Tesar GE, Murray GB, Cassem NH: Use of high-dose intravenous haloperidol in the treatment of agitated cardiac patients. J Clin Psychopharmacol 5:344–347, 1985

Thomas H, Schwartz E, Petrilli R: Droperidol versus haloperidol for chemical restraint of agitated and combative patients. Ann Emerg Med 21:407–413, 1992

Thomas RI, Cameron DJ, Fahs MC: A prospective study of delirium and prolonged hospital stay. Arch Gen Psychiatry 45:937–946, 1988

Timmers JFM, Kalisvaart KJ, Schuurmans M, et al: A review of assessment scales for delirium, in Primary Prevention of Delirium in the Elderly. Edited by Kalisvaart K. Amsterdam, The Netherlands, Academisch Proefschrift, University of Amsterdam, 2005, pp 21–39

Toda H, Kusumi I, Sasaki Y, et al: Relationship between plasma concentration levels of risperidone and clinical effects in the treatment of delirium. Int Clin Psychopharmacol 20:331–333, 2005

Tokita K, Tanaka H, Kawamoto M, et al: Patient-controlled epidural analgesia with bupivacaine and fentanyl suppresses postoperative delirium following hepatectomy. Masui 50:742–746, 2001

Tollefson GD, Montague-Clouse J, Lancaster SP: The relationship of serum anticholinergic activity to mental status performance in an elderly nursing home population. J Neuropsychiatry Clin Neurosci 3:314–319, 1991

Treloar AJ, MacDonald AJ: Outcome of delirium, I: outcome of delirium diagnosed by DSM III-R, ICD-10 and CAMDEX and derivation of the Reversible Cognitive Dysfunction Scale among acute geriatric inpatients. Int J Geriatr Psychiatry 12:609–613, 1997

Trzepacz PT: Neuropathogenesis of delirium: a need to focus our research. Psychosomatics 35:374–391, 1994a

Trzepacz PT: A review of delirium assessment instruments. Gen Hosp Psychiatry 16:397–405, 1994b

Trzepacz PT: Anticholinergic model for delirium. Semin Clin Neuropsychiatry 1:294–303, 1996

Trzepacz PT: The Delirium Rating Scale: its use in consultation/liaison research. Psychosomatics 40:193–204, 1999a

Trzepacz PT: Update on the neuropathogenesis of delirium. Dement Geriatr Cogn Disord 10:330–334, 1999b

Trzepacz PT: Is there a final common neural pathway in delirium? Focus on acetylcholine and dopamine. Semin Clin Neuropsychiatry 5:132–148, 2000

Trzepacz PT, Dew MA: Further analyses of the Delirium Rating Scale. Gen Hosp Psychiatry 17:75–79, 1995

Trzepacz PT, Francis J: Low serum albumin and risk of delirium (letter). Am J Psychiatry 147:675, 1990

Trzepacz PT, Teague GB, Lipowski ZJ: Delirium and other organic mental disorders in a general hospital. Gen Hosp Psychiatry 7:101–106, 1985

Trzepacz PT, Baker RW, Greenhouse J: A symptom rating scale for delirium. Psychiatry Res 23:89–97, 1988a

Trzepacz PT, Brenner R, Coffman G, et al: Delirium in liver transplantation candidates: discriminant analysis of multiple test variables. Biol Psychiatry 24:3–14, 1988b

Trzepacz PT, Sclabassi R, Van Thiel D: Delirium: a subcortical mechanism? J Neuropsychiatry Clin Neurosci 1:283–290, 1989

Trzepacz PT, Leavitt M, Ciongoli K: An animal model for delirium. Psychosomatics 33:404–415, 1992

Trzepacz PT, Ho V, Mallavarapu H: Cholinergic delirium and neurotoxicity associated with tacrine for Alzheimer's dementia. Psychosomatics 37:299–301, 1996

Trzepacz PT, Mulsant BH, Dew MA, et al: Is delirium different when it occurs in dementia? A study using the Delirium Rating Scale. J Neuropsychiatry Clin Neurosci 10:199–204, 1998

Trzepacz PT, Mittal D, Torres R, et al: Validation of the Delirium Rating Scale—Revised-98: comparison to the Delirium Rating Scale and Cognitive Test for Delirium. J Neuropsychiatry Clin Neurosci 13:229–242, 2001

Trzepacz PT, Mittal D, Torres R, et al: Delirium vs dementia symptoms: Delirium Rating Scale—Revised (DRS-R-98) and Cognitive Test for Delirium (CTD) item comparisons. Psychosomatics 43:156–157, 2002

Tsutsui S, Kitamura M, Higachi H, et al: Development of postoperative delirium in relation to a room change in the general surgical unit. Surg Today 26:292–294, 1996

Tune LE, Dainloth NF, Holland A, et al: Association of postoperative delirium with raised serum levels of anticholinergic drugs. Lancet 2:651–653, 1981

Tune L[E], Carr S, Hoag E, et al: Anticholinergic effects of drugs commonly prescribed for the elderly: potential means for assessing risk of delirium. Am J Psychiatry 149:1393–1394, 1992

Turkel SB, Braslow K, Tavare CJ, et al: The delirium rating scale in children and adolescents. Psychosomatics 44:126–129, 2003

Turkel SB, Trzepacz PT, Tavare CJ: Comparison of delirium in adults and children. Psychosomatics 47:320–324, 2006

Turnheim K: When drug therapy gets old: pharmacokinetics and pharmacodynamics in the elderly. Exp Gerontol 38:843–853, 2003

Uchikado H, Akiyama H, Kondo H, et al: Activation of vascular endothelial cells and perivascular cells by systemic inflammation: an immunohistochemical study of postmortem human brain tissues. Acta Neuropathol 107:341–351, 2004

Uchiyama M, Tanaka K, Isse K, et al: Efficacy of mianserin on symptoms of delirium in the aged: an open trial study. Prog Neuropsychopharmacol Biol Psychiatry 20:651–656, 1996

van der Mast RC: Detecting and measuring the severity of delirium with the symptom rating scale for delirium, in Delirium After Cardiac Surgery. Thesis, Erasmus University Rotterdam, Benecke Consultants, Amsterdam, The Netherlands, 1994, pp 78–89

van der Mast RC, Fekkes D: Serotonin and amino acids: partners in delirium pathophysiology? Semin Clin Neuropsychiatry 5:125–131, 2000

van der Mast RC, Fekkes D, van den Broek WW, et al: Reduced cerebral tryptophan availability as a possible cause for post-cardiotomy delirium (letter). Psychosomatics 35:195, 1994

van Hemert AM, van der Mast RC, Hengeveld MW, et al: Excess mortality in general hospital patients with delirium: a 5-year follow-up study of 519 patients seen in psychiatric consultation. J Psychosom Res 38:339–346, 1994

van Leeuwen AMH, Molders J, Sterkmans P, et al: Droperidol in acutely agitated patients: a double-blind placebo-controlled study. J Nerv Ment Dis 164:280–283, 1977

van Munster BC, Korevaar JC, de Rooij SE, et al: The association between delirium and APOE–epsilon 4 allele in the elderly. Int Psychogeriatrics 17 (suppl 2):149, 2005

Vaphiades MS, Celesia GG, Brigell MG: Positive spontaneous visual phenomena limited to the hemianopic field in lesions of central visual pathways. Neurology 47:408–417, 1996

Voyer P, Cole MG, McCusker J, et al: Prevalence and symptoms of delirium superimposed on dementia. Clin Nurs Res 15:46–66, 2006

Wahlund B, Grahn H, Saaf J, et al: Affective disorder subtyped by psychomotor symptoms, monoamine oxidase, melatonin and cortisol: identification of patients with latent bipolar disorder. Eur Arch Psychiatry Clin Neurosci 248:215–224, 1998

Wahlund LA, Bjorlin GA: Delirium in clinical practice: experiences from a specialized delirium ward. Dement Geriatr Cogn Disord 10:389–392, 1999

Wanich CK, Sullivan-Marx EM, Gottlieb GL, et al: Functional status outcomes of a nursing intervention in hospitalized elderly. Image J Nurs Sch 24:201–207, 1992

Webster R, Holroyd S: Prevalence of psychotic symptoms in delirium. Psychosomatics 41:519–522, 2000

Weddington WW: The mortality of delirium: an underappreciated problem? Psychosomatics 23:1232–1235, 1982

Wengel SP, Roccaforte WH, Burke WJ: Donepezil improves symptoms of delirium in dementia: implications for future research. J Geriatr Psychiatry Neurol 11:159–161, 1998

Wengel SP, Burke WJ, Roccaforte WH: Donepezil for postoperative delirium associated with Alzheimer's disease. J Am Geriatr Soc 47:379–380, 1999

Wernicke C, Smolka M, Gallinat J, et al: Evidence for the importance of the human dopamine transporter gene for withdrawal symptomatology of alcoholics in a German population. Neurosci Lett 333:45–48, 2002

Wetli CV, Mash D, Karch SB: Cocaine-associated agitated delirium and the neuroleptic malignant syndrome. Am J Emerg Med 14:425–428, 1996

White S, Calver BL, Newsway V, et al: Enzymes of drug metabolism during delirium. Age Ageing 34:603–608, 2005

Willard LB, Hauss-Wegrzyniak B, Wenk GL: Pathological and biochemical consequences of acute and chronic neuroinflammation within the basal forebrain cholinergic system of rats. Neuroscience 88:193–200, 1999

Williams MA, Campbell EB, Raynor WJ, et al: Reducing acute confusional states in elderly patients with hip fractures. Res Nurs Health 8:329–337, 1985

Williams PD, Helton DR: The proconvulsive activity of quinolone antibiotics in an animal model. Toxicol Lett 58:23–28, 1991

Wilson K, Broadhurst C, Diver M, et al: Plasma insulin growth factor-1 and incident delirium. Int J Geriatr Psychiatry 20:154–159, 2005

Wilson LM: Intensive care delirium: the effect of outside deprivation in a windowless unit. Arch Intern Med 130:225–226, 1972

Wilt JL, Minnema AM, Johnson RF, et al: Torsades de pointes associated with the use of intravenous haloperidol. Ann Intern Med 119:391–394, 1993

Wolff HG, Curran D: Nature of delirium and allied states: the dysergastic reaction. Arch Neurol Psychiatry 33:1175–1215, 1935

Wong AHC, Buckle CE, van Tol HHM: Polymorphisms in dopamine receptors: what do they tell us? Eur J Pharmacol 410:183–203, 2000

World Health Organization: International Statistical Classification of Diseases and Related Health Problems, 10th Revision. Geneva, Switzerland, World Health Organization, 1992

Wu CL, Hsu W, Richman JM, et al: Postoperative cognitive function as an outcome of regional anesthesia and analgesia. Reg Anesth Pain Med 29:257–268, 2004

Yamamoto T, Lyeth BG, Dixon CE, et al: Changes in regional brain acetylcholine content in rats following unilateral and bilateral brainstem lesions. J Neurotrauma 5:69–79, 1988

Yokota H, Ogawa S, Kurokawa A, et al: Regional cerebral blood flow in delirious patients. Psychiatry Clin Neurosci 57:337–339, 2003

Young LJ, George J: Do guidelines improve the process and outcomes of care in delirium? Age Ageing 32:525–528, 2003

Zee-Cheng C-S, Mueller CE, Siefert CF, et al: Haloperidol and torsades de pointes (letter). Ann Intern Med 102:418, 1985

6

NEUROPSYCHIATRIC ASPECTS OF TRAUMATIC BRAIN INJURY

Jonathan M. Silver, M.D.
Robert E. Hales, M.D., M.B.A.
Stuart C. Yudofsky, M.D.

E ach year in the United States, more than 2 million people sustain a traumatic brain injury (TBI); 300,000 of these persons require hospitalization, and more than 80,000 of the survivors are afflicted with the chronic sequelae of such injuries (J.F. Kraus and Sorenson 1994). In this population, psychosocial and psychological deficits are commonly the major source of disability for the victims and of stress for their families. The psychiatrist, neurologist, and neuropsychologist are often called on by other medical specialists or the families to treat these patients. In this chapter, we review the role these professionals play in the prevention, diagnosis, and treatment of the cognitive, behavioral, and emotional aspects of TBI.

EPIDEMIOLOGY

It is commonly taught in introductory courses in psychiatry that suicide is the second most common cause of death among persons under age 35. What is often not stated is that the most common cause is injuries incurred during motor vehicle accidents. TBI accounts for 2% of all deaths and 26% of all injury deaths (Sosin et al. 1989). A conservative estimate of the annual incidence of individuals hospitalized with TBI is approximately 120 per 100,000 (J.F. Kraus and Chu 2005). There are almost 100,000 new disabilities from TBI per year (J.F. Kraus and Chu 2005). In the United States, between 2.5 million and 6.5 million individuals live with the long-term consequences of TBI (NIH Consensus Development Panel 1999). Disorders arising from traumatic injuries to the brain are more common than any other neurological disease, with the exception of headaches (Kurtzke 1984).

Those at the highest risk for brain injury are males ages 15–24 years. Alcohol use is common in brain injury; a positive blood alcohol concentration was demonstrated in 56% of one sample of victims (J.F. Kraus et al. 1989). Motor vehicle accidents account for approximately one-half of traumatic brain injuries; other common causes are falls (21%), assaults and violence (20%), and accidents associated with sports and recreation (3%) (although as many as 90% of injuries in this category may be unreported) (NIH Consensus Development Panel 1999). Children are highly vulnerable to accidents as passengers, to falls as pedestrians, to impact from moving objects (e.g., rocks or baseballs), and to sports injuries. In the United States, as many as 5 million children sustain head injuries each year, and of this group 200,000 are hospitalized (Raphaely et al. 1980). As a result of bicycle accidents alone, 50,000 children sustain head injuries, and 400 children die each year (U.S. Department of Health and Human Services 1989). Tragically, among infants, most head injuries are the result of child abuse (64%) (U.S. Department of Health and Human Services 1989).

NEUROANATOMY OF TRAUMATIC BRAIN INJURY

The patient who sustains brain injury from trauma may incur damage through several mechanisms, which are listed in Table 6–1. Contusions affect specific areas of the brain and usually occur as the result of low-velocity injuries, such as falls. Courville (1945) examined the neuroanatomical sites of contusions and found that most injuries were in the basal and polar portions of the temporal and frontal lobes. Most of these lesions were the result of the location of bony prominences that surround the orbital, frontal, and temporal areas along the base of the skull. Coup injuries occur at the site of impact due to local tissue strain. Contrecoup injuries occur away from the site of impact during sudden deceleration and translational and angular movements of the head. Impact is not required for contrecoup injuries to occur, and they usually occur in frontal and temporal areas (Gennarelli and Graham 1998).

TABLE 6–1.   Mechanisms of neuronal damage in traumatic brain injury

Primary effects

   Contusions

   Diffuse traumatic axonal injury

Secondary effects

   Hematomas

      Epidural effects

      Subdural effects

      Intracerebral effects

   Cerebral edema

   Hydrocephalus

   Increased intracranial pressure

   Infection

   Hypoxia

   Neurotoxicity

   Inflammatory response

   Protease activation

   Calcium influx

   Excitotoxin and free radical release

   Lipid peroxidation

   Phospholipase activation

Diffuse axonal injury refers to mechanical or chemical damage to the axons in cerebral white matter that commonly occurs with lateral angular or rotational acceleration. The axon is vulnerable to injury during high-velocity accidents when there is twisting and turning of the brain around the brain stem (as can occur in "whiplash" car accidents). Axons are stretched, causing delayed (hours) disruption of the cytoskeleton and impaired axoplasm transport. This results in axoplasmic swelling and detachment, changes in membrane structure, disruption in neurofilaments, and wallerian degeneration of the distal stump of the axon (Gennarelli and Graham 2005). The disruption of axons can occur as long as 2 weeks after the injury (Gennarelli and Graham 1998). Chemically, metabolic changes occur, leading to axonal damage. The most vulnerable sites in the brain to axonal injury are the reticular formation, superior cerebellar peduncles, regions of the basal ganglia, hypothalamus, limbic fornices, and corpus callosum (Cassidy 1994).

Subdural hematomas (acute, subacute, and chronic) and intracerebral hematomas have effects that are specific to their locations and degree of neuronal damage. In general, subdural hematomas affect arousal and cognition.

NEUROPSYCHIATRIC ASSESSMENT OF TRAUMATIC BRAIN INJURY

Assessment of TBI has multiple components. Measures and techniques that may be employed are listed in Table 6–2.

HISTORY TAKING

Although brain injuries subsequent to serious automobile, occupational, or sports accidents may not result in diagnostic enigmas for the psychiatrist, less severe trauma may first present as relatively subtle behavioral or affective change. Patients may fail to associate the traumatic event with subsequent symptoms. Prototypic examples include the alcoholic man who is amnestic for a fall that occurred while he was inebriated, the 10-year-old boy who falls from his bicycle and hits his head but fails to inform his parents, and the wife who was beaten by her husband but who is either fearful or ashamed to report the injury to her family physician. Confusion, intellectual changes, affective lability, or psychosis may occur directly after the trauma or as long as many years afterward. Individuals who present for emergency treatment for blunt trauma may not be adequately screened for TBI (Chambers et al. 1996). Even individuals who identified themselves as "nondisabled" but who had experienced a blow to the head that left them at a minimum dazed and confused had symptoms and emotional distress similar to a group of individuals with known mild TBI (Gordon et al. 1998).

For all psychiatric patients, the clinician must specifically inquire whether the patient has been involved in situations that are associated with head trauma. The practitioner should ask about automobile, bicycle, or motorcycle accidents; falls; assaults; playground accidents; and participation in sports that are frequently associated with brain injury (e.g., football, soccer, rugby, and boxing). Patients must be asked whether there was any alteration in consciousness after they were injured, including feeling dazed or confused, losing consciousness, or experiencing a period of amnesia after the accident. The clinician should inquire as to whether the patients were hospitalized and whether they had posttraumatic symptoms, such as headache, dizziness, irritability, problems with concentration, and sensitivity to noise or light. Most patients will not volunteer this information without direct inquiry. Patients are usually unaware of the phenomenon of posttraumatic amnesia and may confuse posttraumatic amnesia with loss of consciousness (LOC). They assume that if they are unable to recall events, they must have been unconscious. Therefore, care must be taken to document the source of this observation (e.g., whether there were observers who witnessed the period of unconsciousness).

Because many patients are unaware of, minimize, or deny the severity of behavioral changes that occur after TBI, family members also must be asked about the effects of injury on the behavior of their relative. For example, in evaluating the social adjustment of patients years after severe brain injury, Oddy et al. (1985) compared symptoms reported by both patients and their relatives. Forty percent of relatives of 28 patients with TBI reported that their relative behaved childishly. However, this symptom was not reported by the patients themselves. Although 28% of the patients complained of problems with their vision after the injury, this difficulty was not reported by relatives. Patients overestimate their level of functioning compared with the reporting of relatives, and they report more physical than nonphysical impairment (Sherer et al. 1998).

TABLE 6–2.   Assessment of traumatic brain injury

Behavioral assessment

Structured interviews (e.g., Structured Clinical Interview for DSM-IV Diagnoses [SCID], Mini-International Neuropsychiatric Inventory [MINI])

Neurobehavioral Rating Scale (NBRS)

Positive and Negative Syndrome Scale (PANSS)

Glasgow Coma Scale (GCS; Table 6–3)

Galveston Orientation and Amnesia Test (GOAT)

Rancho Los Amigos Cognitive Scale (Table 6–4)

Rating scales for depression (Hamilton)

Rating scales for aggression (Overt Aggression Scale/Agitated Behavior Scale)

Neuropsychiatric Inventory/Neuropsychiatric Inventory Questionnaire

Brain Injury Screening Questionnaire

Rivermead Post Concussion Symptoms Questionnaire

Brain imaging

Computed tomography (CT)

Magnetic resonance imaging (MRI) with fluid-attenuated inversion recovery (FLAIR)

Functional magnetic resonance imaging (fMRI)

Single-photon emission computed tomography (SPECT)

Regional cerebral blood flow (rCBF)

Positron emission tomography (PET)

Proton magnetic resonance spectroscopy (MRS)

Diffusion tensor imaging (DTI)

Electrophysiological assessment

Electroencephalography (EEG), including special leads

Computerized EEG

Brain electrical activity mapping (BEAM)

Neuropsychological assessment

Attention and concentration

Premorbid intelligence

Memory

Executive functioning

Verbal capacity

Problem-solving skills

TABLE 6–3. Glasgow Coma Scale

Eye opening

None	1.	Not attributable to ocular swelling
To pain	2.	Pain stimulus is applied to chest or limbs
To speech	3.	Nonspecific response to speech or shout, does not imply the patient obeys command to open eyes
Spontaneous	4.	Eyes are open, but this does not imply intact awareness

Motor response

No response	1.	Flaccid
Extension	2.	"Decerebrate." Adduction, internal rotation of shoulder, and pronation of the forearm
Abnormal flexion	3.	"Decorticate." Abnormal flexion, adduction of the shoulder
Withdrawal	4.	Normal flexor response; withdraws from pain stimulus with adduction of the shoulder
Localizes pain	5.	Pain stimulus applied to supraocular region or fingertip causes limb to move so as to attempt to remove it
Obeys commands	6.	Follows simple commands

Verbal response

No response	1.	(Self-explanatory)
Incomprehensible	2.	Moaning and groaning, but no recognizable words
Inappropriate	3.	Intelligible speech (e.g., shouting or swearing), but no sustained or coherent conversation
Confused	4.	Patient responds to questions in a conversational manner, but the responses indicate varying degrees of disorientation and confusion
Oriented	5.	Normal orientation to time, place, and person

Source. Adapted from Teasdale and Jennett 1974.

Family members also are more aware of emotional changes than are the victims of brain injury. Whereas individuals with TBI tend to view the cognitive difficulties as being more severe than the emotional changes (Hendryx 1989), mood disorders and frustration intolerance are viewed by family members as being more disabling than cognitive disabilities (Rappaport et al. 1989).

In severe TBI, posttraumatic amnesia or LOC may persist for at least 1 week or longer or, in extreme cases, may last weeks to months. Glasgow Coma Scale (GCS) scores for severe TBI are less than 10. Mild head injury is usually defined as LOC for less than 15–20 minutes, GCS score of 13–15, brief or no hospitalization, and no prominent residual neurobehavioral deficits. LOC is not required for the diagnosis of traumatic brain injury; however, there must be some evidence of alteration in consciousness, including feeling dazed or experiencing a period of posttraumatic amnesia (Committee on Head Injury Nomenclature 1966; Quality Standards Subcommittee 1997). Operationalized diagnostic criteria for mild TBI have been proposed (Table 6–5) (Mild Traumatic Brain Injury Committee 1993). A specific grading scale has been devel-

---

TABLE 6–4.   Rancho Los Amigos Cognitive Scale

I.   **No response:** Unresponsive to any stimulus

II.   **Generalized response:** Limited, inconsistent, nonpurposeful responses, often to pain only

III.   **Localized response:** Purposeful responses; may follow simple commands; may focus on presented object

IV.   **Confused, agitated:** Heightened state of activity; confusion, disorientation; aggressive behavior; unable to do self-care; unaware of present events; agitation appears related to internal confusion

V.   **Confused, inappropriate:** Nonagitated; appears alert; responds to commands; distractible; does not concentrate on task; agitated responses to external stimuli; verbally inappropriate; does not learn new information

VI.   **Confused, appropriate:** Good directed behavior, needs cueing; can relearn old skills as activities of daily living (ADL); serious memory problems; some awareness of self and others

VII.   **Automatic, appropriate:** Appears appropriate, oriented; frequently robotlike in daily routine; minimal or absent confusion; shallow recall; increased awareness of self, interaction in environment; lacks insight into condition; decreased judgment and problem solving; lacks realistic planning for future

VIII.   **Purposeful, appropriate:** Alert, oriented; recalls and integrates past events; learns new activities and can continue without supervision; independent in home and living skills; capable of driving; defects in stress tolerance, judgment, abstract reasoning persist; may function at reduced levels in society

---

Source.   Reprinted with permission of the Adult Brain Injury Service of the Rancho Los Amigos Medical Center, Downey, California.

oped for concussions that occur during sports: Grade 1—confusion without amnesia and no LOC; Grade 2—confusion with amnesia and no LOC; and Grade 3—LOC (Kelly 1995).

LABORATORY EVALUATION

Imaging Techniques

Brain imaging techniques are frequently used to demonstrate the location and extent of brain lesions (Belanger et al. 2007). Computed tomography (CT) is used for the acute assessment of the patient with head trauma to document hemorrhage, edema, midline shifts, herniation, fractures, and contusions. The timing of such imaging is important because this establishes a baseline day of injury scan, since lesions may be visualized months after the injury that cannot be seen during the acute phase (Bigler 2005). Thus, for a significant number of patients with severe brain injury, initial CT evaluations may not detect lesions that are observable on CT scans performed at

1 and 3 months after the injury (Cope et al. 1988).

Magnetic resonance imaging (MRI) has been shown to detect clinically meaningful lesions in patients with severe brain injury when CT scans have not demonstrated anatomical bases for the degree of coma (Levin et al. 1987a; Wilberger et al. 1987). MRI is especially sensitive in detecting lesions in the frontal and temporal lobes that are not visualized by CT, and these loci are frequently related to the neuropsychiatric consequences of the injury (Levin et al. 1987a). MRI has been found to be more sensitive for the detection of contusions, shearing injury, and subdural and epidural hematomas (Orrison et al. 1994), and it has been able to document evidence of diffuse axonal injury in patients who have a normal CT scan after experiencing mild TBI (Mittl et al. 1994). When MRI is used, fluid-attenuated inversion recovery (FLAIR) is superior to T2-weighted spin-echo technique, especially in visualizing central diffuse axonal injury of the

TABLE 6–5.   Definition of mild traumatic brain injury

A patient with mild traumatic brain injury is a person who has had a traumatically induced physiological disruption of brain function, as manifested by **at least** one of the following:

1. Any period of loss of consciousness;

2. Any loss of memory for events immediately before or after the accident;

3. Any alteration in mental state at the time of the accident (e.g., feeling dazed, disoriented, or confused); and

4. Focal neurological deficit(s) that may or may not be transient; but where the severity of the injury does not exceed the following: loss of consciousness of approximately 30 minutes or less; after 30 minutes, an initial Glasgow Coma Scale (GCS) score of 13–15; and posttraumatic amnesia (PTA) not greater than 24 hours.

Source. Reprinted from Mild Traumatic Brain Injury Committee of the Head Injury Interdisciplinary Special Interest Group of the American Congress of Rehabilitation Medicine: "Definition of Mild Traumatic Brain Injury." *Journal of Head Trauma Rehabilitation* 8:86–87, 1993. Used with permission.

fornix and corpus callosum (Ashikaga et al. 1997). MRI in the chronic stage is better correlated with neuropsychiatric symptoms (Bigler 2005). Quantitative analyses of individuals with TBI have revealed multiple affected brain structures, including the frontal and temporal lobes, thalamus, hippocampus, and basal ganglia (Bigler 2005).

Functional techniques in brain imaging, such as regional cerebral blood flow (rCBF) and positron emission tomography (PET), can detect areas of abnormal function when even CT and MRI scans fail to show any abnormalities of structure (Anderson et al. 2005). Single-photon emission computed tomography (SPECT) also shows promise in documenting brain damage after TBI. Abnormalities are visualized in patients who have experienced mild TBI (Gross et al. 1996; Masdeu et al. 1994; Nedd et al. 1993) or who have chronic TBI (Nagamachi et al. 1995), even in the presence of normally appearing areas on CT scans. Abnormalities on SPECT appear to correlate with the severity of trauma (Jacobs et al. 1994). These techniques were utilized in examining a group of individuals with late whiplash syndrome (Bicik et al. 1998). Although there was significant frontopolar hypometabolism, it correlated significantly with scores on the Beck Depression Inventory (Beck et al. 1961). However, in individual cases, the reliability of the depiction of hypo-

metabolism was low. A "normal" SPECT scan does not imply normal pathology; in addition, SPECT abnormalities after TBI have not been shown to correlate with cognitive deficits or behavioral symptoms (Anderson et al. 2005). SPECT abnormalities can also be seen in many of the concurrent problems experienced by those with TBI, including depression and substance use. Although some studies have found correlations between neuropsychological deficits and abnormalities on PET, other studies have found no relation between lesion location and deficits (Anderson et al. 2005).

Proton magnetic resonance spectroscopy (MRS), which provides information on intracellular function, has been investigated for the detection of abnormalities in TBI. *N*-acetylaspartate (NAA) is associated with neuronal or axonal loss. Cecil et al. (1998) examined 35 patients with TBI and found that a majority of those with mild TBI as well as those with severe TBI showed abnormal levels of NAA in the splenium, consistent with diffuse axonal injury. Early changes in NAA concentrations in gray matter were predictive of outcome in a group of 14 patients after TBI (Friedman et al. 1999). Ariza et al. (2004) found a correlation between performance on neuropsychological tests and NAA concentrations. Even in mild TBI, abnormalities may be found in areas that are frequent sites of diffuse axonal injury (Inglese 2005).

McAllister et al. (1999, 2001) used functional MRI to assess patterns of regional brain activation in response to working memory loads in a group of individuals 1 month after they had sustained mild TBI. This group demonstrated significantly increased activation during a high-load task, particularly in the right parietal and right dorsolateral frontal regions. However, there were no differences in task performance compared with the control group. This study appears to correlate with the complaints of patients who state that they have to "work harder" to recall things but in whom no deficits are found on objective testing. Other studies (Christodoulou et al. 2001; Easdon et al. 2004) suggest that there is impairment in brain structures required for appropriate responding to stimuli.

Caution must be observed in applying the findings in this literature to a clinical population. We are unable to determine the presence of abnormalities before the accident. Abnormalities on SPECT or PET have been demonstrated in individuals with no history of brain injury who have psychiatric disorders, including posttraumatic stress disorder (PTSD) (Rauch et al. 1996), somatization disorder (Lazarus and Cotterell 1989), major depression (Dolan et al. 1992), and chronic alcoholism (Kuruoglu et al. 1996). When the evidence was reviewed in 1996, the American Academy of Neurology concluded that there currently was insufficient evidence for the use of SPECT to diagnose TBI, and its use in this condition should be considered investigational (Therapeutics and Technology Assessment Subcommittee 1996). With the present state of the art, functional imaging results can only be used as part of an overall evaluation to confirm findings documented elsewhere (Silver and McAllister 1997).

Electrophysiological Techniques

Electrophysiological assessment of the patient after TBI may also assist in the evaluation. Electroencephalography can detect the presence of seizures or abnormal areas of function-

ing. To enhance the sensitivity of this technique, the electroencephalogram (EEG) should be performed after sleep deprivation, with photic stimulation and hyperventilation and with anterotemporal and/or nasopharyngeal leads (Goodin et al. 1990). Computed interpretation of the EEG and brain electrical activity mapping (BEAM) may be useful in detecting areas of dysfunction not shown in the routine EEG (Watson et al. 1995). There is controversy regarding the usefulness of these techniques. The American Academy of Neurology and the American Clinical Neurophysiology Society have concluded that "the evidence of clinical usefulness or consistency of results [is] not considered sufficient for us to support [the] use [of quantitative electroencephalography] in diagnosis of patients with postconcussion syndrome, or minor or moderate head injury" (Nuwer 1997). However, the EEG and Clinical Neuroscience Society addressed significant concerns regarding the interpretation of this report (Thatcher et al. 1999). Their opinion is that there is significant scientific literature on the use and interpretation of quantitative electroencephalography, and that several findings have been consistent (reduced amplitude of high-frequency electroencephalography, especially in the frontal lobes; a shift toward lower increased electroencephalographic frequencies; and changes in electroencephalographic coherence) (Thatcher et al. 1999). A detailed discussion of electrophysiological techniques can be found elsewhere (Arciniegas et al. 2005).

Neuropsychological Testing

Neuropsychological assessment of the patient with TBI is essential to document cognitive and intellectual deficits and strengths. Tests are administered to assess the patient's attention, concentration, memory, verbal capacity, and executive functioning. This latter capacity is the most difficult to assess and includes problem-solving skills, abstract thinking, planning, and reasoning abilities. A valid interpretation of these tests includes assessment of the

TABLE 6–6.   Major factors affecting neuropsychological test findings

Original endowment

Environment

Motivation (effort)

Physical health

Psychological distress

Psychiatric disorders

Medications

Qualifications and experience of
   neuropsychologist

Errors in scoring

Errors in interpretation

Source.   Reprinted from Simon RI: "Ethical and Legal Issues," in *Textbook of Traumatic Brain Injury.* Edited by Silver JM, McAllister TM, Yudofsky SC. Washington, DC, American Psychiatric Publishing, 2005, pp. 583–605. Used with permission.

patient's preinjury intelligence and other higher levels of functioning. Because multiple factors affect the results of testing (Table 6–6), tests must be performed and interpreted by a clinician with skill and experience.

Patients' complaints may not be easily or accurately categorized as either functional (i.e., primarily due to a psychiatric disorder) or neurological (i.e., primarily caused by the brain injury). Nonetheless, outside agencies (e.g., insurance companies and lawyers) may request a neuropsychiatric evaluation to assist with this "differential." In reality, most symptoms result from the interaction of many factors, including neurological, social, emotional, educational, and vocational. Because important insurance and other reimbursement decisions may hinge on whether or not disabilities stem from brain injury, the clinician should take care that his or her impressions are based on data and are not misapplied to deprive the patient of deserved benefits. For example, mood disorders and cognitive sequelae of brain injury are often miscategorized as "mental illnesses" that are not covered by some insurance policies.

TABLE 6–7.   Factors influencing outcome after brain injury

Severity of injury

Type of injury

Anosmia

Intellectual functioning

Psychiatric diagnosis

Sociopathy

Premorbid behavioral problems (children)

Social support

Substance use

Neurological disorder

Age

Apolipoprotein E status

CLINICAL FEATURES

The neuropsychiatric sequelae of TBI include problems with attention and arousal, concentration, and executive functioning; intellectual changes; memory impairment; personality changes; affective disorders; anxiety disorders; psychosis; posttraumatic epilepsy; sleep disorders; aggression; and irritability. Physical problems such as headache, chronic pain, vision impairment, and dizziness complicate recovery. The severity of the neuropsychiatric sequelae of the brain injury is determined by multiple factors existing before, during, and after the injury (Dikmen and Machamer 1995) (Table 6–7). In general, prognosis is associated with the severity of injury. Although duration of posttraumatic amnesia correlates with subsequent cognitive recovery (Levin et al. 1982), in an analysis of 1,142 patients assessed after hospitalization for TBI, the simple presence or absence of LOC was not significantly related to performance on neuropsychological tests (Smith-Seemiller et al. 1996). There is a lack of correlation between the occurrence of LOC and neuropsychological test results in patients with mild brain injury (Lovell et al. 1999). In addition, the symptoms of injury are correlated with the type of damage sustained. For example, those with diffuse axonal injury often experience arousal problems, attention problems, and slow cognitive processing. The presence of total anosmia in a group of patients with closed head injury predicted major vocational problems at least 2 years after these patients had been given medical clearance to return to work (Varney 1988). Posttraumatic anosmia may occur as a result of damage to the olfactory nerve, which is located adjacent to the orbitofrontal cortex, although there may be peripheral nerve involvement that results in anosmia. Impairment in olfactory naming and recognition frequently occurs in patients with moderate or severe brain injury and is related to frontal and temporal lobe damage (Levin et al. 1985).

In a review by J. D. Corrigan (1995), victims of TBI who were intoxicated with alcohol at the time of the injury had longer periods of hospitalization, had more complications during hospitalization, and had a lower level of functioning at the time of discharge from the hospital compared with patients with TBI who had no detectable blood alcohol level at the time of hospitalization. One factor complicating the interpretation of these data is the fact that intoxication may produce decreased responsiveness even without TBI, which can result in a GCS score that indicates greater severity of injury than is actually present. Furthermore, even a history of substance abuse is associated with increased morbidity and mortality rates.

Morbidity and mortality rates after brain injury increase with age. Elderly persons who experience TBI have longer periods of agitation and greater cognitive impairment and are more likely to develop mass lesions and permanent disability than are younger victims (Kim 2005). Individuals who have had a previous brain injury do not recover as well from subsequent injuries (Carlsson et al. 1987).

The interaction between the brain injury and the psychosocial factors cannot be underestimated. Demographic factors have been found to predict cognitive dysfunction after TBI (Smith-Seemiller et al. 1996). Preexisting emotional and behavioral problems are exacer-

bated after injury. It also appears that having a preexisting psychiatric disorder increases the risk of TBI (Fann et al. 2002). Social conditions and support networks that existed before the injury affect the symptoms and course of recovery. In general, individuals with greater preinjury intelligence recover better after injury (G. Brown et al. 1981). Factors such as level of education, level of income, and socioeconomic status are positive factors in the ability to return to work after minor head injury (Rimel et al. 1981).

PERSONALITY CHANGES

Unlike many primary psychiatric illnesses that have gradual onset, TBI often occurs suddenly and devastatingly. Although some patients recognize that they no longer have the same abilities and potential that they had before the injury, many others with significant disabilities deny that there have been any changes. Prominent behavioral traits such as disorderliness, suspiciousness, argumentativeness, isolativeness, disruptiveness, social inappropriateness, and anxiousness often become more pronounced after brain injury.

In a study of children with head injury, G. Brown et al. (1981) found that disinhibition, social inappropriateness, restlessness, and stealing were associated with injuries in which there was LOC extending for more than 7 days. In a survey of the relatives of victims of severe TBI, McKinlay et al. (1981) found that 49% of 55 patients had developed personality changes 3 months after the injury. After 5 years, 74% of these patients were reported to have changes in their personality (N. Brooks et al. 1986). More than one-third of these patients had problems of "childishness" and "talking too much" (N. Brooks et al. 1986; McKinlay et al. 1981).

Thomsen (1984) found that 80% of 40 patients with severe TBI had personality changes that persisted for 2 to 5 years, and 65% had changes lasting 10–15 years after the injury. These changes included childishness (60% and 25%, respectively), emotional lability (40%

and 35%, respectively), and restlessness (25% and 38%, respectively). Approximately two-thirds of patients had less social contact, and one-half had loss of spontaneity and poverty of interests after 10–15 years.

Because of the vulnerability of the prefrontal and frontal regions of the cortex to contusions, injury to these regions is common and gives rise to changes in personality known as the frontal lobe syndrome. For the prototypic patient with frontal lobe syndrome, the cognitive functions are preserved while personality changes abound. Psychiatric disturbances associated with frontal lobe injury commonly include impaired social judgment, labile affect, uncharacteristic lewdness, inability to appreciate the effects of one's behavior or remarks on others, a loss of social graces (such as eating manners), a diminution of attention to personal appearance and hygiene, and boisterousness. Impaired judgment may take the form of diminished concern for the future, increased risk taking, unrestrained drinking of alcohol, and indiscriminate selection of food. Patients may appear shallow, indifferent, or apathetic, with a global lack of concern for the consequences of their behavior.

Certain behavioral syndromes have been related to damage to specific areas of the frontal lobe (Auerbach 1986). The orbitofrontal syndrome is associated with behavioral excesses, such as impulsivity, disinhibition, hyperactivity, distractibility, and mood lability. Injury to the dorsolateral frontal cortex may result in slowness, apathy, and perseveration. This may be considered similar to the negative (deficit) symptoms associated with schizophrenia, wherein the patient may exhibit blunted affect, emotional withdrawal, social withdrawal, passivity, and lack of spontaneity (S.R. Kay et al. 1987). As with TBI, deficit symptoms in patients with schizophrenia are thought to result from disordered functioning of the dorsolateral frontal cortex (Berman et al. 1988). Outbursts of rage and violent behavior occur after damage to the inferior orbital surface of the frontal lobe and anterior temporal lobes.

Patients also develop changes in sexual behavior after brain injury, most commonly decreased sex drive, erectile function, and frequency of intercourse (Zasler 1994). Kleine-Levin syndrome—characterized by periodic hypersomnolence, hyperphagia, and behavioral disturbances that include hypersexuality—has also been reported to occur subsequent to brain injury (Will et al. 1988).

Although there have been studies examining personality changes after TBI, few have focused on Axis II psychopathology in individuals with TBI. In utilizing a structured clinical interview to diagnose personality disorders in 100 individuals with TBI, Hibbard et al. (2000) found that several personality disorders developed after TBI that were reflective of persistent challenges and compensatory coping strategies facing these individuals. Whereas before TBI, 24% of the sample population had personality disorders, 66% of the sample met criteria for personality disorders after TBI. The most common personality disorders were borderline, avoidant, paranoid, obsessive-compulsive, and narcissistic. Koponen et al. (2002), in a 30-year follow-up study of 60 patients with TBI, found that the most frequent personality disorders were paranoid, schizoid, avoidant, and organic personality disorders.

In DSM-IV-TR (American Psychiatric Association 2000), these personality changes would be diagnosed as personality change due to traumatic brain injury. Specific subtypes are provided as the most significant clinical problems (Table 6–8).

INTELLECTUAL CHANGES

Problems with intellectual functioning may be among the most subtle manifestations of brain injury. Changes can occur in the ability to attend, concentrate, remember, abstract, calculate, reason, plan, and process information (McCullagh and Feinstein 2005). Problems with arousal can take the form of inattentiveness, distractibility, and difficulty switching and dividing attention (Ponsford and Kinsella 1992). Mental sluggishness, poor concentra-

---

TABLE 6–8.   DSM-IV-TR diagnostic criteria for personality change due to traumatic brain injury

---

A.   A persistent personality disturbance that represents a change from the individual's previous characteristic personality pattern. (In children, the disturbance involves a marked deviation from normal development or a significant change in the child's usual behavior patterns lasting at least 1 year).

B.   There is evidence from the history, physical examination, or laboratory findings that the disturbance is the direct physiological consequence of a general medical condition.

C.   The disturbance is not better accounted for by another mental disorder (including other mental disorders due to a general medical condition).

D.   The disturbance does not occur exclusively during the course of a delirium.

E.   The disturbance causes clinically significant distress or impairment in social, occupational, or other important areas of functioning.

Specify type:

>   **Labile Type:**   if the predominant feature is affective lability
>
>   **Disinhibited Type:**   if the predominant feature is poor impulse control as evidenced by sexual indiscretions, etc.
>
>   **Aggressive Type:**   if the predominant feature is aggressive behavior
>
>   **Apathetic Type:**   if the predominant feature is marked apathy and indifference
>
>   **Paranoid Type:**   if the predominant feature is suspiciousness or paranoid ideation
>
>   **Other Type:**   if the presentation is not characterized by any of the above subtypes
>
>   **Combined Type:**   if more than one feature predominates in the clinical picture
>
>   **Unspecified Type**

Source.   Reprinted from American Psychiatric Association: *Diagnostic and Statistical Manual of Mental Disorders,* 4th Edition, Text Revision. Washington, DC, American Psychiatric Association, 2000. Used with permission.

---

tion, and memory problems are common complaints of both patients and relatives (N. Brooks et al. 1986; McKinlay et al. 1981; Thomsen 1984). High-level cognitive functions, termed *executive functions*, are frequently impaired, although such impairments are difficult to detect and diagnose with cursory cognitive testing (Table 6–9) (McCullagh and Feinstein 2005). Only specific tests that mimic real-life decision-making situations may objectively demonstrate the problems encountered in daily life (Bechara et al. 1994).

Children who survive head trauma often return to school with behavioral and learning problems (Mahoney et al. 1983). Children with behavioral disorders are much more likely to have a history of prior head injury (Michaud et al. 1993). In addition, children who sustained injury at or before age 2 years had significantly lower IQ scores (Michaud et al. 1993). The risk factors for the sequelae of TBI in children are controversial (Max 2005). In a study of 43 children and adolescents who had sustained TBI, Max et al. (1998b) found that preinjury family functioning was a significant predictor of psychiatric disorders after 1 year. Whereas some investigators have demonstrated neuropsychological sequelae after mild TBI when careful testing is done (Gulbrandsen 1984), others have shown that mild TBI produces virtually no clinically significant long-term deficits (Fay et al. 1993). In patients who survive moderate to severe brain injury, the degree of memory impairment often exceeds the level of intellectual dysfunction (Levin et al. 1988). The following case example illustrates a typical presentation of an adolescent with TBI presenting with behavioral and academic problems.

TABLE 6–9.   **Aspects of executive functions potentially impaired after traumatic brain injury**

Goal establishment, planning, and anticipation of consequences

Initiation, sequencing, and inhibition of behavioral responses

Generation of multiple response alternatives (in contrast to perseverative or stereotyped responses)

Conceptual/inferential reasoning, problem solving

Mental flexibility/ease of mental and behavioral switching

Transcending the immediately salient aspects of a situation (in contrast to "stimulus-bound behavior" or "environmental dependency")

Executive attentional processes

Executive memory processes

Self-monitoring and self-regulation, including emotional responses

Social adaptive functioning: sensitivity to others, using social feedback, engaging in contextually appropriate social behavior

---

Source.   Reprinted from McCullagh S, Feinstein A: "Cognitive Changes," in *Textbook of Traumatic Brain Injury.* Edited by Silver JM, McAllister TW, Yudofsky SC. Washington, DC, American Psychiatric Publishing, 2005, pp. 321–335. Used with permission.

CASE EXAMPLE

A 17-year-old girl was referred by her father for neuropsychiatric evaluation because of many changes that were observed in her personality during the past 2 years. Whereas she had been an A student and had been involved in many extracurricular activities during her sophomore year in high school, there had been a substantial change in her behavior during the past 2 years. She was barely able to maintain a C average, was "hanging around with the bad kids," and was frequently using marijuana and alcohol. A careful history revealed that 2 years earlier, her older brother had hit her in the forehead with a rake, which stunned her, but she did not lose consciousness. Although she had a headache after the accident, no psychiatric or neurological follow-up was pursued.

Neuropsychological testing at the time of evaluation revealed a significant decline in intellectual functioning from her "preinjury" state. Testing revealed poor concentration, attention, memory, and reasoning abilities. Academically, she was unable to "keep up" with the friends she had before her injury, and she began

to socialize with a group of students with little interest in academics and began to conceptualize herself as being a rebel. When neuropsychological testing results were explained to the patient and her family as a consequence of the brain injury, she and her family were able to understand the "defensive" reaction to her changed social behavior.

PSYCHIATRIC DISORDERS

Studies that utilize standard psychiatric diagnostic criteria have found that several psychiatric disorders are common in individuals with TBI (Deb et al. 1999; Fann et al. 1995; Hibbard et al. 1998a; Jorge et al. 1993; van Reekum et al. 2000). In a group of patients referred to a brain injury rehabilitation center, Fann et al. (1995) found that 26% had current major depression, 14% had current dysthymia, 24% had current generalized anxiety disorder, and 8% had current substance abuse. There was a 12% occurrence of pre-TBI depression. Deb et al. (1999) performed a psychiatric evaluation of 196 individuals who were hospitalized after TBI. They found that a psychiatric disorder was present in 21.7% versus 16.4% of a control population of individuals hospitalized for other reasons. Compared with the control group, the individuals with TBI had a higher rate of depression (13.9% vs. 2.1%) and panic disorder (9.0% vs. 0.8%). Factors associated with these psychiatric disorders included a history of psychiatric illness, preinjury alcohol use, unfavorable outcome, lower Mini-Mental State Exam scores, and fewer years of education. Hibbard et al. (1998a) administered a structured psychiatric interview to 100 individuals with TBI. Major depression (61%), substance use disorder (28%), and PTSD (19%) were the most common psychiatric diagnoses elicited. Jorge et al. (1993) found that 26% of individuals had major depression 1 month after injury; 11% had comorbid generalized anxiety disorder.

Several studies suggest that individuals who experience TBI have a higher than expected rate of preinjury psychiatric disorders. Histories of prior psychiatric disorders in individuals with TBI have varied between 17% and 44%, and pre-TBI substance use figures have ranged from 22% to 30% (Jorge et al. 1994; van Reekum et al. 1996). Fann et al. (1995) found that 50% of individuals who had sustained TBI reported a history of psychiatric problems prior to the injury. The Research and Training Center for the Community Integration of Individuals with TBI at Mt. Sinai Medical Center in New York found that in a group of 100 individuals with TBI, 51% had pre-TBI psychiatric disorders, most commonly major depression or substance use disorders, and these occurred at rates more than twice those reported in community samples (Hibbard et al. 1998a). Fann et al. (2002) analyzed a health maintenance organization's database of 450,000 members for the occurrence of a TBI and evidence of a psychiatric condition. They found that the relative risk for TBI was 1.3- to 4-fold higher in individuals with a preceding psychiatric diagnosis (24.2% vs. 14.3%). Interestingly, this held true for all psychiatric disorders except attention-deficit/hyperactivity disorder.

AFFECTIVE CHANGES

Depression occurs frequently after TBI. There are several diagnostic issues that must be considered in the evaluation of the patient who appears depressed after TBI. Sadness is a common reaction after TBI, as patients describe "mourning" the loss of their "former selves," often a reflection of deficits in intellectual functioning and motoric abilities. Careful psychiatric evaluation is required to distinguish grief reactions, sadness, and demoralization from major depression.

The clinician must distinguish mood lability that occurs commonly after brain injury from major depression. Lability of mood and affect may be caused by temporal limbic and basal forebrain lesions (Ross and Stewart 1987) and has been shown to be responsive to standard pharmacological interventions of depression (discussion follows in the subsection "Affective Illness"). In addition, apathy (diminished motivation) secondary to brain injury (which includes decreased motivation, decreased pursuit of pleasurable activities, or schizoid behavior) and complaints of slowness in thought and cognitive processing may resemble depression (Marin and Chakravorty 2005).

The clinician should endeavor to determine whether a patient may have been having an episode of major depression before an accident. Traumatic injury may occur as a result of the depression and suicidal ideation. Alcohol use, which frequently occurs with and complicates depressive illness, is also a known risk factor for motor vehicle accidents. One common scenario is depression leading to poor concentration, to substance abuse, and to risk taking (or even overt suicidal behavior), which together contribute to the motor vehicle accident and brain injury.

Prevalence of Depression After TBI

The prevalence of depression after brain injury has been assessed through self-report questionnaires, rating scales, and assessments by relatives. For mild TBI, estimates of depressive complaints range from 6% to 39%. For depression after severe TBI, in which patients often have concomitant cognitive impairments, reported rates of depression vary from 10% to 77%.

Robert Robinson and his colleagues have performed prospective studies of the occurrence of depression after brain injury (Federoff et al. 1992; Jorge et al. 1993). They evaluated 66 hospitalized patients who sustained acute TBI and followed the course of their mood over 1 year. Diagnoses were made using structured interviews and DSM-III-R (American Psychiatric Association 1987) criteria. The patients were evaluated at 1 month, 3 months, 6 months, and 1 year after injury. At each period, approximately 25% of patients fulfilled criteria for major depressive disorder. The mean duration of depression was 4.7 months, with a range of 1.5–12 months. Of the entire group of patients, 42% developed major depression during the first year after injury. The researchers also found that patients with generalized anxiety disorder and comorbid major depression have longer lasting mood problems than do those patients with depression and no anxiety (Jorge et al. 1993). More recently, this group extended their observations to another group of 91 patients (Jorge et al. 2004). During the first year after TBI, 33% developed depression, significantly more than the "other injury" control group. In those depressed individuals, there was a high rate of comorbid anxiety (75%), aggression (56%), and reduced executive and social functioning.

Studies consistently report increased risk of suicide subsequent to TBI (Tate et al. 1997). Data from a follow-up study (N. Brooks, personal communication, 1990) of 42 patients with severe TBI showed that 1 year after injury, 10% of those surveyed had spoken about suicide and 2% had made suicide attempts. Five years after the traumatic event, 15% of the patients had made suicide attempts. In addition, many other patients expressed hopelessness about their condition and a belief that life was not worth living. Silver et al. (2001) found that those with brain injury reported a higher frequency of suicide attempts than individuals without TBI (8.1% vs. 1.9%). This remained significant even after controlling for socio-

demographic factors, quality-of-life variables, and presence of any coexisting psychiatric disorder. Mann et al. (1999) found an increased occurrence of TBI in individuals who had made suicide attempts. Simpson and Tate (2002) evaluated 172 outpatients with TBI who were in a brain injury rehabilitation unit. Hopelessness was found in 35%, suicidal ideation was found in 23%, and a suicide attempt was found in 18%. The relationship between suicidal behavior and TBI is complicated. Oquendo et al. (2004) evaluated the predictors of suicidal ideation in 340 patients with major depression. Subjects with TBI reported more aggressive behavior during childhood compared with subjects without TBI. Twenty percent of suicide attempters with TBI made their first suicide attempt prior to their brain injury. In addition, there were higher levels of aggressive behavior that antedated the TBI. It appeared that both suicidal behavior and TBI share an antecedent risk factor: aggression. Thus, it appears that the high incidence of suicide attempts in this population is caused by the combination of several factors, namely, major depression with disinhibition secondary to frontal lobe injury and preexisting risk factors such as aggressive behavior. The medical team, family, and other caregivers must work closely together, on a regular and continuing basis, to gauge suicide risk.

Mania After TBI

Manic episodes and bipolar disorder have also been reported to occur after TBI (Burstein 1993), although the occurrence is less frequent than that of depression after brain injury (Bakchine et al. 1989; Bamrah and Johnson 1991; Bracken 1987; Clark and Davison 1987; Nizamie et al. 1988). In the New Haven Epidemiologic Catchment Area2 (ECA) sample, bipolar disorder occurred in 1.6% of those with brain injury, although the odds ratio was no longer significant when sociodemographic factors and quality of life were controlled (Silver et al. 2001). Predisposing factors for the development of mania after brain injury include damage to the basal region of the right temporal lobe (Starkstein et al. 1990) and right orbitofrontal cortex (Starkstein et al. 1988) in patients who have family histories of bipolar disorder.

DELIRIUM

When a psychiatrist is consulted during the period when a patient with a brain injury is emerging from coma, the usual clinical picture is one of delirium with restlessness, agitation, confusion, disorientation, delusions, and/ or hallucinations. As Trzepacz and Kennedy (2005) observed, this period of recovery is often termed *posttraumatic amnesia* in the brain injury literature and is classified as Rancho Los Amigos Cognitive Scale Level IV or V (see Table 6–4). Although delirium in patients with TBI is most often the result of the effects of the injury on brain tissue chemistry, the psychiatrist should be aware that there may be other causes for the delirium (such as side effects of medication, withdrawal, or intoxication from drugs ingested before the traumatic event) and environmental factors (such as sensory monotony). Table 6–10 lists common factors that can result in posttraumatic delirium.

PSYCHOTIC DISORDERS

Psychosis can occur either immediately after brain injury or after a latency of many months of normal functioning (Corcoran et al. 2005). McAllister (1998) observed that psychotic symptoms may result from a number of different post-TBI disorders, including mania, depression, and epilepsy. The psychotic symptoms may persist despite improvement in the cognitive deficits caused by trauma (Nasrallah et al. 1981). Review of the literature published between 1917 and 1964 (Davison and Bagley 1969) revealed that 1%–15% of schizophrenic inpatients have histories of brain injury. Violon and De Mol (1987) found that of 530 head injury patients, 3.4% developed psychosis 1 to 10 years after the injury. Wilcox and Nasrallah (1987) found that a group of patients diagnosed with schizophrenia had a significantly greater history of brain injury with LOC before age 10 than did patients who were diagnosed with mania or depression or patients who were

TABLE 6–10.   Causes of delirium in patients with traumatic brain injury

Mechanical effects (acceleration or deceleration, contusion, and others)

Cerebral edema

Hemorrhage

Infection

Subdural hematoma

Seizure

Hypoxia (cardiopulmonary or local ischemia)

Increased intracranial pressure

Alcohol intoxication or withdrawal, Wernicke's encephalopathy

Reduced hemoperfusion related to multiple trauma

Fat embolism

Change in pH

Electrolyte imbalance

Medications (barbiturates, steroids, opioids, and anticholinergics)

Source.   Reprinted from Trzepacz PT, Kennedy RE: "Delirium and Posttraumatic Amnesia," in *Textbook of Traumatic Brain Injury.* Edited by Silver JM, McAllister TW, Yudofsky SC. Washington, DC, American Psychiatric Publishing, 2005, pp. 175–200. Used with permission.

hospitalized for surgery. Achté et al. (1991) reported on a sample of 2,907 war veterans in Finland who had sustained brain injury. They found that 26% of these veterans had psychotic disorders. In a detailed evaluation of 100 of these veterans, the authors found that 14% had paranoid schizophrenia. In a comparison of patients who developed symptoms of schizophrenia or schizoaffective disorder subsequent to TBI, left temporal lobe abnormalities were found only in the group who developed schizophrenia (Buckley et al. 1993). The rate of schizophrenia in the group of individuals with a history of TBI in the New Haven group in the ECA study was 3.4% (Silver et al. 2001). However, after controlling for alcohol abuse and dependence, the risk for the occurrence of schizophrenia was of borderline significance.

Patients with schizophrenia may have had brain injury that remains undetected unless the clinician actively elicits a history specific for the occurrence of brain trauma. One high-risk group is homeless mentally ill individuals. To examine the relationship of TBI to schizophrenia and homelessness, Silver et al. (1993) conducted a case–control study of 100 homeless and 100 never-homeless indigent schizophrenic men, and a similar population of women. In the group of men, 55 patients had a prior TBI (36 homeless, 19 domiciled, $P < 0.01$). In the group of women, 35 had previous TBI (16 homeless, 19 domiciled, $P =$ not significant). We believe that the cognitive deficits subsequent to TBI in conjunction with psychosis increase the risk for becoming homeless; in addition, being homeless, and living in a shelter, carries a definite risk for trauma (Kass and Silver 1990).

POSTTRAUMATIC EPILEPSY

A varying percentage of patients, depending on the location and severity of injury, will have seizures during the acute period after the trauma. Posttraumatic epilepsy, with repeated seizures and the requirement for anticonvulsant medication, occurs in approximately 12%, 2%, and 1% of patients with severe, moderate, and mild head injuries, respectively, within 5 years of the injury (Annegers et al. 1980). Risk factors for posttraumatic epilepsy include skull fractures and wounds that penetrate the brain, a history of chronic alcohol use, intracranial hemorrhage, and increased severity of injury (Yablon 1993).

Salazar et al. (1985) studied 421 Vietnam veterans who had sustained brain-penetrating injuries and found that 53% had posttraumatic epilepsy. In 18% of these patients, the first seizure occurred after 5 years; in 7%, the first seizure occurred after 10 years. In addition, 26% of the patients with epilepsy had an organic mental syndrome as defined in DSM-III (American Psychiatric Association 1980). In a study of World War II veterans, patients with

brain-penetrating injuries who developed posttraumatic epilepsy had a decreased life expectancy compared with patients with brain-penetrating injuries without epilepsy or compared with patients with peripheral nerve injuries (Corkin et al. 1984). Patients who develop posttraumatic epilepsy have also been shown to have more difficulties with physical and social functioning and to require more intensive rehabilitation efforts (Armstrong et al. 1990).

Posttraumatic epilepsy is associated with psychosis, especially when seizures arise from the temporal lobes. Brief episodic psychoses may occur with epilepsy; about 7% of patients with epilepsy have persistent psychoses (McKenna et al. 1985). These psychoses exhibit a number of atypical features, including confusion and rapid fluctuations in mood. Psychiatric evaluation of 101 patients with epilepsy revealed that 8% had organic delusional disorder that, at times, was difficult to differentiate symptomatically from schizophrenia (Garyfallos et al. 1988). Phenytoin has more profound effects on cognition than does carbamazepine (Gallassi et al. 1988), and negative effects on cognition have been found in patients who received phenytoin after traumatic injury (Dikmen et al. 1991). Minimal impairment in cognition was found with both valproate and carbamazepine in a group of patients with epilepsy (Prevey et al. 1996). Dikmen et al. (2000) found no adverse cognitive effects of valproate when it was administered for 12 months after a TBI was sustained. The effects of phenytoin and carbamazepine in patients recovering from TBI were compared by Smith et al. (1994). They found that both phenytoin and carbamazepine had negative effects on cognitive performance, especially those that involved motor and speed performance. Intellectual deterioration in children undergoing long-term treatment with phenytoin or phenobarbital also has been documented (Corbett et al. 1985). Treatment with more than one anticonvulsant (polytherapy) has been associated with increased adverse neuropsychiatric reactions (Reynolds and Trimble 1985). Of the newer anticonvulsant medications, topiramate, but not gabapentin or lamotrigine, demonstrated adverse cognitive effects in healthy young adults (Martin et al. 1999; Salinsky et al. 2005). Hoare (1984) found that the use of multiple anticonvulsant drugs to control seizures resulted in an increase in disturbed behavior in children. Any patient with TBI who is treated with anticonvulsant medication requires regular reevaluations to substantiate continued clinical necessity.

ANXIETY DISORDERS

Several anxiety disorders may develop after TBI (Warden and Labatte 2005). Jorge et al. (1993) found that 11% of 66 patients with TBI developed generalized anxiety disorder in addition to major depression. Fann et al. (1995) evaluated 50 outpatients with TBI and found that 24% had generalized anxiety disorder. Deb et al. (1999) evaluated 196 individuals who were hospitalized after TBI. Panic disorder developed in 9%. Salazar et al. (2000) evaluated 120 military members after moderate to severe TBI. At 1 year after enrollment to the study of cognitive rehabilitation, 15% met criteria for generalized anxiety disorder. Hibbard et al. (1998a) found that 18% developed PTSD, 14% developed obsessive-compulsive disorder, 11% developed panic disorder, 8% developed generalized anxiety disorder, and 6% developed phobic disorder. All of these were more frequent after TBI compared with before TBI. In analysis of data from the New Haven portion of the ECA study, Silver et al. (2001) found that of individuals with a history of brain injury during their lifetime, the incidences of anxiety disorders were 4.7% for obsessive-compulsive disorder, 11.2% for phobic disorder, and 3.2% for panic disorder. Dissociative disorders, including depersonalization (Grigsby and Kaye 1993) and dissociative identity disorder (Sandel et al. 1990), may occur. It is our clinical observation that patients with histories of prior trauma are at higher risk for developing these disorders.

Because of the potential life-threatening nature of many of the causes of TBI, including motor vehicle accidents and assaults, one would expect that these patients are at increased risk of developing PTSD. There is a 9.2% risk of developing PTSD after exposure to trauma, highest for assaultive violence (Breslau et al. 1998). PTSD and acute stress response, including symptoms of peritraumatic dissociation (Ursano et al. 1999b), are not uncommon after serious motor vehicle accidents (Koren et al. 1999; Ursano et al. 1999a).

PTSD has been found in individuals with TBI (Bryant 1996; McMillan 1996; Ohry et al. 1996; Parker and Rosenblum 1996; Rattok 1996; Silver et al. 1997). In utilizing the SCID in evaluating 100 individuals with a history of TBI, Hibbard et al. (1998a) found that 18% met criteria for PTSD. Harvey and Bryant conducted a 2-year study of 79 survivors of motor vehicle accidents who sustained mild TBI. They found that acute stress disorder developed in 14% of these patients at 1 month. After 2 years, 73% of the group with acute stress disorder developed PTSD (Harvey and Bryant 2000). Six months after severe TBI, 26 of 96 individuals (27.1%) developed PTSD (Bryant et al. 2000). Although few patients had intrusive memories (19.2%), 96.2% reported emotional reactivity. Max et al. (1998a) evaluated 50 children who were hospitalized after TBI. Although only 4% of subjects developed PTSD, 68% had one PTSD symptom after 3 months, suggesting subsyndromal PTSD despite neurogenic amnesia.

Because of the overlap among symptoms of PTSD and mild TBI, it can be difficult to ascribe specific symptoms to the brain injury or to the circumstances of the accident. In studies of patients with PTSD, memory deficits consistent with temporal lobe injury have been demonstrated (Bremner et al. 1993). Imaging studies have shown smaller hippocampal volumes with PTSD (Bremner et al. 1995, 1997). It is therefore apparent that exposure to extreme stressors results in brain dysfunction that may be similar to that found after TBI.

We present the following case illustration.

CASE EXAMPLE

While Mr. A was working, a machine was activated accidentally, and his head was crushed. He had full recall of the sound of his skull cracking and the sensation of blood coming down his forehead. It was several hours before he was transported to a hospital, but he never lost consciousness. His EEG revealed irregular right cerebral activity, and MRI was compatible with contusion and infarction of the right temporal parietal region.

After the accident, Mr. A developed the full syndrome of PTSD; he experienced flashbacks, mood lability, sensitivity to noise, decreased interest, distress when looking at pictures of the accident, and problems with concentration.

SLEEP DISORDERS

It is common for individuals with traumatic brain injury to complain of disrupted sleep patterns, ranging from hypersomnia to difficulty maintaining sleep (Rao et al. 2005). Fichtenberg and colleagues (2000) assessed 91 individuals with TBI who were admitted to an outpatient neurorehabilitation clinic. The presence of depression (as indicated by scores on the Beck Depression Inventory) and mild severity of the TBI were correlated with the occurrence of insomnia. Guilleminault and co-workers (2000) assessed 184 patients with head trauma and hypersomnia. Abnormalities were demonstrated on the multiple sleep latency test. Sleep-disordered breathing was common (occurring in 59 of 184 patients). Hypersomnia must be differentiated from lack of motivation and apathy. In addition, the contribution of pain to disruption of sleep must be considered. Although depression and sleep disorders can be related and have similarities in the sleep endocrine changes (Frieboes et al. 1999), in our experience with depressed individuals after TBI, the sleep difficulties persist after successful treatment of the mood disorder. In addition, we have seen patients who have developed sleep apnea or nocturnal myoclonus subsequent to TBI.

TABLE 6–11. Postconcussion syndrome

Somatic symptoms

  Headache

  Dizziness

  Fatigue

  Insomnia

Cognitive symptoms

  Memory difficulties

  Impaired concentration

Perceptual symptoms

  Tinnitus

  Sensitivity to noise

  Sensitivity to light

Emotional symptoms

  Depression

  Anxiety

  Irritability

Source. Adapted from Lishman 1988.

MILD TRAUMATIC BRAIN INJURY AND POSTCONCUSSION SYNDROME

Patients with mild TBI may present with somatic, perceptual, cognitive, and emotional symptoms that have been characterized as the postconcussion syndrome (Table 6–11). By definition, mild TBI is associated with a brief duration of LOC (less than 20 minutes) or no LOC, and posttraumatic amnesia of less than 24 hours; the patient usually does not require hospitalization after the injury (see Table 6–5). For each patient hospitalized with mild TBI, probably four to five others sustain mild TBIs but receive treatment as outpatients or perhaps get no treatment at all. The psychiatrist is often called to assess the patient years after the injury, and the patient may not associate brain-related symptoms such as depression and cognitive dysfunction with the injury. The results of laboratory tests, such as structural brain imaging studies, often do not reveal significant abnormalities. However, as discussed previously, functional imaging studies such as SPECT (Masdeu et al. 1994; Nedd et al. 1993) and computerized electroencephalography and brain stem auditory evoked potential recordings have demonstrated abnormal findings (Watson et al. 1995). Diffuse axonal injury may occur with mild TBI, as demonstrated in the pathological examination of brains from patients who have died from systemic injuries (Oppenheimer 1968), as well as in nonhuman primates (Gennarelli et al. 1982). In addition, the balance between cellular energy demand and supply can be disrupted (McAllister 2005).

Most studies of cognitive function subsequent to mild TBI suggest that patients report trouble with memory, attention, concentration, and speed of information processing, and patients can in fact be shown to have deficits in these areas shortly after their injury (1 week to 1 month) (S.J. Brown et al. 1994; McAllister 2005; McMillan and Glucksman 1987). In an evaluation of neuropsychological deficits in 53 patients who were experiencing postconcussive problems from 1 to 22 months after injury, Leininger et al. (1990) detected significantly poorer performance ($P < 0.05$) on tests of reasoning, information processing, and verbal learning than that found in a control population. Hugenholtz et al. (1988) reported that significant attentional and information processing impairment ($P < 0.01$) occurred in a group of adults after mild concussion. Although there was improvement over time, the patient group continued to have abnormalities 3 months after the injury. Warden et al. (2001) found that even in previously high-functioning individuals who sustained mild concussion (West Point cadets), there was impairment in processing speed several days after the injury.

Individuals with mild TBI have an increased incidence of somatic complaints, including headache, dizziness, fatigue, sleep disturbance, and sensitivity to noise and light (S. J. Brown et al. 1994; Dikmen et al. 1986; Levin et al. 1987b; Rimel et al. 1981). In the behavioral domain, the most common problems include irritability, anxiety, and depression (Dikmen et al. 1986; Fann et al. 1995; Hibbard et al.

1998a). McAllister (2005) has opined that it may be more accurate to discuss postconcussive symptoms rather than a syndrome.

The majority of individuals with mild TBI recover quickly, with significant and progressive reduction of complaints in all three domains (cognitive, somatic, and behavioral) at 1, 3, and certainly 6 months from the injury (Bernstein 1999). Unfortunately, good recovery is not universal. A significant number of patients continue to complain of persistent difficulties 6–12 months and even longer after their injury. For example, Keshavan et al. (1981) found that 40% of their patients had significant symptoms 3 months after injury. Levin et al. (1987b), in a multicenter study, found that 3 months postinjury, 47% complained of headache, 22% of decreased energy, and 22% of dizziness. In a review of this topic, Bohnen et al. (1992) found a range of 16%–49% of patients with persistent symptoms at 6 months and 1%–50% with persistent symptoms at 1 year. Those with persistent symptoms have been found to have impaired cognitive function (Leininger et al. 1990). S.J. Brown et al. (1994) suggest that if symptoms are present at 3–6 months subsequent to injury, they tend to persist. Alves et al. (1993) prospectively assessed 587 patients with uncomplicated mild TBI for 1 year. The most frequent symptoms were headache and dizziness. The researchers found that fewer than 6% of these subjects complained of multiple symptoms consistent with postconcussion syndrome.

Therefore, there may be two groups of mild TBI patients: those who recover by 3 months and those who have persistent symptoms. It is not known whether the persistent symptoms are part of a cohesive syndrome or simply represent a collection of loosely related symptoms resulting from the vagaries of an individual injury (Alves et al. 1986). However, it is increasingly recognized that "mild" TBI and concussions that occur in sports injuries result in clinically significant neuropsychological impairment (Freeman et al. 2005).

In an extensive review of the literature, Alexander (1995) highlighted several important aspects regarding patients who develop prolonged postconcussion syndrome: 1) they are more likely to have been under stress at the time of the accident, 2) they develop depression and/or anxiety soon after the accident, 3) they have extensive social disruption after the accident, and 4) they have problems with physical symptoms such as headache and dizziness.

The treatment of patients with mild TBI involves initiating several key interventions (T. Kay 1993). In the early phase of treatment, the major goal is prevention of the postconcussion syndrome. This involves providing information and education about understanding and predicting symptoms and their resolution and actively managing a gradual process of return to functioning. Education about the postconcussion syndrome and its natural history improves prognosis (Wade et al. 1998). It is important to involve the patient's family or significant other, so that they understand the disorder and predicted recovery. After the postconcussion syndrome has developed, the clinician must develop an alliance with the patient and validate his or her experience of cognitive and emotional difficulties while not prematurely confronting emotional factors as primary. A combined treatment strategy is required that addresses the emotional problems along with cognitive problems.

AGGRESSION

Individuals who have TBI may experience irritability, agitation, and aggressive behavior (Silver et al. 2005b). These episodes range in severity from irritability to outbursts that result in damage to property or assaults on others. In severe cases, affected individuals cannot remain in the community or with their families and often are referred to long-term psychiatric or neurobehavioral facilities. Increased isolation and separation from others often occur.

In the acute recovery period, 35%–96% reportedly exhibit agitated behavior (Silver et al. 2005b). After the acute recovery phase, irritability or bad temper is common. There has been only one prospective study of the occurrence of agitation and restlessness that has been monitored by an objective rating instrument, the Overt Aggression Scale (OAS; Brooke et al. 1992b). These authors found that of 100 patients with severe TBI (GCS score less than 8, more than 1 hour of coma, and more than 1 week of hospitalization), only 11 patients exhibited agitated behavior. Only 3 patients manifested these behaviors for more than 1 week. However, 35 patients were observed to be restless but not agitated. In a prospective sample of 100 patients admitted to a brain injury rehabilitation unit, 42% exhibited agitated behavior during at least one nursing shift (Bogner and Corrigan 1995). In follow-up periods ranging from 1 to 15 years after injury, these behaviors occurred in 31%–71% of patients who experienced severe TBI (Silver et al. 2005b). Studies of mild TBI have evaluated patients for much briefer periods; 1-year estimates from these studies range from 5% to 70% (Silver et al. 2005b). Tateno et al. (2003), studying an inpatient TBI population, found that aggression was associated with the presence of major depression, frontal lobe lesions, poor premorbid social functioning, and a history of alcohol and substance abuse.

Carlsson et al. (1987) examined the relationship between the number of traumatic brain injuries associated with LOC and various symptoms, and they demonstrated that irritability increases with subsequent injuries. Of the men who did not have head injuries with LOC, 21% reported irritability, whereas 31% of men with one injury with LOC and 33% of men with two or more injuries with LOC admitted to this symptom ($P < 0.0001$).

Explosive and violent behaviors have long been associated with focal brain lesions as well as with diffuse damage to the central nervous system (Anderson and Silver 1999). The current diagnostic category in DSM-IV-TR is personality change due to a general medical condition (American Psychiatric Association 2000) (see Table 6–8). Patients with aggressive behavior would be specified as aggressive type, whereas those with mood lability are specified as labile type. Characteristic behavioral features occur in many individuals who exhibit aggressive behavior after brain injury (Yudofsky et al. 1990). Typically, violence seen in these patients is *reactive* (i.e., triggered by modest or trivial stimuli). It is *nonreflective*, in that it does not involve premeditation or planning, and *nonpurposeful*, in the sense that the aggression serves no obvious long-term aims or goals. The violence is *periodic*, with brief outbursts of rage and aggression interspersed between long periods of relatively calm behavior. The aggression is *ego-dystonic*, such that the individual is often upset or embarrassed after the episode. Finally, it is generally *explosive*, occurring suddenly with no apparent buildup.

PHYSICAL PROBLEMS

Coldness

Complaints of feeling cold, without actual alteration in body temperature, are occasionally seen in patients who have sustained brain injury. This feeling can be distressing to those who experience it. Patients may wear excessive amounts of clothing and may adjust the thermostat so that other members of the family are uncomfortable. Although this is not a commonly reported symptom of TBI, Hibbard et al. (1998b) found that in a sample of 331 individuals with TBI, 27.9% complained of changes in body temperature, and 13% persistently felt cold. Eames (1997), while conducting a study of the cognitive effects of vasopressin nasal spray in patients with TBI, reported incidentally that 13 patients had the persistent feeling of coldness, despite normal sublingual temperature. All were treated with nasal vasopressin spray for 1 month. Eleven of these patients stopped complaining of feeling cold after 1 month of treatment, and 1 other patient had improvement in the symptom, without complete relief. We describe below a series of 6 patients with brain injury whose subsequent complaints of feeling cold were treated with 1-desamino-8-D-arginine vasopressin (DDAVP) (intranasal vasopressin or desmopressin acetate).

In a pilot study, 6 patients who complained of persisting coldness after brain injury were treated with DDAVP twice daily for 1 month (Silver and Anderson 1999). Response was assessed after 1 month of treatment. DDAVP was discontinued, and reassessment was done 1 month later. Five of the 6 patients had a dramatic response to DDAVP, as soon as 1 week after initiating treatment, and no longer complained of feeling cold. Response persisted even after discontinuation of treatment. Patients denied any side effects from treatment with DDAVP. The experience of persisting coldness can respond dramatically to brief treatment with intranasal DDAVP. It is striking that the beneficial effects of DDAVP persisted after the treatment period ended. DDAVP may reverse physiological effects of a relative deficit in vasopressin in the hypothalamus, caused by injury to the vasopressin precursor–producing cells in the anterior hypothalamus, and corrects an internal temperature set point disrupted by the brain injury.

Other Somatic Problems

The psychiatrist treating an individual who has sustained TBI should be aware of many other somatic problems that interfere with functioning and may exacerbate emotional problems. This includes chronic pain (Zasler et al. 2005), headaches (including recurrence of migraines) (Ward and Levin 2005), dizziness from vestibular disorders (Richter 2005), and visual problems (Kapoor and Ciuffreda 2005). There are specific modalities (such as vestibular therapy and vision therapy) that can alleviate these problems and improve quality of ife.

THERAPEUTIC STRATEGIES

There are many useful therapeutic approaches available for people who have brain injuries. Brain-injured patients may develop neuropsychiatric symptoms based on the location of their injury, the emotional reaction to their injury, their preexisting strengths and difficulties, and their social expectations and supports. Comprehensive rehabilitation centers address many of these issues with therapeutic strategies that are developed specifically for this population (Ben-Yishay and Lakin 1989; Binder and Rattok 1989; Pollack 1989; Prigatano 1989).

Although these programs meet many of the needs of patients with TBI, comprehensive neuropsychiatric evaluation (including the daily evaluation and treatment of the patient by a psychiatrist) is rarely available. Although we propose a multifactorial, multidisciplinary, collaborative approach to treatment, for purposes of exposition we have divided treatment into psychopharmacological, behavioral, psychological, and social interventions.

PSYCHOPHARMACOLOGICAL TREATMENT

It is critical to conduct a thorough assessment of the patient before any intervention is initiated. Two issues require particular attention in the evaluation of the potential use of medication. First, the presenting complaints must be carefully assessed and defined. Second, the current treatment must be reevaluated. Although consultation may be requested to decide whether medication would be helpful, it is often the case that 1) other treatment modalities have not been properly applied, 2) there has been misdiagnosis of the problem, or 3) there has been poor communication among treating professionals. On occasion, a potentially effective medication has not been beneficial because it has been prescribed in a dose that is too low or for a period of time that is too brief. In other instances, the most appropriate pharmacological recommendation is that no medication is required and that other therapeutic modalities need to be reassessed. In reviewing the patient's current medication regimen, two key issues should be addressed: 1) the indications for all drugs prescribed and whether they are still necessary, and 2) the potential side effects of these medications. Patients who have had a severe brain trauma may be receiving many medications that result in psychiatric symptoms such as depression, mania, hallucinations, insomnia, nightmares, cognitive impairments, restlessness, paranoia, or aggression.

Few controlled clinical trials have been conducted to assess the effects of medication in patients with brain injury. Unfortunately, there are few rigorous studies that provide guidelines for treatment (Neurobehavioral Guidelines Working Group 2006). Therefore, the decision regarding which medication (if any) to prescribe is based on 1) current knowledge of the efficacy of these medications in other psychiatric disorders, 2) side-effect profiles of the medications, 3) the increased sensitivity to side effects shown by patients with brain injury, 4) analogies from the brain injury symptoms to the recognized psychiatric syndromes (e.g., amotivational syndrome after TBI may be analogous to the deficit syndrome in schizophrenia), and 5) hypotheses regarding how the neurochemical changes after TBI may affect the proposed mechanisms of action of psychotropic medications.

There are several general guidelines that should be followed in the pharmacological treatment of the psychiatric syndromes that occur after TBI: 1) start low, go slow; 2) conduct a therapeutic trial of all medications; 3) maintain continuous reassessment of clinical condition; 4) monitor drug-drug interactions; 5) augment partial response; and 6) discontinue or lower the dose of the most recently prescribed medication if there is a worsening of the treated symptom soon after the medication had been initiated (or increased). In our experience, patients with brain injury of any type are far more sensitive to the side effects of medications than are patients who do not have brain injury. As we explain below, doses of psychotropic medications must be raised and lowered in small increments over protracted periods of time, although patients ultimately may require the same doses and serum levels that are therapeutically effective for patients without brain injury.

When medications are prescribed, it is important that they be given in a manner that enhances the probability of benefit and reduces the possibility of adverse reactions. Medications often should be initiated at dosages that are lower than those usually administered to patients without brain injury. However, comparable doses to those used to treat primary psychiatric disorders may be necessary to treat TBI-related neuropsychiatric conditions effectively. Dose increments should be made gradually, to minimize side effects and enable the clinician to observe adverse consequences. It is important that such medications be given sufficient time to impart their full effects. Thus, when a decision is made to administer a medication, the patient must receive an adequate therapeutic trial of that medication in terms of dosage and duration of treatment.

Because of frequent changes in the clinical status of patients after TBI, continuous reassessment is necessary to determine whether each prescribed medication is still required. For depression following TBI, the standard guidelines for the treatment of major depression offered by the American Psychiatric Association (2000) may offer a reasonable framework within which to develop a working treatment plan, including continuation of medication for a minimum of 16–20 weeks following complete remission of depressive symptoms. For this and all other neuropsychiatric sequelae of TBI, however, no formal treatment guidelines specific to this population are available. Although there is increasingly useful literature regarding the types and doses of medications useful for the treatment of such problems, there are few if any studies regarding the optimal duration of treatment and/or the issues pertaining to treatment discontinuation and relapse risk. In general, if the patient has responded favorably to initial medication treatment for one or another neuropsychiatric problem after TBI, the clinician must use sound judgment and apply risk-benefit determinations to each specific case in deciding whether and/or when to taper and attempt to discontinue the medication following TBI. Continuous reassessment is necessary because spontaneous remission of some symptoms may occur, in which case the medication can be permanently discontinued, or a carryover effect of

the medication may occur (i.e., its effects may persist after the duration of treatment), in which case a reinstatement of the medication may not be required.

When a new medication is initiated in combination with medications previously prescribed, the clinician must be vigilant for the development of drug-drug interactions. These interactions may include alteration of pharmacokinetics that result in increased half-lives and serum levels of medications, as can occur with the use of multiple anticonvulsants. Additionally, alterations of pharmacodynamics may develop during the administration of medications with additive or synergistic clinical effects (e.g., increased sedative effects when several sedating medications are administered simultaneously).

If a patient does not respond favorably to the initial medication prescribed, several alternatives are available. If there has been no response, changing to a medication with a different mechanism of action is suggested, much as is done in the treatment of depressed patients without brain injury. If there has been a partial response to the initial medication, addition of another medication may be useful. The selection of a second supplementary or augmenting medication should be based on consideration of the possible complementary or contrary mechanisms of action of such agents and on the individual and combined side-effect profiles of the initial and secondary agents and their potential pharmacokinetic and pharmacodynamic interactions.

Although individuals after TBI may experience multiple concurrent neuropsychiatric symptoms (e.g., depressed mood, irritability, poor attention, fatigue, and sleep disturbances), suggesting a single "psychiatric diagnosis" such as major depression, we have found that some of these symptoms often persist despite treatment of the apparent "diagnosis." In other words, diagnostic parsimony should be sought but may not always be the best or most accurate diagnostic approach in this population. For this reason, the neuropsychiatric approach of evaluating and monitoring individual symptoms is necessary and differs from the usual "syndromal" approach of the present conventional psychiatric paradigm. Several medications may be required to alleviate several distinct symptoms following TBI, although it is prudent to initiate each treatment one at a time to determine the efficacy and side effects of each prescribed drug.

Studies of the effects of psychotropic medications in patients with TBI are few, and rigorous double-blind, placebo-controlled studies are rare (see Arciniegas et al. 2000). The recommendations contained in this chapter represent a synthesis of the available treatment literature on TBI, the extensions of the known uses of these medications in phenotypically similar psychiatric populations of patients with other types of brain injury (stroke, multiple sclerosis, etc.), and the opinions of the authors of this chapter. We recognize that the pathophysiology of these symptoms may differ in patients with TBI; thus, generalization of response to treatment seen in the context of other forms of brain dysfunction (e.g., stroke, Alzheimer's disease) to TBI may not always be valid. Where there are treatment studies in the TBI population to offer guidance regarding medication treatments, these are noted and referenced for further consideration by interested readers.

AFFECTIVE ILLNESS

Depression

Affective disorders subsequent to brain damage are common and are usually highly detrimental to a patient's rehabilitation and socialization. However, the published literature is sparse regarding the effects of antidepressant agents and/or electroconvulsive therapy (ECT) in the treatment of patients with brain damage in general and TBI in particular (Arciniegas et al. 1999; Bessette and Peterson 1992; Cassidy 1989; Saran 1985; Varney et al. 1987) (see Silver et al. 2005a for review).

Guidelines for using antidepressants for patients with TBI. The choice of an antidepressant depends predominantly on the desired side-effect profile. Usually, antidepressants with the fewest sedative, hypotensive, and anticholinergic side effects are preferred. Thus, the selective serotonin reuptake inhibitors (SSRIs) are usually the first-line medications prescribed. Fann and colleagues performed a single-blind placebo run-in trial of sertraline in 15 patients with major depression after TBI. Two-thirds of these patients achieved a Hamilton Rating Scale for Depression score consistent with remission by 2 months (Fann et al. 2000). In addition, those patients showed improvements in psychomotor speed, recent verbal memory, recent visual memory, and general cognitive efficiency (Fann et al. 2001). In a study comparing nortriptyline and fluoxetine in poststroke depression, nortriptyline was superior in efficacy to fluoxetine, and fluoxetine demonstrated no benefit above placebo (Robinson et al. 2000). If a heterocyclic antidepressant (HCA) is chosen, we suggest nortriptyline or desipramine and careful plasma monitoring to achieve plasma levels in the therapeutic range for the parent compound and its major metabolites (e.g., nortriptyline levels 50–100 ng/mL; desipramine levels greater than 125 ng/mL) (American Psychiatric Association Task Force 1985).

ECT remains a highly effective and underused modality for the treatment of depression overall, and ECT can be used effectively after acute or severe TBI (Kant et al. 1999; Ruedrich et al. 1983). If the patient has preexisting memory impairment, nondominant unilateral ECT should be used.

Side effects. The most common and disabling antidepressant side effects in patients with TBI are the anticholinergic effects, especially with the older HCAs. These medications may impair attention, concentration, and memory, especially in patients with brain lesions. SSRIs, venlafaxine, and bupropion all have minimal or no anticholinergic action.

In some individuals, SSRIs may result in word-finding problems or apathy. This may be due to the effects of SSRIs in decreasing dopaminergic functioning, and it may be reversible with the addition of a dopaminergic or stimulant medication.

The choice of SSRI may require similar consideration. Schmitt et al. (2001) demonstrated that healthy middle-aged adults experienced significantly greater impairments of delayed recall in a word-learning test during treatment with paroxetine 20–40 mg per day than during treatment with placebo, an effect attributed to paroxetine's nontrivial antimuscarinic properties. This study also demonstrated significant improvements in verbal fluency among healthy middle-aged adults treated with sertraline 50–100 mg when compared with treatment with placebo, an effect attributed to sertraline's dopamine reuptake inhibition. Whether similar differences in cognitive profiles distinguish between these and other SSRIs in the TBI population is not yet clear. Nonetheless, observations of distinct cognitive profiles among these agents may merit consideration when selecting an agent in this population.

The available evidence suggests that, overall, antidepressants may be associated with a greater frequency of seizures in patients with brain injury. The antidepressants maprotiline and bupropion may be associated with a higher incidence of seizures (Davidson 1989; Pinder et al. 1977). Although there have been reports of seizures occurring with fluoxetine, Favale et al. (1995) demonstrated an anticonvulsant effect in patients with seizures. In our experience, few patients have experienced seizures during treatment with SSRIs and other newer antidepressants. Although antidepressants should be used with continuous monitoring in patients with severe TBI, we also believe that antidepressants can be used safely and effectively in patients with TBI.

Mania

Manic episodes that occur after TBI have been successfully treated with lithium carbonate, carbamazepine (Stewart and Nemsath 1988), valproic acid (Pope et al. 1988), clonidine (Bakchine et al. 1989), and ECT (Clark and Davison 1987). Lamotrigine and gabapentin are other options, although evidence as to efficacy, especially in individuals with TBI, is sparse. Because of the increased incidence of side effects when lithium is used in patients with brain lesions, we limit the use of lithium in patients with TBI to those with mania or with recurrent depressive illness that preceded their brain damage.

Lithium has been reported to aggravate confusion in patients with brain damage (Schiff et al. 1982), as well as to induce nausea, tremor, ataxia, and lethargy in this population. In addition, lithium may lower seizure threshold (Massey and Folger 1984). Hornstein and Seliger (1989) reported on a patient with preexisting bipolar disorder who experienced a recurrence of mania after experiencing closed head injury. Before the injury, this patient's mania was controlled with lithium carbonate without side effects. However, after the brain injury, dysfunctions of attention and concentration emerged that reversed with lowering of the lithium dosage.

Lability of Mood and Affect

In contrast to mood disorders—conditions in which the baseline emotional state is pervasively disturbed over a relatively long period of time (i.e., weeks)—disorders of affect denote conditions in which the more moment-to-moment variation and regulation of emotion are disturbed. The classic disorder of affective dysregulation is pathological laughing and/or crying (PLC), also sometimes referred to as "emotional incontinence" or "pseudobulbar affect." Patients with this condition experience episodes of involuntary crying and/or laughing that may occur many times per day, are often provoked by trivial (i.e., not sentimental) stimuli, are quite stereotyped in their presentation, are uncontrollable, do not evoke a concordant subjective affective experience, and do not produce a persistent change in the prevailing mood (Poeck 1985). In this classic presentation, PLC appears to be a relatively infrequent (5.3%) consequence of TBI (Zeilig et al. 1996). Affective lability differs from PLC in that both affective expression and experience are episodically dysregulated, the inciting stimulus may be relatively minor but is often somewhat sentimental, and the episodes are somewhat more amenable to voluntary control and are less stereotyped. However, these episodes do not produce a persistent change in mood and are often sources of significant distress and embarrassment to patients that otherwise (quite correctly) report their mood as "fine" (euthymic). The prevalence of affective lability following TBI is not clear, but it is a commonly observed acute and chronic problem after TBI at all levels of severity.

Antidepressants may be used to treat the labile mood that frequently occurs with neurological disease. However, it appears that the control of lability of mood and affect may differ from that of depression, and the mechanism of action of antidepressants in treating mood lability in those with brain injuries may differ from that in the treatment of patients with "uncomplicated" depression (Lauterbach and Schweri 1991; Panzer and Mellow 1992; Ross and Rush 1981; Schiffer et al. 1985; Seliger et al. 1992; Sloan et al. 1992). Schiffer et al. (1985) conducted a double-blind crossover study with amitriptyline and placebo in 12 patients with pathological laughing and weeping secondary to multiple sclerosis. Eight patients experienced a dramatic response to amitriptyline at a maximum dose of 75 mg/day.

There have been several reports of the beneficial effects of fluoxetine for "emotional incontinence" secondary to several neurological disorders (K. W. Brown et al. 1998; Nahas et al. 1998; Panzer and Mellow 1992; Seliger et al. 1992; Sloan et al. 1992). K. W. Brown et al. (1998) treated 20 patients with poststroke emotionalism with fluoxetine in a double-blind, placebo-controlled study. The individuals receiving fluoxetine exhibited statistically and clinically significant improvement. In our experience, all SSRIs can be effective, and the dosage guidelines are similar to those used in the treatment of depression. In addition, other antidepressants, such as nortriptyline, can also be effective for emotional lability. We emphasize that for many patients it may be necessary to administer these medications at standard antidepressant dosages to obtain full therapeutic effects, although response may occur for others within days of initiating treatment at relatively low doses. Preliminary data suggest that dextromethorphan may improve this syndrome in certain neurological disorders (B. R. Brooks et al. 2004).

COGNITIVE FUNCTION AND AROUSAL

Stimulants, such as dextroamphetamine and methylphenidate, and dopamine agonists, such as amantadine and bromocriptine, may be beneficial in treating the patient with apathy and impaired concentration to increase arousal and to diminish fatigue. These medications all act on the catecholaminergic system but in different ways. Dextroamphetamine blocks the reuptake of norepinephrine and in higher doses also blocks the reuptake of dopamine. Methylphenidate has a similar mechanism of action. Amantadine acts both presynaptically and postsynaptically at the dopamine receptor and may also increase cholinergic and GABAergic activity (Cowell and Cohen 1995). In addition, amantadine is an N-methyl-D-aspartate (NMDA) glutamate receptor antagonist (Weller and Kornhuber 1992). Bromocriptine is a dopamine type 1 receptor antagonist and a dopamine type 2 receptor agonist. It appears to be a dopamine agonist at midrange doses (Berg et al. 1987). Assessment of improvement in attention and arousal may be difficult (Whyte 1992), and further work needs to be conducted in this area to determine whether these medications affect outcome. Therefore, careful objective assessment with appropriate neuropsychological tests may be helpful in determining response to treatment.

Dextroamphetamine and Methylphenidate

Several reports have indicated that impairments in verbal memory and learning, attention, and behavior are alleviated with either dextroamphetamine or methylphenidate

(Bleiberg et al. 1993; Evans et al. 1987; Kaelin et al. 1996; Lipper and Tuchman 1976; Weinberg et al. 1987; Weinstein and Wells 1981). When used, methylphenidate should be initiated at 5 mg twice daily and dextroamphetamine at 2.5 mg twice daily. Maximum dosage of each medication is usually 60 mg/day, administered twice daily or three times daily. However, we have seen some patients who have required higher dosages of methylphenidate to obtain a reasonable serum level of 15 mg/mL.

Sinemet and Bromocriptine

Lal et al. (1988) reported on the use of L-dopa/carbidopa (Sinemet) in the treatment of 12 patients with brain injury (including anoxic damage). With treatment, patients exhibited improved alertness and concentration; decreased fatigue, hypomania, and sialorrhea; and improved memory, mobility, posture, and speech. Dosages administered ranged from 10/100 to 25/250 four times daily. Eames (1989) suggests that bromocriptine may be useful in treating cognitive initiation problems of brain-injured patients at least 1 year after injury. He recommended starting at 2.5 mg/day and administering treatment for at least 2 months at the highest dose tolerated (up to 100 mg/day). Other investigators have found that patients with nonfluent aphasia (Gupta and Mlcoch 1992), akinetic mutism (Echiverri et al. 1988), or apathy (Catsman-Berrevoets and Harskamp 1988) have improved after treatment with bromocriptine. Parks et al. (1992) suggest that bromocriptine exerts specific effects on the frontal lobe and increases goal-directed behaviors.

Amantadine

Amantadine may be beneficial in the treatment of anergia, abulia, mutism, and anhedonia subsequent to brain injury (Chandler et al. 1988; Cowell and Cohen 1995; Gualtieri et al. 1989; Nickels et al. 1994). M. F. Kraus and Maki (1997) administered amantadine at a dosage of 400 mg/day to six patients with TBI. Improvement was found in motivation, atten-

tion, and alertness, as well as executive function and dyscontrol. Dosage should be initially 50 mg twice daily and should be increased every week by 100 mg/day to a maximum dosage of 400 mg/day.

Tricyclic Antidepressants

Although the drugs involved are not in the category of stimulants or dopamine agonists, Reinhard et al. (1996) administered amitriptyline (1 patient) and desipramine (2 patients) and found improvement in arousal and initiation after TBI. The authors hypothesize that the improvement is from the noradrenergic effects of the HCA.

Side Effects of Medications for Impaired Concentration and Arousal

Adverse reactions to medications for impaired concentration and arousal are most often related to increases in dopamine activity. Dexedrine and methylphenidate may lead to paranoia, dysphoria, agitation, and irritability. Depression often occurs on discontinuation, so stimulants should be discontinued using a slow regimen. Interestingly, there may be a role for stimulants to increase neuronal recovery subsequent to brain injury (Crisostomo et al. 1988). Side effects of bromocriptine include sedation, nausea, psychosis, headaches, and delirium. Amantadine may cause confusion, hallucinations, edema, and hypotension; these reactions occur more often in elderly patients.

There is often concern that stimulant medications may lower seizure threshold in patients with TBI who are at increased risk for posttraumatic seizures. Wroblewski and colleagues (1992) reviewed their experience with methylphenidate in 30 patients with severe brain injury and seizures and examined the changes in seizure frequency after initiation of methylphenidate. The number of seizures was monitored for 3 months before treatment with methylphenidate, for 3 months during treatment, and for 3 months after treatment was discontinued. The researchers found that only 4 patients experienced more seizures during methylphenidate treatment, whereas 26 had either fewer seizures or the same number of seizures during treatment. The authors concluded that there is no significant risk in lowering seizure threshold with methylphenidate treatment in this high-risk group.

PROBLEMS WITH PROCESSING MULTIPLE STIMULI

Although individuals with traumatic brain injury may have difficulty with maintaining attention on single tasks, they can also have difficulty in processing multiple stimuli. This difficulty has been called an abnormality in auditory gating, and it is consistent with an abnormal response in processing auditory stimuli that are given 50 ms apart (P50 response) (Arciniegas et al. 2000). Preliminary evidence suggests that this response normalizes after treatment with donep-ezil 5 mg, which also results in symptomatic improvement (Arciniegas et al. 2001).

FATIGUE

Stimulants (methylphenidate and dextroamphetamine) and amantadine can diminish the profound daytime fatigue experienced by patients with TBI. Dosages utilized would be similar to those used for treatment of diminished arousal and concentration. Modafinil, a medication for the treatment of excessive daytime somnolence in patients with narcolepsy, also may have a role in treatment of post-TBI fatigue. There have been studies specifically in patients with multiple sclerosis that have shown benefit (Rammahan et al. 2000; Terzoudi et al. 2000), whereas another controlled study showed no benefit (Stankoff et al. 2005). Teitelman (2001) described his use of modafinil among 10 outpatients with nonpenetrating TBI and functionally significant excessive daytime sleepiness and in 2 patients with somnolence caused by sedating psychiatric medications. Dosages should start with 100 mg in the morning and can be increased to up to 600 mg/day administered in two doses (i.e., 400 mg in the morning and 200 mg in the afternoon).

COGNITION

Cholinesterase Inhibitors

TBI may produce cognitive impairments via disruption of cholinergic function (Arciniegas et al. 1999), and the relative sensitivity of TBI patients to medications with anticholinergic agents has prompted speculation that cognitively impaired TBI patients may have a relatively reduced reserve of cholinergic function. This has prompted trials of procholinergic agents, and in particular physostigmine, to treat behavioral dyscontrol and impaired cognition in TBI survivors (Eames and Sutton 1995). However, the significant peripheral effects and narrow margin of safety of physostigmine have made treatment with this agent impractical. With the advent of relatively centrally selective acetylcholinesterase inhibitors such as donepezil, the issue of cholinergic augmentation strategies in the treatment of cognitive impairment following TBI is currently being revisited, and preliminary reports suggest that donepezil may improve memory and global functioning (Kaye et al. 2003; Morey et al. 2003; Taverni et al. 1998; Whelan et al. 2000; Zhang et al. 2004). Doses of donepezil range from 5 mg to 10 mg per day. A report of rivastigmine (3–12 mg/day) used in a double-blind randomized, placebo-controlled multicenter study of 154 patients suggested improvements in cognition in those individuals with the most significant memory problems (Silver et al. 2006). The most common side effects include sedation, insomnia, diarrhea, and dizziness, which are minimized by starting with the lower dosage and adjusting upward slowly. Although these adverse effects are generally transient, a few patients will be unable to tolerate the medication due to persistent severe diarrhea.

PSYCHOSIS

The psychotic ideation resulting from TBI is generally responsive to treatment with antipsychotic medications. However, side effects such as hypotension, sedation, and confusion are common. Also, brain-injured patients are particularly subject to dystonia, akathisia, and other parkinsonian side effects—even at relatively low doses of antipsychotic medications (Wolf et al. 1989). Antipsychotic medications have also been reported to impede neuronal recovery after brain injury (Feeney et al. 1982). Therefore, we advise that antipsychotics be used sparingly during the acute phases of recovery after the injury. Of the newer "atypical" antipsychotic medications, quetiapine has the fewest extrapyramidal effects. Risperidone, olanzapine, aripiprazole, and ziprasidone may all have a role in the treatment of post-TBI psychosis, although published literature is limited. Therapeutic effect may not be evident for 3 weeks after treatment at each dosage. In general, we recommend a low-dose neuroleptic strategy for all patients with neuropsychiatric disorders. Clozapine is a novel and effective antipsychotic medication that does not produce extrapyramidal side effects. Although its use in patients with neuropsychiatric disorders has yet to be investigated fully, its side-effect profile poses many potential disadvantages. It is highly anticholinergic, produces significant sedation and hypotension, lowers seizure threshold profoundly, and is associated with a 1% risk of agranulocytosis that requires lifetime weekly monitoring of blood counts. Clozapine treatment is associated with a significant dose-related incidence of seizures (ranging from 1% to 2% of patients who receive doses below 300 mg/day and 5% of patients who receive 600–900 mg/day); thus, in patients with TBI it must be used with extreme caution and for most carefully considered indications (Lieberman et al. 1989).

SLEEP

Sleep patterns of patients with brain damage are often disordered, with impaired rapid eye movement (REM) recovery and multiple nocturnal awakenings (Prigatano et al. 1982). Hypersomnia that occurs after severe missile head injury most often resolves within the first year after injury, whereas insomnia that occurs in patients with long periods of coma and diffuse injury has a more chronic course (Aske-

nasy et al. 1989). Barbiturates and long-acting benzodiazepines should be prescribed for sedation with great caution, if at all. These drugs interfere with REM and Stage IV sleep patterns and may contribute to persistent insomnia (Buysse and Reynolds 1990). Clinicians should warn patients of the dangers of using over-the-counter preparations for sleeping and for colds because of the prominent anticholinergic side effects of these agents.

Trazodone, a sedating antidepressant medication that is devoid of anticholinergic side effects, may be used for nighttime sedation. A dose of 50 mg should be administered initially; if this is ineffective, doses up to 150 mg may be prescribed.

Nonpharmacological approaches should be considered. These include minimizing daytime naps, adhering to regular sleep times, and engaging in regular physical activity during the day.

AGGRESSION AND AGITATION

Although there is no medication approved by the U.S. Food and Drug Administration (FDA) that is specifically for the treatment of aggression, medications are widely used (and commonly misused) in the management of patients with acute or chronic aggression. After appropriate assessment of possible etiologies of these behaviors, treatment is focused on the occurrence of comorbid neuropsychiatric conditions (depression, psychosis, insomnia, anxiety, delirium) (see Figure 6–1), whether the treatment is in the acute (hours to days) or chronic (weeks to months) phase, and the severity of the behavior (mild to severe). The clinician must be aware that patients may not respond to just one medication but may require combination treatment, similar to the pharmacotherapeutic treatment for refractory depression.

Chronic Aggression

If a patient continues to exhibit periods of agitation or aggression beyond several weeks, the use of specific antiaggressive medications should be initiated to prevent these episodes from occurring. Because no medication has been approved by the FDA for treatment of

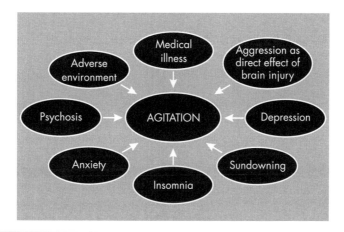

FIGURE 6–1.   Factors associated with agitation in brain injury.

aggression, the clinician must use medications that may be antiaggressive but that have been approved for other uses (e.g., seizure disorders, depression, hypertension) (Silver and Yudofsky 1994; Yudofsky et al. 1998).

Antipsychotic medications.   If, after thorough clinical evaluation, it is determined that the aggressive episodes result from psychosis, such as paranoid delusions or command hallucinations, then antipsychotic medications will be the treatment of choice. Risperidone has been used to treat agitation in elderly patients with dementia with good results (Goldberg and Goldberg 1995). Olanzapine appears to be more sedating, and quetiapine may have fewer extrapyramidal symptoms than risperidone. Clozapine may have greater antiaggressive effects than other antipsychotic medications (Michals et al. 1993; Ratey et al. 1993). The increased risk of seizures, however, must be carefully assessed.

Antianxiety medications.   Serotonin appears to be a key neurotransmitter in the modulation of aggressive behavior. In preliminary reports, buspirone, a serotonin type 1A agonist, has been reported to be effective in the management of aggression and agitation for patients with head injury, dementia, developmental disabilities, or autism (Silver and Yudofsky 1994; Yudofsky et al. 1998). In rare

instances, some patients become more aggressive when treated with buspirone. Therefore, buspirone should be initiated at low dosages (i.e., 5 mg twice daily) and increased by 5 mg every 3–5 days. Dosages of 45–60 mg/day may be required before there is improvement in aggressive behavior, although we have noted dramatic improvement within 1 week.

Clonazepam may be effective in the long-term management of aggression, although controlled, double-blind studies have not yet been conducted. We use clonazepam when pronounced aggression and anxiety occur together or when aggression occurs in association with neurologically induced tics and similarly disinhibited motor behaviors. Dosages should initially be 0.5 mg twice daily and may be increased to as high as 2–4 mg twice daily, as tolerated. Sedation and ataxia are frequent side effects.

Anticonvulsive medications.   The anticonvulsant carbamazepine has been demonstrated to be effective for treatment of bipolar disorders and has also been advocated for control of aggression in both epileptic and nonepileptic populations. Reports indicate that the antiaggressive response of carbamazepine can be found in patients with and without electroencephalographic abnormalities (Silver and Yudofsky 1994; Yudofsky et al. 1998). Azouvi et al. (1999) found that 8 of 10 patients with aggressive behavior after TBI responded to carbamazepine.

In our experience and that of others, the anticonvulsant valproic acid may also be helpful to some patients with organically induced aggression (Geracioti 1994; Giakas et al. 1990; Horne and Lindley 1995; Mattes 1992; Wroblewski et al. 1997). For patients with aggression and epilepsy whose seizures are being treated with anticonvulsant drugs such as phenytoin and phenobarbital, switching to carbamazepine or to valproic acid may treat both conditions.

Gabapentin may be beneficial for the treatment of agitation in patients with dementia (Herrmann et al. 2000; Roane et al. 2000). Dosages have ranged from 200–2,400 mg/day. However, Childers and Holland (1997) report an increase in anxiety and restlessness (i.e., agitation) in two cognitively impaired TBI patients for whom gabapentin was prescribed to reduce chronic pain.

Antimanic medications. Although lithium is known to be effective in controlling aggression related to manic excitement, many studies suggest that it may also have a role in the treatment of aggression in selected nonbipolar patient populations (Yudofsky et al. 1998). Included are patients with TBI (Bellus et al. 1996; Glenn et al. 1989) as well as patients with mental retardation who exhibit self-injurious or aggressive behavior, children and adolescents with behavioral disorders, prison inmates, and patients with other organic brain syndromes.

Patients with brain injury have increased sensitivity to the neurotoxic effects of lithium (Hornstein and Seliger 1989; Moskowitz and Altshuler 1991). Because of lithium's potential for neurotoxicity and its relative lack of efficacy in many patients with aggression secondary to brain injury, we limit the use of lithium in patients whose aggression is related to manic effects or recurrent irritability related to cyclic mood disorders.

Antidepressants. The antidepressants that have been reported to control aggressive behavior are those that act preferentially (amitriptyline) or specifically (trazodone and fluoxetine) on serotonin. Fluoxetine has been reported to be effective in the treatment of aggressive behavior in patients who have sustained brain injury as well as in patients with personality disorders and depression, and adolescents with mental retardation and self-injurious behavior (Silver and Yudofsky 1994; Yudofsky et al. 1998). We have used SSRIs with considerable success in aggressive patients with brain lesions. The dosages used are similar to those for the treatment of mood lability and depression.

We have evaluated and treated many patients with emotional lability that is characterized by frequent episodes of tearfulness and irritability and the full symptomatic picture of neuroaggressive syndrome (Silver and Yudofsky 1994). These patients—who would be diagnosed under DSM-IV-TR with personality change, labile type, due to traumatic brain injury—have responded well to antidepressants. This is discussed above in the section "Lability of Mood and Affect."

Antihypertensive medications: beta-blockers. The first report of the use of β-adrenergic receptor blockers in the treatment of acute aggression appeared in 1977, and within the next 10 years more than 25 articles on this topic appeared in the neurologic and psychiatric literature, reporting experience in using β-blockers with more than 200 patients with aggression (Yudofsky et al. 1987). Most of these patients had been unsuccessfully treated with antipsychotics, minor tranquilizers, lithium, and/or anticonvulsants before being treated with β-blockers. The β-blockers that have been investigated in controlled prospective studies include propranolol (a lipid-soluble, nonselective receptor antagonist), nadolol (a water-soluble, nonselective receptor antagonist), and pindolol (a lipid-soluble, nonselective β receptor antagonist with partial sympathomimetic activity). Evidence suggests

TABLE 6–12. Clinical use of propranolol

1. Conduct a thorough medical evaluation.

2. Exclude patients with the following disorders: bronchial asthma, chronic obstructive pulmonary disease, insulin-dependent diabetes mellitus, congestive heart failure, persistent angina, significant peripheral vascular disease, hyperthyroidism.

3. Avoid sudden discontinuation of propranolol (particularly in patients with hypertension).

4. Begin with a single test dose of 20 mg/day in patients for whom there are clinical concerns with hypotension or bradycardia. Increase dose of propranolol by 20 mg/day every 3 days.

5. Initiate propranolol on a 20-mg-three-times-daily schedule for patients without cardiovascular or cardiopulmonary disorder.

6. Increase the dosage of propranolol by 60 mg/day every 3 days.

7. Increase medication unless the pulse rate is reduced below 50 beats/minute or systolic blood pressure is less than 90 mm Hg.

8. Do not administer medication if severe dizziness, ataxia, or wheezing occurs. Reduce or discontinue propranolol if such symptoms persist.

9. Increase dose to 12 mg/kg of body weight or until aggressive behavior is under control.

10. Doses greater than 800 mg are not usually required to control aggressive behavior.

11. Maintain the patient on the highest dose of propranolol for at least 8 weeks before concluding that the patient is not responding to the medication. Some patients, however, may respond rapidly to propranolol.

12. Use concurrent medications with caution. Monitor plasma levels of all antipsychotic and anticonvulsive medications.

Source. Reprinted from Silver JM, Yudofsky SC: "Pharmacologic Treatment of Aggression." *Psychiatric Annals* 17:397–407, 1987. Used with permission from SLACK Incorporated.

that β-adrenergic receptor blockers are effective agents for the treatment of aggressive and violent behaviors, particularly those related to organic brain syndrome. The effectiveness of propranolol in reducing agitation has been demonstrated during the initial hospitalization after TBI (Brooke et al. 1992a). Guidelines for the use of propranolol are listed in Table 6–12. When a patient requires the use of a once-a-day medication because of compliance difficulties, long-acting propranolol (i.e., Inderal LA) or nadolol (Corgard) can be used. When patients develop bradycardia that prevents prescribing therapeutic dosages of propranolol, pindolol (Visken) can be substituted, using one-tenth the dosage of propranolol. The intrinsic sympathomimetic activity of pindolol stimulates the β receptor and restricts the development of bradycardia.

The major side effects of β-blockers when used to treat aggression are the lowering of blood pressure and pulse rate. Because peripheral β receptors are fully blocked with dosages of 300–400 mg/day, further decreases in these vital signs usually do not occur even when doses are increased to much higher levels. Despite reports of depression with the use of β-blockers, controlled trials and our experience indicate that it is a rare occurrence. Because the use of propranolol is associated with significant increases in plasma levels of thioridazine, which has an absolute dosage ceiling of 800 mg/day, the combination of these two medications should be avoided whenever possible.

Table 6–13 summarizes our recommendations for the use of various classes of medication in the treatment of chronic aggressive disorders associated with TBI. Acute aggression

TABLE 6–13.   Pharmacotherapy of agitation

Acute agitation/severe aggression

  Antipsychotic drugs

  Benzodiazepines

Chronic agitation

  Atypical antipsychotics

  Anticonvulsants (VPA, CBZ, ?gabapentin)

  Serotonergic antidepressants (SSRI, trazodone)

  Buspirone

  β-Blockers

Note.   CBZ=carbamazepine; SSRI=selective serotonin reuptake inhibitor; VPA=valproic acid.

may be treated by using the sedative properties of neuroleptics or benzodiazepines. In treating aggression, the clinician, when possible, should diagnose and treat underlying disorders and should use, when possible, antiaggressive agents specific for those disorders. When there is partial response after a therapeutic trial with a specific medication, adjunctive treatment with a medication with a different mechanism of action should be instituted. For example, a patient with partial response to β-blockers can have additional improvement with the addition of an anticonvulsant.

Acute Aggression and Agitation

In the treatment of agitation and of acute or severe episodes of aggressive behavior, medications that are sedating may be indicated. However, because these drugs are not specific in their ability to inhibit aggressive behavior, there may be detrimental effects on arousal and cognitive function. Therefore, the use of sedation-producing medications must be time limited, to avoid the emergence of seriously disabling side effects ranging from oversedation to tardive dyskinesia.

After the diagnosis and treatment of underlying causes of aggression and the evaluation and documentation of aggressive be-

haviors (such as with the OAS), the use of pharmacological interventions can be considered in two categories: 1) the use of the sedating effects of medications, as required in acute situations, so that the patient does not harm him/herself or others; and 2) the use of nonsedating antiaggressive medications for the treatment of chronic aggression (Silver and Yudofsky 1994; Yudofsky et al. 1995).

Antipsychotic drugs.   Antipsychotics are the most commonly used medications in the treatment of aggression. Although these agents are appropriate and effective when aggression is derivative of active psychosis, the use of neuroleptic agents to treat chronic aggression, especially that secondary to organic brain injury, is often ineffective and entails significant risks that the patient will develop serious complications. Usually, it is the sedative side effects rather than the antipsychotic properties of antipsychotics that are used (i.e., misused) to "treat" (i.e., mask) the aggression. Often, patients develop tolerance to the sedative effects of the neuroleptics and therefore require increasing doses. As a result, extrapyramidal and anticholinergic-related side effects occur. Paradoxically (and frequently), because of the development of akathisia, the patient may become more agitated and restless as the dose of neuroleptic is increased, especially when a high-potency antipsychotic such as haloperidol is administered. The akathisia is often mistaken for increased irritability and agitation, and a vicious cycle of increasing neuroleptics and worsening akathisia occurs.

In patients with brain injury and acute aggression, we recommend starting a neuroleptic such as risperidone at low doses of 0.5 mg orally, with repeated administration every hour until control of aggression is achieved. If after several administrations of risperidone the patient's aggressive behavior does not improve, the hourly dose may be increased until the patient is so sedated that he or she no longer exhibits agitation or violence. Once the patient is not aggressive for 48 hours, the daily dosage should be decreased gradually (i.e., by 25%/

day) to ascertain whether aggressive behavior reemerges. In this case, consideration should then be made about whether it is best to increase the dose of risperidone and/or to initiate treatment with a more specific antiaggressive drug.

Sedatives and hypnotics. There is an inconsistent body of literature on the effects of the benzodiazepines in the treatment of aggression. The sedative properties of benzodiazepines are especially helpful in the management of acute agitation and aggression. Most likely, this is due to the effect of benzodiazepines on increasing the inhibitory neurotransmitter GABA. Paradoxically, several studies report increased hostility and aggression as well as the induction of rage in patients treated with benzodiazepines. However, these reports are balanced by the observation that this phenomenon is rare (Dietch and Jennings 1988). Benzodiazepines can produce amnesia, and preexisting memory dysfunction can be exacerbated by the use of benzodiazepines. Brain-injured patients may also experience increased problems with coordination and balance with benzodiazepine use.

For treatment of acute aggression, lorazepam 1–2 mg may be administered every hour by either oral or intramuscular route until sedation is achieved (Silver and Yudofsky 1994). Intramuscular lorazepam has been suggested as an effective medication in the emergency treatment of the violent patient (Bick and Hannah 1986). Intravenous lorazepam is also effective, although the onset of action is similar when administered intramuscularly. Caution must be taken with intravenous administration, and the drug should be injected in doses less than 1 mg/min to avoid laryngospasm. As with neuroleptics, gradual tapering of lorazepam may be attempted when the patient has been in control for 48 hours. If aggressive behavior recurs, medications for the treatment of chronic aggression may be initiated. Lorazepam in 1- or 2-mg doses, administered either orally or by injection, may be administered, if necessary, in combination with a neuroleptic medication

(haloperidol, 2–5 mg). Other sedating medications such as paraldehyde, chloral hydrate, or diphenhydramine may be preferable to sedative antipsychotic agents.

BEHAVIORAL AND COGNITIVE TREATMENTS

Behavioral treatments are important in the care of patients who have sustained TBI. These programs require careful design and execution by a staff well versed in behavioral techniques. Behavioral methods can be used in response to aggressive outbursts and other maladaptive social behaviors (P. W. Corrigan and Bach 2005). One study (Eames and Wood 1985) found that behavior modification was 75% effective in dealing with disturbed behavior after severe brain injury.

After brain injury, patients may need specific cognitive strategies to assist with impairments in memory and concentration (Cicerone et al. 2005; Gordon and Hibbard 2005). As opposed to earlier beliefs that cognitive therapy should "exercise" the brain to develop skills that have been damaged, current therapies involve teaching the patient new strategies to compensate for lost or impaired functions. Salazar et al. (2000) for the Defense and Veterans Head Injury Program (DVHIP) Study Group compared an intensive 8-week in-hospital cognitive rehabilitation program to a limited home program. Both groups improved, but there was no significant difference between the two treatments. (For more information on cognitive treatments, see Chapter 18 of this book.) We emphasize that for most patients, treatment strategies are synergistic. For example, the use of β-adrenergic receptor antagonists to treat agitation and aggression may enhance a patient's ability to benefit from behavioral and cognitive treatments.

PSYCHOLOGICAL AND SOCIAL INTERVENTIONS

In the broadest terms, psychological issues involving patients who incur brain injury revolve around four major themes: 1) psycho-pathology that preceded the injury, 2) psychological responses to the traumatic event, 3) psychological reactions to deficits brought about by brain injury, and 4) psychological issues related to potential recurrence of brain injury.

Preexisting psychiatric illnesses are most frequently intensified with brain injury. Therefore, the angry, obsessive patient or the patient with chronic depression will exhibit a worsening of these symptoms after brain injury. Specific coping mechanisms that were used before the injury may no longer be possible because of the cognitive deficits caused by the neurological disease. Therefore, patients need to learn new methods of adaptation to stress. In addition, as mentioned above, the social, economic, educational, and vocational status of the patient (and how these are affected by brain lesions) influence the patient's response to the injury.

The events surrounding brain injury often have far-reaching experiential and symbolic significance for the patient. Such issues as guilt, punishment, magical wishes, and fears crystallize about the nidus of a traumatic event. For example, a patient who sustains brain injury during a car accident may view his injury as punishment for long-standing violent impulses toward an aggressive father. In such cases, reassurance and homilies about his lack of responsibility for the accident are usually less productive than psychological exploration.

A patient's reactions to being disabled by brain damage have realistic as well as symbolic significance. When intense effort is required for a patient to form a word or to move a limb, frustration may be expressed as anger, depression, anxiety, or fear. Particularly in cases in which brain injury results in permanent impairment, a psychiatrist may experience counter-transferential discomfort that results in failure to discuss directly with the patient and his or her family the implications of resultant disabilities and limitations. Gratuitous optimism, collaboration with denial of the patient, and facile solutions to complex problems are rarely effec-

tive and can erode the therapeutic alliance and ongoing treatment. Tyerman and Humphrey (1984) assessed 25 patients with severe brain injury for changes in self-concept. Patients viewed themselves as markedly changed after their injury but believed that they would regain preexisting capacities within a year. The authors concluded that these unrealistic expectations may hamper rehabilitation and adjustment of both the patient and his or her relatives. By gently and persistently directing the patient's attention to the reality of the disabilities, the psychiatrist may help the patient begin the process of acceptance and adjustment to the impairment. Clinical judgment will help the psychiatrist in deciding whether and when explorations of the symbolic significance of the patient's brain injury should be pursued.

Families of patients with neurological disorders are under severe stress. The relative with a brain injury may be unable to fulfill his or her previous role or function as parent or spouse, thus significantly affecting the other family members (Cavallo and Kay 2005). Oddy et al. (1978) evaluated 54 relatives of patients with brain injury within 1, 6, and 12 months of the traumatic event. Approximately 40% of the relatives showed depressive symptoms within 1 month of the event; 25% of the relatives showed significant physical or psychological illness within 6–12 months of the brain damage. Mood disturbances, especially anxiety, depression, and social role dysfunction, are also seen within this time (Kreutzer et al. 1994; Linn et al. 1994; Livingston et al. 1985a, 1985b). Family members may experience increased substance use, unemployment, and decreased financial status over time (Hall et al. 1994). By treating the psychological responses of relatives to the brain injury, the clinician can foster a supportive and therapeutic atmosphere for the patient as well as significantly help the relative. For both patients and their families, severe TBI results in multifaceted losses, including the loss of dreams about and expectations for the future. The psychiatrist may be of enormous benefit in treating the family and patient by providing support, insight, and other points of view. Educational and supportive treatment of families can be therapeutic when used together with appropriate social skills training. Patient advocacy groups, such as the National Brain Injury Foundation, can provide important peer support for families. Many patients require clear, almost concrete statements describing their behaviors because insight and judgment may be impaired.

It is a distressing fact that brain injury can and often does recur. With repeated injury, there is an increase in the incidence of neuropsychiatric and emotional symptoms (Carlsson et al. 1987). Patients' fears and anxieties about recurrence of injury are more than simply efforts at magical control over terrifying conditions. Therapeutic emphasis should be placed on actions and activities that will aid in preventing recurrence, including compliance with appropriate medications and abstinence from alcohol and other substances of abuse.

PREVENTION

MOTOR VEHICLE ACCIDENTS

The proper use of seat belts with upper-torso restraints is 45% effective in preventing fatalities, 50% effective in preventing moderate to critical injuries, and 10% effective in preventing minor injuries when used by drivers and passengers (U.S. Department of Transportation 1984). This translates to 12,000–15,000 lives saved per year (National Safety Council 1986). Orsay et al. (1988) noted that victims of motor vehicle accidents who wore seat belts had a 60.1% reduction in injury severity. Without specific legislation, car restraints are used infrequently. Many brain injuries occur in side impacts, when the heads of occupants collide with the structural column between the windshield and the side window. More than 7,000 motor vehicle–related deaths are caused by side impacts, nearly half of which deaths are due to brain trauma (Jagger 1992). In 2003, there were 44,800 motor vehicle accident–related fatalities (National Safety Council 2006). There were 2.2 million disabling injuries

ries from motor vehicle accidents in 1998 (National Safety Council 1999).

The use of safety belts has prevented a significant number of deaths and injuries (Centers for Disease Control 1992; Kaplan and Cowley 1991). Driver and passenger air bags have decreased the number and severity of injuries, although they have not been as effective in controlling severe injuries of the lower extremities (Kuner et al. 1996).

Alcohol dependence is a highly prevalent and destructive illness. In addition, alcohol abuse is a common concomitant of affective and characterological disorders. Alcohol intoxication is frequently found in the patient who has suffered brain injury, whether from violence, falls, or motor vehicle accidents (Brismar et al. 1983). In the United States, the proportion of alcohol involvement in motor vehicle fatalities has been decreasing over the past several years. Whereas during the week, 24% of fatally injured drivers have blood alcohol concentrations (BACs) at or above 0.087%, on weekends, the proportion increases to 45% (Insurance Institute for Highway Safety 2005a). Alcohol-related deaths have been decreased by a combination of "zero tolerance" laws and laws lowering the allowable BAC for impaired driving from 0.10% to 0.08% (Insurance Institute for Highway Safety 2005a).

Drivers in fatal accidents have a more frequent history of alcohol use, previous accidents, moving traffic violations, psychopathology, stress, paranoid thinking, and depression. They often have less control of hostility and anger, with a decreased tolerance for tension, and a history of increased risk taking (Tsuang et al. 1985). Therefore, we strongly advocate that in all psychiatric and other medical histories a detailed inquiry about alcohol use, seat belt use, and driving patterns be present. Examples of driving patterns, accident records, violations, driving while intoxicated, speeding patterns, car maintenance, presence of distractions such as children and animals, and hazardous driving conditions should be included in a complete driving record. The use of illicit substances and medications that may induce sedation, such as antihistamines, antihypertensive agents, anticonvulsants, minor tranquilizers, and antidepressants, should also be assessed and documented. Psychiatric patients are at greater risk for motor vehicle accidents because they often have several of these characteristics (Noyes 1985).

Clearly, motorcycle riding, with or without helmets, and using bicycles for commuting purposes are associated with head injuries, even when safety precautions are taken and when driving regulations are observed. In 2005, there were 4,439 motorcyclist deaths (Insurance Institute for Highway Safety 2005d). It has been estimated that for every motorcycle-related death, there are another 37 injuries and many more that remain unreported to the police (Baker et al. 1987). Helmets can reduce the risk of on-highway motorcycle fatalities by about 37% and are 67% effective in preventing brain injuries (Insurance Institute for Highway Safety 2005d). Death rates from TBI are twice as high in states with weak or nonexistent helmet laws, compared with rates in states with helmet laws that apply to all riders (Sosin et al. 1989). Fewer than half of the states mandate that all riders wear helmets. In 2005, there were 782 bicyclists killed in crashes with motor vehicles, a number that has been decreasing over the years (Insurance Institute for Highway Safety 2005b). Virtually all of those riders were not wearing helmets (Insurance Institute for Highway Safety 2005b). Every year, 1,300 cyclists are killed in the United States (Centers for Disease Control 1988). The use of bicycle helmets can significantly decrease the morbidity and mortality resulting from bicycle-related head injuries (Thompson et al. 1989). However, only 16 states have mandatory helmet laws, and even these apply only to riders under age 18.

Significant preventive measures to reduce head trauma include counseling a patient about risk taking; the treatment of alcoholism and depression; the judicious prescription of medications and full explanations of sedation, cognitive impairment, and other potentially dangerous side effects; and public information activities on topics such as the proper use of seat belts, the dangers of drinking and driving, and automobile safety measures.

PREVENTION OF BRAIN INJURY IN CHILDREN

Beyond nurturance, children rely on their parents or guardians for guidance and protection. Each year in the United States more than 1,500 children under age 13 die as motor vehicle passengers; more than 90% of these children were not using car seat restraints (Insurance Institute for Highway Safety 2005c). Child safety seats have been found to be 80%–90% effective in the prevention of injuries to children (National Safety Council 1985). In a sample of 494 children younger than 4 years old who had suffered motor vehicle accident trauma (Agran et al. 1985), 70% had been unrestrained, 12% were restrained with seat belts, and 22% were restrained in child safety seats. In general, restrained children tended to sustain less serious injuries than the unrestrained children.

Children younger than 4 years old who are not restrained in safety seats are 11 times more likely to be killed in motor vehicle accidents (National Safety Council 1985). It is not safe for the child to sit on the lap of the parent, with or without restraints, because the adult's weight can crush the child during an accident. Young children traveling with drivers who themselves are not wearing seat belts are four times as likely to be left unrestrained (National Safety Council 1985). Legislation in Britain mandating the use of child safety seats has had a significant effect on decreasing fatal and serious injuries to children (Avery and Hayes 1985). In the United States, all 50 states and the District of Columbia have mandatory laws for child safety seats (National Safety Council 1985). Children who ride on bicycle-mounted child seats are highly subject to injuries to the head and face and should wear bicycle helmets. Alcohol use by adults is frequently a factor in child injuries and fatalities (Li 2000). In the majority of drinking driver–related child passenger deaths, the child was an unrestrained passenger (Quinlan et al. 2000).

Children are often involved in sports that carry the risk of brain injury. Sports such as boxing, gymnastics, diving, soccer, football, basketball, and hockey are associated with considerable risk of TBI. It has been estimated that 300,000 cases of TBI occur during sports or recreation (Centers for Disease Control and Prevention 1997). For children ages 10–14 years, sports and recreational activities account for 43% of TBIs (J.F. Kraus and Nourjah 1988). Powell and Barber-Foss (1999) found that 3.9% of 17,815 high school athletes had sustained a mild TBI. Mild brain injury is not uncommon in football and can result in persistent symptoms and disabilities (Gerberich et al. 1983). An estimated 20% of high school football players sustain concussion during a single football season, with some reporting symptoms persisting as long as 6–9 months after the end of the season (Gerberich et al. 1983). Soccer may involve the use of the head with sudden twists to strike the ball that may also result in neuropsychiatric abnormalities (Tysvaer et al. 1989).

The clinician must always be alert to the possibility that parents may be neglectful, may use poor judgment, and may even be directly violent in their treatment of children. Unfortunately, it is not uncommon for head trauma to result from overt child abuse on the part of parents, other adults, and peers. We must always be alert to such possibilities in our patients, and when these problems are discovered, we must take direct actions to address them. We encourage direct counseling of parents who do not consistently use infant and child car seats for their children.

CONCLUSION

Invariably, brain injury leads to emotional damage in the patient and in the family. In this chapter, we have reviewed the most frequently occurring psychiatric symptoms that are associated with TBI. We have emphasized how the informed psychiatrist is not only effective but essential in both the prevention of brain injury and, when it occurs, the treatment of its sequelae. In addition to increased efforts devoted to the prevention of brain injury, we advocate a multidisciplinary and multidimensional approach to the assessment and treatment of neuropsychiatric aspects of brain injury.

RECOMMENDED READING

Silver JM, McAllister TW, Yudofsky SC (eds): Textbook of Traumatic Brain Injury. Washington, DC, American Psychiatric Publishing, 2005

REFERENCES

Achté K, Jarho L, Kyykka T, et al: Paranoid disorders following war brain damage: preliminary report. Psychopathology 24:309–315, 1991

Agran PF, Dunkie DE, Winn DG: Motor vehicle accident trauma and restraint usage patterns in children less than 4 years of age. Pediatrics 76:382–386, 1985

Alexander MP: Mild traumatic brain injury: pathophysiology, natural history, and clinical management. Neurology 45:1253–1260, 1995

Alves WM, Coloban ART, O'Leary TJ, et al: Understanding posttraumatic symptoms after minor head injury. J Head Trauma Rehabil 1:1–12, 1986

Alves W, Macciocchi SN, Barth JT: Postconcussive symptoms after uncomplicated mild head injury. J Head Trauma Rehabil 8:48–59, 1993

American Psychiatric Association: Diagnostic and Statistical Manual of Mental Disorders, 3rd Edition. Washington, DC, American Psychiatric Association, 1980

American Psychiatric Association: Diagnostic and Statistical Manual of Mental Disorders, 3rd Edition, Revised. Washington, DC, American Psychiatric Association, 1987

American Psychiatric Association: Diagnostic and Statistical Manual of Mental Disorders, 4th Edition, Text Revision. Washington, DC, American Psychiatric Association, 2000

American Psychiatric Association Task Force on the Use of Laboratory Tests in Psychiatry: Tricyclic antidepressants: blood level measurements and clinical outcome: an APA Task Force report. Am J Psychiatry 142:155–162, 1985

Anderson KE, Silver JM: Neurological and mental diseases and violence, in Medical Management of the Violent Patient: Clinical Assessment and Therapy. Edited by Tardiff K. New York, Marcel Dekker, 1999, pp 87–124

Anderson KE, Taber KH, Hurley RA: Functional imaging, in Textbook of Traumatic Brain Injury. Edited by Silver JM, McAllister TM, Yudofsky SC. Washington, DC, American Psychiatric Publishing, 2005, pp 107–134

Annegers JF, Grabow JD, Groover RV, et al: Seizures after head trauma: a population study. Neurology 30:683–689, 1980

Arciniegas D, Adler L, Topkoff J, et al: Attention and memory dysfunction after traumatic brain injury: cholinergic mechanisms, sensory gating, and a hypothesis for further investigation. Brain Inj 13:1–13, 1999

Arciniegas DB, Topkoff J, Silver JM: Neuropsychiatric aspects of traumatic brain injury. Curr Treat Options Neurol 2:169–186, 2000

Arciniegas DB, Topkoff JL, Anderson CA, et al: Normalization of P50 physiology by donepezil hydrochloride in traumatic brain injury patients (abstract). J Neuropsychiatry Clin Neurosci 13:140, 2001

Arciniegas DB, Anderson CA, Rojas DC: Electrophysiological techniques, in Textbook of Traumatic Brain Injury. Edited by Silver JM, McAllister TM, Yudofsky SC. Washington, DC, American Psychiatric Publishing, 2005, pp 135–158

Ariza M, Junque C, Mataro M, et al: Neuropsychological correlates of basal ganglia and medial temporal lobe NAA/Cho reductions in traumatic brain injury. Arch Neurol 61:541–544, 2004

Armstrong KK, Sahgal V, Bloch R, et al: Rehabilitation outcomes in patients with posttraumatic epilepsy. Arch Phys Med Rehabil 71:156–160, 1990

Ashikaga R, Araki Y, Ishida O: MRI of head injury using FLAIR. Neuroradiology 39:239–242, 1997

Askenasy JJM, Winkler I, Grushkiewicz J, et al: The natural history of sleep disturbances in severe missile head injury. J Neurol Rehabil 3:93–96, 1989

Auerbach SH: Neuroanatomical correlates of attention and memory disorders in traumatic brain injury: an application of neurobehavioral subtypes. J Head Trauma Rehabil 1:1–12, 1986

Avery JG, Hayes HRM: Death and injury to children in cars: Britain. BMJ 291:515, 1985

Azouvi P, Jokic C, Attal N, et al: Carbamazepine in agitation and aggressive behaviour following severe closed head injury: results of an open trial. Brain Inj 13:797–804, 1999

Bakchine S, Lacomblez L, Benoit N, et al: Manic-like state after bilateral orbitofrontal and right temporoparietal injury: efficacy of clonidine. Neurology 39:777–781, 1989

Baker SP, Whitfield RA, O'Neill B: Geographic variations in mortality from motor vehicle crashes. N Engl J Med 316:1384–1387, 1987

Bamrah JS, Johnson J: Bipolar affective disorder following head injury. Br J Psychiatry 158:117–119, 1991

Bechara A, Damasio AR, Damasio H, et al: Insensitivity to future consequences following damage to human prefrontal cortex. Cognition 50:7–15, 1994

Beck AT, Ward CH, Mendelson M, et al: An inventory for measuring depression. Arch Gen Psychiatry 4:561–571, 1961

Belanger HG, Vanderploeg RD, Curtiss G, et al: Recent neuroimaging techniques in mild traumatic brain injury. J Neuropsychiatry Clin Neurosci 19:5–20, 2007

Bellus SB, Stewart D, Vergo JG, et al: The use of lithium in the treatment of aggressive behaviours with two brain-injured individuals in a state psychiatric hospital. Brain Inj 10:849–860, 1996

Ben-Yishay Y, Lakin P: Structured group treatment for brain-injury survivors, in Neuropsychological Treatment After Brain Injury. Edited by Ellis DW, Christensen A-L. Boston, MA, Kluwer Academic, 1989, pp 271–295

Berg MJ, Ebert B, Willis DK, et al: Parkinsonism—drug treatment: part I. Drug Intell Clin Pharm 21:10–21, 1987

Berman KF, Illowsky BP, Weinberger DR: Physiological dysfunction of dorsolateral prefrontal cortex in schizophrenia, IV: further evidence for regional and behavioral specificity. Arch Gen Psychiatry 45:616–622, 1988

Bernstein DM: Recovery from head injury. Brain Inj 13:151–172, 1999

Bessette RF, Peterson LG: Fluoxetine and organic mood syndrome. Psychosomatics 33:224–225, 1992

Bicik I, Radanov BP, Schafer N, et al: PET with 18-fluorodeoxyglucose and hexamethylpropylene amine oxime SPECT in late whiplash syndrome. Neurology 51:345–350, 1998

Bick PA, Hannah AL: Intramuscular lorazepam to restrain violent patients. Lancet 1:206–207, 1986

Bigler ED: Structural imaging, in Textbook of Traumatic Brain Injury. Edited by Silver JM, McAllister TM, Yudofsky SC. Washington, DC, American Psychiatric Publishing, 2005, pp 79–106

Binder LM, Rattok J: Assessment of the postconcussive syndrome after mild head trauma, in Assessment of the Behavioral Consequences of Head Trauma. Edited by Lezak MD. New York, Alan R Liss, 1989, pp 37–48

Bleiberg J, Garmoe W, Cederquist J, et al: Effects of Dexedrine on performance consistency following brain injury: a double-blind placebo cross-over case study. Neuropsychiatry Neuropsychol Behav Neurol 6:245–248, 1993

Bogner JA, Corrigan JD: Epidemiology of agitation following brain injury. NeuroRehabilitation 5:293–297, 1995

Bohnen N, Twijnstra A, Jolles J: Post-traumatic and emotional symptoms in different subgroups of patients with mild head injury. Brain Inj 6:481–487, 1992

Bracken P: Mania following head injury. Br J Psychiatry 150:690–692, 1987

Bremner JD, Scott TM, Delaney RC, et al: Deficits in short-term memory in posttraumatic stress disorder. Am J Psychiatry 150:1015–1019, 1993

Bremner JD, Randall P, Scott TM, et al: MRI-based measurement of hippocampal volume in patients with combat-related posttraumatic stress disorder. Am J Psychiatry 152:973–981, 1995

Bremner JD, Randall P, Vermetten E, et al: Magnetic resonance imaging–based measurement of hippocampal volume in posttraumatic stress disorder related to childhood physical and sexual abuse: a preliminary report. Biol Psychiatry 41:23–32, 1997

Breslau N, Kessler RC, Chilcoat HD, et al: Trauma and posttraumatic stress disorder in the community: the 1996 Detroit Area Survey of Trauma. Arch Gen Psychiatry 55:626–632, 1998

Brismar B, Engstrom A, Rydberg U: Head injury and intoxication: a diagnostic and therapeutic dilemma. Acta Chir Scand 149:11–14, 1983

Brooke MM, Patterson DR, Questad KA, et al: The treatment of agitation during initial hospitalization after traumatic brain injury. Arch Phys Med Rehabil 73:917–921, 1992a

Brooke MM, Questad KA, Patterson DR, et al: Agitation and restlessness after closed head injury: a prospective study of 100 consecutive admissions. Arch Phys Med Rehabil 73:320–323, 1992b

Brooks BR, Thisted RA, Appel SH, et al: Treatment of pseudobulbar affect in ALS with dextromethorphan/quinidine: a randomized trial. ALS Study Group. Neurology 63:1364–1370, 2004

Brooks N: Personal communication, reported in Eames P, Haffey WJ, Cope DN: Treatment of behavioral disorders, in Rehabilitation of the Adult and Child with Traumatic Brain Injury, 2nd Edition. Edited by Rosenthal M, Griffith ER, Bond MR, et al. Philadelphia, PA, FA Davis, 1990, pp 410–432

Brooks N, Campsie L, Symington C, et al: The five year outcome of severe blunt head injury: a relative's view. J Neurol Neurosurg Psychiatry 49:764–770, 1986

Brown G, Chadwick O, Shaffer D, et al: A prospective study of children with head injuries, III: psychiatric sequelae. Psychol Med 11:63–78, 1981

Brown KW, Sloan RL, Pentland B: Fluoxetine as a treatment for post-stroke emotionalism. Acta Psychiatr Scand 98:455–458, 1998

Brown SJ, Fann JR, Grant I: Postconcussional disorder: time to acknowledge a common source of neurobehavioral morbidity. J Neuropsychiatry Clin Neurosci 6:15–22, 1994

Bryant RA: Posttraumatic stress disorder, flashbacks, and pseudomemories in closed head injury. J Trauma Stress 9:621–629, 1996

Bryant RA, Marosszeky JE, Crooks J, et al: Posttraumatic stress disorder after severe traumatic brain injury. Am J Psychiatry 157:629–631, 2000

Buckley P, Stack JP, Madigan C, et al: Magnetic resonance imaging of schizophrenia-like psychoses associated with cerebral trauma: clinicopathological correlates. Am J Psychiatry 150:146–148, 1993

Burstein A: Bipolar and pure mania disorders precipitated by head trauma. Psychosomatics 34:194–195, 1993

Buysse DJ, Reynolds CF III: Insomnia, in Handbook of Sleep Disorders. Edited by Thorpy MJ. New York, Marcel Dekker, 1990, pp 373–434

Carlsson GS, Svardsudd K, Welin L: Long-term effects of head injuries sustained during life in three male populations. J Neurosurg 67:197–205, 1987

Cassidy JW: Fluoxetine: a new serotonergically active antidepressant. J Head Trauma Rehabil 4:67–69, 1989

Cassidy JW: Neuropathology, in Neuropsychiatry of Traumatic Brain Injury. Edited by Silver JM, Yudofsky SC, Hales RE. Washington, DC, American Psychiatric Press, 1994, pp 43–80

Catsman-Berrevoets CE, Harskamp FV: Compulsive pre-sleep behavior and apathy due to bilateral thalamic stroke: response to bromocriptine. Neurology 38:647–649, 1988

Cavallo MM, Kay T: The family system, in Textbook of Traumatic Brain Injury. Edited by Silver JM, McAllister, Yudofsky SC. Washington, DC, American Psychiatric Publishing, 2005, pp 533–558

Cecil KM, Hills EC, Sandel ME, et al: Proton magnetic resonance spectroscopy for detection of axonal injury in the splenium of the corpus callosum of brain-injured patients. J Neurosurg 88:795–801, 1998

Centers for Disease Control: Bicycle-related injuries: data from the National Electronic Injury Surveillance System. MMWR Morb Mortal Wkly Rep 36:269–271, 1988

Centers for Disease Control: Increased safety-belt use: United States, 1991. MMWR Morb Mortal Wkly Rep 41:421–423, 1992

Centers for Disease Control and Prevention: Sports-related recurrent brain injuries—United States. MMWR Morb Mortal Wkly Rep 46:224–227, 1997

Chambers J, Cohen SS, Hemminger L, et al: Mild traumatic brain injuries in low-risk trauma patients. J Trauma 41:976–979, 1996

Chandler MC, Barnhill JL, Gualtieri CT: Amantadine for the agitated head-injury patient. Brain Inj 2:309–311, 1988

Childers MK, Holland D: Psychomotor agitation following gabapentin use in brain injury. Brain Inj 11:537–540, 1997

Christodoulou C, DeLuca J, Ricker JH, et al: Functional magnetic resonance imaging of working memory impairment after traumatic brain injury. J Neurol Neurosurg Psychiatry 71:161–168, 2001

Cicerone KD, Dahlberg C, Malec JF, et al: Evidence-based cognitive rehabilitation: updated review of the literature from 1998 through 2002. Arch Phys Med Rehabil 86:1681–1692, 2005

Clark AF, Davison K: Mania following head injury: a report of two cases and a review of the literature. Br J Psychiatry 150:841–844, 1987

Committee on Head Injury Nomenclature: Report of the Ad Hoc Committee to study head injury nomenclature: proceedings of the Congress of Neurological Surgeons in 1964. Clin Neurosurg 12:386–394, 1966

Cope DN, Date ES, Mar EY: Serial computerized tomographic evaluations in traumatic head injury. Arch Phys Med Rehabil 69:483–486, 1988

Corbett JA, Trimble MR, Nichol TC: Behavioral and cognitive impairments in children with epilepsy: the long-term effects of anticonvulsant therapy. J Am Acad Child Psychiatry 24:17–23, 1985

Corcoran C, McAllister TW, Malaspina D: Psychotic disorders, in Textbook of Traumatic Brain Injury. Edited by Silver JM, McAllister, Yudofsky SC. Washington, DC, American Psychiatric Publishing, 2005, pp 213–229

Corkin S, Sullivan EV, Carr A: Prognostic factors for life expectancy after penetrating head injury. Arch Neurol 41:975–977, 1984

Corrigan JD: Substance abuse as a mediating factor in outcome from traumatic brain injury. Arch Phys Med Rehabil 76:302–309, 1995

Corrigan PW, Bach PA: Behavioral treatment, in Textbook of Traumatic Brain Injury. Edited by Silver JM, McAllister TW, Yudofsky SC. Washington, DC, American Psychiatric Publishing, 2005, pp 661–678

Courville CB: Pathology of the Nervous System, 2nd Edition. Mountain View, CA, Pacific Press Publications, 1945

Cowell LC, Cohen RF: Amantadine: a potential adjuvant therapy following traumatic brain injury. J Head Trauma Rehabil 10:91–94, 1995

Crisostomo EA, Duncan PW, Propst M, et al: Evidence that amphetamine with physical therapy promotes recovery of motor function in stroke patients. Ann Neurol 23:94–97, 1988

Davidson J: Seizures and bupropion: a review. J Clin Psychiatry 50:256–261, 1989

Davison K, Bagley CR: Schizophrenic-like psychoses associated with organic disorders of the central nervous system: a review of the literature, in Current Problems in Neuropsychiatry: Schizophrenia, Epilepsy, the Temporal Lobe. Edited by Herrington RN. Br J Psychiatry (special publication no 4), 1969, pp 113–184

Deb S, Lyons I, Koutzoukis C, et al: Rate of psychiatric illness 1 year after traumatic brain injury. Am J Psychiatry 156:374–378, 1999

Dietch JT, Jennings RK: Aggressive dyscontrol in patients treated with benzodiazepines. J Clin Psychiatry 49:184–189, 1988

Dikmen S, Machamer JE: Neurobehavioral outcomes and their determinants. J Head Trauma Rehabil 10:74–86, 1995

Dikmen S, McLean A, Temkin N: Neuropsychological and psychosocial consequences of minor head injury. J Neurol Neurosurg Psychiatry 49:1227–1232, 1986

Dikmen SS, Temkin NR, Miller B, et al: Neurobehavioral effects of phenytoin prophylaxis of posttraumatic seizures. JAMA 265:1271–1277, 1991

Dikmen SS, Machamer JE, Win HR, et al: Neuropsychological effects of valproate in traumatic brain injury: a randomized trial. Neurology 54:895–902, 2000

Dolan RJ, Bench CJ, Brown RG, et al: Regional cerebral blood flow abnormalities in depressed patients with cognitive impairment. J Neurol Neurosurg Psychiatry 55:768–773, 1992

Eames P: The use of Sinemet and bromocriptine. Brain Inj 3:319–320, 1989

Eames P: Feeling cold: an unusual brain injury symptom and its treatment with vasopressin. J Neurol Neurosurg Psychiatry 62:198–199, 1997

Eames P, Sutton A: Protracted post-traumatic confusional state treated with physostigmine. Brain Inj 9:729–734, 1995

Eames P, Wood R: Rehabilitation after severe brain injury: a follow-up study of a behavior modification approach. J Neurol Neurosurg Psychiatry 48:613–619, 1985

Easdon C, Levine B, O'Connor C, et al: Neural activity associated with response inhibition following traumatic brain injury: an event-related fMRI investigation. Brain Cogn 54:136–138, 2004

Echiverri HC, Tatum WO, Merens TA, et al: Akinetic mutism: pharmacologic probe of the dopaminergic mesencephalo-frontal activating system. Pediatr Neurol 4:228–230, 1988

Evans RW, Gualtieri CT, Patterson D: Treatment of chronic closed head injury with psychostimulant drugs: a controlled case study and an appropriate evaluation procedure. J Nerv Ment Dis 175:106–110, 1987

Fann JR, Katon WJ, Uomoto JM, et al: Psychiatric disorders and functional disability in outpatients with traumatic brain injuries. Am J Psychiatry 152:1493–1499, 1995

Fann JR, Uomoto JM, Katon WJ: Sertraline in the treatment of major depression following mild traumatic brain injury. J Neuropsychiatry Clin Neurosci 12:226–232, 2000

Fann JR, Uomoto JM, Katon WJ: Cognitive improvement with treatment of depression following mild traumatic brain injury. Psychosomatics 42:48–54, 2001

Fann JR, Leonetti A, Jaffe K, et al: Psychiatric illness and subsequent traumatic brain injury: a case control study. J Neurol Neurosurg Psychiatry 72:615–620, 2002

Favale E, Rubino V, Mainaardi P, et al: Anticonvulsant effect of fluoxetine in humans. Neurology 45:1926–1927, 1995

Fay GC, Jaffe KM, Polissar NL, et al: Mild pediatric brain injury: a cohort study. Arch Phys Med Rehabil 74:895–901, 1993

Federoff PJ, Starkstein SE, Forrester AW, et al: Depression in patients with acute traumatic brain injury. Am J Psychiatry 149:918–923, 1992

Feeney DM, Gonzalez A, Law WA: Amphetamine, haloperidol, and experience interact to affect rate of recovery after motor cortex injury. Science 217:855–857, 1982

Fichtenberg NL, Millis SR, Mann NR, et al: Factors associated with insomnia among post-acute traumatic brain injury survivors. Brain Inj 14:659–667, 2000

Freeman JR, Barth JT, Broshek DK, et al: Sports injuries, in Textbook of Traumatic Brain Injury. Edited by Silver JM, McAllister, Yudofsky SC. Washington, DC, American Psychiatric Publishing, 2005, pp 453–476

Frieboes R-M, Muller U, Murck H, et al: Nocturnal hormone secretion and the sleep EEG in patients several months after traumatic brain injury. J Neuropsychiatry Clin Neurosci 11:354–360, 1999

Friedman SD, Brooks WM, Jung RE, et al: Quantitative proton MRS predicts outcome after traumatic brain injury. Neurology 52:1384–1391, 1999

Gallassi R, Morreale A, Lorusso S, et al: Carbamazepine and phenytoin: comparison of cognitive effects in epileptic patients during monotherapy and withdrawal. Arch Neurol 45:892–894, 1988

Garyfallos G, Manos N, Adamopoulou A: Psychopathology and personality characteristics of epileptic patients: epilepsy, psychopathology and personality. Acta Psychiatr Scand 78:87–95, 1988

Gennarelli TA, Graham DI: Neuropathology of the head injuries. Semin Clin Neuropsychiatry 3:160–175, 1998

Gennarelli TA, Graham DI: Neuropathology, in Textbook of Traumatic Brain Injury. Edited by Silver JM, McAllister TM, Yudofsky SC. Washington, DC, American Psychiatric Publishing, 2005, pp 27–50

Gennarelli TA, Thibault LE, Adams JH, et al: Diffuse axonal injury and traumatic coma in the primate. Ann Neurol 12:564–574, 1982

Geracioti TD: Valproic acid treatment of episodic explosiveness related to brain injury. J Clin Psychiatry 55:416–417, 1994

Gerberich SG, Priest JD, Boen JR, et al: Concussion incidences and severity in secondary school varsity football players. Am J Public Health 73:1370–1375, 1983

Giakas WJ, Seibyl JP, Mazure CM: Valproate in the treatment of temper outbursts (letter). J Clin Psychiatry 51:525, 1990

Glenn MB, Wroblewski B, Parziale J, et al: Lithium carbonate for aggressive behavior or affective instability in ten brain-injured patients. Am J Phys Med Rehabil 68:221–226, 1989

Goldberg RJ, Goldberg JS: Low-dose risperidone for dementia related disturbed behavior in nursing home. Paper presented at the annual meeting of the American Psychiatric Association, Miami, FL, May 20–25, 1995

Goodin DS, Aminoff MJ, Laxer KD: Detection of epileptiform activity by different noninvasive EEG methods in complex partial epilepsy. Ann Neurol 27:330–334, 1990

Gordon WA, Hibbard MR: Cognitive rehabilitation, in Textbook of Traumatic Brain Injury. Edited by Silver JM, McAllister, Yudofsky SC. Washington, DC, American Psychiatric Publishing, 2005, pp 655–660

Gordon WA, Brown M, Sliwinski M, et al: The enigma of "hidden" traumatic brain injury. J Head Trauma Rehabil 13:1–18, 1998

Grigsby J, Kaye K: Incidence and correlates of depersonalization following head trauma. Brain Inj 7:507–513, 1993

Gross H, Kling A, Henry G, et al: Local cerebral glucose metabolism in patients with long-term behavioral and cognitive deficits following mild traumatic brain injury. J Neuropsychiatry Clin Neurosci 8:324–334, 1996

Gualtieri T, Chandler M, Coons TB, et al: Amantadine: a new clinical profile for traumatic brain injury. Clin Neuropharmacol 12:258–270, 1989

Guilleminault C, Yuen KM, Gulevich MG, et al: Hypersomnia after head-neck trauma: a medicolegal dilemma. Neurology 54:653–659, 2000

Gulbrandsen GB: Neuropsychological sequelae of light head injuries in older children 6 months after trauma. J Clin Neuropsychol 6:257–268, 1984

Gupta SR, Mlcoch AG: Bromocriptine treatment of nonfluent aphasia. Arch Phys Med Rehabil 73:373–376, 1992

Hall KM, Karzmark P, Stevens M, et al: Family stressors in traumatic brain injury: a two-year follow-up. Arch Phys Med Rehabil 75:876–884, 1994

Hamm RJ, Dixon CE, Gbadebo DM, et al: Cognitive deficits following traumatic brain produced by controlled cortical impact. J Neurotrauma 9:11–20, 1992

Harvey AG, Bryant RA: Two-year prospective evaluation of the relationship between acute stress disorder and posttraumatic stress disorder following mild traumatic brain injury. Am J Psychiatry 15:626–628, 2000

Hendryx PM: Psychosocial changes perceived by closed-head-injured adults and their families. Arch Phys Med Rehabil 70:526–530, 1989

Herrmann N, Lanctot K, Myszak M: Effectiveness of gabapentin for the treatment of behavioral disorders in dementia. J Clin Psychopharmacol 20:90–93, 2000

Hibbard MR, Uysal S, Kepler K, et al: Axis I psychopathology in individuals with traumatic brain injury. J Head Trauma Rehabil 13:24–39, 1998a

Hibbard MR, Uysal S, Sliwinski M, et al: Undiagnosed health issues in individuals with traumatic brain injury living in the community. J Head Trauma Rehabil 13:47–57, 1998b

Hibbard MR, Bogdany J, Uysal S, et al: Axis II psychopathology in individuals with traumatic brain injury. Brain Inj 14:45–61, 2000

Hoare P: The development of psychiatric disorder among schoolchildren with epilepsy. Dev Med Child Neurol 26:3–13, 1984

Horne M, Lindley SE: Divalproex sodium in the treatment of aggressive behavior and dysphoria in patients with organic brain syndromes. J Clin Psychiatry 56:430–431, 1995

Hornstein A, Seliger G: Cognitive side effects of lithium in closed head injury (letter). J Neuropsychiatry Clin Neurosci 1:446–447, 1989

Hugenholtz H, Stuss DT, Stethem LL, et al: How long does it take to recover from a mild concussion? Neurosurgery 22:853–858, 1988

Inglese M, Makani S, Johnson G, et al: Diffuse axonal injury in mild traumatic brain injury. J Neurosurg 103:298–303, 2005

Insurance Institute for Highway Safety, Highway Loss Data Institute: Fatality facts: alcohol. Washington, DC, Insurance Institute for Highway Safety, Highway Loss Data Institute, 2005a. Available at: http://www.iihs.org/research/fatality_facts/alcohol.html. Accessed January 10, 2007.

Insurance Institute for Highway Safety, Highway Loss Data Institute: Fatality facts: bicycles. Washington, DC, Insurance Institute for Highway Safety, Highway Loss Data Institute, 2005b. Available at: http://www.iihs.org/research/fatality_facts/bicycles.html. Accessed January 10, 2007.

Insurance Institute for Highway Safety, Highway Loss Data Institute: Fatality facts: children. Washington, DC, Insurance Institute for Highway Safety, Highway Loss Data Institute, 2005c. Available at: http://www.iihs.org/research/fatality_facts/children.html. Accessed January 10, 2007.

Insurance Institute for Highway Safety, Highway Loss Data Institute: Fatality facts: motorcycles. Washington, DC, Insurance Institute for Highway Safety, Highway Loss Data Institute, 2005d. Available at: http://www.iihs.org/research/fatality_facts/motorcycles.html. Accessed January 10, 2007.

Jacobs A, Put E, Ingels M, et al: Prospective evaluation of technetium-99m-HMPAO SPECT in mild and moderate traumatic brain injury. J Nucl Med 35:942–947, 1994

Jagger J: Prevention of brain trauma by legislation, regulation, and improved technology: a focus on motor vehicles. J Neurotrauma 9 (suppl): S313–S316, 1992

Jorge RE, Robinson RG, Starkstein SE, et al: Depression and anxiety following traumatic brain injury. J Neuropsychiatry Clin Neurosci 5:369–374, 1993

Jorge RE, Robinson RG, Starkstein SE, et al: Influence of major depression on 1-year outcome in patients with traumatic brain injury. J Neurosurg 81:726–733, 1994

Jorge RE, Robinson RG, Moser D, et al: Major depression following traumatic brain injury. Arch Gen Psychiatry 61:42–50, 2004

Kaelin DL, Cifu DX, Matthies B: Methylphenidate effect on attention deficit in the acutely brain-injured adult. Arch Phys Med Rehabil 77:6–9, 1996

Kant R, Coffey CE, Bogyi AM: Safety and efficacy of ECT in patients with head injury: a case series. J Neuropsychiatry Clin Neurosci 11:32–37, 1999

Kaplan BH, Cowley RA: Seatbelt effectiveness and cost of noncompliance among drivers admitted to a trauma center. Am J Emerg Med 9:4–10, 1991

Kapoor N, Ciuffreda KJ: Vision problems, in Textbook of Traumatic Brain Injury. Edited by Silver JM, McAllister, Yudofsky SC. Washington, DC, American Psychiatric Publishing, 2005, pp 405–417

Kass F, Silver JM: Neuropsychiatry and the homeless. J Neuropsychiatry Clin Neurosci 2:15–19, 1990

Kay SR, Fiszbein A, Opler LA: The Positive and Negative Syndrome Scale (PANSS) for schizophrenia. Schizophr Bull 13:261–276, 1987

Kay T: Neuropsychological treatment of mild traumatic brain injury. J Head Trauma Rehabil 8:74–85, 1993

Kaye NS, Townsend JB 3rd, Ivins R: An open-label trial of donepezil (Aricept) in the treatment of persons with mild traumatic brain injury. J Neuropsychiatry Clin Neurosci 15:383–384, 2003

Kelly JP: Concussion, in Current Therapy in Sports Medicine, 3rd Edition. Edited by Torg JS, Shephard RJ. Philadelphia, PA, CV Mosby, 1995, pp 21–24

Keshavan MS, Channabasavanna SM, Narahana Reddy GN: Post-traumatic psychiatric disturbances: patterns and predictors of outcome. Br J Psychiatry 138:157–160, 1981

Kim E: Elderly, in Textbook of Traumatic Brain Injury. Edited by Silver JM, McAllister TM, Yudofsky SC. Washington, DC, American Psychiatric Publishing, 2005, pp 495–508

Koponen S, Taiminen T, Portin R, et al: Axis I and II psychiatric disorders after traumatic brain injury: a 30 year follow-up study. Am J Psychiatry 159:1315–1321, 2002

Koren D, Arnon I, Klein E: Acute stress response and posttraumatic stress disorder in traffic victims: a one-year prospective, follow-up study. Am J Psychiatry 156:367–373, 1999

Kraus JF, Chu LD: Epidemiology, in Textbook of Traumatic Brain Injury. Edited by Silver JM, McAllister TM, Yudofsky SC. Washington, DC, American Psychiatric Publishing, 2005, pp 3–26

Kraus JF, Nourjah P: The epidemiology of mild, uncomplicated brain injury. J Trauma 28:1637–1643, 1988

Kraus JF, Sorenson SB: Epidemiology, in Neuropsychiatry of Traumatic Brain Injury. Edited by Silver JM, Yudofsky SC, Hales RE. Washington, DC, American Psychiatric Press, 1994, pp 3–41

Kraus JF, Morgenstern H, Fife D, et al: Blood alcohol tests, prevalence of involvement, and outcomes following brain injury. Am J Public Health 79:294–299, 1989

Kraus MF, Maki PM: Effect of amantadine hydrochloride on symptoms of frontal lobe dysfunction in brain injury: case studies and review. J Neuropsychiatry Clin Neurosci 9:222–230, 1997

Kreutzer JS, Gervasio AH, Camplair PS: Primary caregivers' psychological status and family functioning after traumatic brain injury. Brain Inj 8:197–210, 1994

Kuner EH, Schlickewei W, Oltmanns D: Injury reduction by the airbag in accidents. Injury 27:185–188, 1996

Kurtzke JF: Neuroepidemiology. Ann Neurol 16:265–277, 1984

Kuruoglu AC, Arikan Z, Vural G, et al: Single photon emission computerized tomography in chronic alcoholism: antisocial personality disorder may be associated with decreased frontal perfusion. Br J Psychiatry 169:348–354, 1996

Lal S, Merbitz CP, Grip JC: Modification of function in head-injured patients with Sinemet. Brain Inj 2:225–233, 1988

Lauterbach EC, Schweri MM: Amelioration of pseudobulbar affect by fluoxetine: possible alteration of dopamine-related pathophysiology by a selective serotonin reuptake inhibitor. J Clin Psychopharmacol 11:392–393, 1991

Lazarus A, Cotterell KP: SPECT scan reveals abnormality in somatization disorder patient. J Clin Psychiatry 50:475–476, 1989

Leininger BE, Gramling SE, Farrell AD, et al: Neuropsychological deficits in symptomatic minor head injury patients after concussion and mild concussion. J Neurol Neurosurg Psychiatry 53:293–296, 1990

Levin HS, Benton AL, Grossman RG: Neurobehavioral Consequences of Closed Head Injury. New York, Oxford University Press, 1982

Levin HS, High WM, Eisenberg HM: Impairment of olfactory recognition after closed head injury. Brain 108:579–591, 1985

Levin HS, Amparo E, Eisenberg HM, et al: Magnetic resonance imaging and computerized tomography in relation to the neurobehavioral sequelae of mild and moderate head injuries. J Neurosurg 66:706–713, 1987a

Levin HS, Mattis S, Ruff RM, et al: Neurobehavioral outcome following minor head injury: a three-center study. J Neurosurg 66:234–243, 1987c

Levin HS, Goldstein FC, High WM Jr, et al: Disproportionately severe memory deficit in relation to normal intellectual functioning after closed head injury. J Neurol Neurosurg Psychiatry 51:1294–1301, 1988

Li G: Child injuries and fatalities from alcohol-related motor vehicle crashes: call for a zero-tolerance policy. JAMA 283:2291–2292, 2000

Lieberman JA, Kane JM, Johns CA: Clozapine: guidelines for clinical management. J Clin Psychiatry 50:329–338, 1989

Linn RT, Allen K, Willer BS: Affective symptoms in the chronic stage of traumatic brain injury: a study of married couples. Brain Inj 8:135–147, 1994

Lipper S, Tuchman MM: Treatment of chronic post-traumatic organic brain syndrome with dextroamphetamine: first reported case. J Nerv Ment Dis 162:266–371, 1976

Lishman WA: Physiogenesis and psychogenesis in the "post-concussional syndrome." Br J Psychiatry 153:460–469, 1988

Livingston MG, Brooks DN, Bond MR: Patient outcome in the year following severe head injury and relatives' psychiatric and social functioning. J Neurol Neurosurg Psychiatry 48:876–881, 1985a

Livingston MG, Brooks DN, Bond MR: Three months after severe head injury: psychiatric and social impact on relatives. J Neurol Neurosurg Psychiatry 48:870–875, 1985b

Lovell MR, Iverson GL, Collins MW, et al: Does loss of consciousness predict neuropsychological decrements after concussion? Clin J Sport Med 9:193–198, 1999

Mahoney WJ, D'Souza BJ, Haller JA, et al: Long-term outcome of children with severe head trauma and prolonged coma. Pediatrics 71:754–762, 1983

Mann JJ, Waternaux C, Haas GL, et al: Toward a clinical model of suicidal behavior in psychiatric patients. Am J Psychiatry 156:181–189, 1999

Marin RS, Chakravorty S: Disorders of diminished motivation, in Textbook of Traumatic Brain Injury. Edited by Silver JM, McAllister TM, Yudofsky SC. Washington, DC, American Psychiatric Publishing, 2005, pp 337–352

Martin R, Kuzniecky R, Ho S, et al: Cognitive effects of topiramate, gabapentin, and lamotrigine in healthy young adults. Neurology 52:321–327, 1999

Masdeu JC, Van Heertum RL, Kleiman A, et al: Early single-photon emission computed tomography in mild head trauma: a controlled study. J Neuroimaging 4:177–181, 1994

Massey EW, Folger WN: Seizures activated by therapeutic levels of lithium carbonate. South Med J 77:1173–1175, 1984

Mattes JA: Valproic acid for nonaffective aggression in the mentally retarded. J Nerv Ment Dis 180:601–602, 1992

Max JE: Children and adolescents, in Textbook of Traumatic Brain Injury. Edited by Silver JM, McAllister TM, Yudofsky SC. Washington, DC, American Psychiatric Publishing, 2005, pp 477–494

Max JE, Castillo CS, Robin DA, et al: Posttraumatic stress symptomatology after childhood traumatic brain injury. J Nerv Ment Dis 186:589–596, 1998a

Max JE, Robin DA, Lindgren SD, et al: Traumatic brain injury in children and adolescents: psychiatric disorders at one year. J Neuropsychiatry Clin Neurosci 10:290–297, 1998b

McAllister TW: Traumatic brain injury and psychosis: what is the connection? Semin Clin Neuropsychiatry 3:211–223, 1998

McAllister TW: Mild brain injury and the postconcussion syndrome, in Textbook of Traumatic Brain Injury. Edited by Silver JM, McAllister, Yudofsky SC. Washington, DC, American Psychiatric Publishing, 2005, pp 279–308

McAllister TW, Saykin AJ, Flashman LA, et al: Brain activation during working memory 1 month after mild traumatic brain injury: a functional MRI study. Neurology 53:1300–1308, 1999

McAllister TW, Sparling MB, Flashman LA, et al: Differential working memory load effects after mild traumatic brain injury. Neuroimage 14:1004–1012, 2001

McCullagh S, Feinstein A: Cognitive changes, in Textbook of Traumatic Brain Injury. Edited by Silver JM, McAllister TM, Yudofsky SC. Washington, DC, American Psychiatric Publishing, 2005, pp 321–335

McKenna PJ, Kane JM, Parrish K: Psychotic syndromes in epilepsy. Am J Psychiatry 142:895–904, 1985

McKinlay WW, Brooks DN, Bond MR, et al: The short-term outcome of severe blunt head injury as reported by the relatives of the injured person. J Neurol Neurosurg Psychiatry 44:527–533, 1981

McMillan TM: Post-traumatic stress disorder following minor and severe closed head injury: 10 single cases. Brain Inj 10:749–758, 1996

McMillan TM, Glucksman EE: The neuropsychology of moderate head injury. J Neurol Neurosurg Psychiatry 50:393–397, 1987

Michals ML, Crismon ML, Roberts S, et al: Clozapine response and adverse effects in nine brain-injured patients. J Clin Psychopharmacol 13:198–203, 1993

Michaud LJ, Rivara FP, Jaffe KM, et al: Traumatic brain injury as a risk factor for behavioral disorders in children. Arch Phys Med Rehabil 74:368–375, 1993

Mild Traumatic Brain Injury Committee of the Head Injury Interdisciplinary Special Interest Group of the American Congress of Rehabilitation Medicine: Definition of mild traumatic brain injury. J Head Trauma Rehabil 8:86–87, 1993

Mittl RL, Grossman RI, Hiehle JF, et al: Prevalence of MR evidence of diffuse axonal injury in patients with mild head injury and normal head CT findings. AJNR Am J Neuroradiol 15:1583–1589, 1994

Morey CE, Cilo M, Berry J, et al: The effect of Aricept in persons with persistent memory disorder following traumatic brain injury: a pilot study. Brain Inj 17:809–816, 2003

Moskowitz AS, Altshuler L: Increased sensitivity to lithium-induced neurotoxicity after stroke: a case report. J Clin Psychopharmacol 11:272–273, 1991

Nagamachi S, Nichikawa T, Ono S, et al: A comparative study of 123I-IMP SPET and CT in the investigation of chronic-stage head trauma patients. Nucl Med Commun 16:17–25, 1995

Nahas Z, Arlinghaus KA, Kotrla KJ, et al: Rapid response of emotional incontinence to selective serotonin reuptake inhibitors. J Neuropsychiatry Clin Neurosci 10:453–455, 1998

Nasrallah HA, Fowler RC, Judd LL: Schizophrenia-like illness following head injury. Psychosomatics 22:359–361, 1981

National Safety Council: Accident Facts. Chicago, IL, National Safety Council, 1985

National Safety Council: Accident Facts. Chicago, IL, National Safety Council, 1986

National Safety Council: Accident Facts. Chicago, IL, National Safety Council, 1999

National Safety Council: Report on Injuries in America. 2006. Available at: http://www.nsc.org/library/report_injury_usa.htm. Accessed January 15, 2007.

Nedd K, Sfakianakis G, Ganz W, et al: 99mTc-HMPAO SPECT of the brain in mild to moderate traumatic brain injury patients: compared with CT: a prospective study. Brain Inj 7:469–479, 1993

Neurobehavioral Guidelines Working Group; Warden DL, Gordon B, McAllister TW, et al: Guidelines for the pharmacologic treatment of neurobehavioral sequelae of traumatic brain injury. J Neurotrama 23:1468–1501, 2006

Nickels JL, Schneider WN, Dombovy ML, et al: Clinical use of amantadine in brain injury rehabilitation. Brain Inj 8:709–718, 1994

NIH Consensus Development Panel on Rehabilitation of Persons With Traumatic Brain Injury: Rehabilitation of persons with traumatic brain injury. JAMA 282:974–983, 1999

Nizamie SH, Nizamie A, Borde M, et al: Mania following head injury: case reports and neuropsychological findings. Acta Psychiatr Scand 77:637–639, 1988

Noyes R Jr: Motor vehicle accidents related to psychiatric impairment. Psychosomatics 26:569–580, 1985

Nuwer MR: Assessment of digital EEG, quantitative EEG and EEG brain mapping: report of the American Academy of Neurology and the American Clinical Neurophysiology Society. Neurology 49:277–292, 1997

Oddy M, Humphrey M, Uttley D: Stresses upon the relatives of head-injured patients. Br J Psychiatry 133:507–513, 1978

Oddy M, Coughlan T, Tyerman A, et al: Social adjustment after closed head injury: a further follow-up seven years after injury. J Neurol Neurosurg Psychiatry 48:564–568, 1985

Ohry A, Rattok J, Solomon Z: Post-traumatic stress disorder in brain injury patients. Brain Inj 10:687–695, 1996

Oppenheimer DR: Microscopic lesions in the brain following head injury. J Neurol Neurosurg Psychiatry 31:299–306, 1968

Oquendo MA, Friedman JH, Grunebaum MF, et al: Mild traumatic brain injury and suicidal behavior in major depression. J Nerv Ment Dis 192:430–434, 2004

Orrison WW, Gentry LR, Stimac GK, et al: Blinded comparison of cranial CT and MR in closed head injury evaluation. AJNR Am J Neuroradiol 15:351–356, 1994

Orsay EM, Turnbull TL, Dunne M, et al: Prospective study of the effect of safety belts on morbidity and health care costs in motor-vehicle accidents. JAMA 260:3598–3603, 1988

Panzer MJ, Mellow AM: Antidepressant treatment of pathologic laughing or crying in elderly stroke patients. J Geriatr Psychiatry Neurol 4:195–199, 1992

Parker RS, Rosenblum A: IQ loss and emotional dysfunctions after mild head injury in a motor vehicle accident. J Clin Psychol 52:32–43, 1996

Parks RW, Crockett DJ, Manji HK, et al: Assessment of bromocriptine intervention for the treatment of frontal lobe syndrome: a case study. J Neuropsychiatry Clin Neurosci 4:109–110, 1992

Pinder RM, Brogden RN, Speight TM, et al: Maprotiline: a review of its pharmacological properties and therapeutic efficacy in mental states. Drugs 13:321–352, 1977

Poeck K: Pathological laughter and crying, in Handbook of Clinical Neurology, Vol. 45: Clinical Neuropsychology, No 1. Edited by Fredericks JAM. Amsterdam, Elsevier, 1985, pp 219–225

Pollack IW: Traumatic brain injury and the rehabilitation process: a psychiatric perspective, in Neuropsychological Treatment After Brain Injury. Edited by Ellis D, Christensen A-L. Boston, MA, Kluwer Academic, 1989, pp 105–127

Ponsford J, Kinsella G: Attention deficits following closed head injury. J Clin Exp Neuropsychol 14:822–838, 1992

Pope HG Jr, McElroy SL, Satlin A, et al: Head injury, bipolar disorder, and response to valproate. Compr Psychiatry 29:34–38, 1988

Powell JW, Barber-Foss KD: Traumatic brain injury in high school athletes. JAMA 282:958–963, 1999

Prevey ML, Delany RC, Cramer JA, et al: Effect of valproate on cognitive functioning: comparison with carbamazepine. Arch Neurol 53:1008–1016, 1996

Prigatano GP: Work, love, and play after brain injury. Bull Menninger Clin 53:414–431, 1989

Prigatano GP, Stahl ML, Orr WC, et al: Sleep and dreaming disturbances in closed head injury patients. J Neurol Neurosurg Psychiatry 45:78–80, 1982

Quality Standards Subcommittee of the American Academy of Neurology: Practice parameter. Neurobiology (Bp) 48:1–5, 1997

Quinlan KP, Brewer RD, Sleet DA, et al: Characteristics of child passenger deaths and injuries involving drinking drivers. JAMA 283:2249–2252, 2000

Rammahan KW, Rosenberg JH, Pollak CP, et al: Modafinil: efficacy for the treatment of fatigue in patients with multiple sclerosis (abstract). Neurology 54 (suppl 3):A24, 2000

Rao V, Rollings P, Spiro J: Fatigue and sleep problems, in Textbook of Traumatic Brain Injury. Edited by Silver JM, McAllister, Yudofsky SC. Washington, DC, American Psychiatric Publishing, 2005, pp 369–384

Raphaely RC, Swedlow DB, Downes JJ, et al: Management of severe pediatric head trauma. Pediatr Clin North Am 27:715–727, 1980

Rappaport M, Herrero-Backe C, Rappaport ML, et al: Head injury outcome up to ten years later. Arch Phys Med Rehabil 70:885–892, 1989

Ratey JJ, Leveroni C, Kilmer D, et al: The effects of clozapine on severely aggressive psychiatric inpatients in a state hospital. J Clin Psychiatry 54:219–223, 1993

Rattok J: Do patients with mild brain injuries have posttraumatic stress disorder, too? J Head Trauma Rehabil 11:95–97, 1996

Rauch SL, van Der Kolk BA, Fisler RE, et al: A symptom provocation study of posttraumatic stress disorder using positron emission tomography and script-driven imagery. Arch Gen Psychiatry 53:380–387, 1996

Reinhard DL, Whyte J, Sandel ME: Improved arousal and initiation following tricyclic antidepressant use in severe brain injury. Arch Phys Med Rehabil 77:80–83, 1996

Reynolds EH, Trimble MR: Adverse neuropsychiatric effects of anticonvulsant drugs. Drugs 29:570–581, 1985

Richter EF III: Balance problems and dizziness, in Textbook of Traumatic Brain Injury. Edited by Silver JM, McAllister, Yudofsky SC. Washington, DC, American Psychiatric Publishing, 2005, pp 393–404

Rimel RW, Giordani B, Barht JT, et al: Disability caused by minor head injury. Neurosurgery 9:221–228, 1981

Roane DM, Feinberg TE, Meckler L, et al: Treatment of dementia-associated agitation with gabapentin. J Neuropsychiatry Clin Neurosci 12:40–43, 2000

Robinson RG, Schultz SK, Castillo C, et al: Nortriptyline versus fluoxetine in the treatment of depression and in short-term recovery after stroke: a placebo-controlled, double-blind study. Am J Psychiatry 157:351–359, 2000

Ross ED, Rush AJ: Diagnosis and neuroanatomical correlates of depression in brain-damaged patients: implications for a neurology of depression. Arch Gen Psychiatry 38:1344–1354, 1981

Ross ED, Stewart RS: Pathological display of affect in patients with depression and right frontal brain damage. An alternative mechanism. J Nerv Ment Dis 176:165–172, 1987

Ruedrich I, Chu CC, Moore SI: ECT for major depression in a patient with acute brain trauma. Am J Psychiatry 140:928–929, 1983

Salazar AM, Jabbari B, Vance SC, et al: Epilepsy after penetrating head injury, I: clinical correlates: a report of the Vietnam head injury study. Neurology 35:1406–1414, 1985

Salazar AM, Warden DL, Schwab K, et al: Cognitive rehabilitation for traumatic brain injury: a randomized trial. Defense and Veterans Head Injury Program (DVHIP) Study Group. JAMA 283:3075–3081, 2000

Salinsky MC, Storzbach D, Spenceer DC, et al: Effects of topiramate and gabapentin on cognitive abilities in healthy volunteers. Neurology 64:792–798, 2005

Sandel ME, Weiss B, Ivker B: Multiple personality disorder: diagnosis after a traumatic brain injury. Arch Phys Med Rehabil 71:523–535, 1990

Saran AS: Depression after minor closed head injury: role of dexamethasone suppression test and antidepressants. J Clin Psychiatry 46:335–338, 1985

Schiff HB, Sabin TD, Geller A, et al: Lithium in aggressive behavior. Am J Psychiatry 139:1346–1348, 1982

Schiffer RB, Herndon RM, Rudick RA: Treatment of pathologic laughing and weeping with amitriptyline. N Engl J Med 312:1480–1482, 1985

Schmitt JA, Kruizinga MJ, Reidel WJ: Non-serotonergic pharmacological profiles and associated cognitive effects of serotonin reuptake inhibitors. J Psychopharmacol 15:173–179, 2001

Seliger GM, Hornstein A, Flax J, et al: Fluoxetine improves emotional incontinence. Brain Inj 6:267–270, 1992

Sherer M, Boake C, Levin E, et al: Characteristics of impaired awareness after traumatic brain injury. J Int Neuropsychol Soc 4:380–387, 1998

Silver JM, Anderson KA: Vasopressin treats the persistent feeling of coldness after brain injury. J Neuropsychiatry Clin Neurosci 11:248–252, 1999

Silver JM, McAllister TW: Forensic issues in the neuropsychiatric evaluation of the patient with mild traumatic brain injury. J Neuropsychiatry Clin Neurosci 9:102–113, 1997

Silver JM, Yudofsky SC: Pharmacologic treatment of aggression. Psychiatr Ann 17:397–407, 1987

Silver JM, Yudofsky SC: Aggressive disorders, in Neuropsychiatry of Traumatic Brain Injury. Edited by Silver JM, Yudofsky SC, Hales RE. Washington, DC, American Psychiatric Press, 1994, pp 313–356

Silver JM, Caton CM, Shrout PE, et al: Traumatic brain injury and schizophrenia. Paper presented at the annual meeting of the American Psychiatric Association, San Francisco, CA, May 22–27, 1993

Silver JM, Rattok J, Anderson K: Post-traumatic stress disorder and traumatic brain injury. Neurocase 3:151–157, 1997

Silver JM, Weissman M, Kramer R, et al: Association between severe head injuries and psychiatric disorders: findings from the New Haven NIMH Epidemiologic Catchment Area Study. Brain Inj 15:935–945, 2001

Silver JM, Arciniegas DA, Yudofsky SC: Psychopharmacology, in Textbook of Traumatic Brain Injury. Edited by Silver JM, McAllister TM, Yudofsky SC. Washington, DC, American Psychiatric Publishing, 2005a, pp 609–640

Silver JM, Yudofsky SC, Anderson KE: Aggressive disorders, in Textbook of Traumatic Brain Injury. Edited by Silver JM, McAllister TM, Yudofsky SC. Washington, DC, American Psychiatric Publishing, 2005b, pp 259–278

Silver JM, Koumaras B, Chen M, et al: The effects of rivastigmine on cognitive function in patients with traumatic brain injury. Neurology 67:748–755, 2006

Simpson G, Tate R: Suicidality after traumatic brain injury: demographic, injury and clinical correlates. Psychol Med 32:687–697, 2002

Sloan RL, Brown KW, Pentland B: Fluoxetine as a treatment for emotional lability after brain injury. Brain Inj 6:315–319, 1992

Smith KR, Goulding PM, Wilderman D, et al: Neurobehavioral effects of phenytoin and carbamazepine in patients recovering from brain trauma: a comparative study. Arch Neurol 51:653–660, 1994

Smith-Seemiller L, Lovell MR, Smith SS: Cognitive dysfunction after closed head injury: contributions of demographics, injury severity and other factors. Appl Neuropsychol 3:41–47, 1996

Sosin DM, Sacks JJ, Smith SM: Head injury-associated deaths in the United States from 1979–1986. JAMA 262:2251–2255, 1989

Stankoff B, Waubant E, Confavreux C, et al: Modafinil for fatigue in MS: a randomized placebo-controlled double-blind study. French Modafinil Study Group. Neurology 64:1139–1143, 2005

Starkstein SE, Boston JD, Robinson RG: Mechanisms of mania after brain injury: 12 case reports and review of the literature. J Nerv Ment Dis 176:87–100, 1988

Starkstein SE, Mayberg HS, Berthier ML, et al: Mania after brain injury: neuroradiological and metabolic findings. Ann Neurol 27:652–659, 1990

Stewart JT, Nemsath RH: Bipolar illness following traumatic brain injury: treatment with lithium and carbamazepine. J Clin Psychiatry 49:74–75, 1988

Tate R, Simpson G, Flanagan S, et al: Completed suicide after traumatic brain injury. J Head Trauma Rehabil 12:16–20, 1997

Tateno A, Jorge RE, Robinson RG. Clinical correlates of aggressive behavior after traumatic brain injury. J Neuropsychiatry Clin Neurosci 15:155–160, 2003

Taverni JP, Seliger G, Lichtman SW: Donepezil mediated memory improvement in traumatic brain injury during post acute rehabilitation. Brain Inj 12:77–80, 1998

Teasdale G, Jennett B: Assessment of coma and impaired consciousness: a practical scale. Lancet 2:81–84, 1974

Teitelman E: Off-label uses of modafinil. Am J Psychiatry 158:1431, 2001

Terzoudi M, Gavrielidou P, Heilakos G, et al: Fatigue in multiple sclerosis: evaluation of a new pharmacological approach (abstract). Neurology 54 (suppl 3):A61–A62, 2000

Thatcher RW, Moore N, John ER, et al: QEEG and traumatic brain injury: rebuttal of the American Academy of Neurology 1997 Report by the EEG and Clinical Neuroscience Society. Clin Electroencephalogr 30:94–98, 1999

Therapeutics and Technology Assessment Subcommittee of the American Academy of Neurology: Assessment of brain SPECT. Neurology 46:278–285, 1996

Thompson RS, Rivara FP, Thompson DC: A case-control study of the effectiveness of bicycle safety helmets. N Engl J Med 320:1361–1367, 1989

Thomsen IV: Late outcome of very severe blunt head trauma: a 10–15 year second follow-up. J Neurol Neurosurg Psychiatry 47:260–268, 1984

Trzepacz PT, Kennedy RE: Delirium and posttraumatic amnesia, in Textbook of Traumatic Brain Injury. Edited by Silver JM, McAllister TM, Yudofsky SC. Washington, DC, American Psychiatric Publishing, 2005, pp 175–200

Tsuang MT, Boor M, Fleming JA: Psychiatric aspects of traffic accidents. Am J Psychiatry 142:538–546, 1985

Tyerman A, Humphrey M: Changes in self-concept following severe head injury. Int J Rehabil Res 7:11–23, 1984

Tysvaer AT, Storli O, Bachen NI: Soccer injuries to the brain. Acta Neurol Scand 80:151–156, 1989

Ursano RJ, Fullerton CS, Epstein RS, et al: Acute and chronic posttraumatic stress disorder in motor vehicle accident victims. Am J Psychiatry 156:589–595, 1999a

Ursano RJ, Fullerton CS, Epstein RS, et al: Peritraumatic dissociation and posttraumatic stress disorder following motor vehicle accidents. Am J Psychiatry 156:1808–1810, 1999b

U.S. Department of Health and Human Services: Interagency Head Injury Task Force Report. Washington, DC, U.S. Department of Health and Human Services, 1989

U.S. Department of Transportation: Final regulatory impact assessment on amendments to Federal Motor Vehicle Safety Standard 208, Front Seat Occupant Protection (DOT Publ No HS-806-572). Washington, DC, U.S. Department of Transportation, 1984

van Reekum R, Bolago I, Finlayson MA, et al: Psychiatric disorders after traumatic brain injury. Brain Inj 10:319–327, 1996

van Reekum R, Cohen T, Wong J: Can traumatic brain injury cause psychiatric disorders? J Neuropsychiatry Clin Neurosci 12:316–327, 2000

Varney NR: Prognostic significance of anosmia in patients with closed-head trauma. J Clin Exp Neuropsychol 10:250–254, 1988

Varney NR, Martzke JS, Roberts RJ: Major depression in patients with closed head injury. Neuropsychology 1:7–9, 1987

Violon A, De Mol J: Psychological sequelae after head trauma in adults. Acta Neurochir (Wien) 85:96–102, 1987

Wade DT, King NS, Crawford S, et al: Routine follow up after head injury: a second randomised clinical trial. J Neurol Neurosurg Psychiatry 65:177–183, 1998

Ward TM, Levin M: Headaches, in Textbook of Traumatic Brain Injury. Edited by Silver JM, McAllister, Yudofsky SC. Washington, DC, American Psychiatric Publishing, 2005, pp 385–391

Warden DL, Labbate LA: Posttraumatic stress disorder and other anxiety disorders, in Textbook of Traumatic Brain Injury. Edited by Silver JM, McAllister, Yudofsky SC. Washington, DC, American Psychiatric Publishing, 2005, pp 231–243

Warden D, Bleiberg J, Cameron KL, et al: Persistent prolongation of simple reaction time in sports concussion. Neurology 57:524–526, 2001

Watson MR, Fenton GW, McClelland RJ, et al: The post-concussional state: neurophysiological aspects. Br J Psychiatry 167:514–521, 1995

Weinberg RM, Auerbach SH, Moore S: Pharmacologic treatment of cognitive deficits: a case study. Brain Inj 1:57–59, 1987

Weinstein GS, Wells CE: Case studies in neuropsychiatry: post-traumatic psychiatric dysfunction—diagnosis and treatment. J Clin Psychiatry 42:120–122, 1981

Weller M, Kornhuber J: A rationale for NMDA receptor antagonist therapy of the neuroleptic malignant syndrome. Med Hypotheses 38:329–333, 1992

Whelan FJ, Walker MS, Schulz SK: Donepezil in the treatment of cognitive dysfunction associated with traumatic brain injury. Ann Clin Psychiatry 12:131–135, 2000

Whyte J: Neurologic disorders of attention and arousal: assessment and treatment. Arch Phys Med Rehabil 73:1094–1103, 1992

Wilberger JE, Deeb A, Rothfus W: Magnetic resonance imaging in cases of severe head injury. Neurosurgery 20:571–576, 1987

Wilcox JA, Nasrallah HA: Childhood head trauma and psychosis. Psychiatry Res 21:303–306, 1987

Will RG, Young JPR, Thomas DJ: Klein-Levin syndrome: report of two cases with onset of symptoms precipitated by head trauma. Br J Psychiatry 152:410–412, 1988

Wolf B, Grohmann R, Schmidt LG, et al: Psychiatric admissions due to adverse drug reactions. Compr Psychiatry 30:534–545, 1989

Wroblewski BA, Leary JM, Phelan AM, et al: Methylphenidate and seizure frequency in brain-injured patients with seizure disorders. J Clin Psychiatry 53:86–89, 1992

Wroblewski BA, Joseph AB, Kupfer J, et al: Effectiveness of valproic acid on destructive and aggressive behaviours in patients with acquired brain injury. Brain Inj 11:37–47, 1997

Yablon SA: Posttraumatic seizures. Arch Phys Med Rehabil 74:983–1001, 1993

Yudofsky SC, Silver JM, Schneider SE: Pharmacologic treatment of aggression. Psychiatric Annals 17:397–407, 1987

Yudofsky SC, Silver JM, Hales RE: Pharmacologic management of aggression in the elderly. J Clin Psychiatry 51 (suppl 10):22–28, 1990

Yudofsky SC, Silver JM, Hales RE: Psychopharmacology of aggression, in American Psychiatric Press Textbook of Psychopharmacology. Edited by Schatzberg AF, Nemeroff CB. Washington, DC, American Psychiatric Press, 1995, pp 735–751

Yudofsky SC, Silver JM, Hales RE: Treatment of agitation and aggression, in Textbook of Psychopharmacology, 2nd Edition. Edited by Schatzberg AF, Nemeroff CB. Washington, DC, American Psychiatric Press, 1998, pp 881–900

Zasler N: Sexual dysfunction, in Neuropsychiatry of Traumatic Brain Injury. Edited by Silver JM, Yudofsky SC, Hales RE. Washington, DC, American Psychiatric Press, 1994, pp 443–470

Zasler ND, Martelli MF, Nicholson K: Chronic pain, in Textbook of Traumatic Brain Injury. Edited by Silver JM, McAllister, Yudofsky SC. Washington, DC, American Psychiatric Publishing, 2005, pp 419–433

Zeilig G, Drubach DA, Katz-Zeilig M, Karatinos J: Pathological laughter and crying in patients with closed traumatic brain injury. Brain Inj 10:591–597, 1996

Zhang L, Plotkin RC, Wang G, et al: Cholinergic augmentation with donepezil enhances recovery in short-term memory and sustained attention after traumatic brain injury. Arch Phys Med Rehabil 85:1050–1055, 2004

7

NEUROPSYCHIATRIC ASPECTS OF SEIZURE DISORDERS

H. Florence Kim, M.D.

Frank Y. Chen, M.D.

Stuart C. Yudofsky, M.D.

Robert E. Hales, M.D., M.B.A.

Gary J. Tucker, M.D.

Before the development of the electroencephalogram (EEG) by Dr. Hans Berger in the 1930s, all seizure disorders were classified with mental disorders (Berger 1929–1938). Indeed, a strong link between epilepsy and psychiatry has been known for more than a century.

Epilepsy represents one of the more interesting aspects of brain-behavior relations. It is not only an important medical condition but also an important part of the differential diagnosis of behavior disorders. Because of its ability to cause behavioral symptoms without overt classical seizures, epilepsy is an important natural model of behavioral disturbance.

Epilepsy can cause both chronic and episodic behavior disorders. Unfortunately, the cause of the epilepsy itself is often unclear, as laboratory diagnostic evidence may not be present on EEGs or imaging modalities. Thus, the hypothesis about etiology is based solely on the clinical picture.

SEIZURE DISORDERS

SEIZURES AND EPILEPSY

Epilepsy is a term applied to a broad group of disorders. The defining feature of any of the epilepsies is the seizure. A seizure is usually defined as having all or parts of the following: an impairment of consciousness, involuntary movements, behavior changes, and altered perceptual experiences.

The diagnosis of epilepsy is made only when a person has recurrent seizures (a paroxysmal cerebral neuronal firing, which may or may not produce disturbed consciousness and perceptual or motor alterations). *Grand mal* (generalized tonic-clonic) seizures usually involve relatively short (10–30 seconds) tonic movements, with marked extension and flexion of muscles, without shaking. A longer phase (15–60 seconds) involving clonic movements, manifesting as rhythmic muscle group shaking, follows the tonic phase. Tonic phase movements may be associated with laryngeal stridor. Urinary and/or fecal incontinence may occur and may be followed by headache, sleepiness, and confusion. Seizures preceded by perceptual, autonomic, affective, or cognitive alterations (aura) usually indicate a focal onset with secondary generalization. There are many types of seizures that vary markedly from the above description (Chadwick 1993; Engel 1992).

CLASSIFICATION OF SEIZURES

The classification of seizures and epilepsy is constantly evolving. It has shifted away from terms such as *grand mal* in an attempt to correlate clinical seizure type with electroencephalographic ictal (i.e., during the seizure) and interictal (i.e., between seizures) changes. The most recent classification of epileptic seizures by the International League Against Epilepsy (ILAE) in 2001 has moved away from previous phenomenological descriptions to the creation of a list of seizure types that represent diagnostic entities on the basis of common pathophysiology and anatomy (International League Against Epilepsy Commission Report 2001a).

In place of a fixed classification, a diagnostic scheme consisting of five levels or axes to provide a standardized description of epilepsy is now recommended by the International League Against Epilepsy Commission Report (2001b) (Table 7–1). Axis I is a description of the ictal event according to the International League Against Epilepsy Commission Report's (2001a) standardized *Glossary of Descriptive Terminology for Ictal Semiology*. This descrip-

TABLE 7–1. International League Against Epilepsy (ILAE) proposed diagnostic scheme

Axis I: Ictal phenomenology describing the ictal events

Axis II: Seizure type
Specify from ILAE List of Epileptic Seizures. Identify localization within the brain or precipitating stimuli when appropriate.

Axis III: Epileptic syndrome
Specify from ILAE List of Epilepsy Syndromes. Specify only when syndromic diagnosis is possible.

Axis IV: Etiology
Specify genetic defects or specific pathologies from ILAE Classification of Diseases Frequently Associated With Epileptic Seizures or Epilepsy Syndromes. Specify only when etiology is known.

Axis V: Impairment classification derived from World Health Organization (optional)

Source. Adapted from International League Against Epilepsy Commission Report: A proposed diagnostic scheme for people with epileptic seizures and with epilepsy: report of the ILAE Task Force on Classification and Terminology. *Epilepsia* 42:796–803, 2001b. Used with permission.

tion will not reference etiology, anatomy, or mechanisms. Axis II consists of the epileptic seizure type, diagnostic entities denoting therapeutic, prognostic, and etiological mechanisms. If anatomical localization is possible, it should be specified here. For reflex seizures, or seizures precipitated by sensory stimuli, precipitating factors should be specified on this axis as well. These seizure types are separated into self-limited and continuous seizures and further divided into generalized and focal seizures. Axis III is the epileptic syndrome, a constellation of signs and symptoms that define an epileptic condition. It is not necessary to specify a syndromic diagnosis, if one is not known. Axis IV lists the etiology if known, such as a specific disease or a genetic or pathological abnormality. Axis V is a classification of impairment associated with the epileptic condition and is considered optional.

Generalized Seizures

Generalized seizures (generalized attacks) manifest immediately and spread bilaterally through the cerebral cortex. No preceding motor or perceptual experiences occur, and there is almost invariably total loss of consciousness.

Focal (Partial) Seizures

Focal seizures (partial or localization-related) result in epileptic firing in a specific focus in the brain (usually the cerebral cortex). *Simple partial seizures* (previously called *elementary partial seizures*) involve no alteration in consciousness. *Complex partial seizures* (CPSs) involve a defect in consciousness (i.e., confusion, dizziness). Some authors further subdivide CPSs into type 1 (temporal lobe) and type 2 (extratemporal). Forty percent of all patients with epilepsy will have CPSs (International League Against Epilepsy Commission 1985). The terms *simple* and *complex partial seizures* are no longer recommended for use in classification of specific seizure types but may still be used as descriptive terms.

Tonic-Clonic Seizures

Tonic-clonic seizures (grand mal seizures) are the most common form of generalized seizure, with a total loss of consciousness and a tetanic muscular phase lasting usually several seconds (tonic), followed by a phase of repetitive jerking lasting usually 1–2 minutes (clonic). These seizures may be generalized, or they may begin as partial seizures and secondarily generalize.

Partial seizures secondarily generalized start as partial seizures and then spread bilaterally throughout the cerebral cortex, producing secondary generalization. These seizures are distinct from a previous classification of secondary generalized epilepsy, which referred to a kind of epilepsy generalized from the start, with features of a diffuse cerebral pathology.

Absence Seizures

Typical *absence seizures* (*petit mal* seizures) occur primarily in children. These start generalized, with loss of consciousness for a few seconds without any motor phase. Typical electroencephalographic findings are bilateral and synchronous and have spike waves of 3–4 Hz.

Status Epilepticus

Status epilepticus (a continuous seizure state that involves two or more seizures superimposed on each other without total recovery of consciousness) is a true medical emergency. Generalized status epilepticus can be convulsive (tonic-clonic seizures) or nonconvulsive (behavioral or cognitive changes from baseline such as confusion, stupor, or coma, accompanied by continuous or near continuous seizure activity on EEGs). Several other forms of status epilepticus exist, including absence status epilepticus and focal status epilepticus types, when consciousness may be preserved, and the diagnosis is often made by electroencephalography (Novak et al. 1971).

CAUSES OF EPILEPSY

The idiopathic or genetic epilepsies, in which no central nervous system (CNS) pathology is evident, are usually childhood syndromes. In patients older than 30, the onset of epilepsy or recurrent seizures is usually associated with CNS pathology. These syndromes are usually described as symptomatic or secondary seizure disorders, or epilepsy. Conditions such as head injury, encephalitis, birth trauma, or hyperpyrexia represent rather static and permanent lesions that can cause epilepsy or seizures. Conditions that are progressive (change over time) include medication overdose or withdrawal, tumor, infections, metabolic disease (e.g., hypoglycemia and uremia), and endocrine diseases. Alzheimer's disease and other dementias, multiple sclerosis, cerebral arteriopathy, and other degenerative or infiltrative conditions can all lead to a progressive and changing picture of seizures.

Seizures can also be a reaction to various medical or physiological stresses. This fact is particularly evident at both ends of the age spectrum. For example, febrile conditions are more likely to cause seizures in young people and older people.

TEMPORAL LOBE EPILEPSY

Temporal lobe epilepsy is no longer recognized by the ILAE, but we utilize the term in the descriptive sense, implying both complex and simple partial seizures, including psychomotor automatisms and tonic-clonic seizures that may originate from the temporal lobe. Many such phenomena interpreted as having originated in the temporal lobe may, in fact, be extratemporal.

Although the term *temporal lobe epilepsy* has formally become an anachronism, in practice it is still commonly used in the absence of an adequate alternative. The phenomena of temporal lobe epilepsy are *not* synonymous with those of its proposed nonanatomical replacement, CPSs, because CPSs are restricted to patients who have focal firing with defects of consciousness.

In practice, many patients with temporal lobe epilepsy have no defect of consciousness and have simple partial seizures (e.g., olfactory hallucinations). In addition, they may have simple partial seizures with psychic symptomatology (e.g., cognitive alterations, such as flashbacks or déjà vu experiences occurring in clear consciousness). Temporal lobe epilepsy may also manifest with the *temporal lobe absence* or behavioral arrest that is associated with a brief loss of consciousness of 10–30 seconds. These episodes may be associated with minor automatisms (e.g., chewing movements) and with "drop attacks" (the falling associated with loss of muscle tone). Patients with temporal lobe epilepsy often appear to be staring and after the episode may be aware that they had a loss of consciousness. They may experience postictal features such as headache and sleepiness. Thus, the temporal lobe absence differs from petit mal because the latter is a shorter episode, without muscle movements and postictal features (Fenton 1986).

Temporal lobe epilepsy may manifest with psychomotor automatisms alone, which are no longer regarded as a form of CPS. Psychomotor automatisms may involve a psychic (cognitive-affective, somatosensory, or perceptual) phase followed by a motor phase. The psychic phase may be brief and amnestic. Associated perceptual alterations (auditory buzz or hum, complex verbalizations, or aphasias) may occur. Visual abnormalities include diplopia, misperceptions of movement, and changes in perceived object size or shape. Other alterations may include illusions, tactile distortions, olfactory phenomena (e.g., generally unpleasant, burning, or rotting smells), gustatory phenomena (e.g., metallic tastes), and somatosensory autonomic symptoms (e.g., piloerection, gastric sensations, or nausea). Flashbacks and alterations of consciousness (*jamais vu*, depersonalization, derealization, and déjà vu) may occur. These are followed by automatisms of various degrees of complexity. There may be simple buttoning or unbuttoning or masticatory movements, more complex "wandering" fugue states, furor-type anger (which is very rare), or speech automatisms (which are far more common than is recognized).

The features of temporal lobe epilepsy are varied and protean (Bear 1986; Blumer 1975). Table 7–2 describes some of the symptoms that have often been associated with temporal lobe disturbances.

EPIDEMIOLOGY OF SEIZURE DISORDERS

It is often difficult to get a clear idea of the epidemiology of epilepsy. Prevalence is 5–40 per 1,000 people. The incidence is 40–70 per 100,000 people per year in industrialized countries and more than twice as high in developing countries. Worldwide, 50 million people are affected by epilepsy, with 2.4 million new cases occurring every year (GCAE Secretariat 2003). The incidence of epilepsy is highest in young children, decreases in adults, and peaks again in the elderly (Dekker 2002).

TABLE 7–2.   Behavioral symptoms often associated with seizures, particularly temporal lobe epilepsy

Hallucinations: all sensory modalities

Illusions

Déjà vu

Jamais vu

Depersonalization

Repetitive thoughts and nightmares

Flashbacks and visual distortions

Epigastric sensations

Automatisms

Affective and mood changes

Catatonia

Cataplexy

Amnestic episodes

PSYCHOSOCIAL FACETS OF EPILEPSY

The epileptic patient encounters major psychosocial stressors, including chronic illness. Studies comparing the epileptic patient with groups of patients with other chronic illnesses, such as rheumatic heart disease, diabetes mellitus, and cancer, have concluded that each of these conditions has its own special stressors (Dodrill and Batzel 1986). However, in comparing any of these populations with patients with organic brain disease, specific unique problems arise (Szatmari 1985).

A special difficulty of the epileptic patient is the often paroxysmal (episodic) element to the illness. Between episodes, the person with epilepsy may be functioning normally. Substantial covert stress leads the person with epilepsy to be afraid of performing normal social activities, such as dating during adolescence. The fear of a seizure is greater than the occurrence. In addition, the witnessing of an actual tonic-clonic seizure is a frightening experience for many members of the general population, and much folklore is associated with seizures (Temkin 1979). Consequently, conceptions of epilepsy may be distorted thereafter, and even an isolated seizure may have grave consequences on interpersonal relationships.

Within American culture, persons with epilepsy are perceived as an inferior minority group. In some preliterate subcultures, an epileptic seizure is often regarded as a type of communication with ancestors or with higher beings, and epileptic individuals may be perceived as having special powers. Many of them become shamans or witch doctors and are highly respected members of their culture (Temkin 1979). Also, the disorders create limitations on the patient's activities (i.e., epileptic individuals cannot operate complex machinery, work in jobs that expose them to dangers, swim alone, or even bathe autonomously). Not being allowed to drive is a major obstacle in our society. These functional limitations are often disregarded by the patient (e.g., driving), and may create additional guilt, moral and ethical consequences, and legal complications. Frequently, in families with epileptic members, abnormal relationships develop, leading to increased dependency or isolation. Patterns of dependency can be difficult to dislodge, and it may be easier to remain ill than to become seizure-free and healthy. The epileptic patient needs to learn to develop independence and a sense of self-care and to create constructive relationships that promote health. These psychological factors and their effect on epilepsy should not be underestimated (Hoare 1984; Stevens 1988; Ziegler 1982).

DIAGNOSIS

Epilepsy diagnosis is clinical, similar to schizophrenia. Although an EEG can be confirmatory, 20% of patients with epilepsy will have a normal EEG, and 2% of patients without epilepsy will have spike and wave formations (Engel 1992). The best diagnostic test for seizures is the observation of a seizure or the report of someone who has observed the seizure. Thus, history is crucial. Important information includes age at onset of seizures, history of illness or trauma to the nervous system, a family history, and some idea of whether the condition is progressive or static. Attempts should be made to determine whether the seizures are idiopathic or secondary. Certainly, these descriptions are most helpful in the diagnosis of major motor or generalized seizures. They are also useful in determining the relation between the seizures and various behavioral disturbances. Because the seizure focus can reside in any location in the brain, the number of behavioral symptoms associated with seizures is considerable (see Table 7–2).

Laboratory

An elevated prolactin level is the only major laboratory value used in the diagnostic workup of seizure disorders. Serum prolactin is released by epileptic activity spreading from the temporal lobe to the hypothalamic-pituitary axis (Bauer 1996). A 3- to 4-fold rise in prolactin levels occurs within 15–20 minutes of a generalized tonic-clonic seizure. Since prolactin level normalizes within 60 minutes, blood should be drawn 15–20 minutes after the seizure. In a study of 200 consecutive patients seen in the emergency department setting with a diagnosis of seizure followed by syncope, the sensitivity of serum prolactin level was 42%, specificity was 82%, positive predictive value was 74%, negative predictive value was 54%, and overall diagnostic accuracy was 60% (Vukmir 2004). Furthermore, elevated prolactin levels have not been helpful in differentiating true seizures from nonepileptic or pseudoseizures (G. Shukla et al. 2004; Willert et al. 2004). Some data indicate that repeated seizures and shorter seizure-free periods decrease the prolactin response (Malkowicz et al. 1995). Prolactin levels also may be elevated by neuroleptic use. Thus, elevated serum prolactin levels may be helpful as a confirmatory test for suspected seizure but not as a singular diagnostic test.

Imaging

Structural imaging techniques such as magnetic resonance imaging and computed tomography scans are crucial for the evaluation of symptomatic epilepsies. Both structural and functional imaging modalities are also useful for localization of seizure foci to evaluate candidates for surgical intervention. Functional imaging such as single-photon emission computed tomography (SPECT) and positron emission tomography (PET) has been valuable in evaluating ictal events and blood flow to focal lesions during a seizure. Postictal and interictal evaluations are much less informative. SPECT studies are very reliable for localizing ictal events. PET is better in the detection of interictal temporal lobe hypermetabolism (Ho et al. 1995). As these instruments become more sensitive, their use will increase in the clinical evaluation of seizure disorders.

EEG

The EEG is one of the most important tests in the evaluation of seizures, suspected seizures, or episodic behavioral disturbances. Paroxysmal interictal EEGs with spikes and wave complexes can confirm the clinical diagnosis of a seizure disorder. The EEG can, when positive, differentiate between seizure types (e.g., absence seizures from generalized seizures) and indicate the possibility of a structural lesion when there are focal findings in the EEG. A normal EEG result does not eliminate the possibility of a seizure disorder being present. The EEG is a reflection of surface activity in the cortex and may not reflect seizure activity deep in the brain. Most clinicians, when confronted with a behavior disorder that does not fit the usual clinical picture of a schizophrenic psychosis (particularly if the disorder is episodic), will obtain an EEG. A negative EEG result may deter further seizure workup. The diagnosis of epilepsy (as with schizophrenia) is a clinical one and although the EEG can confirm the diagnosis, it cannot exclude it. Even with elaborate recordings (24-hour EEGs) and concomitant videotaping, a seizure disorder cannot always be diagnosed.

Special techniques such as use of nasopharyngeal electrodes (Bickford 1979), sphenoidal electrodes (Ebersole and Leroy 1983), buccal skin electrodes (Sadler and Goodwin

1986), or cerebral cortical placements (Heath 1982) may assist with diagnosis by EEG.

Medications that should be avoided include benzodiazepines, which may have, by virtue of their strong antiepileptic effects, profound effects in normalizing the EEG. Because effects on receptor activity may last weeks, even with the short-acting benzodiazepines, demonstration of abnormal activity after administration of benzodiazepines may decrease substantially. L-Tryptophan should also be avoided. Adamec and Stark (1983) found that L-tryptophan has some effect in raising the seizure threshold during electroconvulsive therapy (ECT). Some psychotropic medications, such as neuroleptics, tricyclic and heterocyclic antidepressants, and benzodiazepines (Pincus and Tucker 1985), also may increase synchronization of the EEG (leading to a seizurelike pattern). One report (Ryback and Gardner 1991) described a small series in which procaine activation of the EEG was useful in identifying patients with episodic behavior disorders responsive to anticonvulsants.

Recent advances in electroencephalographic technology may ultimately change the whole perspective of its use in psychiatry. Evoked potentials and quantitative electroencephalography are promising research tools that have yet to show specific clinical utility in the diagnosis and treatment of neuropsychiatric disorders.

DIFFERENTIAL DIAGNOSIS OF BEHAVIORAL SYMPTOMS ASSOCIATED WITH EPILEPSY

Medical conditions must be distinguished from seizures: panic disorder, hyperventilation, hypoglycemia, various transient cerebral ischemias, migraine, narcolepsy, malingering, and conversion reactions. Characteristics of temporal lobe epilepsy are subjective experiences or feelings, automatisms, and, more rarely, catatonia or cataplexy. Because the symptoms are usually related to a focal electrical discharge in the brain, they are generally consistent and few in number. Although the

list of possible symptoms may be quite large (see Table 7–2), each patient will have a limited number of specific symptoms—for example, auditory hallucinations (usually voices), repetitive sounds, or visual hallucinations and misperceptions of a consistent type that includes a visual disturbance. The automatisms are simple (e.g., chewing, swallowing, pursing of the lips, looking around, smiling, grimacing, crying). Other types of automatisms are attempting to sit up, examining or fumbling with objects, and buttoning or unbuttoning clothes. Complex, goal-directed behavior is unusual during these episodes. Aggressive behavior is also rare. The only time the patient will sometimes become aggressive is when an attempt is made to restrain or prevent ambulation (Rodin 1973). Typical attacks usually consist of a cessation of activity, followed by automatism and impairment of consciousness. The entire episode usually lasts from 10 seconds to as long as 30 minutes. The motor phenomena and postural changes, such as catatonia, are rarer (Fenton 1986; Kirubakaran et al. 1987).

The profile of patients who present primarily with behavioral symptoms is usually of episodic "brief" disturbances lasting for variable time periods (hours to days). The patient often states that such episodes have occurred once a month or once every 3 months. The patient seeks psychiatric attention when the frequency of the episodes increases to daily or several per day with resultant impairment of functioning. Critical factors helpful in the diagnosis of temporal lobe epilepsy are shown in Table 7–3.

A final term that requires clarification does not refer to epileptic seizures. *Pseudoseizure* is used synonymously with *nonepileptic seizure* or *conversion reaction*. The differentiation of this condition from true seizures is at times extremely difficult (Table 7–4), often complicated by the fact that the person who is suspected of having "seizures," primarily related to psychological reasons, often has a history of true seizures. Devinsky and Gordon (1998) noted that nonepileptic seizures often can follow epileptic seizures. They postulated that

TABLE 7–3.   Factors helpful in the diagnosis of temporal lobe epilepsy

Does the patient describe typical subjective alterations?

Has the patient been observed performing characteristic automatisms?

Was the patient confused during the episode?

Is the patient's memory for events that occurred impaired?

Did the patient experience postictal depression?

Has the patient had other lapses during which he or she engaged in nearly identical behavior?

TABLE 7–4.   General features of nonepileptic seizures ("pseudoseizures")

Setting

Environmental gain (audience usually present)

Seldom sleep related

Often triggered (e.g., by stress)

Suggestive profile on Minnesota Multiphasic Personality Inventory (Hathaway and McKinley 1989)

Attack

Atypical movements, often bizarre or purposeful

Seldom results in injury

Often starts and ends gradually

Out-of-phase movements of extremities

Side-to-side movements

Examination

Restraint accentuates the seizure

Inattention decreases over time

Plantar flexor reflexes

Reflexes intact (corneal, pupillary, and blink)

Consciousness preserved

Autonomic system uninvolved

Autonomically intact

After attack

No postictal features (lethargy, tiredness, abnormal electroencephalogram findings)

Prolactin normal (after 30 minutes)

No or little amnesia

Memory exists (hypnosis or amobarbital sodium)

the epileptic seizure, particularly the CPS, leads to possible loss of inhibition of impulses and emotions. The patients with nonepileptic seizures differ from seizure disorder patients in that they may have significantly more stress, more negative life events, and a history of child abuse, and more somatic symptoms and awareness of their bodies (Arnold and Privitera 1996; Tojek et al. 2000). Most of the nonepileptic seizure patients have somatoform disorders, particularly conversion, rather than dissociative disorders. Interestingly, the patients with nonepileptic seizures who did not fit the criteria for conversion had a high incidence of anxiety and psychotic disorders (Alper et al. 1995; Kuyk et al. 1999). A significant number of patients with nonepileptic seizures also have concomitant mood and anxiety disorders. Therefore, combination treatment with psychotropic medications such as selective serotonin reuptake inhibitors (SSRIs), benzodiazepines, or atypical antipsychotics and individual psychotherapy can be extremely helpful in decreasing the frequency and morbidity associated with nonepileptic seizures (M. Thomas and Jankovic 2004).

Frontal lobe epilepsy can also present with bizarre behavioral symptoms and can be confused with nonepileptic seizures. Laskowitz et al. (1995) noted that the symptoms often appear as spells with an aura of panic symptoms, with weird vocalizations and with bilateral limb movements but no periods of postictal tired-ness and no confusion; also, no oral or alimentary movements occur. These spells last about 60–70 seconds. Fortunately, most of these seizures are symptomatic of a CNS lesion, and usually the correct diagnosis is made with the EEG or imaging studies. P. Thomas et al. (1999) described a form of nonconvulsive status epilepticus of frontal origin. These patients often presented with a mood disturbance similar to hypomania, subtle cognitive impairments, some disinhibition, and some indifference.

ETIOLOGICAL LINKS OF SEIZURES TO PSYCHOPATHOLOGY

The increased incidence of psychopathology and seizure disorders is clear and evident, but the exact etiology of this increased incidence is unclear. There have been two major theories historically. One is an affinity theory, best exemplified by the classic articles of Slater et al. (1963), which described a group of patients with epilepsy and psychosis. An opposing theory was first postulated by Von Meduna (1937), who observed (incorrectly) that the schizophrenic patients under his care had few epileptic conditions (Fink 1984). He then hypothesized that the induction of a seizure in a psychotic patient might be therapeutic. Landolt (1958) observed a group of patients whose EEG results seemed to normalize during a psychotic episode. This has been called "forced normalization." This inverse relation between seizures and behavioral disturbances has been noted by many clinicians. For example, it is not uncommon for a patient with epilepsy to have a marked decrease in seizures for a prolonged time and then later to have an increase in behavioral disturbances. After a seizure, the behavior seems to normalize again. Although these observations are clinically and statistically apparent (Schiffer 1987), their exact etiological importance to all patients with epilepsy and behavioral disturbance is unclear. The relation between psychopathology and seizures is further complicated by whether the behavioral disturbance is a preictal event, an ictal event, or a postictal event. *Kindling*, a pathophysiological event, is the sequence whereby repetitive subthreshold electrical or chemical stimuli to specific brain areas eventually induce a seizure or a behavioral disturbance that persists, but it has never been demonstrated in humans (Adamec and Stark 1983). This process has been hypothesized as one of the possible causes of psychopathology.

Other hypotheses about the cause of the psychopathology have been that seizures create a type of organic brain syndrome related to some underlying diffuse process or are caused by active focal damage (Pincus and Tucker 1985). Toxicity of the medicines used to treat seizure disorders also has been implicated, and although most anticonvulsant drugs cause significant cognitive impairment, they do not seem to be associated with the development of major psychopathology (Dodrill and Troupin 1991; Meador et al. 1993; Moehle et al. 1984; Trimble 1988).

TEMPORAL LOBE SPECIFICITY AND PSYCHOPATHOLOGY

A major question about the behavior changes in epilepsy is whether behavioral disturbances occur more commonly in patients with temporal lobe epilepsy specifically or whether the behavioral disturbances are related to seizure disorders in general.

This issue is complex, with many confounding variables. For example, more complicated patients gravitate toward university hospitals, where studies are usually undertaken (Currie et al. 1970). Another confounding variable is the age at onset of psychomotor epilepsy, which is similar to that of schizophrenia. Moreover, three-quarters of patients with psychomotor seizures or CPSs are older than 16 years at the onset of the seizure disorder (Stevens 1988).

The vast majority of patients with seizure disorders will have temporal lobe foci on EEG at some point during their illness. Kristensen and Sindrup (1978) compared CPS patients with psychosis with CPS patients without psychosis and could find little difference in the two groups with regard to age at onset, laterality of focus, and interval between epilepsy onset and time of examination. The patients with psychosis had significantly more neurological signs, spike EEGs, a history of brain damage, and no family history of seizure disorders, suggesting that these patients may have had other associated organic brain syndromes.

Additionally, patients with CPSs and secondary generalization are often more difficult to keep seizure-free than are those with generalized seizures. Their greater number of seizures and the frequent evidence of associated organic brain syndromes further confound the relation to behavioral disturbance.

The confounding variables include increased seizures, increased amounts of anticonvulsants, and increased numbers of different types of seizures. The temporal lobe constitutes 40% of the cerebral cortex (Stevens 1988).

Despite these confounding factors and limited available data, it appears that patients with temporal lobe epilepsy and other focal epilepsies are at greater risk for developing psychiatric disorders than are patients with primary generalized seizure disorders (Edeh and Toone 1987). Poor response to treatment is also related to increased psychiatric comorbidity. Patients with treatment-refractory epilepsy quite often have temporal lobe epilepsy. In one study, patients awaiting temporal lobectomy had a lifetime prevalence of psychiatric disorders of 75% (Glosser et al. 2000). Thus, epilepsy patients most at risk for developing psychiatric comorbidity are those with localization-related epilepsies and a chronic, treatment-resistant course (Blumer et al. 1995; Cockerell et al. 1996; Fiordelli et al. 1993; Glosser et al. 2000).

COMORBID PSYCHIATRIC SYNDROMES

The relation of psychopathology and seizure disorders is difficult to establish. Most of the studies rest at the level of case report, and even large-scale studies usually deal with populations that have come to psychiatric attention rather than community-based samples (Popkin and Tucker 1994). The following question constantly arises: Are we dealing with behavior associated with a seizure disorder, or is the behavior associated with another underlying disease of the CNS that can cause seizures? At the symptom level, we are frequently dealing with general symptoms related to damage of the CNS and not specific to any one condition or region of the brain. The symptoms can be episodic changes in mood, irritability or impulsiveness, psychosis, anxiety disorders, or confusional syndromes. The other major types of symptoms usually seen with CNS dysfunction are related to more insidious disorders, such as dementia, depression, various motor diseases, or distinctive personality changes such as those seen after head trauma (Popkin and Tucker 1994).

The temporal relation of mood or psychotic symptoms to seizure episodes is also important and thus has been classified into peri-ictal, ictal, postictal, and interictal episodes. The term *peri-ictal* (or premonitory) refers to psychiatric symptoms immediately before and after the seizure. These symptoms may last hours to days and may resolve when the seizure itself occurs. *Ictal* symptoms are affective or psychotic symptoms that occur during the seizure itself. *Postictal* psychiatric symptoms begin shortly after the cessation of seizure activity. And *interictal* refers to chronic psychiatric symptoms that appear during seizure-free periods. This classification is important in that each type appears to follow a differing constellation and severity of symptoms and thus may require different treatment approaches.

PSYCHOSIS

It is clear that *all* of the symptoms described in schizophrenic patients can occur in patients with seizure disorders (Toone et al. 1982). Seizure disorders and schizophrenia have many empirical similarities that also make the differential diagnosis difficult. The peak age at onset is similar. Both disorders may occur in early to late adolescence, although epilepsy often presents in childhood and may occur at any age. The neurotransmitter dopamine is somehow related in both conditions because dopamine antagonists are antipsychotic and mildly epileptogenic. Dopamine agonists are psychotogenic and mildly antiepileptic (Trimble 1977). The family history can be of help in that the genetic frequencies are similar for both conditions, with 10%–13% of the offspring of parents with either schizophrenia or epilepsy having the same condition (Metrakos and Metrakos 1961), but this leaves most cases without a family history of either condition.

Clinically, there seem to be three psychotic presentations that one sees with seizure disorders. One is an episodic course that is usually related to seizure activity, manifested by perceptual changes, alterations in consciousness, and poor memory for the events. Periictal, ictal, and postictal psychoses often follow this episodic course. A chronic interictal psychotic condition also occurs in which the patient may have simple auditory hallucinations, paranoia, or other perceptual changes, and this condition closely resembles schizophrenia. The third type is simply a variation in which the patient usually has some type of persistent experience of depersonalization or visual distortion that, for lack of a better name, is usually labeled as psychotic. This third type is probably a variant of the chronic psychotic state.

Although Slater et al. (1963) postulated a long period between the onset of seizures and subsequent psychosis, it is not uncommon for a clinician to treat a patient for "schizophrenia" who is often completely unresponsive to antipsychotic medications. During the course of this treatment, the patient has a grand mal seizure. An EEG is then obtained that confirms the diagnosis of epilepsy.[1] The patient is then given anticonvulsant medication, and a marked decrease in the "psychotic" symptoms occurs.

Many of these patients seem quite intact even when experiencing the symptoms, particularly so between episodes. Their mental status examinations seem to show no evidence of other schizophrenic symptoms. During the episode, what is often seen is a confusional state and an alteration in consciousness rather than an inability to communicate. What they and their families describe is an abrupt change in personality, mood, or ability to function. It is

TABLE 7–5. Diagnostic clues indicating psychosis may be due to lesion of the central nervous system or seizures
Presentation that does not meet DSM-IV-TR criteria
Good premorbid social history
Abrupt change in personality, mood, or ability to function
Rapid fluctuations in mental status
Unresponsiveness to usual biological or psychological interventions

important to remain suspicious of altered perceptual experiences that do not completely meet DSM-IV-TR (American Psychiatric Association 2000) criteria for schizophrenia and to reevaluate patients whose symptoms do not respond to antipsychotic medication (Table 7–5).

Treatment of Psychotic Conditions

The major treatment of the episodic psychotic conditions is usually the appropriate use of anticonvulsant medications. The treatment of chronic conditions involves both anticonvulsant and antipsychotic medications. In general, the use of medication in these patients is difficult in that very small doses of any medication often cause an increase in symptoms that diminishes over time. Consequently, very small doses and infrequent changes seem to be the major guidelines in treating these conditions. Although all of the neuroleptics can lower the seizure threshold, the rate of seizures with atypical antipsychotic agents is quite low, and their use is increasing in patients with seizures and psychosis, despite lack of controlled clinical trials as to their efficacy in treating seizure-related psychosis. Of the traditional neuroleptics, haloperidol, fluphenazine, molindone, pimozide, and trifluoperazine

---

[1]It is important to note that although neuroleptics may lower the seizure threshold, they do not usually cause seizures in patients who are not predisposed to them. Among inpatients taking psychotropic medication, seizures were infrequent, occurring in 0.03% of psychiatric inpatients (Popli et al. 1995).

seem to lower the seizure threshold the least. The propensity for clozapine to lower the seizure threshold is quite well known, so it is only used in patients whose symptoms do not respond to all other antipsychotic medications. Furthermore, the use of clozapine and carbamazepine is contraindicated because of the risk of agranulocytosis.

ANXIETY DISORDERS

The correspondence between seizure disorders and anxiety disorders is a fascinating topic, and the substantial overlapping of symptoms (Table 7–6) often makes differentiation between these classes of disorders complex. Either type of syndrome can be confused with the other, and the same class of medications (benzodiazepines) helps to reduce the symptoms and subsequent impairment of both types. Panic disorder and CPSs are each included in the differential diagnosis of the other. Although many symptoms overlap, evidence of neurophysiological linkage between anxiety and seizure disorder remains tenuous, except that both involve underlying limbic dysfunction (Fontaine et al. 1990). This connection appears to be more relevant between partial seizure and CPS than other seizure disorders, and it has been speculated that a subgroup of patients exists who have panic disorder that has a pathophysiological relation to epilepsy (Dantendorfer et al. 1995). This relation is not surprising given that modulation of fear is associated with the temporal lobes; others have hypothesized relations between the parietal and the frontal lobe neural circuits and panic attacks (Alemayehu et al. 1995; McNamara and Fogel 1990).

Roth and Harper (1962) have pointed out some of the similarities between epilepsy and anxiety disorders. Both are episodic disorders with sudden onset without a precipitating event; both sometimes present with dissociative symptoms: depersonalization, derealization, and déjà vu; both often present with abnormal perceptual and emotional disturbances, such as intense fear and terror; and both have associated physical symptoms. Sig-

TABLE 7–6.   Anxiety disorder symptoms that overlap with those of seizure disorder

Panic disorder

 Fear

 Depersonalization

 Derealization

 Déjà vu

 Jamais vu

 Misperceptions

 Illusions

 Dizziness

 Paresthesias

 Chills or hot flashes

Obsessive-compulsive disorder

 Obsessions, forced or intrusive

Posttraumatic stress disorder

 Recurrent memories or distressing
  recollections

 Flashback-like episodes

 Irritability

 Difficulty concentrating

Agoraphobia

 Fear of recurrent episodes that leads to
  restriction of activities

nificant clinical differences between panic disorder and CPS help to differentiate the two: in panic disorders, consciousness is usually preserved, olfactory hallucinations are unusual, the patient has a positive family history, EEG results are usually normal, and many patients do not respond well to anticonvulsants (Handal et al. 1995).

Treatment of Comorbid Anxiety

Patients with seizure disorders and comorbid anxiety disorder should receive treatment for their anxiety. Clinical experience indicates that SSRIs (first-line treatments for primary anxiety disorders) are helpful in the treatment of anxiety disorders in epilepsy patients. SSRIs can cause potential interactions with hepatically metabolized antiepileptic medications because they can inhibit various cytochrome P450 enzymes. Benzodiazepines such as clonazepam and alprazolam also can be helpful in the treatment of anxiety disorders in epilepsy patients. Psychotherapeutic approaches such as cognitive-behavioral therapy, behavioral modification, short-term symptom-focused therapies, and psychoeducation may be helpful.

MOOD DISORDERS

CNS disorders and chronic medical illnesses, including epilepsy, are frequently associated with increased incidence of mood disorders (Silver et al. 1990). Suicide is of special concern because its prevalence is greater in patients with epilepsy than in the general population (Gehlert 1994; Nilsson et al. 2002). Suicide is the cause of death in 10% of all patients with epilepsy, compared with 1% in the general population (Jones et al. 2003).

Patients with uncontrolled seizures have a prevalence of depression up to 10 times greater than in the general population and up to 5 times greater than in patients with controlled seizures (Harden and Goldstein 2002; Hermann et al. 2000; Lambert and Robertson 1999). Depressed epilepsy patients had twice as many emergency department and nonpsychiatric office visits as did their nondepressed counterparts (Cramer et al. 2004).

Little is known about the prevalence of other mood disorders such as mania and dysthymia in patients with seizure disorders.

Several features of depression in epilepsy require special consideration before one diagnoses a comorbid mood disorder. Peri-ictal depression or premonitory dysphoria may occur before or after the seizure, lasting hours to days. Depressive or dysphoric symptoms of this type may stop when the seizure occurs or may continue for days after the seizure. Ictal depressive symptoms occur during the seizure and are characterized by sudden onset of symptoms without precipitating factors and can even manifest as impulsive suicidality (Prueter and Norra 2005). Postictal depressive episodes oc-

cur after seizure activity resolves and may last for up to 2 weeks. The most common type of depression in epilepsy is interictal depression, which may manifest as major depressive or dysthymic episodes. Interictal depression does not fit DSM-IV-TR classification well because it tends to have a chronic course and atypical mood symptoms of pain, mixed phases of euphoria and dysphoria, and short intervals without affective symptoms (Kanner 2003).

In evaluating depression in a patient with epilepsy, it is very important to examine the medications the patient is taking. Anticonvulsants have been identified as causal agents of depression and cognitive impairments; phenobarbital, the anticonvulsant vigabatrin, and multiple combinations of anticonvulsants appear to contribute to mood disturbance (Bauer and Elger 1995; Brent et al. 1990; Levinson and Devinsky 1999; Mendez et al. 1993). Other anticonvulsants have minimal effect, and some, such as carbamazepine and lamotrigine, may have beneficial effects on mood.

Treatment of Comorbid Mood Disorders

Data on the treatment of depression in seizure patients are extremely limited. In general, pre-ictal and ictal depressive symptoms may not require antidepressant treatment because these episodes are often self-limited, and improved seizure control will reduce their occurrence (Lambert and Robertson 1999). However, postictal and interictal depressions require treatment with antidepressant medication.

When depression does occur, the clinician should determine whether the patient has had a recent change in antiepileptic medication regimen. If the patient is taking an antiepileptic medication with known depressogenic effects, it should be replaced, if possible, by one with mood-stabilizing effects such as carbamazepine, valproate, or lamotrigine. For patients with a bipolar diathesis or suspected mood lability, monotherapy with carbamazepine or valproic acid (or now lamotrigine) may suffice to prevent episodes, decrease severity of symptoms, and minimize overall decompensation.

All antidepressants, including the SSRI antidepressants, are proconvulsive, although the incidence of seizures in healthy individuals is low (Alldredge 1999). Despite few controlled clinical data on the efficacy of SSRI antidepressants in the treatment of mood disorders in epilepsy patients, SSRIs are generally recommended as first-line treatments (Kanner and Nieto 1999). Citalopram and sertraline are often used because of their minimal interactions with antiepileptic medications. It is important to start any medication with smaller doses than are conventionally given for primary psychiatric disorders, with gradual dose increases over time. Regular monitoring of interval EEGs and antiepileptic medication levels is recommended. Of the older antidepressant medications, most of the tricyclic antidepressants are known to lower the seizure threshold. This is particularly true of amitriptyline, maprotiline, and clomipramine. Bupropion is also very likely to cause seizures. However, doxepin, trazodone, and the monoamine oxidase inhibitors have less of a tendency to lower the seizure threshold (Rosenstein et al. 1993). Most of the seizures reported with any of these medications are dose related; therefore, blood level monitoring in these patients can be quite useful.

In most cases, treating the depression often improves seizure control. In an open study evaluating the use of fluoxetine as an adjunctive medication in patients with CPSs, 6 of 17 patients showed a dramatic improvement, and the others had a 30% reduction in their seizure frequency over 14 months (Favale et al. 1995). To date, no evidence shows that any one particular antidepressant is more effective than another, and the choice should be made on clinical grounds. Epileptic patients with refractory or severe depression and even mania should be considered for ECT because it is not contraindicated in people with epilepsy. ECT raises the seizure threshold by more than 50% (Sackeim 1999). However, controlled clinical trials with ECT are lacking in epilepsy patients as well (Zwil and Pelchat 1994).

The role of psychotherapeutic approaches seems intuitively beneficial, but few empirical studies have evaluated this topic (Fenwick 1994; Mathers 1992; Regan et al. 1993). A study by Gillham (1990) reported that psychological intervention with education to improve coping skills could be helpful in reducing seizure frequency and psychological symptoms (as well as depressive symptoms) in patients with refractory seizures.

Vagus nerve stimulation is a well-tolerated, efficacious treatment for refractory epilepsy. Its efficacy in the treatment of mood disorders is not conclusively established, although results from open, long-term studies of treatment-resistant depression are promising. Repetitive transcranial magnetic stimulation is currently being investigated as a treatment for epilepsy and mood disorders but is not recommended for clinical use at this time.

BEHAVIORAL AND PERSONALITY DISTURBANCES

The literature and clinical experience clearly point to an association between seizure disorders and behavioral disturbances (Blumer 1999; Blumer et al. 1995; Neppe and Tucker 1988). Most of our knowledge in this area comes from cross-sectional case–control studies, case reports, and tertiary centers that treat the most severe cases. Several factors, such as stigma of the illness, adverse social factors, level of social support, cultural acceptability, consequences of the illness on psychosocial adaptation, and interpersonal relationships, play an important role in shaping patterns of behavior and have a significant effect on the integrity of personality development. Factors that may assume a role in the pathogenesis of personality and behavioral disturbance are the age at onset of the seizure disorder, the type of seizure disorder, the location and the laterality, the frequency of the seizures, the etiology, the presence of a structural lesion, the presence of another medical illness or behavioral dysfunction, and the ongoing administration of anticonvulsants.

An increase in episodic and impulsive aggression also has been associated with seizure disorders, particularly CPS (Blake et al. 1995;

Mann 1995). Following the postictal period, uncooperative and aggressive behavior may occur when a confused patient is restrained or may occur in a patient who develops a postictal paranoid psychosis (Rodin 1973). Aggressive behavior during a seizure is very unusual, and aggressive activity is usually carried out in a disordered, uncoordinated, and nondirected way (Fenwick 1986). The prevalence of interictal aggression is increased in some seizure disorders, CPS, and generalized seizure disorders but may be an epiphenomenon of epilepsy. This probably can be accounted for by other factors associated with violence and aggression: exposure to violence as a child, male sex, low IQ, low socioeconomic status, adverse social factors, focal or diffuse neurological lesions, refractory seizures, cognitive impairment, history of institutionalization, and drug use (Devinsky and Vazquez 1993).

The manner in which a particular seizure disorder promotes psychopathic behavioral syndromes is not well understood. Auras have been hypothesized as manifestations of an underlying mechanism that contributes to the development of personality disturbance (Mendez et al. 1993). Evidence indicates that patients with chronic seizure disorders develop brain neuropathology, and histological studies of the temporal lobes in CPS show neuronal loss (Sloviter and Tamminga 1995).

Devinsky and Vazquez (1993) emphasized the diversity of symptoms, behaviors, and profiles and that the most important characteristic of patients with a seizure disorder is the tendency for extremes of behavior to be accentuated in numerous manners. It is the maladaptive consequences and dysfunctional traits that should be of paramount importance in treatment.

COGNITIVE DISORDERS

Cognitive function in patients with epilepsy is highly variable, often related to the pathogenesis or etiology of the seizure disorder, anatomical localization of seizure foci, and severity and clinical course of the disorder. Results from several studies suggested that cognitive deficits

may be apparent at disease onset (Aikia et al. 2001; Elger et al. 2004; Pulliainen et al. 2000). No controlled, long-term studies of idiopathic generalized tonic-clonic seizures and absence seizures are available. Temporal lobe epilepsy, a focal or localization-related epilepsy, is often associated with memory impairment. Left-sided temporal lobe epilepsy is often characterized by verbal memory deficits because of the language-dominant hemisphere being affected. However, right-sided temporal lobe epilepsy is not necessarily characterized by nonverbal memory impairment.

Generalized tonic-clonic seizures are more likely to cause cognitive impairment than are focal seizures. Status epilepticus, convulsive or nonconvulsive, can lead to severe and persistent amnesia (Dietl et al. 2004; Oxbury et al. 1997). However, the long-term cognitive effects of status epilepticus have not been comprehensively studied (Dodrill and Wilensky 1990).

Thus, it appears that cognitive function is compromised at disease onset in adult epilepsy patients and that cognitive function is fairly stable early in the disease course. Further cognitive impairment is modulated by the clinical course of the disease, with seizure remission resulting in arrest or even reversal of cognitive decline. However, the long-term cognitive outcome of epilepsy patients is largely unknown (Elger et al. 2004).

OVERALL GUIDELINES FOR TREATMENT OF COMORBID PSYCHIATRIC SYNDROMES

With any chronic illness, basic principles should be applied in developing a treatment plan. Seizure disorders are no exception, and guidelines for treatment are summarized in Table 7–7. A thorough assessment of premorbid functioning, past episodes, previous trials and responses, duration of the current episode, and level of impairment and psychosocial dysfunction facilitates proper intervention and guides subsequent management. Given that insults to the CNS produce only a limited amount of symptom expression, the mood, anxiety, psychotic, cognitive, and behavioral

TABLE 7–7. Basic principles of treating patients with a seizure disorder and concomitant psychiatric symptoms

1. Perform a thorough assessment of biopsychosocial factors that aggravate neuropsychiatric symptoms.

2. Evaluate the need for adjustment of the anticonvulsant.

3. Consider psychotherapeutic approaches (individual, group, family) that are specific for the syndrome or that target behaviors or stressors.

4. Preferably—but not always—use anticonvulsant monotherapy.

5. Optimize the addition of psychotropic medication by targeting specific psychiatric symptoms.

6. Start with smaller than usual dose and wait until symptoms stabilize (often weeks) before changing doses.

7. Anticipate interactions between anticonvulsant and psychotropic medications.

8. Collaborate with other caregivers.

symptoms and signs associated with seizure disorders do not fit neatly into the DSM-IV-TR psychiatric categories (Tucker 1996). The neuropsychiatrist may elect to treat patients with a suspected seizure disorder empirically. These patients, including those with refractory psychiatric illness, may find benefit with an anticonvulsant (Post et al. 1985). In a few patients with concomitant psychiatric illness, anticonvulsant monotherapy for the seizure disorder may suffice (Neppe et al. 1988). Patients taking anticonvulsants should have serum blood levels checked at the first indication of incipient or worsening psychiatric symptoms or signs. An increase in the dosage of an anticonvulsant may be all that is necessary to diminish symptoms and prevent decompensation. Conversely, patients with complex medication regimens may realize symptom improvement after dosage reduction (Trimble and Thompson 1983).

Most patients will require treatment of psychiatric syndromes. Individual, group, family, or couples therapies can provide specific syndrome-focused treatments. Psychotherapeutic approaches have many advantages. They avoid drug interactions, circumvent the tendency of psychotropic medications to alter seizure thresholds, and can teach patients behavior and coping skills that may have a positive effect on symptoms and dysfunction.

Many patients will require pharmacotherapy, either combined with psychotherapeutic approaches or alone. Patients with temporal lobe epilepsy have a wide variety of mood, anxiety, dissociative, psychotic, and behavioral disturbances that frequently resemble psychiatric disorders. Discriminating the symptoms of previous seizures from target psychiatric symptoms will ensure a greater likelihood of response to medication.

Although we recommend an aggressive approach for the treatment of comorbid psychiatric syndromes, we are judicious with the dosing of psychotropics and prefer gradual increases. Clinical experience shows that many patients with seizure disorders seem to respond to smaller doses. When a new drug is added, it is mandatory for the clinician to be aware of potential drug interactions.

Many anticonvulsants will lower the serum drug level of psychotropics through enzyme induction (Perucca et al. 1985), and psychotropics may increase the levels of anticonvulsants secondary to increased P450 hepatic enzyme competition (Cloyd et al. 1986). For patients receiving tricyclic antidepressants, monitoring of serum levels is recommended (Preskorn and Fast 1992). Initially, anticonvulsant blood levels should be monitored weekly and then monthly, after the addition of a psychotropic. After a few months, serum levels can be checked less frequently. Thereafter, any changes in the dosage of medications require reexamination of serum blood levels.

Finally, the importance of coordinating care with other professionals and health care providers cannot be overemphasized. It behooves the psychiatrist to work with a neurologist (if available) to develop a long-term strategy. Often, psychiatrists will assume the role of supervising all treatment planning (Schoenenberger et al. 1995).

SPECIFIC ASPECTS OF ANTICONVULSANT USE

MANAGEMENT

In many of the patients who have suspected seizure disorders, the psychiatrist will be left to manage the anticonvulsants. Until the psychiatrist is comfortable with these medications, collaboration with a neurologist is helpful and a good learning technique. However, as valproic acid and carbamazepine have become more common in the treatment of bipolar illness, the basic principles are known to most psychiatrists (McElroy et al. 1988; Neppe et al. 1988).

PHARMACOKINETIC INTERACTIONS

Anticonvulsant administration is particularly important and particularly difficult by virtue of enzyme induction and inhibition occurring in the liver. This enzyme induction tends to affect predominantly the cytochrome P450 enzyme system in the liver. This implies that both the metabolism of anticonvulsants (particularly carbamazepine) and the metabolism of other lipid-soluble compounds are accelerated (Alldredge 1999; Post et al. 1985). However, some of the new anticonvulsants—oxcarbazepine, gabapentin, and vigabatrin—have few drug interactions (Dichter and Brodie 1996).

Of the major anticonvulsants, phenobarbital, phenytoin, carbamazepine, lamotrigine, topiramate, and tiagabine have potent drug interactions. Table 7–8 indicates what is known about some interactions and shows the com-

TABLE 7–8. Known interactions between carbamazepine and other drugs

Drugs that increase carbamazepine level

　Carbamazepine epoxide only

　Cimetidine

　Erythromycin

　Isoniazid

　Nicotinamide

　Propoxyphene

　Troleandomycin

　Valproic acid

　Viloxazine

Drugs that decrease carbamazepine level

　Alcohol (chronic use)

　Carbamazepine itself (autoinduction)

　Cigarettes

　Phenobarbital

　Phenytoin

　Primidone and phenobarbital (as metabolite)

Conditions caused by carbamazepine

　Escape from dexamethasone suppression

　Oral contraceptive failure

　Pregnancy test failure

Substances whose effects are decreased by carbamazepine

　Clonazepam

　Dicumarol

　Doxycycline

　Ethosuximide

　Haloperidol

　Isoniazid

　Phenytoin

　Sodium valproate

　Theophylline

　Vitamin D, calcium, and folate

Note. Because enzyme induction is the mechanism in most of these interactions, it can be hypothesized that similar effects occur with phenytoin, phenobarbital, and primidone.

plexity of these drug interactions (Bertilsson 1978; Birkhimer et al. 1985; Bramhall and Levine 1988; Dichter and Brodie 1996; Dorn 1986; Jann et al. 1985; Kidron et al. 1985; S. Shukla et al. 1984; Zimmerman 1986).

Phenobarbital

Phenobarbital is the most potent of the enzyme inducers; when it is used in combination, it reduces levels of other anticonvulsants. In addition, phenobarbital may cause psychological depression and may lead to addiction, or to lethal overdose, which was a major cause of death in the 1950s. It also produces a cognitive impairment, which may explain the rigidity of personality observed in patients with seizure disorders taking phenobarbital.

There is little role for barbiturates in the outpatient management of seizure disorders except in patients who are already taking and tolerating them. Side effects may include CNS depression, psychological depression, and cognitive impairments. It is extremely difficult to taper off barbiturates without inducing an epileptic seizure.

Phenytoin

Diphenylhydantoin sodium (or phenytoin) has limited use in the neuropsychiatric patient, despite being an outstanding anticonvulsant in controlling generalized tonic-clonic and partial seizures. The side-effect profile (Pulliainen and Jokelainen 1994) includes mild cognitive impairment. Because phenytoin has a small therapeutic range, patients can easily become drug toxic, and, ironically, may experience seizures or worsening of them (petit mal). Gum hyperplasia is a classic finding (Trimble 1979, 1988).

Carbamazepine

The increasing use of carbamazepine rather than phenytoin is due to fewer side effects, psychotropic properties, and proven value in severe disorders and bipolar illness. It is as effective as phenytoin in both generalized tonic-clonic seizures and partial seizures and thus is the drug of choice for such conditions.

It is ineffective in petit mal absences, for which sodium valproate or ethosuximide is preferred.

Carbamazepine may be used in treating nonresponsive psychotic or atypical psychotic patients with any temporal lobe abnormalities on EEG, with episodic hostility, or with affective lability (Blumer et al. 1988; Cowdry and Gardner 1988; Neppe et al. 1991).

Carbamazepine and the other anticonvulsants involved in enzyme induction can cause many unanticipated side effects (Cloyd et al. 1986) (e.g., patients taking oral contraceptives may have their steroid levels lowered, patients may become vitamin D deficient, folic acid may be depleted). Elevation in hepatic enzyme levels (γ-glutamyl transferase) commonly occurs; this does not imply that the anticonvulsant drugs should be stopped.

Patients taking neuroleptics who are given carbamazepine may have more side effects as a consequence of raised levels from competition at enzyme system pathways.

In addition to the phenomenon of induction of hepatic enzymes, a second phenomenon of deinduction of hepatic enzyme systems occurs (Neppe and Kaplan 1988).

Valproate

Sodium valproate is useful in combined tonic-clonic and petit mal seizures. It also appears to be effective against CPSs.

Valproate does not induce enzymes but metabolically competes; it raises levels of psychotropics and itself. It is safe, relatively nontoxic, and generally well tolerated. The major concern is potentially fatal, rare hepatotoxicity in young children, particularly with other anticonvulsants (McElroy et al. 1988).

New Antiepileptic Drugs

There are many new antiepileptic drugs: gabapentin, felbamate, oxcarbazepine, tiagabine, topiramate, vigabatrin, levetiracetam, and lamotrigine. Most of these drugs for which the actions are known affect either the inhibitory γ-aminobutyric acid system (gabapentin, tiagabine, vigabatrin) or the excitatory glutaminergic system (felbamate, lamotrigine). These drugs have been well studied and all have various mild to serious side effects (Table 7–9) (Dichter and Brodie 1996; Ketter et al. 1999). Gabapentin, lamotrigine, and topiramate have been increasingly used in psychiatry for bipolar disorder and anxiety disorders and may have uses for similar disorders in seizure disorder patients (Ghaemi and Gaughan 2000; Ketter et al. 1999).

CONCLUSION

Psychopathology occurs in only a minority of persons with epilepsy. Attempted etiological explanations such as kindling, lateralization, localization, and biochemical changes are all, therefore, explanations for a small proportion of the epileptic population. Medications used to treat seizure disorders often do not alleviate behavior changes, and at times agents such as neuroleptics and antidepressants help behavior change but not seizure disturbances. The exact etiology of these conditions remains to be determined. Clinical judgment in the individual case remains the essential standard of care in the absence of solid evidence for specific indications and protocols for the use of anticonvulsant/psychotropic combinations in specific populations.

RECOMMENDED READING

Trimble M, Schmitz B (eds): The Neuropsychiatry of Epilepsy. Cambridge, UK, Cambridge University Press, 2002

REFERENCES

Adamec RE, Stark AC: Limbic kindling and animal behavior: implications for human psychopathology associated with complex partial seizures. Biol Psychiatry 18:269–293, 1983

Aikia M, Salmenpera T, Partanen K, et al: Verbal memory in newly diagnosed patients and patients with chronic left temporal lobe epilepsy. Epilepsy Behav 2:20–27, 2001

Alemayehu S, Bergey GK, Barry E, et al: Panic attacks as ictal manifestations of parietal lobe seizures. Epilepsia 36:824–830, 1995

TABLE 7–9. Selected clinical aspects of the newer anticonvulsants

Felbamate[a,b]

  Irritability, insomnia, stimulant effects

  Aplastic anemia, hepatitis

Gabapentin

  Weight gain

  Few drug interactions

  Anxiolytic

Lamotrigine[a,b]

  No weight gain

  Occasional tourettism

  Rash

  Does not induce P450 system

  Can increase neurotoxicity of carbamazepine

Levetiracetam

  Increased incidence of depression and behavioral disturbance

Oxcarbazepine

  Few drug interactions (not affected by enzyme inducers)

  Induces 3A family of P450 system weakly

  Hyponatremia

Tiagabine

  Confusion, fatigue

  Does not induce P450 system

Topiramate[a]

  Hyperammonemic encephalopathy when combined with valproate

  Cognitive impairments

  Weak effect on P450 system

Vigabatrin[a]

  Increased incidence of depression and psychosis

  Weight gain

  Possible retinal damage

  No drug interactions

[a]Can affect phenytoin, carbamazepine, or phenobarbital levels.
[b]Valproate decreases levels of this compound.

Alldredge BK: Seizure risk associated with psychotropic drugs: clinical and pharmacokinetic considerations. Neurology 53 (suppl 2):S68–S75, 1999

Alper K, Devinsky O, Perrine K, et al: Psychiatric classification of nonconversion nonepileptic seizures. Arch Neurol 52:199–201, 1995

American Psychiatric Association: Diagnostic and Statistical Manual of Mental Disorders, 4th Edition, Text Revision. Washington, DC, American Psychiatric Association, 2000

Arnold LM, Privitera MD: Psychopathology and trauma in epileptic and psychogenic seizure patients. Psychosomatics 37:438–443, 1996

Bauer J: Epilepsy and prolactin in adults: a clinical review. Epilepsy Res 24:1–7, 1996

Bauer J, Elger CE: Anticonvulsive drug therapy: historical and current aspects. Nervenarzt 66:403–411, 1995

Bear DM: Behavioural changes in temporal lobe epilepsy: conflict, confusion challenge, in Aspects of Epilepsy and Psychiatry. Edited by Trimble ME, Bolwig TG. London, England, Wiley, 1986, pp 19–29

Berger H: Ueber das Elektrenkephalogramm des Menschen. Arch Psychiatr Nervenkr I–XIV:87–108, 1929–1938

Bertilsson L: Clinical pharmacokinetics of carbamazepine. Clin Pharmacokinet 3:128–143, 1978

Bickford RG: Activation procedures and special electrodes, in Current Practice of Unusual Electroencephalography. Edited by Kass D, Daly DD. New York, Raven, 1979, pp 269–306

Birkhimer LJ, Curtis JL, Jann MW: Use of carbamazepine in psychiatric disorders. Clin Pharm 4:425–434, 1985

Blake P, Pincus J, Buckner C: Neurologic abnormalities in murderers. Neurology 45:1641–1647, 1995

Blumer D: Temporal lobe epilepsy and its psychiatric significance, in Psychiatric Aspects of Neurological Disease. Edited by Benson FD, Blumer D. New York, Grune & Stratton, 1975, pp 171–198

Blumer D: Evidence supporting the temporal lobe epilepsy personality syndrome: Neurology 53 (suppl 2):S9–S12, 1999

Blumer D, Heilbronn M, Himmelhoch J: Indications for carbamazepine in mental illness: atypical psychiatric disorder or temporal lobe syndrome? Compr Psychiatry 29:108–122, 1988

Blumer D, Montouris G, Hermann B: Psychiatric morbidity in seizure patients on a neurodiagnostic monitoring unit. J Neuropsychiatry Clin Neurosci 7:445–456, 1995

Bramhall D, Levine M: Possible interaction of ranitidine with phenytoin. Drug Intell Clin Pharm 22:979–980, 1988

Brent DA, Crumrine PK, Varma R, et al: Phenobarbital treatment and major depressive disorder in children with epilepsy: a naturalistic follow-up. Pediatrics 85:1086–1091, 1990

Chadwick D: Seizures, epilepsy, and other episodic disorders, in Brain's Diseases of the Nervous System, 10th Edition. Edited by Walton J. London, England, Oxford University Press, 1993, pp 697–733

Cloyd JC, Levy RH, Wedlund RH: Relationship between carbamazepine concentration and extent of enzyme autoinduction (abstract). Epilepsia 27:592, 1986

Cockerell OC, Moriarty J, Trimble M, et al: Acute psychological disorders in patients with epilepsy: a nationwide study. Epilepsy Res 25:119–131, 1996

Cowdry R, Gardner DL: Pharmacotherapy of borderline personality disorder. Arch Gen Psychiatry 45:111–119, 1988

Cramer JA, Blum D, Fanning K, et al: The impact of comorbid depression on health resource utilization in a community sample of people with epilepsy. Epilepsy Behav 5:337–342, 2004

Currie S, Heathfield RWG, Henson RA, et al: Clinical course and prognosis of temporal lobe epilepsy: a survey of 666 patients. Brain 94:173–190, 1970

Dantendorfer K, Amering M, Baischer W, et al: Is there a pathophysiological and therapeutic link between panic disorder and epilepsy? Acta Psychiatr Scand 91:430–432, 1995

Dekker PA: Epilepsy: A Manual for Medical and Clinical Officers in Africa. Geneva, World Health Organization, 2002

Devinsky O, Gordon E: Epileptic seizures progressing into nonepileptic conversion seizures. Neurology 51:1293–1296, 1998

Devinsky O, Vazquez B: Behavioral changes associated with epilepsy. Neurol Clin 11:127–149, 1993

Dichter M, Brodie M: New antiepileptic drugs. N Engl J Med 334:1583–1590, 1996

Dietl T, Urbach H, Helmstaedter C, et al: Persistent severe amnesia due to seizure recurrence after unilateral temporal lobectomy. Epilepsy Behav 6:394–400, 2004

Dodrill CB, Batzel LW: Interictal behavioral features of patients with epilepsy. Epilepsia 27 (suppl 2):S64–S76, 1986

Dodrill CB, Troupin AS: Neuropsychological effects of carbamazepine and phenytoin. Neurology 41:141–143, 1991

Dodrill CB, Wilensky AJ: Intellectual impairment as an outcome of status epilepticus. Neurology 40 (suppl 2):23–27, 1990

Dorn JM: A case of phenytoin toxicity possibly precipitated by trazodone. J Clin Psychiatry 47:89–90, 1986

Ebersole JS, Leroy RJ: Evaluation of ambulatory EEG monitoring. Neurology 33:853–860, 1983

Edeh J, Toone B: Relationship between interictal psychopathology and the type of epilepsy: results of a survey in general practice. Br J Psychiatry 151:95–101, 1987

Elger CE, Helmstaedter C, Kurthen M: Chronic epilepsy and cognition. Lancet Neurol 3:663–672, 2004

Engel J: The epilepsies, in Cecil's Textbook of Medicine, 19th Edition. Edited by Wyngoorden J, Smith L, Bennet C. Philadelphia, PA, WB Saunders, 1992, pp 2202–2213

Favale E, Rubino P, Mainardi P, et al: Anticonvulsant effect of fluoxetine in humans. Neurology 45:1926–1927, 1995

Fenton GW: The EEG, epilepsy and psychiatry, in What Is Epilepsy? Edited by Trimble MR, Reynolds EH. Edinburgh, UK, Churchill Livingstone, 1986, pp 139–160

Fenwick P: In dyscontrol epilepsy, in What Is Epilepsy? Edited by Trimble MR, Reynolds EH. Edinburgh, UK, Churchill Livingstone, 1986, pp 161–182

Fenwick P: The behavioral treatment of epilepsy generation and inhibition of seizures. Neurol Clin 12:175–202, 1994

Fink M: Meduna and the origins of convulsive therapy. Am J Psychiatry 141:1034–1041, 1984

Fiordelli E, Beghi E, Bogliun G, et al: Epilepsy and psychiatric disturbance: a cross-sectional study. Br J Psychiatry 163:446–450, 1993

Fontaine R, Breton G, Déry R, et al: Temporal lobe abnormalities in panic disorder: an MRI study. Biol Psychiatry 27:304–310, 1990

GCAE Secretariat: Epilepsy: Out of the Shadows. ILAE/IBE/WHO Global Campaign Against Epilepsy. Heemstede, The Netherlands, World Health Organization, 2003

Gehlert S: Perceptions of control in adults with epilepsy. Epilepsia 35:81–88, 1994

Ghaemi S, Gaughan S: Novel anticonvulsants: a new generation of mood stabilizers. Harv Rev Psychiatry 8:1–7, 2000

Gillham RA: Refractory epilepsy: an evaluation of psychological methods in outpatient management. Epilepsia 31:427–432, 1990

Glosser G, Zwil AS, Glosser DS, et al: Psychiatric aspects of temporal lobe epilepsy before and after anterior temporal lobectomy. J Neurol Neurosurg Psychiatry 68:53–58, 2000

Handal N, Masand P, Weilburg J: Panic disorder and complex partial seizures: a truly complex relationship. Psychosomatics 36:498–502, 1995

Harden CL, Goldstein MA: Mood disorders in patients with epilepsy: epidemiology and management. CNS Drugs 16:291–302, 2002

Hathaway SR, McKinley JC: Minnesota Multiphasic Personality Inventory—2. Minneapolis, University of Minnesota, 1989

Heath RG: Psychosis and epilepsy: similarities and differences in the anatomic-physiologic substrate. Advances in Biological Psychiatry 8:106–116, 1982

Hermann BP, Seidenberg M, Bell B: Psychiatric comorbidity in chronic epilepsy: identification, consequences, and treatment of major depression. Epilepsia 41 (suppl 2):S31–S41, 2000

Ho S, Berkovic S, Berlangieri S, et al: Comparison of ictal SPECT and interictal PET in the presurgical evaluation of TLE. Ann Neurol 37:738–745, 1995

Hoare P: Does illness foster dependency? Dev Med Child Neurol 26:20–24, 1984

International League Against Epilepsy Commission: Proposal for classification of epilepsies and epileptic syndromes. Epilepsia 26:268–278, 1985

International League Against Epilepsy Commission Report: Glossary of descriptive terminology for ictal semiology: report of the ILAE task force on classification and terminology. Epilepsia 42:1212–1218, 2001a

International League Against Epilepsy Commission Report: A proposed diagnostic scheme for people with epileptic seizures and with epilepsy: report of the ILAE Task Force on Classification and Terminology. Epilepsia 42:796–803, 2001b

Jann MW, Ereshefsky L, Saklad SR, et al: Effects of carbamazepine on plasma haloperidol levels. J Clin Psychopharmacol 5:106–109, 1985

Jones JE, Hermann BP, Barry JJ, et al: Rates and risk factors for suicide, suicidal ideation, and suicide attempts in chronic epilepsy. Epilepsy Behav 4:S31–S38, 2003

Kanner AM: Depression in epilepsy: a frequently neglected multifaceted disorder. Epilepsy Behav 4:S11–S19, 2003

Kanner AM, Nieto JC: Depressive disorders in epilepsy. Neurology 53 (5 suppl 2):S26–S32, 1999

Ketter T, Post R, Theodore W: Positive and negative psychiatric effects of antiepileptic drugs in patients with seizure disorders. Neurology 53 (suppl 2):S53–S67, 1999

Kidron R, Averbuch I, Klein E, et al: Carbamazepine-induced reduction of blood levels of haloperidol in chronic schizophrenia. Biol Psychiatry 20:219–222, 1985

Kirubakaran V, Sen S, Wilkinson C: Catatonic stupor: unusual manifestation of TLE. Psychiatr J Univ Ott 12:244–246, 1987

Kristensen O, Sindrup EH: Psychomotor epilepsy and psychosis, II: electroencephalographic findings. Acta Neurol Scand 57:370–379, 1978

Kuyk J, Spinhoven P, Boas W, et al: Dissociation in temporal lobe epilepsy and pseudo-epileptic seizure patients. J Nerv Ment Dis 187:713–720, 1999

Lambert MV, Robertson MM: Depression in epilepsy: etiology, phenomenology, and treatment. Epilepsia 40 (suppl 10):S21–S47, 1999

Landolt H: Serial encephalographic investigations during psychotic episodes in epileptic patients and during schizophrenic attacks, in Lectures on Epilepsy. Edited by Lorentz de Haas AM. London, England, Elsevier, 1958, pp 91–133

Laskowitz D, Sperling M, French J, et al: The syndrome of frontal lobe epilepsy. Neurology 45:780–787, 1995

Levinson D, Devinsky O: Psychiatric events during vigabatrin therapy. Neurology 53:1503–1511, 1999

Malkowicz D, Legido A, Jackel R, et al: Prolactin secretion following repetitive seizures. Neurology 45:448–452, 1995

Mann JJ: Violence and aggression, in Psychopharmacology: The Fourth Generation of Progress. Edited by Bloom FE, Kupfer DJ. New York, Raven, 1995, pp 1919–1928

Mathers CB: Group therapy in the management of epilepsy. Br J Med Psychol 65:279–287, 1992

McElroy S, Keck P, Pope H, et al: Valproate in primary psychiatric disorders, in Use of Anticonvulsants in Psychiatry. Edited by McElroy S, Pope H. Clifton, NJ, Oxford Health Care, 1988, pp 25–42

McNamara ME, Fogel BS: Anticonvulsant-responsive panic attacks with temporal lobe EEG abnormalities. J Neuropsychiatry Clin Neurosci 2:193–196, 1990

Meador KJ, Loring DW, Abney OL, et al: Effects of carbamazepine and phenytoin on EEG and memory in healthy adults. Epilepsia 34:153–157, 1993

Mendez MF, Doss RC, Taylor JL, et al: Depression in epilepsy: relationship to seizures and anticonvulsant therapy. J Nerv Ment Dis 181:444–447, 1993

Metrakos K, Metrakos JD: Genetics of convulsive disorders, II: genetics and encephalographic studies in centrencephalic epilepsy. Neurology 11:454–483, 1961

Moehle KA, Bolter JF, Long CJ: The relationship between neuropsychological functioning and psychopathology in temporal lobe epileptic patients. Epilepsia 25:418–422, 1984

Neppe VM, Kaplan C: Short-term treatment of atypical spells with carbamazepine. Clin Neuropharmacol 11:287–289, 1988

Neppe VM, Tucker GJ: Modern perspectives on epilepsy in relation to psychiatry: behavioral disturbances of epilepsy. Hosp Community Psychiatry 39:389–396, 1988

Neppe VM, Tucker GJ, Wilensky AJ: Fundamentals of carbamazepine use in neuropsychiatry. J Clin Psychiatry 49 (suppl 4):4–6, 1988

Neppe VM, Bowman B, Sawchuk KSLJ: Carbamazepine for atypical psychosis with episodic hostility: a preliminary study. J Nerv Ment Dis 179:339–340, 1991

Nilsson L, Ahlbom A, Farahmand BY, et al. Risk factors for suicide in epilepsy: a case control study. Epilepsia 43:664–651, 2002

Novak J, Corke P, Fairley N: "Petit mal status" in adults. Dis Nerv Syst 32:245–248, 1971

Oxbury S, Oxbury J, Renowden S, et al: Severe amnesia: an unusual late complication after temporal lobectomy. Neuropsychologia 35:975–988, 1997

Perucca E, Manzo L, Crema A: Pharmacokinetic interactions between antiepileptic and psychotropic drugs, in The Psychopharmacology of Epilepsy. Edited by Trimble M. Chichester, UK, Wiley, 1985, pp 95–105

Pincus JH, Tucker GJ: Behavioral Neurology, 3rd Edition. New York, Oxford University Press, 1985

Popkin M, Tucker GJ: Mental disorders due to a general medical condition and substance-induced disorders: mood, anxiety, psychotic, catatonic, and personality disorders, in DSM-IV Source Book. Edited by Widiger T, Frances J, Pincus HA, et al. Washington, DC, American Psychiatric Press, 1994, pp 243–276

Popli A, Kando J, Pillay S, et al: Occurrence of seizures related to psychotropic medication among psychiatric inpatients. Psychiatr Serv 46:486–488, 1995

Post RM, Uhde TW, Joffe RT, et al: Anticonvulsant drugs in psychiatric illness: new treatment alternatives and theoretical implications, in The Psychopharmacology of Epilepsy. Edited by Trimble MR. Chichester, UK, Wiley, 1985, pp 141–171

Preskorn SH, Fast GA: Tricyclic antidepressant-induced seizures and plasma drug concentration. J Clin Psychiatry 53:160–162, 1992

Prueter C, Norra C: Mood disorders and their treatment in patients with epilepsy. J Neuropsychiatry Clin Neurosci 17:20–28, 2005

Pulliainen V, Jokelainen M: Effects of phenytoin and carbamazepine on cognitive functions in newly diagnosed epileptic patients. Acta Neurol Scand 89:81–86, 1994

Pulliainen V, Kuikka P, Jokelainen M: Motor and cognitive functions in newly diagnosed adult seizure patients before antiepileptic medication. Acta Neurol Scand 101:73–78, 2000

Regan KJ, Banks GK, Beran RG: Therapeutic recreation programmes for children with epilepsy. Seizure 2:195–200, 1993

Rodin EA: Psychomotor epilepsy and aggressive behavior. Arch Gen Psychiatry 28:210–213, 1973

Rosenstein DL, Nelson JC, Jacobs SC, et al: Seizures associated with antidepressants: a review. J Clin Psychiatry 54:289–299, 1993

Roth M, Harper M: Temporal lobe epilepsy and the phobic anxiety-depersonalization syndrome, II: practical and theoretical considerations. Compr Psychiatry 3:215–226, 1962

Ryback R, Gardner E: Limbic system dysrhythmia: a diagnostic EEG procedure utilizing procaine activation. J Neuropsychiatry Clin Neurosci 3:321–329, 1991

Sackeim HA: The anticonvulsant hypothesis of the mechanisms of action of ECT: current status. J ECT 15:5–26, 1999

Sadler M, Goodwin J: The sensitivity of various electrodes in the detection of epilepsy from potential patients with partial complex seizures (letter). Epilepsia 27:627, 1986

Schiffer R: Epilepsy, psychosis, and forced normalization (editorial). Arch Neurol 44:253, 1987

Schoenenberger R, Tonasijevic M, Jha A, et al: Appropriateness of antiepileptic drug level monitoring. JAMA 274:1622–1626, 1995

Shukla G, Bhatia M, Vivekanandhan S: Serum prolactin levels for differentiation of nonepileptic versus true seizures: limited utility. Epilepsy Behav 5:517–521, 2004

Shukla S, Godwin CD, Long LE, et al: Lithium-carbamazepine neurotoxicity and risk factors. Am J Psychiatry 141:1604–1606, 1984

Silver JM, Hales RE, Yudofsky SC: Psychopharmacology of depression in neurologic disorders. J Clin Psychiatry 51:33–39, 1990

Slater E, Beard AW, Glithero E: The schizophrenia-like psychoses of epilepsy. Br J Psychiatry 109:95–150, 1963

Sloviter RS, Tamminga CA: Cortex, VII: the hippocampus in epilepsy (letter). Am J Psychiatry 152:659, 1995

Stevens JR: Psychiatric aspects of epilepsy. J Clin Psychiatry 49 (suppl 4):49–57, 1988

Szatmari P: Some methodologic criteria for studies in developmental neuropsychiatry. Psychiatr Dev 3:153–170, 1985

Temkin O: The Falling Sickness, 2nd Edition. Baltimore, MD, Johns Hopkins University Press, 1979

Thomas M, Jankovic J: Psychogenic movement disorders: diagnosis and management. CNS Drugs 18:437–452, 2004

Thomas P, Zifkin B, Migneco O, et al: Nonconvulsive status epilepticus of frontal origin. Neurology 52:1174–1183, 1999

Tojek TM, Lumley M, Barkley G, et al: Stress and other psychosocial characteristics of patients with psychogenic nonepileptic seizures. Psychosomatics 41:221–226, 2000

Toone BK, Garralda ME, Ron MA: The psychoses of epilepsy and the functional psychoses: a clinical and phenomenological comparison. Br J Psychiatry 141:256–261, 1982

Trimble MR: The relationship between epilepsy and schizophrenia: a biochemical hypothesis. Biol Psychiatry 12:299–304, 1977

Trimble MR: The effects of anticonvulsant drugs on cognitive abilities. Pharmacol Ther 4:677–685, 1979

Trimble MR: Cognitive hazards of seizure disorders. Epilepsia 29 (suppl 1):S19–S24, 1988

Trimble MR, Thompson PJ: Anticonvulsant drugs, cognitive impairment, and behavior. Epilepsia 24 (suppl):S55–S63, 1983

Tucker GJ: Current diagnostic issues in neuropsychiatry, in Neuropsychiatry. Edited by Fogel BS, Schiffer RB. Baltimore, MD, Williams & Wilkins, 1996, pp 1009–1014

Von Meduna L: Die Konvulsionstherapie der Schizophrenia. Halle, Germany, Marhold, 1937

Vukmir RB: Does serum prolactin indicate the presence of seizure in the emergency department patient? J Neurol 251:736–739, 2004

Willert C, Spitzer C, Kusserow S, et al: Serum neuron-specific enolase, prolactin, and creatine kinase after epileptic and psychogenic non-epileptic seizures. Acta Neurol Scand 109:318–323, 2004

Ziegler R: Epilepsy: individual illness, human prediscontent and family dilemma. Fam Relat 31:435–444, 1982

Zimmerman AW: Hormones and epilepsy. Neurol Clin 4:853–861, 1986

Zwil AS, Pelchat RJ: ECT in the treatment of patients with neurological and somatic disease. Int J Psychiatry Med 24:1–29, 1994

8

NEUROPSYCHIATRIC ASPECTS OF CEREBROVASCULAR DISORDERS

Robert G. Robinson, M.D.
Sergio E. Starkstein, M.D., Ph.D.

Stroke is the most common serious neurological disorder in the world and is the leading cause of long-term disability. Stroke accounts for half of all the acute hospitalizations for neurological disease and according to the American Heart Association, there are 700,000 new strokes annually and 5.5 million survivors of stroke in the United States, with 10% of individuals over age 75 years being stroke survivors (Thom et al. 2006).

The neuropsychiatric complications of cerebrovascular disease include a wide range of emotional and cognitive disturbances. In this chapter we present the latest research on many of the emotional disorders associated with stroke.

CLASSIFICATION OF CEREBROVASCULAR DISEASE

Although there are many ways to classify the wide range of disorders that constitute cerebrovascular disease from the perspective of its neuropsychiatric complications, probably the most pragmatic way of classifying this disease is to examine the means by which parenchymal changes in the brain occur. The first of these, ischemia, may occur either with or without infarction of parenchyma and includes transient ischemic attacks, atherosclerotic thrombosis, cerebral embolism, and hemorrhage. The last of these, hemorrhage, may cause either direct parenchymal damage by extravasation of blood into the surrounding brain tissue, as in intracerebral hemorrhage, or indirect damage by hemorrhage into the ventricles, subarachnoid space, extradural area, or subdural area. These changes result in a common mode of expression, defined by Adams and Victor (1985) as a sudden, convulsive, focal neurological deficit, or stroke.

To expand slightly on this categorization (i.e., the means by which parenchymal changes occur), there are four major categories of cerebrovascular disease. These include 1) atherosclerotic thrombosis, 2) cerebral embolism, 3) lacunae, and 4) intracranial hemorrhage. In various studies of the incidence of cerebrovascular disease (e.g., Wolf et al. 1977), the ratio of infarcts to hemorrhages has been shown to be about 5:1. Atherosclerotic thrombosis and cerebral embolism each account for approximately one-third of all incidents of stroke.

NEUROPSYCHIATRIC SYNDROMES ASSOCIATED WITH CEREBROVASCULAR DISEASE

A number of emotional disorders, many of which are discussed in this section, have been associated with cerebrovascular disease. The neuropsychiatric disorder that has received the greatest amount of investigation, however, is poststroke depression (PSD).

POSTSTROKE DEPRESSION

Diagnosis

Although strict diagnostic criteria have not been used in some studies of emotional disorders associated with cerebrovascular disease (Andersen et al. 1993), most studies have used structured interviews and diagnostic criteria defined by DSM-IV-TR (American Psychiatric Association 2000) or Research Diagnostic Criteria (Aben et al. 2002; E. Cassidy et al. 2004; Morris et al. 1990). Poststroke major depression is now categorized in DSM-IV-TR (American Psychiatric Association 2000) as "mood disorder due to stroke with major depressive-like episode" (pp 404–405). For patients with less severe forms of depression, there are

"research criteria" in DSM-IV-TR for minor depression (i.e., subsyndromal major depression; depression or anhedonia with at least one but fewer than four additional symptoms of major depression) or, alternatively, a diagnosis of mood disorder due to stroke with depressive features (i.e., depressed mood but criteria for major depression not met).

Phenomenology

Lipsey et al. (1986) examined the frequency of depressive symptoms in a group of 43 patients with major PSD compared with that in a group of 43 age-matched patients with "functional" (i.e., no known brain pathology) depression. The main finding was that both groups showed almost identical profiles of symptoms, including those that were not part of the diagnostic criteria. More than 50% of the patients who met the diagnostic criteria for major PSD reported sadness, anxiety, tension, loss of interest and concentration, sleep disturbances with early morning awakening, loss of appetite with weight loss, difficulty concentrating and thinking, and thoughts of death.

Prevalence

In recent years there have been a large number of studies around the world examining the prevalence of PSD. These publications indicate an increasing interest among clinicians caring for poststroke patients in the frequency and significance of depression following stroke. The findings of many of these studies are shown in Table 8–1. In general, these studies have found similar rates of major and minor depression among patients hospitalized for acute stroke, in rehabilitation hospitals, and in outpatient clinics. The mean frequency of major depression among patients in acute and rehabilitation hospitals was 21.6% for major depression and 20% for minor depression (Robinson 2006). Among patients studied in community settings, however, the mean prevalence of major depression was 14% and minor depression was 9.1% (Robinson 2006). Thus, PSD is common both among patients who are receiving treatment for stroke and among community samples. The higher rates of depression among patients who were receiving treatment for stroke are probably related to the greater severity of stroke seen in treatment settings compared with community settings, in which many patients have no physical or intellectual impairment.

Duration

A series of 142 acute stroke patients was prospectively studied in a 2-year longitudinal study of PSD (Robinson 2006). At the time of the initial in-hospital evaluation, 19% of the patients had the DSM-IV-TR symptom cluster of major depression, whereas 25% had the symptom cluster of minor depression. Of those with major depression, 47% still had major depression at the 6-month follow-up evaluation, whereas only 11% of the original group still had major depression at 1-year follow-up, and none were still depressed at 2 years (Figure 8–1). In contrast, however, patients with minor depression had a less favorable prognosis; more than 50% of the patients with in-hospital minor depression continued to have major or minor depression throughout the 2-year follow-up. In addition, about 30% of patients who were not depressed in the hospital became depressed after discharge. Thus, the natural course of major depression appeared to be between 6 months and 1 year, whereas the duration of minor depression was more variable, and in many cases the patients appeared to be chronically depressed.

Morris et al. (1990) found that among a group of 99 patients in a stroke rehabilitation hospital in Australia, those with major depression had a mean duration of major depression of 40 weeks, whereas those with adjustment disorders (minor depression) had a duration of depression of only 12 weeks. These findings confirm that major depression has a duration of approximately 9 months to 1 year but suggest that among 80 patients with acute stroke, 27 (34%) developed major depression in the hospital or at 3-month follow-up. Of these patients with major depression, 15 (60%) had re-

covered by 1-year follow-up, but by 3-year follow-up, only 1 more patient had recovered.

Although all studies found that the majority of depressions were less than 1 year in duration, the mean frequency of major depression that was persistent beyond 1 year was 26%.

Relationship to Lesion Variables

Relationship between depressive disorder and lesion location has been perhaps the most controversial area of research in the field of post-stroke mood disorder. Although establishing an association between specific clinical symptoms and lesion location is one of the fundamental goals of clinical practice in neurology, this has rarely been the case with psychiatric disorders. Cognitive impairment, speech impairment, and the extent and severity of motor or sensory impairment are all symptoms of stroke that are commonly used by clinicians to localize lesions to particular brain regions. There is, however, no known neuropathology consistently associated with primary mood disorders (i.e., mood disorders without known brain injury) or secondary mood disorders (i.e., mood disorders associated with a physical illness). The idea that there may be a neuropathology associated with a development of major depression has led to both surprise and skepticism.

The first study to report a significant correlation of clinical to pathological variables in PSD was an investigation by Robinson and Szetela (1981) of 29 patients with left hemisphere brain injury secondary to stroke ($n = 18$) or to traumatic brain injury ($n = 11$). Based on localization of the lesion by computed tomography (CT), there was a significant inverse correlation between the severity of depression and the distance of the anterior border of the lesion from the frontal pole ($r = 0.76$). This surprising finding led to a number of subsequent examinations of this phenomenon in other populations. A meta-analysis by Narushima et al. (2003) found eight independent studies of severity of depression and proximity of the stroke lesion to the right or left frontal pole done within the first 6 months

TABLE 8–1. Prevalence studies of poststroke depression

Study	Patient population	N	Criteria	% Major	% Minor	Total %
Finset et al. 1989	Rehab hospital	42	Cutoff score			36
Morris et al. 1990	Rehab hospital	99	CIDI, DSM-III	14	21	35
Schubert et al. 1992	Rehab hospital	18	DSM-III-R	28	44	72
Gainotti et al. 1999	Rehab hospital	153	DSM-III-R	31	NR	31+
Schwartz et al. 1993	Rehab hospital	91	DSM-III	40		40[a]
E. Cassidy et al. 2004	Rehab hospital	91	DSM-IV	20	NR	20
Spalletta et al. 2005	Rehab hospital	200	SCID, DSM IV	25	31	56
Feibel and Springer 1982	Outpatient (6 months)	91	Nursing evaluation			26
Robinson and Price 1982	Outpatient (6 months–10 years)	103	Cutoff score			29
Collin et al. 1987	Outpatient	111	Cutoff score			42
Astrom et al. 1993a, 1993b	Outpatient					
	(3 months)	73	DSM-III	31	NR	31[a]
	(1 year)	73	DSM-III	16	NR	16[a]
	(2 years)	57	DSM-III	19	NR	19[a]
	(3 years)	49	DSM-III	29	NR	29[a]
Castillo et al. 1995	Outpatient					
	(3 months)	77	PSE, DSM-III	20	13	33
	(6 months)	80	PSE, DSM-III	21	21	42
	(1 year)	70	PSE, DSM-III	11	16	27
	(2 years)	67	PSE, DSM-III	18	17	35
Pohjasvaara et al. 1998	Outpatient	277	DSM-III-R	26	14	40
Dennis et al. 2000	Outpatient (6 months)	309	Cutoff score			38
N. Herrmann et al. 1998	Outpatient					
	(3 months)	150	Cutoff score			27
	(1 year)	136				22

TABLE 8–1. Prevalence studies of poststroke depression (continued)

Study	Patient population	N	Criteria	% Major	% Minor	Total %
Kotila et al. 1998	Outpatient					
	(3 months)	321	Cutoff score			47
	(1 year)	311				48
Wade et al. 1987	Community	379	Cutoff score			30
House et al. 1991	Community	89	PSE, DSM-III	11	12	23
Burvill et al. 1995	Community	294	PSE, DSM-III	15	8	23
Ebrahim et al. 1987	Acute hospital	149	Cutoff score			23
Fedoroff et al. 1991	Acute hospital	205	PSE, DSM-III	22	19	41
Castillo et al. 1995	Acute hospital	291	PSE, DSM-III	20	18	38
Starkstein et al. 1992	Acute hospital	80	PSE, DSM-III	16	13	29
Astrom et al. 1993a, 1993b	Acute hospital	80	DSM-III	25	NR	25[a]
M. Herrmann et al. 1993	Acute hospital	21	RDC	24	14	38
Andersen et al. 1994a	Acute hospital or outpatient	285	Ham-D cutoff	10	11	21
Aben et al. 2002	Acute hospital	190	SCID, DSM-IV	23	16	39
			Mean	20	21	34[a]

Note. CIDI = Composite International Diagnostic Interview; DSM-III = *Diagnostic and Statistical Manual of Mental Disorders, 3rd Edition*; DSM-III-R = *Diagnostic and Statistical Manual of Mental Disorders, 3rd Edition, Revised*; DSM-IV = *Diagnostic and Statistical Manual of Mental Disorders, 4th Edition*; Ham-D = Hamilton Rating Scale for Depression; NR = not reported; PSE = Present State Examination; RDC = Research Diagnostic Criteria; SADS = Schedule for Affective Disorders and Schizophrenia; SCID = Structured Clinical Interview for DSM-IV.
[a]Because depression was not included, these values may be low.

Source. Reprinted from Robinson RG: *The Clinical Neuropsychiatry of Stroke*, 2nd Edition. Cambridge, UK, Cambridge University Press, 2006. Used with permission.

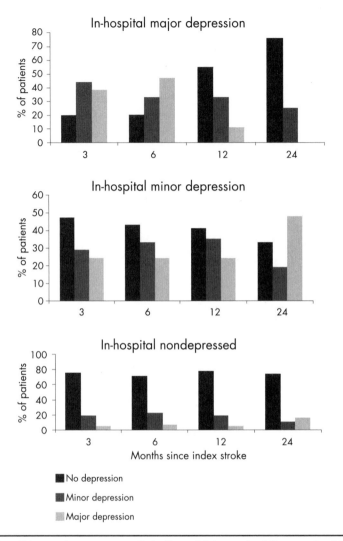

FIGURE 8–1. Diagnostic outcome at 3, 6, 12, and 24 months follow-up for 142 patients based on their in-hospital diagnoses of DSM-IV major depression (n=27), DSM-IV minor depression (n=36), or no mood disorder (n=79).

Among the patients with in-hospital major depression (*top panel*), note the increase in the nondepressed group at 12 and 24 months. This is not seen in the minor depression patients (*middle panel*). About 25% of the initially nondepressed patients were found to have a depression diagnosis at follow-up.

Source.   Reprinted from Robinson RG: *The Clinical Neuropsychiatry of Stroke*, 2nd Edition. Cambridge, UK, Cambridge University Press, 2006. Used with permission.

following stroke. In total, 163 patients had an overall correlation coefficient of –0.53 using fixed and –0.59 using random model assumptions ($P < 0.001$). In the right hemisphere, however, a total of 106 patients had nonsignificant correlations between severity of depression and distance of the lesions from the right

frontal pole ($r = -0.20$, fixed model; $r = -0.23$, random model) (Narushima et al. 2003).

In addition, however, lesion location also influences the frequency of depression. In a study of 45 patients who were on average 2–3 weeks poststroke with single lesions restricted to either cortical or subcortical structures in the left or right hemisphere, Starkstein et al. (1987b) found that 44% of patients with left cortical lesions were depressed, whereas 39% of patients with left subcortical lesions, 11% of patients with right cortical lesions, and 14% of patients with right subcortical lesions were depressed. When patients were further divided into those with anterior and those with posterior lesions, 5 of 5 patients with left cortical lesions involving the frontal lobe had depression compared with 2 of 11 patients with left cortical posterior lesions. Moreover, 4 of the 6 patients with left subcortical anterior lesions had depression compared with 1 of 7 patients with left subcortical posterior lesions.

Based on the finding that PSD and lesion location were dependent on time since stroke, Robinson (2003) conducted a meta-analysis of studies conducted within 2 months following stroke, comparing the frequency of major depression among patients with left anterior versus left posterior lesions and left anterior versus right anterior lesions (Table 8–2). There were 128 patients in the left anterior–left posterior comparison, with a fixed model odds ratio (OR) of 2.29 (95% confidence interval [CI] 1.6–3.4, $P < 0.001$) and random model OR of 2.29 (95% CI 1.5–3.4, $P < 0.001$). Similarly, the comparison of left and right anterior lesions had an OR of 2.18 (fixed model: 95% CI 1.4–3.3, $P < 0.001$) and 2.16 (random model: 95% CI 1.3–3.6, $P < 0.004$), respectively.

This study suggests that the failure of other investigators to replicate the association of left anterior lesion location with increased frequency of depression may in most cases be related to time since stroke. The lateralized effect of left anterior lesions on both major and minor depression is a phenomenon of the acute poststroke period when the patients are less than 2 months poststroke. The most recent review by Bhogal al. (2004) concluded that the association between left hemisphere lesion location and PSD was dependent on whether the patients were inpatients or community patients (OR = 1.36, 95% CI 1.05–1.76, $P < 0.05$) or acute patients versus chronic patients (OR acute = 2.14, 95% CI 1.5–3.04, $P < 0.05$).

Premorbid Risk Factors

The studies just reviewed indicate that although a significant proportion of patients with left anterior or right posterior lesions develop PSD, not every patient with a lesion in these locations developed a depressive mood. This observation raises the question of why clinical variability occurs and why some but not all patients with lesions in these locations develop depression.

Starkstein et al. (1988b) examined these questions by comparing 13 patients with major PSD with 13 stroke patients without depression, all of whom had lesions of the same size and location. Eleven pairs of patients had left hemisphere lesions; two pairs had right hemisphere lesions. Damage was cortical in 10 pairs and subcortical in 3 pairs. The groups did not differ on important demographic variables, such as age, sex, socioeconomic status, or education. They also did not differ on family or personal history of psychiatric disorders or neurological deficits. Patients with major PSD, however, had significantly more subcortical atrophy ($P < 0.05$), as measured both by the ratio of third ventricle to brain (i.e., the area of the third ventricle divided by the area of the brain at the same level) and by the ratio of lateral ventricle to brain (i.e., the area of the body of the lateral ventricle contralateral to the brain lesion divided by the brain area at the same level). It is likely that the subcortical atrophy preceded the stroke. Thus, a mild degree of subcortical atrophy may be a premorbid risk factor that increases the risk of developing major depression following a stroke.

In summary, lesion location is not the only factor that influences the development of PSD. Subcortical atrophy that probably precedes the stroke and a family or personal history of affective disorders also seem to play an important role. The most consistently identified risk factor for depression, however, is severity of functional physical impairment.

Relationship to Physical Impairment

Numerous investigators have reported a significant association between depression and func-

TABLE 8–2.   Meta-analysis of the relationship of depression to lesion location

Study	N	L ant.	L post.	RR	95% CI	P	N	L ant.	R ant.	RR	95% CI	P
Astrom et al. 1993b	21	12/14	2/7	2.62*	1.20–8.63	0.017	25	12/13	2/12	5.54*	1.55–19.82	0.000
Morris et al. 1996	20	9/10	3/10	3.00*	1.14–7.91	0.006	29	9/14	3/15	3.21*	1.08–9.51	0.016
Robinson et al. 1984	18	6/7	4/11	2.36*	1.02–5.45	0.040	16	6/6	4/10	2.27*	1.09–4.75	0.028
Robinson et al. 1986b	15	6/7	2/8	2.35*	1.16–9.54	0.019	11	6/6	2/5	2.23	0.85–5.87	0.46
House et al. 1990	13	1/1	7/12	1.3	0.52–3.28	0.642	15	1/1	7/14	1.50	0.58–3.87	0.506
M. Herrmann 1995	17	7/7	3/10	2.95*	1.21–7.13	0.007	NA	NA	NA	NA	NA	NA
Gainotti et al. 1999	22	1/4	8/18	0.56	0.95–3.32	0.474	16	1/4	8/12	0.38	0.07–2.15	0.146
Fixed combined	128	42/50	29/76	2.29*	1.6–3.4	0.000	112	35/44	26/68	2.18*	1.4–3.3	0.000
Random combined	126	42/50	29/76	2.29*	1.5–3.4	0.000	112	35/44	26/68	2.16*	1.3–3.6	0.004

Note.   Major depression was significantly more frequent following left anterior (L ant.) lesions than right anterior (R ant.) or left posterior (L post.) lesions. CI = confidence interval; NA = not applicable; RR = relative risk.
*$P < 0.05$.

Source.   Reprinted from Robinson RG: "The Controversy Over Post-Stroke Depression and Lesion Location." *Psychiatric Times* 20:39–40, 2003. Used with permission.

tional physical impairment (i.e., activities of daily living [ADL]). Of 18 studies involving 3,281 patients, 15 (83%) found a statistically significant relationship between PSD and severity of impairment in ADL. This association, however, might be construed as the severe functional impairment producing depression or, alternatively, the severity of depression influencing the severity of functional impairment. Studies, in fact, support both interpretations.

Narushima and Robinson (2003) compared 34 patients who received antidepressant treatment with either nortriptyline (100 mg/day) or fluoxetine (40 mg/day) for 12 weeks beginning 19–25 days after stroke with 28 patients who received the same antidepressant treatment but began at 140 (± 28 SD) days poststroke. During the period from 6 to 24 months following stroke, with the two groups matched for time since stroke, there was a significant group by time interaction using either intention-to-treat or efficacy analysis (Figure 8–2). The early-treatment group continued to show gradual recovery in ADL over 2 years, whereas the late-treatment group showed gradual deterioration between the 12- and 24-month follow-ups. A logistic regression analysis examining the effects of diagnosis (depressed or nondepressed), medication (fluoxetine or nortriptyline), presence of severe motor impairment (National Institutes of Health stroke scale rating), presence of prior psychiatric history, use of antidepressants beyond the 12-week study period, and use of early versus late antidepressant treatment showed that only the use of early versus late antidepressants predicted ADL scores at 2-year follow-up (Narushima and Robinson 2003).

Relationship to Cognitive Impairment

Numerous investigators have reported that elderly patients with functional major depression have intellectual deficits that improve with treatment of depression (Robinson et al. 1986a). This issue was first examined in patients with PSD by Robinson et al. (1986a).

Patients with major depression after a left hemisphere infarct were found to have significantly lower (more impaired) scores on the Mini-Mental State Examination (MMSE) (Folstein et al. 1975) than did a comparable group of nondepressed patients. Both the size of patients' lesions and their depression scores correlated independently with severity of cognitive impairment.

In a second study (Starkstein et al. 1988b), stroke patients with and without major depression were matched for lesion location and volume. Of 13 patients with major PSD, 10 had an MMSE score lower than that of their matched control subjects, 2 had the same score, and only 1 patient had a higher score ($P < 0.001$). Thus, even when patients were matched for lesion size and location, depressed patients were more cognitively impaired.

In a follow-up study, Bolla-Wilson et al. (1989) administered a comprehensive neuropsychological battery and found that patients with major depression and left hemisphere lesions had significantly greater cognitive impairments than did nondepressed patients with comparable left hemisphere lesions ($P < 0.05$). These cognitive deficits involved tasks of temporal orientation, language, and executive motor and frontal lobe functions. On the other hand, among patients with right hemisphere lesions, patients with major depression did not differ from nondepressed patients on any of the measures of cognitive impairment.

Spalletta et al. (2002) examined 153 patients with first-ever stroke lesions of the left ($n = 87$) or right ($n = 66$) hemisphere who were less than 1 year poststroke. Patients with left hemisphere lesions and major depression ($n = 30$) showed significantly more impairment on the MMSE than nondepressed patients with left hemisphere lesions ($n = 27$) (MMSE scores: 12.3 ± 9 [SD], major depression; 18.9 ± 8.5 [SD], nondepressed; $P < 0.001$) (Figure 8–3).

Treatment studies of PSD have generally failed to show an improvement in cognitive function even when poststroke mood disorders responded to antidepressant therapy (Andersen et al. 1996). Kimura et al. (2000) exam-

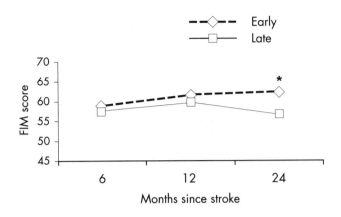

FIGURE 8–2.   Recovery in activities of daily living as measured by the Functional Independence Measure (FIM) over 2 years of follow-up.

All patients were treated for 12 weeks in a double-blind study with fluoxetine or nortriptyline. Patients who received treatment within 1 month poststroke (mean = 2 weeks, "Early") improved significantly more than those who received treatment after the first month poststroke (mean = 12 weeks, "Late"). FIM scores were measured at the same times following stroke to control for group differences in time since stroke when the 3-month treatment was given.
*Intention to treat, $P = 0.02$. Efficacy, $P = 0.02$.

Source.   Reprinted from Robinson RG: *The Clinical Neuropsychiatry of Stroke,* 2nd Edition. Cambridge, UK, Cambridge University Press, 2006. Used with permission.

ined this issue in a study comparing nortriptyline and placebo using a double-blind treatment methodology among patients with major ($n = 33$) or minor ($n = 14$) PSD. Although the groups showed no significant differences in the change in MMSE scores from beginning to end of the treatment study, when patients were divided into those who responded to treatment (i.e., greater than 50% decline in Hamilton Rating Scale for Depression [Ham-D] [Hamilton 1960] score and no longer meeting depression diagnosis criteria) and those who did not respond, there was a significantly greater improvement in MMSE scores among patients who responded to treatment ($n = 24$) compared with patients who did not ($n = 23$) (Figure 8–4). There were no significant differences between the two groups in their baseline Ham-D scores, demographic characteristics, stroke characteristics, or neurological findings. A repeated-measures analysis of variance (ANOVA) demonstrated significant group by time interaction ($P = 0.005$), and planned post hoc comparisons dem-

onstrated that the responders had significantly less impaired MMSE scores than did the nonresponders, at nortriptyline doses of 75 mg ($P = 0.036$) and 100 mg ($P = 0.024$).

Mechanism of Poststroke Depression

Although the cause of PSD remains unknown, one of the mechanisms that has been hypothesized to play an etiological role is dysfunction of the biogenic amine system. The noradrenergic and serotonergic cell bodies are located in the brain stem and send ascending projections through the median forebrain bundle to the frontal cortex. The ascending axons then arc posteriorly and run longitudinally through the deep layers of the cortex, arborizing and sending terminal projections into the superficial cortical layers (Morrison et al. 1979). Lesions that disrupt these pathways in the frontal cortex or the basal ganglia may affect many downstream fibers. On the basis of these neuroanatomical facts and the clinical findings that the severity of depression correlates with the prox-

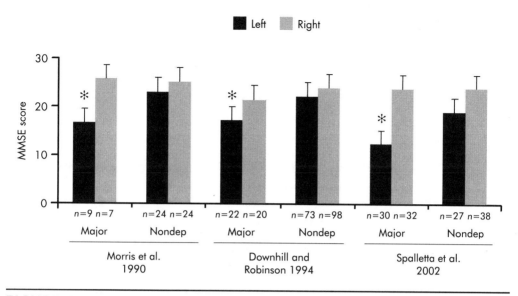

FIGURE 8–3. Mini-Mental State Examination (MMSE) scores following acute stroke in three studies among patients with major or no mood disturbance grouped according to the hemisphere of ischemia.

In all three studies, there was a significant difference between patients with major depression (Major) after left hemisphere stroke and nondepressed (Nondep) patients with similar lesions. Major depression after right hemisphere lesions did not lead to the same phenomenon. Error bars represent the standard deviation divided by the square root of N.
*$P = 0.001$.

Source. Reprinted from Robinson RG: *The Clinical Neuropsychiatry of Stroke, 2nd Edition.* Cambridge, UK, Cambridge University Press, 2006. Used with permission.

imity of the lesion to the frontal pole, Robinson et al. (1984) suggested that PSD may be the consequence of depletions of norepinephrine and/or serotonin produced by lesions in the frontal lobe or basal ganglia.

A hypothesis by Spalletta et al. (2006) suggested that proinflammatory cytokines due to ischemic brain damage may lead to PSD. Stroke is known to produce cytokine release such as intracellular anthocyanin 1 (AN1) or interleukin-1β (IL-1β), which have been found to be elevated in deceased individuals over age 60 years who had a history of major depression compared with control subjects. Cytokines might then activate the enzyme indole-2,3 dioxygenase (IDO), which catabolizes tryptophan, leading to decreased levels of serotonin (Capuron and Dantzer 2003). Thus, depletion of serotonin may trigger depressions following stroke.

Treatment of Poststroke Depression

At the time of this writing, there were eight placebo-controlled, randomized, double-blind treatment studies on the efficacy of single-antidepressant treatment of PSD (Table 8–3). In the first study, Lipsey et al. (1984) examined 14 patients treated with nortriptyline and 20 patients given placebo. The 11 patients treated with nortriptyline who completed the 6-week study showed significantly greater improvement in their Ham-D scores than did 15 placebo-treated patients ($P < 0.01$). In another double-blind controlled trial in which the selective serotonin reuptake inhibitor (SSRI) citalopram was used, improvement in Ham-D scores was significantly greater over 6 weeks in patients receiving active treatment ($n = 27$ completers) than in the placebo group ($n = 32$ completers) (Andersen et al. 1994a).

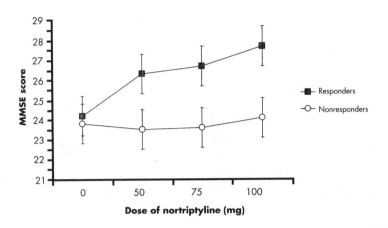

FIGURE 8–4.   Change of Mini-Mental State Examination (MMSE) scores in patients with post-stroke major depression during a double-blind treatment study of nortriptyline versus placebo.

Treatment responders ($n = 15$) showed significantly greater improvement in cognitive function than nonresponders ($n = 18$) ($P = 0.0087$). Error bars represent standard error of the mean (SE).

Source.   Reprinted from Kimura M, Robinson RG, Kosier T: "Treatment of Cognitive Impairment After Poststroke Depression." *Stroke* 31:1482–1486, 2000. Used with permission.

At both 3 and 6 weeks, the group receiving active treatment had significantly lower Ham-D scores than did the group receiving placebo. This study established for the first time the efficacy of an SSRI in the treatment of PSD.

Electroconvulsive therapy has also been reported to be effective for treating PSD (Murray et al. 1986). It causes few side effects and no neurological deterioration. Psychostimulants have also been reported in open-label trials to be effective for the treatment of PSD. Finally, psychological treatment using cognitive-behavioral therapy (CBT) in 123 stroke patients has been found by Lincoln and Flannaghan (2003) to be no more effective than an attention (i.e., placebo) treatment ($n = 39$, CBT completers; $n = 43$, placebo completers).

Psychosocial Adjustment

Thompson et al. (1989) examined 40 stroke patients and their caregivers at an average of 9 months after the occurrence of stroke. They found that a lack of meaningfulness in life and overprotection by the caregiver were independent predictors of depression. Kotila et al. (1998) examined depression after stroke as part of the FINNSTROKE Study. This study examined the effect of active rehabilitation programs after discharge together with support and social activities on the frequency of depression among patients and caregivers at 3 months and 1 year after stroke. At both 3 months and 1 year, the frequency of depression was significantly lower among patients receiving active outpatient treatment (at 3 months, 41% vs. 54% among patients without active rehabilitation programs; at 1 year, 42% vs. 55%). The rate of depression among caregivers was significantly greater at 1 year in districts without active rehabilitation programs than in districts with them ($P = 0.036$). Greater severity of impairment as measured by the Rankin Scale (Rankin 1957) was also associated with increased depression among caregivers at 3 months after stroke.

POSTSTROKE MANIA

Among 366 patients with bipolar disorder, F. Cassidy and Carroll (2002) found that late-onset mania (i.e., after age 47) was significantly associated with risk factors for vascular disease.

TABLE 8–3. Treatment studies of poststroke depression

Study	N	Medication (n) (max dose)	Duration	Evaluation method	Results	Response rate	Completion rate
Double-blind placebo-controlled studies							
Lipsey et al. 1984	34	Nortriptyline (14) (100 mg), placebo (20)	6 weeks	Ham-D, ZDS	Nortriptyline > placebo, intention to treat and efficacy	100% nortriptyline, 33% placebo	11 of 14 nortriptyline, 15 of 20 placebo
Reding et al. 1986	27	Trazodone (7) (200 mg), placebo (9)	32 ± 6 days	ZDS	Trazodone > placebo on Barthel ADL scores for patients with abnormal DST	NR	NR
Andersen et al. 1994b	66	Citalopram (33) (20 mg, 10 mg > 65 years), placebo (33)	6 weeks	Ham-D, MES	Intention-to-treat response rates: citalopram > placebo	61% citalopram, 29% placebo	26 of 33 citalopram, 31 of 33 placebo
Grade et al. 1998	21	Methylphenidate (10) (30 mg), placebo (11)	3 weeks	Ham-D	Intention-to-treat response rates: methylphenidate > placebo	NR	9 of 10 methylphenidate, 10 of 11 placebo
Wiart et al. 2000	31	Fluoxetine (16) (20 mg) placebo (15)	6 weeks	MADRS	Intention-to-treat response rates: fluoxetine > placebo	62% fluoxetine, 33% placebo	14 of 16 fluoxetine, 15 of 15 placebo
Robinson et al. 2000	56	Fluoxetine (23) (40 mg), nortriptyline (16) (100 mg), placebo (17)	12 weeks	Ham-D	Intention-to-treat response rates: nortriptyline > placebo = fluoxetine = placebo	14% fluoxetine, 77% nortriptyline, 31% placebo	14 of 23 fluoxetine, 13 of 16 nortriptyline, 13 of 17 placebo
Fruehwald et al. 2003	54	Fluoxetine (28) (20 mg), placebo (26)	12 weeks	BDI, Ham-D	Ham-D > 15 fluoxetine = placebo Ham-D scores	69% fluoxetine Ham-D < 13, 75% placebo	26 of 28 fluoxetine, 24 of 26 placebo
Rampello et al. 2005	31	Reboxetine (16) (4 mg), placebo (15)	16 weeks	BDI, Ham-D	Reboxetine > placebo for PSD patients with retardation	NR	NR

TABLE 8–3. Treatment studies of poststroke depression (continued)

Study	N	Medication (n) (max dose)	Duration	Evaluation method	Results	Response rate	Completion rate
Double-blind studies without placebo control							
Miyai et al. 2000	24	Desipramine (13) (100 mg), trazodone (6) (100 mg), fluoxetine (5) (20 mg)	4 weeks	Ham-D	Desipramine=trazodone= fluoxetine, no placebo comparison	NR	8 of 13 desipramine, 6 of 6 trazodone, 4 of 5 fluoxetine
Lauritzen et al. 1994	20	Imipramine (mean 75 mg) and mianserin (mean = 25 mg); desipramine (mean 66 mg) and mianserin (mean 27 mg)	6 weeks	Ham-D, MES	Intention-to-treat response rates: imipramine+mianserin >desipramine and mianserin on MES but not Ham-D	Ham-D no different than MES, 81% imipramine + mianserin, 13% desipramine + mianserin	8 of 10 imipramine + mianserin, 5 of 10 desipramine + mianserin

Note. ADL = activities of daily living; BDI = Beck Depression Inventory; DST = dexamethasone suppression test; Ham-D = Hamilton Rating Scale for Depression; MADRS = Montgomery-Åsberg Depression Rating Scale; MES = Melancholia Scale; NR = not reported; PSD = poststroke depression; ZDS = Zung Self-Rating Depression Scale.

Phenomenology of Secondary Mania

Starkstein et al. (1988a) examined a series of 12 consecutive patients who met DSM-III (American Psychiatric Association 1980) criteria for an organic affective syndrome, manic type. These patients, who developed mania after a stroke, traumatic brain injury, or tumors, were compared with patients with functional (i.e., no known neuropathology) mania (Starkstein et al. 1987a). The two groups of patients showed similar frequencies of elation, pressured speech, flight of ideas, grandiose thoughts, insomnia, hallucinations, and paranoid delusions. Thus, the symptoms of mania that occurred after brain damage (secondary mania) appeared to be the same as those found in patients with mania without brain damage (primary mania).

Lesion Location

Several studies of patients with brain damage have found that patients who develop secondary mania have a significantly greater frequency of lesions in the right hemisphere than patients with depression or no mood disturbance. The right hemisphere lesions that lead to mania tend to be in specific right hemisphere structures that have connections to the limbic system. The right basotemporal cortex appears to be particularly important, because direct lesions as well as distant hypometabolic effects (diaschisis) of this cortical region are frequently associated with secondary mania.

Robinson and colleagues (1988) reported on 17 patients with secondary mania. Most had right hemisphere lesions involving either cortical limbic areas, such as the orbitofrontal cortex and the basotemporal cortex, or subcortical nuclei, such as the head of the caudate or the thalamus. The frequency of right hemisphere lesions was significantly greater than in patients with major depression, who tended to have left frontal or basal ganglia lesions.

Risk Factors

Not every patient with a lesion in limbic areas of the right hemisphere will develop secondary mania. Therefore, there must be risk factors for this disorder.

Studies thus far have identified two such factors. One is a genetic vulnerability for affective disorder (Robinson et al. 1988), and the other is a mild degree of subcortical atrophy. The subcortical atrophy probably preceded the stroke, but its cause remains unknown (Starkstein et al. 1987a).

A case report by Starkstein et al. (1989a) suggested that the mechanism of secondary mania is not related to the release of transcallosal inhibitory fibers (i.e., the release of left limbic areas from tonic inhibition due to a right hemisphere lesion). A patient who developed secondary mania after bleeding from a right basotemporal arteriovenous malformation underwent a Wada test before the therapeutic embolization of the malformation. Injection of amobarbital in the left carotid artery did not abolish the manic symptoms (which would be expected if the "release" theory were correct).

Although the mechanism of secondary mania remains unknown, both lesion studies and metabolic studies suggest that the right basotemporal cortex may play an important role. A combination of biogenic amine system dysfunction and release of tonic inhibitory input into the basotemporal cortex and lateral limbic system may lead to the production of mania.

Treatment of Secondary Mania

Although no systematic treatment studies of secondary mania have been conducted, one report suggested several potentially useful treatment modalities. Bakchine et al. (1989) carried out a double-blind, placebo-controlled treatment study in a single patient with secondary mania. Clonidine (0.6 mg/day) rapidly reversed the manic symptoms, whereas carbamazepine (1,200 mg/day) was associated with no mood changes and levodopa (375 mg/day) was associated with an increase in manic symptoms. In other treatment studies, however, the anticonvulsants valproic acid and carbamazepine as well as neuroleptics and lithium therapy have been reported to be useful in treating secondary mania (Starkstein et al. 1991). None of these treatments, however, have been evaluated in double-blind, placebo-controlled studies.

POSTSTROKE BIPOLAR DISORDER

Although some patients have one or more manic episodes after brain injury, other manic patients also have depression after brain injury. In an effort to examine the crucial factors in determining which patients have bipolar as opposed to unipolar disorder, Starkstein et al. (1991) examined 19 patients with the diagnosis of secondary mania. The bipolar (manic-depressive) group consisted of patients who, after the occurrence of the brain lesion, met DSM-III-R (American Psychiatric Association 1987) criteria for organic mood syndrome, mania, followed or preceded by organic mood syndrome, depressed. The unipolar-mania group consisted of patients who met the criteria for mania described previously (i.e., DSM-III-R organic mood syndrome, mania), not followed or preceded by depression. All patients had CT scan evidence of vascular, neoplastic, or traumatic brain lesion and no history of other neurological, toxic, or metabolic conditions.

Patients in the bipolar group were found to have significantly greater intellectual impairment as measured by MMSE scores ($P < 0.05$). Almost half of the patients in the bipolar group had recurrent episodes of depression, whereas approximately one-fourth of patients in both the unipolar and bipolar groups had recurrent episodes of mania.

Of the 7 patients with bipolar disorder, 6 had lesions restricted to the right hemisphere, which involved the head of the caudate nucleus (2 patients); the thalamus (3 patients); and the head of the caudate nucleus, the dorsolateral frontal cortex, and the basotemporal cortex (1 patient). The remaining patient developed bipolar illness after surgical removal of a pituitary adenoma. In contrast to the primarily subcortical lesions in the bipolar group, 8 of 12 patients in the unipolar-mania group had lesions restricted to the right hemisphere, which involved the basotemporal cortex (6 patients), orbitofrontal cortex (1 patient), and head of the caudate nucleus (1 patient). The remaining 4 patients had bilateral lesions involving the orbitofrontal cortex (3 patients) and the orbitofrontal white matter (1 patient) (Starkstein et al. 1991).

This study suggests that a prior episode of depression may have occurred in about one-third of patients with secondary mania. Patients with bipolar disorder tend to have subcortical lesions (mainly involving the right head of the caudate or the right thalamus), whereas patients with pure mania tend to show a higher frequency of cortical lesions (particularly in the right orbitofrontal and right basotemporal cortices). Finally, bipolar patients tend to have greater cognitive impairment than do patients with unipolar mania, which may either reflect differences in lesion location or suggest that the presence of a previous episode of depression may produce residual cognitive effects.

POSTSTROKE ANXIETY DISORDER

Castillo et al. (1993, 1995) found that 78 patients (27%) of a group of 288 patients hospitalized with an acute stroke met DSM-III-R criteria for generalized anxiety disorder (GAD) (excluding the 6-month duration criteria). Most patients with GAD also had major or minor depression (i.e., 58 of 78 patients with GAD also had depression). Depression plus anxiety was associated with left cortical lesions, whereas anxiety alone was associated with right hemisphere lesions. In a 2-year follow-up in a subgroup of 142 of these 288 patients, it was found that 32 (23%) developed GAD after the initial in-hospital evaluation (i.e., between 3 and 24 months after stroke). Early-onset but not late-onset GAD was associated with a history of psychiatric disorder, including alcohol abuse, and early-onset anxiety had a mean duration of 1.5 months, whereas delayed-onset GAD had a mean duration of 3 months (Castillo et al. 1995).

Astrom (1996) examined 71 acute stroke patients for anxiety disorder and followed these patients over 3 years. The strongest correlates of GAD were the absence of social contacts outside the family and dependence of patients on others to perform their primary ADL. These factors were significantly more common in the GAD compared with the non-

GAD population at 3 months, 1 year, 2 years, and 3 years after stroke. At 3-year follow-up, however, GAD was associated with both cortical atrophy (7 of 7 GAD patients had cortical atrophy vs. 19 of 39 non-GAD patients) and greater subcortical atrophy (as measured by frontal horn ratios on CT scan, $P = 0.03$).

Shimoda and Robinson (1998) examined the effect of GAD on outcome in patients with stroke. A group of 142 patients examined during hospitalization for acute stroke and followed for 2 years were diagnosed with GAD ($n = 9$), major depressive disorder alone ($n = 10$), both GAD and major depression ($n = 10$), or neither GAD nor depression ($n = 36$). An examination of the effect of GAD and major depression at the time of the initial hospital evaluation on recovery in ADL at short-term follow-up (3–6 months) demonstrated a significant effect of major depression but no significant effect of GAD and no interaction. At long-term follow-up (1–2 years), however, there was a significant interaction between major depression and GAD to inhibit recovery in ADL.

Similarly, an analysis of social functioning at short-term follow-up showed significant main effects of both major depression and GAD but no interaction (Shimoda and Robinson 1998). At long-term follow-up there were significant interactions between GAD and time as well as between major depression, GAD, and time. These findings indicate that patients with GAD were more impaired in their social functioning over the entire 2-year follow-up period and that patients with major depression plus GAD had the most severe impairment in social functioning of any group. Perhaps the most significant finding from this study, however, was that major depressive disorder and anxiety disorder diagnosed at the time of the initial in-hospital evaluation had a greater effect on impairment in ADL at 1-year and 2-year follow-up than major depression alone, anxiety disorder alone, or no mood or anxiety disturbance. These findings suggest that anxiety disorder is an important variable affecting long-term prognosis after stroke.

A treatment study has examined the effect of nortriptyline on GAD that is comorbid with PSD (Kimura and Robinson 2003). The study included 29 patients who met criteria for GAD (17 with comorbid major depression, 10 with minor depression, and 2 with no depression). Analysis of the 27 GAD patients with comorbid depression used an intention-to-treat analysis that included 4 patients who dropped out of the study. There were no significant differences between nortriptyline and the placebo-treated patients in background characteristics, including age, education, and time since stroke. There were also no significant differences between actively treated and placebo-treated patients in their neurological findings or the nature of the stroke lesion. In the group treated with nortriptyline, 54% of the patients had right hemisphere lesion; 64% of the placebo group had similar lesions. Motor impairments were present in 77% of the nortriptyline-treated patients and in 86% of the placebo-treated patients. Aphasia was found in 23% of the nortriptyline-treated patients and in 14% of the placebo patients. Because some patients in the study had been treated for 6 weeks whereas others had been treated for 12 weeks, they were combined based on the dose of nortriptyline that they were receiving (Kimura and Robinson 2003).

A repeated-measures ANOVA of Hamilton Anxiety Scale (Ham-A) (Hamilton 1959) scores using an intention-to-treat analysis demonstrated a significant group by time interaction ($P = 0.002$) (i.e., the nortriptyline group improved more quickly than the placebo group) (Figure 8–5). Planned comparisons revealed that the nortriptyline group was significantly more improved than the placebo group at nortriptyline doses of 50 mg, 75 mg, and 100 mg. Nine of 13 (69%) in the nortriptyline-treated group had a greater than 50% reduction in Ham-A scores, whereas only 3 of 14 placebo-treated patients (21%) had a similar reduction ($P = 0.017$). To determine whether depression and anxiety symptoms were responding independently, the rate of change in symptom severity was compared between a Ham-A and a Ham-D measurement. At

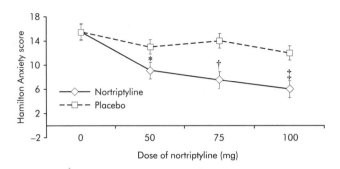

FIGURE 8–5.   Mean Hamilton Anxiety Scale scores among patients with generalized anxiety disorder and comorbid depression after stroke following treatment with nortriptyline and placebo.

The nortriptyline group ($n = 13$) showed significantly greater improvement in anxiety symptoms than the placebo group ($n = 14$) ($P = 0.002$). Error bars represent standard error of the mean (SE).
*$P < 0.05$; †$P < 0.01$; ‡$P < 0.02$.

Source.   Reprinted from Kimura M, Robinson RG: "Treatment of Poststroke Generalized Anxiety Disorder Comorbid With Poststroke Depression: Merged Analysis of Nortriptyline Trials." *American Journal of Geriatric Psychiatry* 11:320–327, 2003. Used with permission.

50 mg of nortriptyline (i.e., 2–3 weeks), there was a 39% improvement in Ham-A scores and only a 14% improvement in Ham-D scores ($P = 0.03$). This suggests that anxiety symptoms were responding more rapidly than depressive symptoms with nortriptyline therapy. This was the first study using double-blind, placebo-controlled methodology to demonstrate that GAD following stroke can be effectively treated with the tricyclic antidepressant nortriptyline.

POSTSTROKE PSYCHOSIS

The phenomenon of hallucinations and delusions in patients who have experienced stroke has been called agitated delirium, acute atypical psychosis, peduncular hallucinosis, release hallucinations, and acute organic psychosis. In a study of acute organic psychosis occurring after stroke lesions, Rabins et al. (1991) found a very low prevalence of psychosis among stroke patients (only 5 in more than 300 consecutive admissions). All 5 of these patients, however, had right hemisphere lesions, primarily involving frontoparietal regions. When compared with 5 age-matched patients with cerebrovascular lesions in similar locations but no psychosis, patients with secondary psychosis had significantly greater subcortical atro-

phy, as manifested by significantly larger areas of both the frontal horn of the lateral ventricle and the body of the lateral ventricle (measured on the side contralateral to the brain lesion) (Rabins et al. 1991). Several investigators have also reported a high frequency of seizures among patients with secondary psychosis (Levine and Finklestein 1982). These seizures usually started after the occurrence of the brain lesion but before the onset of psychosis. The study by Rabins et al. (1991) found seizures in 3 of 5 patients with poststroke psychosis, compared with 0 of 5 poststroke, nonpsychiatric control subjects.

It has been hypothesized that three factors may be important in the mechanism of organic hallucinations, namely 1) a right hemisphere lesion involving the temporoparietal cortex, 2) seizures, and/or 3) subcortical brain atrophy (Rabins et al. 1991).

APATHY

Apathy is the absence or lack of motivation as manifested by decreased motor function, cognitive function, emotional feeling, and interest. It has been reported frequently among patients with brain injury. Using the Apathy Scale, Starkstein et al. (1993a) examined a consecutive series of 80 patients with single-stroke lesions and no significant impairment in comprehension. Of 80 patients, 9 (11%) showed apathy as their only psychiatric disorder, whereas another 11% had both apathy and depression. The only demographic correlate of apathy was age, as apathetic patients (with or without depression) were significantly older than nonapathetic patients. In addition, apathetic patients showed significantly more severe deficits in ADL, and a significant interaction was noted between depression and apathy on ADL scores, with the greatest impairment found in patients who were both apathetic and depressed.

CATASTROPHIC REACTION

Catastrophic reaction is a term coined by Goldstein (1939) to describe the "inability of the organism to cope when faced with physical or cognitive deficits" and is expressed by anxiety, tears, aggressive behavior, swearing, displacement, refusal, renouncement, and sometimes compensatory boasting. Starkstein et al. (1993b) assessed a consecutive series of 62 patients using the Catastrophic Reaction Scale, which was developed to assess the existence and severity of catastrophic reactions. The Catastrophic Reaction Scale has been demonstrated to be a reliable instrument in the measurement of symptoms of catastrophic reaction.

Catastrophic reactions occurred in 12 of 62 (19%) consecutive patients with acute stroke lesions (Starkstein et al. 1993b). Three major findings emerged from this study. First, patients with catastrophic reactions were found to have a significantly higher frequency of familial and personal history of psychiatric disorders (mostly depression) than were patients without catastrophic reactions. Second, catastrophic reaction was not significantly more frequent among aphasic (33%) than non-aphasic (66%) patients. This finding does not support the contention that catastrophic reactions are an understandable psychological response of "frustrated" aphasic patients (Gainotti 1972). Third, 9 of the 12 patients with

catastrophic reaction also had major depression, 2 had minor depression, and only 1 was not depressed. On the other hand, among the 50 patients without catastrophic reactions, 7 had major depression, 6 had minor depression, and 37 were not depressed. Thus, catastrophic reaction was significantly associated with major depression, but the findings do not support the proposal by Gainotti et al. (1999) that the catastrophic reaction is an integral part of PSD. It is rather a comorbid condition that occurs in some but not all patients with PSD or that may characterize a subgroup of PSD.

PATHOLOGICAL EMOTIONS

Emotional lability is a common complication of stroke lesions. It is characterized by sudden, easily provoked episodes of crying that, although frequent, generally occur in appropriate situations and are accompanied by a congruent mood change. Pathological laughing and crying is a more severe form of emotional lability and is characterized by episodes of laughing and/or crying that are not appropriate to the context. They may appear spontaneously or may be elicited by nonemotional events and do not correspond to underlying emotional feelings. These disorders have also been termed *emotional incontinence, pathologic emotions,* and *involuntary emotional expression disorder.*

Robinson et al. (1993) examined the clinical correlates and treatment of emotional lability (including pathological laughter and crying) in 28 patients with either acute or chronic stroke. A Pathological Laughter and Crying Scale (PLACS) (Robinson et al. 1993) was developed to assess the existence and severity of emotional lability.

The doses of nortriptyline were 25 mg for 1 week, 50 mg for 2 weeks, 70 mg for 1 week, and 100 mg for the last 2 weeks of the study. One patient dropped out during the study, 2 patients withdrew before initiation of the study, and 28 completed the 6-week protocol. Patients receiving nortriptyline showed significant improvements in PLACS scores compared with the placebo-treated patients. These differences became statistically significant at

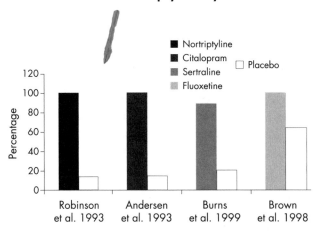

FIGURE 8–6.   Comparison of double-blind treatment studies using nortriptyline, citalopram, sertraline, or fluoxetine in patients with pathological crying.

Percentage of patients with > 50% reduction in severity score or crying episodes. The mean pooled data response rates were 96% for active medication and 27.5% for placebo. These findings suggest that all of these medications are effective in the treatment of poststroke pathological crying.

Source.   Reprinted from Robinson RG: *The Clinical Neuropsychiatry of Stroke*, 2nd Edition. Cambridge, UK, Cambridge University Press, 2006. Used with permission.

4 and 6 weeks. Although a significant improvement in depression scores was also observed, improvements in PLACS scores were significant for both depressed and nondepressed patients with pathological laughing and crying, indicating that treatment response was not simply related to an improvement in depression (Robinson et al. 1993).

There have now been four double-blind treatment studies of pathological emotion, and both fluoxetine (Brown et al. 1998) and sertraline (Burns et al. 1999) have been shown to significantly reduce the frequency of crying episodes (see Figure 8–6). These findings have supported the conclusion that SSRI antidepressant medications are rapidly effective in reducing the number of crying episodes in patients with poststroke pathological emotions.

APROSODY

Ross and Mesulam (1979) have described aprosody as abnormalities in the affective components of language, encompassing prosody and emotional gesturing. Prosody can be defined as the "variation of pitch, rhythm, and stress of pronunciation that bestows certain semantic and emotional meaning to speech" (Ross and Mesulam 1979, p. 144).

Starkstein et al. (1994) examined prosody comprehension in 59 patients with acute stroke lesions. With the use of tapes expressing verbal emotion and photos of emotional facial expression, impaired comprehension of emotion was found in a mild form in 10 patients (17%) and in a severe form in 19 (32%). Severe aprosody was associated with the following three clinical variables: 1) neglect for tactile stimulation, 2) lesions of the right hemisphere, including the basal ganglia and temporoparietal cortex, and 3) significantly larger third ventricle–to-brain ratio. Although Ross and Rush (1981) suggested that patients with sensory aprosody might not be able to recognize their own depressed mood, major depression was found in 2 of 19 patients (11%) with severe aprosody and in 7 of 30 (23%) without aprosody (not significant) (Starkstein et al. 1994).

CONCLUSION

There are numerous emotional and behavioral disorders that occur after cerebrovascular lesions. Depression occurs in about 40% of stroke patients, with approximately equal distributions of major depression and minor depression. Major depression is significantly associated with left frontal and left basal ganglia lesions during the acute stroke period and may be successfully treated with nortriptyline or citalopram. Treatment of depression has also been shown to improve poststroke cognitive function.

Mania is a rare complication of stroke and is strongly associated with right hemisphere damage involving the orbitofrontal cortex, basal temporal cortex, thalamus, or basal ganglia. Risk factors for mania include a family history of psychiatric disorders and subcortical atrophy. Bipolar disorders are associated with subcortical lesions of the right hemisphere, whereas right cortical lesions lead to mania without depression.

GAD, which is present in about 27% of stroke patients, is associated with depression in the majority of cases. Among the few patients with poststroke anxiety and no depression, there is a high frequency of alcoholism and lesions of the right hemisphere. Apathy is present in about 20% of stroke patients. It is associated with older age, more severe deficits in ADL, and a significantly higher frequency of lesions involving the posterior limb of the internal capsule. A controlled treatment study demonstrated that poststroke GAD can be treated effectively with nortriptyline.

Psychotic disorders are rare complications of stroke lesions. Poststroke hallucinations are associated with right hemisphere temporoparietal lesions, subcortical brain atrophy, and seizures.

Catastrophic reactions occur in about 20% of stroke patients. These reactions are not related to the severity of impairments or the presence of aphasia but may represent a symptom for one clinical type of poststroke major depression. Catastrophic reactions are associated with anterior subcortical lesions and may result from a "release" of emotional display in a subgroup of depressed patients. Pathological laughing and crying is another common complication of stroke lesions that may sometimes coexist with depression and may be successfully treated with nortriptyline, citalopram, fluoxetine, or sertraline.

RECOMMENDED READINGS

Robinson RG: The Clinical Neuropsychiatry of Stroke, 2nd Edition. Cambridge, UK, Cambridge University Press, 2006

Whyte EM, Mulsant BH: Poststroke depression: epidemiology, pathophysiology and biological treatment. Biol Psychiatry 52:253–264, 2002

REFERENCES

Aben I, Verhey F, Lousberg R, et al: Validity of the Beck Depression Inventory, Hospital Anxiety and Depression Scale, SCL-90, and Hamilton Depression Rating Scale as screening instruments for depression in stroke patients. Psychosomatics 43:386–393, 2002

Adams RD, Victor M: Principles of Neurology. New York, McGraw-Hill, 1985

American Psychiatric Association: Diagnostic and Statistical Manual of Mental Disorders, 4th Edition, Text Revision. Washington, DC, American Psychiatric Press, 2000

Andersen G, Vestergaard K, Riis J: Citalopram for post-stroke pathological crying. Lancet 342: 837–839, 1993

Andersen G, Vestergaard K, Lauritzen L: Effective treatment of poststroke depression with the selective serotonin reuptake inhibitor citalopram. Stroke 25:1099–1104, 1994a

Andersen G, Vestergaard K, Riis JO, et al: Incidence of post-stroke depression during the first year in a large unselected stroke population determined using a valid standardized rating scale. Acta Psychiatr Scand 90:190–195, 1994b

Andersen G, Vestergaard K, Riis JO, et al: Dementia of depression or depression of dementia in stroke? Acta Psychiatr Scand 94:272–278, 1996

Astrom M: Generalized anxiety disorder in stroke patients: a 3-year longitudinal study. Stroke 27:270–275, 1996

Astrom M, Adolfsson R, Asplund K: Major depression in stroke patients: a 3-year longitudinal study. Stroke 24:976–982, 1993a

Astrom M, Olsson T, Asplund K: Different linkage of depression to hypercortisolism early versus late after stroke: a 3-year longitudinal study. Stroke 24:52–57, 1993b

Bakchine S, Lacomblez L, Benoit N, et al: Manic-like state after orbitofrontal and right temporo-parietal injury: efficacy of clonidine. Neurology 39:778–781, 1989

Bhogal SK, Teasell R, Foley N, et al: Lesion location and poststroke depression: systematic review of the methodological limitations in the literature. Stroke 35:794–802, 2004

Bolla-Wilson K, Robinson RG, Starkstein SE, et al: Lateralization of dementia of depression in stroke patients. Am J Psychiatry 146:627–634, 1989

Brown KW, Sloan RL, Pentland B: Fluoxetine as a treatment for post-stroke emotionalism. Acta Psychiatr Scand 98:455–458, 1998

Burns A, Russell E, Stratton-Powell H, et al: Sertraline in stroke-associated lability of mood. Int J Geriatr Psychiatry 14:681–685, 1999

Burvill PW, Johnson GA, Jamrozik KD, et al: Prevalence of depression after stroke: the Perth Community Stroke Study. Br J Psychiatry 166:320–327, 1995

Capuron L, Dantzer R: Cytokines and depression: the need for a new paradigm. Brain Behav Immun 17 (suppl 1):S119–S124, 2003

Cassidy E, O'Connor R, O'Keane V: Prevalence of post-stroke depression in an Irish sample and its relationship with disability and outcome following inpatient rehabilitation. Disabil Rehabil 26:71–77, 2004

Cassidy F, Carroll BJ: Vascular risk factors in late onset mania. Psychol Med 32:359–362, 2002

Castillo CS, Starkstein SE, Fedoroff JP, et al: Generalized anxiety disorder after stroke. J Nerv Ment Dis 181:100–106, 1993

Castillo CS, Schultz SK, Robinson RG: Clinical correlates of early onset and late-onset poststroke generalized anxiety. Am J Psychiatry 152:1174–1179, 1995

Collin J, Tinson D, Lincoln NB: Depression after stroke. Clin Rehabil 1:27–32, 1987

Dennis M, O'Rourke S, Lewis S, et al: Emotional outcomes after stroke: factors associated with poor outcome. J Neurol Neurosurg Psychiatry 68:47–52, 2000

Downhill JE Jr, Robinson RG: Longitudinal assessment of depression and cognitive impairment following stroke. J Nerv Ment Dis 182:425–431, 1994

Ebrahim S, Barer D, Nouri F: Affective illness after stroke. Br J Psychiatry 151:52–56, 1987

Fedoroff JP, Lipsey JR, Starkstein SE, et al: Phenomenological comparisons of major depression following stroke, myocardial infarction or spinal cord lesions. J Affect Disord 22:83–89, 1991

Feibel JH, Springer CJ: Depression and failure to resume social activities after stroke. Arch Phys Med Rehabil 63:276–277, 1982

Finset A, Goffeng L, Landro NI, et al: Depressed mood and intra-hemispheric location of lesion in right hemisphere stroke patients. Scand J Rehabil Med 21:1–6, 1989

Folstein MF, Folstein SE, McHugh PR: Mini-Mental State: a practical method for grading the cognitive state of patients for the clinician. J Psychiatr Res 12:189–198, 1975

Fruehwald S, Gatterbauer E, Rehak P, et al: Early fluoxetine treatment of post-stroke depression: a three-month double-blind placebo-controlled study with an open-label long-term follow up. J Neurol 250:347–351, 2003

Gainotti G: Emotional behavior and hemispheric side of the brain. Cortex 8:41–55, 1972

Gainotti G, Azzoni A, Marra C: Frequency, phenomenology and anatomical-clinical correlates of major post-stroke depression. Br J Psychiatry 175:163–167, 1999

Goldstein K: The Organism: A Holistic Approach to Biology Derived From Pathological Data in Man. New York, American Books, 1939

Grade C, Redford B, Chrostowski J, et al: Methylphenidate in early poststroke recovery: a double-blind, placebo-controlled study. Arch Phys Med Rehabil 79:1047–1050, 1998

Hamilton M: The assessment of anxiety states by rating. Br J Med Psychol 32:50–55, 1959

Hamilton MA: A rating scale for depression. J Neurol Neurosurg Psychiatry 23:56–62, 1960

Herrmann M, Bartels C, Wallesch CW: Depression in acute and chronic aphasia: symptoms, patho-anatomical-clinical correlations and functional implications. J Neurol Neurosurg Psychiatry 56:672–678, 1993

Herrmann M, Bartels C, Schumacher M, et al: Post-stroke depression: is there a pathoanatomic correlate for depression in the postacute stage of stroke? Stroke 26:850–856, 1995

Herrmann N, Black SE, Lawrence J, et al: The Sunnybrook Stroke Study: a prospective study of depressive symptoms and functional outcome. Stroke 29:618–624, 1998

House A, Dennis M, Warlow C, et al: Mood disorders after stroke and their relation to lesion location: a CT scan study. Brain 113:1113–1130, 1990

House A, Dennis M, Mogridge L, et al: Mood disorders in the year after first stroke. Br J Psychiatry 158:83–92, 1991

Kimura M, Robinson RG: Treatment of poststroke generalized anxiety disorder comorbid with poststroke depression: merged analysis of nortriptyline trials. Am J Geriatr Psychiatry 11:320–327, 2003

Kimura M, Robinson RG, Kosier T: Treatment of cognitive impairment after poststroke depression. Stroke 31:1482–1486, 2000

Kotila M, Numminen H, Waltimo O, et al: Depression after stroke: results of the FINNSTROKE study. Stroke 29:368–372, 1998

Lauritzen L, Bendsen BB, Vilmar T, et al: Post-stroke depression: combined treatment with imipramine or desipramine and mianserin: a controlled clinical study. Psychopharmacology 114:119–122, 1994

Levine DN, Finklestein S: Delayed psychosis after right temporoparietal stroke or trauma: relation to epilepsy. Neurology 32:267–273, 1982

Lincoln NB, Flannaghan T: Cognitive behavioral psychotherapy for depression following stroke: a randomized controlled trial. Stroke 34:111–115, 2003

Lipsey JR, Robinson RG, Pearlson GD, et al: Nortriptyline treatment of post-stroke depression: a double-blind study. Lancet 1:297–300, 1984

Lipsey JR, Spencer WC, Rabins PV, et al: Phenomenological comparison of functional and post-stroke depression. Am J Psychiatry 143:527–529, 1986

Miyai I, Suzuki T, Kang J, et al: Improved functional outcome in patients with hemorrhagic stroke in putamen and thalamus compared with those with stroke restricted to the putamen or thalamus. Stroke 31:1365–1369, 2000

Morris PLP, Robinson RG, Raphael B: Prevalence and course of depressive disorders in hospitalized stroke patients. Int J Psychiatry Med 20:349–364, 1990

Morris PLP, Robinson RG, Raphael B, et al: Lesion location and post-stroke depression. J Neuropsychiatry Clin Neurosci 8:399–403, 1996

Morrison JH, Molliver ME, Grzanna R: Noradrenergic innervation of the cerebral cortex: widespread effects of local cortical lesions. Science 205:313–316, 1979

Murray GB, Shea V, Conn DK: Electroconvulsive therapy for poststroke depression. J Clin Psychiatry 47:258–260, 1986

Narushima K, Robinson RG: The effect of early versus late antidepressant treatment on physical impairment associated with poststroke depression: is there a time-related therapeutic window? J Nerv Ment Dis 191:645–652, 2003

Narushima K, Kosier JT, Robinson RG: A reappraisal of post-stroke depression, intra and inter-hemispheric lesion location using meta-analysis. J Neuropsychiatry Clin Neurosci 15:422–430, 2003

Pohjasvaara T, Leppavuori A, Siira I, et al: Frequency and clinical determinants of poststroke depression. Stroke 29:2311–2317, 1998

Rabins PV, Starkstein SE, Robinson RG: Risk factors for developing atypical (schizophreniform) psychosis following stroke. J Neuropsychiatry Clin Neurosci 3:6–9, 1991

Rampello L, Alvano A, Chiechio S, et al: An evaluation of efficacy and safety of reboxetine in elderly patients affected by "retarded" post-stroke depression: a random, placebo-controlled study. Arch Gerontol Geriatr 40:275–285, 2005

Rankin J: Cerebral vascular accidents in patients over the age of 60, III: diagnosis and treatment. Scott Med J 2:254–268, 1957

Reding MJ, Orto LA, Winter SW, et al: Antidepressant therapy after stroke: a double-blind trial. Arch Neurol 43:763–765, 1986

Robinson RG: The controversy over post-stroke depression and lesion location. Psychiatric Times 20:39–40, 2003

Robinson RG: The Clinical Neuropsychiatry of Stroke, 2nd Edition. Cambridge, UK, Cambridge University Press, 2006

Robinson RG, Price TR: Post-stroke depressive disorders: a follow-up study of 103 patients. Stroke 13:635–641, 1982

Robinson RG, Szetela B: Mood change following left hemispheric brain injury. Ann Neurol 9:447–453, 1981

Robinson RG, Kubos KL, Starr LB, et al: Mood disorders in stroke patients: importance of location of lesion. Brain 107:81–93, 1984

Robinson RG, Bolla-Wilson K, Kaplan E, et al: Depression influences intellectual impairment in stroke patients. Br J Psychiatry 148:541–547, 1986a

Robinson RG, Lipsey JR, Rao K, et al: Two-year longitudinal study of post-stroke mood disorders: comparison of acute-onset with delayed-onset depression. Am J Psychiatry 143:1238–1244, 1986b

Robinson RG, Boston JD, Starkstein SE, et al: Comparison of mania with depression following brain injury: causal factors. Am J Psychiatry 145:172–178, 1988

Robinson RG, Parikh RM, Lipsey JR, et al: Pathological laughing and crying following stroke: validation of a measurement scale and a double-blind treatment study. Am J Psychiatry 150:286–293, 1993

Robinson RG, Schultz SK, Castillo C, et al: Nortriptyline versus fluoxetine in the treatment of depression and in short term recovery after stroke: a placebo controlled, double-blind study. Am J Psychiatry 157:351–359, 2000

Ross ED, Mesulam MM: Dominant language functions of the right hemisphere? Prosody and emotional gesturing. Arch Neurol 36:144–148, 1979

Ross ED, Rush AJ: Diagnosis and neuroanatomical correlates of depression in brain-damaged patients: implications for a neurology of depression. Arch Gen Psychiatry 38:1344–1354, 1981

Schubert DS, Burns R, Paras W, et al: Increase of medical hospital length of stay by depression in stroke and amputation patients: a pilot study. Psychother Psychosom 57:61–66, 1992

Schwartz JA, Speed NM, Brunberg JA, et al: Depression in stroke rehabilitation. Biol Psychiatry 33:694–699, 1993

Shimoda K, Robinson RG: Effect of anxiety disorder in impairment and recovery from stroke. J Neuropsychiatry Clin Neurosci 10:34–40, 1998

Spalletta G, Guida G, De Angelis D, et al: Predictors of cognitive level and depression severity are different in patients with left and right hemispheric stroke within the first year of illness. J Neurol 249:1541–1551, 2002

Spalletta G, Ripa A, Caltagirone C: Symptom profile of DSM-IV major and minor depressive disorders in first-ever stroke patients. Am J Geriatr Psychiatry 13:108–115, 2005

Spalletta G, Bossù P, Ciaramella A, et al: The etiology of post-stroke depression: a review of the literature and a new hypothesis involving inflammatory cytokines. Mol Psychiatry 11:984–991, 2006

Starkstein SE, Pearlson GD, Boston J, et al: Mania after brain injury: a controlled study of causative factors. Arch Neurol 44:1069–1073, 1987a

Starkstein SE, Robinson RG, Price TR: Comparison of cortical and subcortical lesions in the production of post-stroke mood disorders. Brain 110:1045–1059, 1987b

Starkstein SE, Boston JD, Robinson RG: Mechanisms of mania after brain injury: 12 case reports and review of the literature. J Nerv Ment Dis 176:87–100, 1988a

Starkstein SE, Robinson RG, Price TR: Comparison of patients with and without post-stroke major depression matched for size and location of lesion. Arch Gen Psychiatry 45:247–252, 1988b

Starkstein SE, Berthier PL, Lylyk A, et al: Emotional behavior after a WADA test in a patient with secondary mania. J Neuropsychiatry Clin Neurosci 1:408–412, 1989

Starkstein SE, Fedoroff JP, Berthier MD, et al: Manic depressive and pure manic states after brain lesions. Biol Psychiatry 29:149–158, 1991

Starkstein SE, Robinson RG, Berthier ML: Poststroke hallucinatory delusional syndromes. Neuropsychiatry Neuropsychol Behav Neurol 5:114–118, 1992

Starkstein SE, Fedoroff JP, Price TR, et al: Apathy following cerebrovascular lesions. Stroke 24:1625–1630, 1993a

Starkstein SE, Fedoroff JP, Price TR, et al: Catastrophic reaction after cerebrovascular ledions: frequency, correlates, and validation of a scale. J Neurol Neurosurg Psychiatry 5:189–194, 1993b

Starkstein SE, Federoff JP, Price TR, et al: Neuropsychological and neuroradiologic correlates of emotional prosody comprehension. Neurology 44:515–522, 1994

Thom T, Haase N, Rosamond W, et al: Heart disease and stroke statistics—2006 update: a report from the American Heart Association Statistics Committee and Stroke Statistics Subcommittee. Circulation 113:e85–e151, 2006

Thompson SC, Sobolew-Shobin A, Graham MA, et al: Psychosocial adjustment following stroke. Soc Sci Med 28:239–247, 1989

Wade DT, Legh-Smith J, Hewer RA: Depressed mood after stroke: a community study of its frequency. Br J Psychiatry 151:200–205, 1987

Wiart L, Petit H, Joseph PA, et al: Fluoxetine in early poststroke depression: a double-blind placebo-controlled study. Stroke 31:1829–1832, 2000

Wolf PA, Dawber TR, Thomas HE, et al: Epidemiology of stroke, in Advances in Neurology. Edited by Thompson RA, Green R. New York, Raven, 1977, pp 5–19

9

NEUROPSYCHIATRIC ASPECTS OF BRAIN TUMORS

Trevor R. P. Price, M.D.
Kenneth L. Goetz, M.D.
Mark R. Lovell, Ph.D.

The annual incidence of primary brain tumors is 9.0 per 100,000 and that of metastatic brain tumors is 8.3 per 100,000. Evidence suggests that the overall incidence of brain tumors and the proportion of brain tumors that are malignant have been increasing over the past two decades in industrialized countries (Jukich et al. 2001; Olney et al. 1996).

Brain tumors are typically classified according to whether they are primary or metastatic, as well as by location and histological cell type. Most primary tumors are either meningiomas or more frequently gliomas. The most common metastatic lesions are from lung and breast malignancies. Seventy percent of all tumors are supratentorial, with occurrence by lobe as indicated in Figure 9–1. This distribution is influenced to some degree by tumor histology (Figure 9–2).

Age is also a determining factor for the frequency of various tumor types. In children, astrocytomas are most common, followed by medulloblastomas (Radhakrishnan et al. 1994). Gliomas are more often seen in the middle-aged population, and meningiomas increase in incidence among the elderly (Radhakrishnan et al. 1994). Metastatic tumors are more frequent in the elderly and occur with greater frequency than primary brain tumors.

It has been reported that primary brain tumors are up to 10 times more common among psychiatric patients than among psychiatrically healthy control subjects and that mental changes and behavioral symptoms, including confusion and various other neuropsychiatric symptoms, are more frequent early indicators of primary brain tumors than are classic physical manifestations such as headaches, seizures,

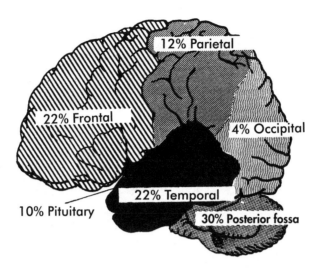

FIGURE 9–1.   Relative frequency of intracranial brain tumors according to location in the adult.

Source.   Reprinted from Lohr JB, Cadet JL: "Neuropsychiatric Aspects of Brain Tumors," in *The American Psychiatric Press Textbook of Neuropsychiatry.* Edited by Talbott JA, Hales RE, Yudofsky SC. Washington, DC, American Psychiatric Press, 1987, p. 355. Used with permission.

and focal neurological signs (Kocher et al. 1984).

Although the various tumor classifications may eventually turn out to be important in understanding the occurrence of neuropsychiatric symptoms associated with brain tumors, no large-scale, detailed studies have yet carefully examined correlations between such symptoms and various tumor characteristics. Our knowledge of the neuropsychiatric and neuropsychological concomitants of brain tumors is based on a relatively small number of clinical case reports and uncontrolled case series from the older neurological and neurosurgical literature. Much of the discussion that follows draws on these sources.

FREQUENCY OF NEUROPSYCHIATRIC SYMPTOMS IN PATIENTS WITH BRAIN TUMORS

Unfortunately, and surprisingly, few recent studies have examined the frequency of psychiatric symptoms in patients with brain tumors. The studies that are available tend to

be large autopsy studies, predominantly from the first half of the twentieth century.

For example, Keschner et al. (1938) noted psychiatric symptoms in 413 (78%) of 530 patients with brain tumors, and Schlesinger (1950) found behavior changes in 301 (51%) of his series of 591 patients. Although tumor-associated, complex neuropsychiatric symptoms may occur along with focal neurological signs and symptoms, often they may be the first clinical indication of a tumor, as was the case in 18% of the patients examined by Keschner et al. (1938). In a study of 4 patients with intracranial tumors, Ko and Kok (1989) noted that 3 patients had initially presented to psychiatrists for diagnosis and treatment. Another more recent analysis of a group of patients with meningiomas indicated that 21% of them had initially presented with psychiatric symptoms in the absence of neurological signs or symptoms (Gupta and Kumar 2004). Taken together, these studies underscore the need for primary care physicians and psychiatrists to be alert to the potential presence of neurological abnormalities in patients who present with psychiatric and behavioral symptoms.

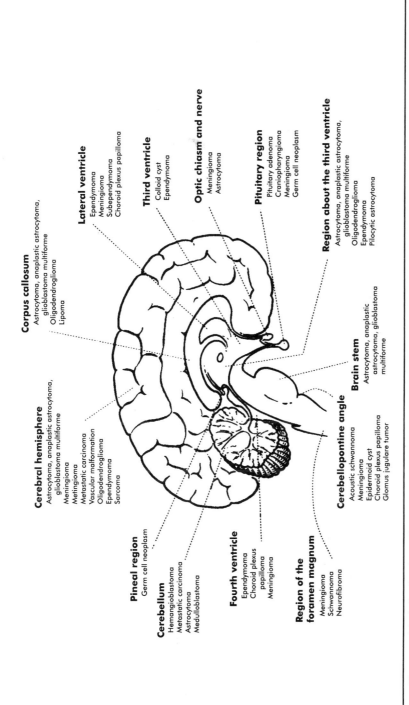

Corpus callosum
Astrocytoma, anaplastic astrocytoma,
glioblastoma multiforme
Oligodendroglioma
Lipoma

Lateral ventricle
Ependymoma
Meningioma
Subependymoma
Choroid plexus papilloma

Third ventricle
Colloid cyst
Ependymoma

Optic chiasm and nerve
Meningioma
Astrocytoma

Pituitary region
Pituitary adenoma
Craniopharyngioma
Meningioma
Germ cell neoplasm

Region about the third ventricle
Astrocytoma, anaplastic astrocytoma,
glioblastoma multiforme
Oligodendroglioma
Ependymoma
Pilocytic astrocytoma

Cerebral hemisphere
Astrocytoma, anaplastic astrocytoma,
glioblastoma multiforme
Meningioma
Metingioma
Metastatic carcinoma
Vascular malformation
Oligodendroglioma
Ependymoma
Sarcoma

Brain stem
Astrocytoma, anaplastic
astrocytoma, glioblastoma
multiforme

Cerebellopontine angle
Acoustic schwannoma
Meningioma
Epidermoid cyst
Choroid plexus papilloma
Glomus jugulare tumor

Pineal region
Germ cell neoplasm

Cerebellum
Hemangioblastoma
Metastatic carcinoma
Astrocytoma
Medulloblastoma

Fourth ventricle
Ependymoma
Choroid plexus
papilloma
Meningioma

**Region of the
foramen magnum**
Meningioma
Schwannoma
Neurofibroma

FIGURE 9–2. Topographical distribution of intracranial tumors in the adult.

Source. Reprinted from Burger PC, Scheithauer BW, Vogel FS: *Surgical Pathology of the Nervous System and Its Coverings,* 3rd Edition. New York, Churchill Livingstone, 1991. Copyright Elsevier 1991. Used with permission.

Minski (1933) studied 58 patients with cerebral tumors and, in addition to reporting that the psychiatric symptomatology of 25 of these patients simulated "functional psychoses," noted that 19 had actually attributed the onset of their behavioral symptoms to various stresses, including financial worries and the deaths of relatives. This underscores the difficulty that clinicians face in making an appropriate diagnosis early in the course of disease. It may be impossible on purely clinical grounds to determine the organic basis of the patient's complaints until progression of the tumor has resulted in the emergence of more typical and unmistakable neurological signs and symptoms.

Despite the high prevalence of psychiatric symptoms in patients with brain tumors, the prevalence of intracranial tumors in psychiatric patients, compiled from autopsy data from mental hospitals, is only about 3%. This rate is similar to that found in autopsy series in general hospitals (Galasko et al. 1988). In a study by J.K.A. Roberts and Lishman (1984), only 1 of 323 psychiatric patients who had computed tomography (CT) scans done as part of the diagnostic evaluation was found to have a tumor. Hollister and Boutros (1991) evaluated CT or magnetic resonance imaging (MRI) studies performed on 337 psychiatric patients. Only 2 patients were found to have brain tumors, and both had significant neurological findings on physical examination. Other studies suggest that the risk of an occult neoplasm in patients presenting with purely psychiatric complaints may be as low as 0.1% (Hobbs 1963; Remington and Robert 1962).

Two large autopsy studies (Klotz 1957; Selecki 1965) of psychiatric patients have suggested that approximately half of all tumors had gone undiagnosed before postmortem examination. Of interest is another autopsy study, by Percy et al. (1972), which reported that before the advent of modern imaging techniques, 37% of brain tumors in an unselected population had been first diagnosed at autopsy. Most of these patients were asymptomatic during their lifetimes. Undoubtedly, sophisticated brain imaging, which was un-available at the time these series were done, would have diminished the likelihood of missing a tumor.

GENERAL NEUROPSYCHIATRIC AND NEUROPSYCHOLOGICAL CONSIDERATIONS

GENERAL NEUROPSYCHIATRIC CONSIDERATIONS

Patients with CNS tumors can present with mental symptoms that are virtually indistinguishable from those found in patients with primary psychiatric disorders (Jarquin-Valdivia 2004; Madhusoodanan et al. 2004). These symptoms run the gamut from major depression and schizophrenia to personality disorders and conversion syndromes. Over the years, many clinicians and researchers have hypothesized the existence of a predictable relation between tumor location and neuropsychiatric phenomenology. Some studies have supported the generally held belief that depression is more common in frontal lobe tumors and psychosis is more common with temporal lobe neoplasms (Filley and Klein-schmidt-DeMasters 1995; Wellisch et al. 2002). Most of the older, autopsy-related studies did not strongly support this hypothesis and often concluded that observed behavior changes were of no localizing value (Keschner et al. 1938; Selecki 1965). The nature and severity of psychiatric dysfunction accompanying tumors are probably determined by other factors that are of as great as or of even greater importance than anatomical location. The reason that this is the case may be that neuroanatomical substrates of particular behaviors tend not to be localized to single lobes or specific anatomical locations.

The best examples of these nonlocalized substrates are behaviors mediated by tumors involving the limbic system, which includes the temporal lobes and portions of the frontal lobes, the hypothalamus, and the midbrain. Tumors affecting any of these structures may produce similar psychopathology. Furthermore, even lesions outside the limbic system may produce similar behavior changes, attributable to limbic release or disinhibition, through diaschisis or disconnection syndromes (see subsection "General Neuropsychological Considerations" later in this chapter). Limbic tumors often have been associated with depression, affective flattening, apathy, agitation, assaultive behavior, and even a variety of psychotic symptoms. In one study of patients with tumors in or near limbic system structures who had initially been admitted to psychiatric hospitals (Malamud 1967), it was found that the patients shared similar psychopathology regardless of the actual structures involved.

A study (Starkstein et al. 1988) of patients who developed mania after a variety of brain lesions, including tumors, also illustrates the difficulty of trying to associate specific kinds of psychiatric symptoms with the anatomical location of tumors. Although there was an overall predominance of right-sided involvement, lesions occurred in the frontal, temporoparietal, and temporo-occipital lobes, as well as in the cerebellum, thalamus, and pituitary. The authors concluded that the unifying aspect in all of these lesions was not their anatomical location but rather the interconnection of the involved structures with the orbitofrontal cortex. This finding underscores the need for formulating more sophisticated localization models in which both neuroanatomical location and connectivity are considered as they relate to focal brain lesions.

Other factors also may influence presenting symptoms and thereby diminish the localizing value of a particular behavior change. Increased intracranial pressure is a nonspecific consequence of CNS tumors in general and has been implicated in behavior changes such as apathy, depression, irritability, agitation, and changes in consciousness. In one study of lesions involving the occipital lobes, it was concluded that most observed mental changes were due to increases in intracranial pressure rather than to effects of the tumors themselves (Allen 1930).

Another factor is the patient's premorbid level of functioning, which often has a significant effect on the nature of the clinical presentation. Tumors often cause an exaggeration of the individual's previous predominant character traits and coping styles. The behavior changes associated with a brain tumor usually represent a complex combination of the patient's premorbid psychiatric status, tumor-associated mental symptoms, and adaptive or maladaptive responses to the psychological stress of having been diagnosed with a brain tumor.

It has been noted that rapidly growing tumors are more commonly associated with severe, acute psychiatric symptoms, such as agitation or psychosis, as well as with more obvious cognitive dysfunctions. Patients with slow-growing tumors are more likely to present with vague personality changes, apathy, or depression, often without associated cognitive changes (Lishman 1987). Multiple tumor foci also tend to produce behavioral symptoms with greater frequency than do single lesions.

In general, the factors that most significantly influence symptom formation appear to be the extent of tumor involvement, the rapidity of its growth, and its propensity to cause increased intracranial pressure. In addition, the patient's premorbid psychiatric history, level of functioning, and characteristic psychological coping mechanisms may play a significant contributing role in determining the nature of a patient's particular symptoms. Lesion location may often, in fact, play a relatively minor role.

While lesion location is probably not the most important factor in determining the occurrence of specific types of neuropsychiatric symptoms, there have been some reports that brain lesions in certain locations may be associated with increased frequency of psychiatric symptoms. For example, although Keschner et al. (1936) found no overall difference in the types of behavioral symptoms associated with tumors of the frontal and temporal lobes, they did find that, to a small degree, complex visual and auditory hallucinations were more common among patients with tumors of the temporal lobe and that "facetiousness" was more

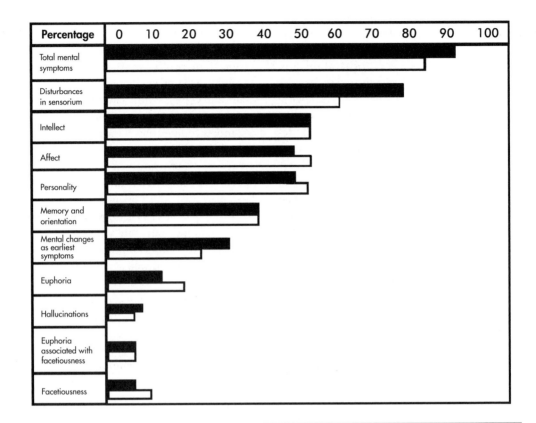

FIGURE 9–3.   Comparison of incidence of mental symptoms in 110 patients with tumors of the temporal lobe (*solid bars*) and in 64 patients with tumors of the frontal lobe (*open bars*).

Source.   Reprinted from Keschner M, Bender MB, Strauss I: "Mental Symptoms in Cases of Tumor of the Temporal Lobe." *Archives of Neurology and Psychiatry* 35:572–596, 1936. Copyright 1936, American Medical Association. Used with permission.

frequently found among those with tumors of the frontal lobe (Figure 9–3). Behavior changes are twice as likely to occur among patients with supratentorial tumors as among those with infratentorial tumors (Keschner et al. 1938). Likewise, mental changes tend to be early symptoms in 18% of the patients with supratentorial tumors but in only 5% of those with infratentorial tumors. Psychiatric disturbances also were found to be more common among patients with tumors of the frontal and temporal lobes than in those with tumors of the parietal or occipital lobes.

Psychotic symptoms tend to be particularly frequent among patients with tumors of the temporal lobes and pituitary gland and much less common among those with occipital and cerebellar tumors, although this finding seems to depend on the particular study being reviewed (Davison and Bagley 1969).

Despite limitations, the literature taken as a whole seems to support a higher frequency of behavior changes among patients with lesions of the frontal and temporal lobes, as well as those with lesions involving deep midline structures. Similarly, bilateral tumors and those with multifocal involvement appear to be more frequently associated with neuropsychiatric symptoms.

GENERAL NEUROPSYCHOLOGICAL CONSIDERATIONS

Neuropsychological testing is often useful in patients with CNS neoplasms. Currently, neuropsychological testing is most often used to determine the extent of cognitive dysfunction associated with a tumor, to provide a preoperative baseline measure of cognitive or memory functioning, or to monitor the efficacy and progress of cognitive rehabilitation efforts after treatment.

The histological type and rate of growth of a tumor may affect the nature and severity of cognitive symptoms. For example, rapidly growing, invasive tumors, such as glioblastoma multiforme, have long been thought to cause obvious cognitive dysfunction, whereas slower-growing, noninvasive tumors, such as meningiomas, have not as frequently been associated with obvious cognitive changes (Reitan and Wolfson 1985). However, a more recent, well-controlled study did not find significant differences between patients with glioblastomas and those without glioblastomas on a battery of neuropsychological tests (Scheibel et al. 1996). In patients with slower-growing tumors, the degree to which cognitive deficits will become clinically apparent is substantially affected by the individual's level of intelligence and adaptive functioning before the development of the tumor. Thus, patients with higher premorbid IQs, who tend to have greater cognitive and intellectual reserves, as well as a broader range of coping and adaptive skills, tend to compensate for and conceal emerging cognitive impairments more successfully for longer periods. In addition, younger patients may be less likely than older patients to manifest cognitive and behavioral deficits (Bigler 1984).

Specific patterns of deficits may be linked to anatomical location (Scheibel et al. 1996), and the tumor also may produce disruption of brain function in nonadjacent regions. According to Lezak (1995), several types of "distance effects" may be important in determining the types of deficits found on neuropsychological testing in brain tumor patients. First, *diaschisis* refers to impairment of neuronal activity in a functionally related but distant region of the brain (von Monakow 1914). Second, disconnection of a given region of the brain from a more distant region by a structural lesion can

also produce cognitive symptoms. This has been dramatically demonstrated in patients who have undergone surgical sectioning of the corpus callosum as treatment for intractable seizures. In keeping with the foregoing, Hahn et al. (2003) reported that on a battery of standardized neuropsychological tests, patients with left hemisphere tumors had significantly more depressive symptoms and reported more problems with memory, inattentiveness, distractibility, and verbal fluency. Recognition of the localizing value of these associations may lead the clinician to consider organic pathology more strongly in certain patients and perhaps to pursue more vigorously the diagnosis of a previously unsuspected brain tumor.

SPECIFIC NEUROPSYCHIATRIC AND NEUROPSYCHOLOGICAL SYMPTOMS AND BRAIN TUMOR LOCATION

In the discussion that follows, we review the range of neuropsychiatric and neuropsychological signs and symptoms that have been reported to co-occur preferentially with brain tumors involving various anatomical structures, including the frontal, temporal, parietal, and occipital lobes; the diencephalon; the corpus callosum; the pituitary; and the posterior fossa.

TUMORS OF THE FRONTAL LOBE

Neuropsychiatric and Behavioral Manifestations

Tumors of the frontal lobes are frequently associated with behavioral symptoms. One study reported mental changes in as many as 90% of cases (Strauss and Keschner 1935). Of these patients, 43% manifested such changes early in the course of their illness.

Injuries to the frontal lobes have been associated with three kinds of clinical syndromes (Cummings 1993). The orbitofrontal syndrome is characterized by changes in personality. These patients typically present with irritability and lability. Cognitively, patients with this syndrome often have poor judgment and a lack of insight into their behavior.

Conversely, patients with injury to the frontal convexities, the so-called dorsolateral prefrontal syndrome, often present with apathy, indifference, and psychomotor retardation. Cognitively, such patients have difficulty initiating or persisting in behavioral activities, have problems with sustained attention and/or sequencing, and may show perseverative behavior (Goldberg 1986). These deficits may not be apparent on standard intellectual or neuropsychological assessments but usually become apparent with more specific tests of executive functioning, such as the Wisconsin Card Sorting Test (Goldberg 1986; Heaton 1985).

Finally, an anterior cingulate syndrome has been described. Patients with this syndrome may be akinetic, with mutism and an inability to respond to commands.

Most patients with tumors of the frontal lobe present with combinations of symptoms. This is probably due in part to the fact that tumors of the frontal lobe are rarely confined to a single subregion and may be causing effects on other areas, both directly and indirectly via pressure effects and edema, as well as by diaschisis and disconnection. It is therefore difficult to find descriptions of these three syndromes in pure form when reviewing the literature on neoplasms of the frontal lobe. Psychiatric symptoms also appear to be more common in patients with lesions of the anterior frontal lobe than in those with lesions of the posterior frontal lobe, suggesting that tumor location on the anteroposterior gradient within the frontal lobe may play a role in determining clinical presentation (Gautier-Smith 1970).

Anxiety has been described and has been noted to increase with frontal tumor progression (Kaplan and Miner 1997). Affective symptoms are common and can include depression, irritability, apathy, and euphoria. Often psychomotor retardation with aspontaneity, hypokinesia, or akinesia is present. In one study of 25 patients with frontal lobe tumors (Direkze

et al. 1971), 5 (20%) had initially presented to psychiatric units with what appeared to be mood disturbances. In their study of 85 patients, Strauss and Keschner (1935) reported affective symptoms in 63%, of whom 30% presented with euphoria and 4% presented with hypomania. Although these authors found no correlation between clinical presentations and laterality of lesions, Belyi (1987) noted a tendency for patients with right frontal lesions to present with euphoria, whereas those with left frontal lesions tended to present with akinesia, abulia, and depressed affect. Another study reported psychiatric symptoms only in patients with right frontal as opposed to left frontal meningiomas (Lampl et al. 1995). A study by Burns and Swerdlow (2003) reported pedophilia and constructional apraxia signs and symptoms occurring in association with a right orbitofrontal tumor.

Changes in personality have been found in as many as 70% of patients with frontal lobe tumors (Strauss and Keschner 1935). These changes, which have been described as "characteristic" of frontal lobe disease (Pincus and Tucker 1978), include irresponsibility, childishness, facetiousness, disinhibition, and indifference toward others, as well as inappropriate sexual behavior. Although these behaviors are consistent with descriptions of the characteristic features of orbitofrontal syndrome, it should be noted that similar "frontal lobe" personality changes have been described in patients with temporal lobe and diencephalic lesions, probably as a result of the rich, reciprocal interconnections that link the temporal, limbic, and frontal regions.

Psychotic symptoms occur with some regularity in patients with frontal lobe tumors. Strauss and Keschner (1935) reported a 10% incidence of both delusions and hallucinations in their series. Other psychotic symptoms reported in patients with frontal lobe tumors have included paranoid ideation and ideas of reference. Typically, delusions secondary to intracranial tumors are less complex than those that occur as part of the delusional systems of schizophrenic patients. Likewise, simple rather than complex hallucinations and visual rather than auditory hallucinations tend to occur in patients with brain tumors.

Neuropsychological Manifestations

Cognitively, patients with tumors of the frontal region of the brain, and of the prefrontal area in particular, often present with significant behavior changes in the absence of obvious intellectual decline or focal neurological dysfunction. In such patients, previously acquired cognitive skills are often preserved, and performance on formal intelligence testing may be quite adequate. More sophisticated neuropsychological assessment of executive functioning, however, often detects profound deficits in the individual's ability to organize, initiate, and direct personal behavior (Lezak 1995; Teuber 1972).

Tumors of the frontal lobes also can result in significant deficits in attentional processes. In addition, tumors of the posterior frontal lobe can lead to expressive (Broca's) aphasia, when the lesion is localized to the dominant hemisphere (Benson 1979), or aprosody, when it is localized to the anterior nondominant hemisphere (Ross 1988).

TUMORS OF THE TEMPORAL LOBE

Neuropsychiatric and Behavioral Manifestations

In any discussion of the psychiatric and behavioral symptoms associated with tumors of the temporal lobe, it is important to distinguish between seizure-associated and non-seizure-associated symptoms and, within the former category, ictal and interictal phenomena. Ictal phenomena are discussed by Kim et al. in Chapter 7 of this book. In this section, we confine our discussion to non-seizure-associated and interictal symptoms due to temporal lobe tumors.

Patients with temporal lobe tumors have been noted to have a high frequency of schizophrenia-like illnesses. Malamud (1967) reported that 6 (55%) of 11 patients with temporal lobe tumors initially presented with a

diagnosis of schizophrenia. Selecki (1965) reported that an initial diagnosis of schizophrenia had been made in 2 of his 9 patients with temporal lobe tumors, and he reported auditory hallucinations in 5. More recently, G. W. Roberts et al. (1990) reported that gangliogliomas, neoplastic hamartomatous lesions that preferentially involve the left medial temporal lobes, are frequently found in patients with delayed-onset, schizophrenia-like psychoses associated with chronic temporal lobe epilepsy.

Patients with temporal lobe dysfunction due to tumors or other causes often present with psychotic symptoms that are somewhat atypical for classic schizophrenia. Supporting the association between psychotic symptomatology and temporal lobe tumors is the work of Davison and Bagley (1969), who reviewed 77 psychotic patients with known brain neoplasms and found that tumors of the temporal lobes were most frequent.

Other studies, however, have not confirmed the apparent high frequency of psychotic syndromes in patients with temporal lobe tumors. Keschner et al. (1936) studied 110 such patients and found that only 2 had complex hallucinations. In another study (Mulder and Daly 1952), only 4 (4%) of 100 patients with temporal lobe tumors had psychotic symptoms. Strobos (1953) noted complex auditory hallucinations in only 1 (1.6%) of his 62 patients with temporal lobe tumors. He found complex visual hallucinations in 5 (8%) and simple olfactory or gustatory hallucinations in 19 (31%), although these almost invariably immediately preceded the onset of seizures.

Neuropsychiatric symptoms associated with temporal lobe tumors tend to be similar to those seen in patients with frontal lobe tumors and may include depressed mood with apathy and irritability or euphoric, expansive mood with hypomania or mania.

Personality change has been described in more than 50% of patients with temporal lobe tumors and may be an early symptom thereof (Keschner et al. 1936). Personality changes caused by brain tumors, including affective lability, episodic behavioral dyscontrol, intermittent anger, irritability, euphoria, and facetiousness, are also commonly seen (Lishman 1987).

Anxiety symptoms appear to be commonly associated with temporal lobe tumors. Mulder and Daly (1952) noted anxiety in 36 (36%) of their 100 patients. Two cases of panic attacks in patients with right temporal lobe tumors have been reported (Drubach and Kelly 1989; Ghadirian et al. 1986).

Neuropsychological Manifestations

Tumors of the temporal lobes can also result in neuropsychological and cognitive deficits. First, verbal or nonverbal memory functioning may be affected, depending on the cerebral hemisphere involved. Dysfunction of the dominant temporal lobe is often associated with deficits in the ability to learn and remember verbal information, whereas that of the nondominant temporal lobe is often associated with deficits in acquiring and retaining nonverbal (i.e., visuospatial) information (Bauer et al. 1993; Butters and Milotis 1979). Tumors of the dominant temporal lobe also may result in receptive (Wernicke's) aphasia, whereas tumors of the nondominant lobe may lead to disruption of the discrimination of nonspeech sounds (Spreen et al. 1965).

TUMORS OF THE PARIETAL LOBE

Neuropsychiatric and Behavioral Manifestations

In general, tumors of the parietal lobe are relatively "silent" with respect to psychiatric symptoms (Critchley 1964). Schlesinger (1950) found affective symptoms in only 5 (16%) of 31 patients with parietal lobe tumors. The affective symptoms in these patients were predominantly depression and apathy, rather than euphoria or mania. Case studies also have reported depression in a woman with a left parietal lesion (Madhusoodanan et al. 2004) and mania in patients with right parietal tumors (Khouzam et al. 1994; Salazar-Calderon Perriggo et al. 1993).

Psychotic symptoms also appear to be less common in patients with parietal lobe tumors.

Selecki (1965), however, reported episodes of "paranoid psychosis" in 2 of the 7 patients with parietal lobe tumors in his series. Cotard's syndrome, involving the denial of one's own existence, has been reported in a patient with a left parietal astrocytoma (Bhatia 1993).

Neuropsychological Manifestations

In general, parietal lobe tumors are more likely to lead to cognitive than to psychiatric symptoms.

Tumors of the anterior parietal lobes may result in abnormalities of sensory perception in the contralateral hand. Inability of the individual to perceive objects placed in the hand (astereognosis) is common and may have localizing value to the contralateral parietal cortex. Difficulty in recognizing shapes, letters, and numbers drawn on the hand (agraphesthesia) is common and may aid in localizing neoplasms to the parietal lobes. Apraxias also may be present. Parietal lobe tumors may interfere with the ability to decipher visuospatial information, particularly when they are localized to the nondominant hemisphere (Warrington and Rabin 1970).

Tumors of the dominant parietal lobe may lead to dysgraphia, acalculia, finger agnosia, and right-left confusion (Gerstmann's syndrome) and often affect reading and spelling. Individuals with parietal lobe tumors often present with a marked lack of awareness or even frank denial of their neurological and neuropsychiatric difficulties. Such phenomena are referred to as *anosognosia* or *neglect syndromes*. Because of the often bizarre neurological complaints and atypical symptoms that may accompany parietal lobe tumors, patients with these lesions are often thought to have psychiatric problems and often initially receive misdiagnoses of either a conversion disorder or some other type of somatization disorder (Jones and Barklage 1990).

TUMORS OF THE OCCIPITAL LOBE

Neuropsychiatric and Behavioral Manifestations

Patients with tumors of the occipital lobe also may present with psychiatric symptoms, but they have been reported to be less likely to do so than those with tumors of the frontal or temporal lobes (Keschner et al. 1938). In 1930, Allen found psychiatric symptoms in 55% of a large series (N = 40) of patients with occipital lobe tumors. In 17% of these patients, behavioral symptoms had been the presenting complaint. The most characteristic finding was visual hallucinations, which were present in 25%. These hallucinations tended to be simple and unformed and were frequently merely flashes of light. Only 2 patients had complex visual hallucinations.

Other symptoms that have been observed in patients with occipital lobe tumors include agitation, irritability, suspiciousness, and fatigue. Keschner et al. (1938) observed affective symptoms in 5 (45%) of 11 patients with occipital lobe tumors. Three (27%) of these patients were dysphoric, and 2 (18%) presented with euphoria or facetiousness.

Neuropsychological Manifestations

Tumors of the occipital lobes may cause significant and characteristic difficulties in cognitive and perceptual functions. A typical finding in patients with occipital lobe neoplasms is homonymous hemianopsia. Inability to recognize items visually (visual agnosia) also may be seen (Lezak 1995). Inability to recognize familiar faces, a condition known as *prosopagnosia*, also may accompany neoplastic lesions in the occipital lobes, particularly when they are bilateral (Meadows 1974).

DIENCEPHALIC TUMORS

Neuropsychiatric and Behavioral Manifestations

Tumors of the diencephalon typically involve regions that are part of or closely contiguous to the limbic system. These lesions also interrupt the various cortical-striatal-pallidal-thalamic-cortical loops, which affect many frontal lobe functions (Alexander and Crutcher 1990). It is therefore not surprising that these lesions are often associated with psychiatric and behavioral disturbances. For example, Malamud (1967)

reported diagnoses of schizophrenia in 4 of 7 patients with tumors involving structures near the third ventricle. Cairns and Mosberg (1951) reported "emotional instability" and psychosis in patients with colloid cysts of the third ventricle. Burkle and Lipowski (1978) also reported depression, affective flattening, and withdrawal in a patient with a colloid cyst of the third ventricle. Personality changes similar to those seen in patients with frontal lobe disease (Gutmann et al. 1990), akinetic mutism (Cairns et al. 1941), catatonia (Neuman et al. 1996), or obsessive-compulsive disorder (Gamazo-Garran et al. 2002) have all been reported in patients with diencephalic or deep midline tumors.

Hypothalamic tumors have been associated with disorders of eating behavior, including hyperphagia (Coffey 1989), and with symptoms indistinguishable from those of anorexia nervosa (Lin et al. 2003). Chipkevitch (1994) reported on 21 cases in the literature in which patients with brain lesions presented with symptoms consistent with a diagnosis of anorexia nervosa. Eleven (52%) of these patients had tumors of the hypothalamus. In 8 of these patients, surgical resection or radiation treatment led to improvement in the symptoms of anorexia. Patients with lesions of the hypothalamus also can present with hypersomnia and daytime somnolence.

Neuropsychological Manifestations

Neoplasms originating in subcortical brain regions often have their most significant effects on memory. These lesions often result in significant impairment in the retrieval of learned material. Detailed neuropsychological evaluations of patients with subcortical tumors may identify a pattern of "subcortical dementia" characterized by a general slowing of thought processes, forgetfulness, apathy, abulia, and depression and an impaired ability to manipulate acquired knowledge (Cummings 1990). Tumors in this area also may lead indirectly to more diffuse, generalized cognitive dysfunction by interfering with the normal circulation of cerebrospinal fluid (CSF), causing hydrocephalus.

TUMORS OF THE CORPUS CALLOSUM

Tumors of the corpus callosum, especially involving the the genu and splenium (Schlesinger 1950), have been associated with behavioral symptoms in as many as 90% of patients (Selecki 1964). Although a broad array of behavior changes, including psychosis and personality changes, have been reported, affective symptoms appear to be particularly common with tumors involving this area. In one study, patients with corpus callosum tumors were compared with patients with other types of tumors. Significantly more depression was found in the group with tumors of the corpus callosum (Nasrallah and McChesney 1981). Tanaghow et al. (1989) also described a patient with a corpus callosum tumor without focal neurological findings who had initially presented with atypical features of depression and prominent cognitive deficits.

PITUITARY TUMORS

Patients with pituitary tumors often present with behavior changes resulting from upward extension of the tumor to other structures, particularly those in the diencephalon. This is a common occurrence in patients with craniopharyngiomas, who sometimes present with disorders of sleep or temperature regulation, clinical phenomena that are ordinarily more common with tumors of the hypothalamus. Anorexia nervosa syndromes also have been reported in patients with craniopharyngiomas (Chipkevitch 1994).

Tumors of the pituitary also can result in endocrine disturbances, which can cause neuropsychiatric symptoms. Basophilic adenomas are commonly associated with Cushing's syndrome, which is likewise often associated with affective lability, depression, or psychotic symptoms. Patients with acidophilic adenomas often present with acromegaly, which has been associated, although infrequently, with both anxiety and depression (Avery 1973).

As with brain tumors involving other anatomical locations, the entire spectrum of psychiatric symptoms, from depression and apathy (Weitzner et al. 2005) to paranoia, has

been reported to occur in patients with pituitary tumors. One review of 5 patients with pituitary lesions reported delusions and hallucinations in 3 (60%) (White and Cobb 1955). In a study by Russell and Pennybacker (1961), 8 (33%) of 24 patients had severe mental disturbances that dominated their clinical picture, and 3 (13%) had initially presented to psychiatric hospitals for diagnosis and treatment.

TUMORS OF THE POSTERIOR FOSSA

Although they are less common overall, all of the psychiatric and behavioral disturbances that have been described in patients with supratentorial tumors also have been reported in patients with infratentorial and posterior fossa lesions.

In one series, psychiatric and behavioral symptoms were found in 76% of the patients with lesions of the posterior fossa and included paranoid delusions and affective disorders (Wilson and Rupp 1946). Pollack et al. (1996) also reported affective disorders, psychosis, personality change, and somatization in their small series. Cases of mania also have been noted (e.g., Greenberg and Brown 1985). Tumors of the posterior fossa have been reported to be associated with irritability, apathy, hypersomnolence, and auditory hallucinations (Cairns 1950). Visual hallucinations have been reported in conjunction with tumors compressing the midbrain (Dunn and Weisberg 1983; Nadvi and van Dellen 1994), and manic or mixed states have been described in 3 adults with acoustic neuroma (Kalayam et al. 1994). Overanxious disorder of childhood with school phobia was reported in a 12-year-old boy with a fourth-ventricle tumor (Blackman and Wheler 1987). The anxiety symptoms were alleviated by surgical removal of the tumor.

LATERALITY OF BRAIN TUMORS AND CLINICAL MANIFESTATIONS

Although few reports have specifically addressed laterality issues with brain tumors, studies reviewing cases of mania secondary to mixed CNS lesions, including tumors, have found a preponderance of right hemisphere lesions (Cummings and Mendez 1984; Jamieson and Wells 1979; Starkstein et al. 1988). A study of unilateral frontal tumors (Belyi 1987) reported that left-sided lesions were commonly associated with akinesia and depression, whereas right-sided lesions were more often associated with euphoria and underestimation of the seriousness of their illnesses by the patients in the study. Pringle et al. (1999) also reported a higher incidence of psychiatric disturbances overall in women with left-sided lesions. Anxiety, on the other hand, may be more common with right hemisphere tumors (Mainio et al. 2003).

These studies suggest that lesion laterality may be a more important factor in symptom formation than had previously been thought. In addition, overall, the available literature suggests the need to reevaluate tumor location and its implications for neuropsychiatric and neuropsychological symptomatology from a different, more topographical perspective. Investigators should consider not only specific regional anatomical localization but also factors such as laterality, anterior/posterior and cortical/subcortical location, and afferent and efferent projections between the region directly involved with the tumor and distant anatomical regions. More important, such a perspective will provide a more clinically relevant, although necessarily more complex, theoretical framework from which to approach the study of psychopathological symptoms and syndromes associated with brain tumors.

CLINICAL DIAGNOSIS

GENERAL CLINICAL CHARACTERISTICS OF BRAIN TUMORS

The most characteristic clinical feature of CNS tumors is the progressive appearance of focal neurological signs and symptoms in addition to neuropsychiatric symptoms. The latter are actually more frequent than the neurological signs and symptoms in early brain tumors

and may include changes in personality and affect, altered sensorium, and cognitive and memory dysfunction. The specific constellation of clinical phenomena encountered and how rapidly they progress depend on the type, size, location, and rate of growth of the tumor; whether it is benign or malignant; and, if the latter, how aggressive it is and whether there is associated cerebral edema, increased intracranial pressure, and hydrocephalus.

Typical neurological signs and symptoms associated with brain tumors include headaches (25%–35%), nausea and vomiting (33%), seizures (20%–50%), papilledema, and visual changes, including field cuts and diplopia. Focal motor and sensory changes are of considerable value in localizing the tumor.

WHEN TO SUSPECT A BRAIN TUMOR IN A PSYCHIATRIC PATIENT

Although recognition of brain tumors in patients presenting with characteristic focal neurological signs and symptoms should not ordinarily be problematic, it may be quite difficult to diagnose a brain tumor promptly and accurately in a patient presenting with predominantly psychiatric and behavioral symptoms. However, the occurrence of one or more of the following five signs and symptoms in a known psychiatric patient or in a patient presenting for the first time with psychiatric symptoms should heighten the clinician's index of suspicion regarding the possibility of a brain tumor:

1. Seizures, especially if of new onset in an adult and if focal or partial, with or without secondary generalization; seizures may be the initial neurological manifestation of a tumor in as many as 50% of cases
2. Headaches, especially if of new onset; generalized and dull (i.e., nonspecific); of increasing severity and/or frequency; or positional, nocturnal, or present immediately on awakening
3. Nausea and vomiting, especially in conjunction with headaches
4. Sensory changes: visual changes such as loss or diminution of vision, visual field

defects, or diplopia; auditory changes such as tinnitus or hearing loss, especially when unilateral; and vertigo

5. Other focal neurological signs and symptoms, such as localized weakness, localized sensory loss, paresthesias or dysesthesias, ataxia, and incoordination

The clinician should bear in mind that nausea and vomiting, visual field defects, papilledema, and other focal neurological signs and symptoms may not be seen until very late, especially with "silent" tumors, such as meningiomas or slow-growing astrocytomas, and other kinds of tumors occurring in relatively "silent" locations (see subsection "Physical and Neurological Examinations" later in this chapter).

DIAGNOSTIC EVALUATION

A comprehensive, careful, and detailed history of the nature and time course of both psychiatric and neurological signs and symptoms is the cornerstone of diagnosis. This should be supplemented by careful physical and neurological examinations, appropriate brain imaging and electrodiagnostic studies, and bedside neurocognitive assessment, including the Mini-Mental State Examination (MMSE), as well as formal neuropsychological testing.

Physical and Neurological Examinations

All psychiatric patients, and particularly those in whom the psychiatrist is considering a brain tumor in the differential diagnosis, should have full and careful physical, neurological, and mental status examinations. It is important to be aware that even despite repeated careful clinical examinations, some brain tumors may not become clinically apparent until relatively late in their course. Such tumors often involve the anterior frontal lobes, corpus callosum, nondominant parietal and temporal lobes, and posterior fossa, the so-called silent regions.

CT Scans

In the 1970s, the CT scan largely replaced plain skull films, radioisotope brain scans, elec-troencephalography, echoencephalography, and pneumoencephalography in the diagnosis of brain tumors because it provided far greater resolution of anatomical brain structures and was much more able to identify small soft-tissue mass lesions. The capacity of the CT scan to detect neoplasms has been further enhanced by the concomitant use of intravenous iodinated contrast materials, such as iohexol, that highlight tumors when they are present. CT scans can also suggest the presence of tumors by showing calcifications, cerebral edema, obstructive hydrocephalus, a shift in midline structures, or other abnormal changes in the ventricular system. Although they are extremely useful, CT scans may not identify very small tumors, tumors in the posterior fossa, tumors that are isodense with respect to brain tissue and/or CSF, and tumors diffusely involving the meninges (i.e., carcinomatosis).

MRI Scans

In general, MRI is superior to CT scanning in the diagnosis of brain tumors and other soft-tissue lesions in the brain because of its higher degree of resolution and greater ability to detect very small lesions. In addition, MRI does not involve exposure to radiation. Its chief drawbacks are its cost and its inability to detect calcified lesions. It also cannot be used in patients in whom ferrometallic foreign objects are present. Enhancement of MRI with gadolinium further increases its diagnostic sensitivity.

Cisternography

CT cisternography, a radiographic technique for evaluating the ventricular system, subarachnoid spaces, and basilar cisterns, may be helpful in the differential diagnosis of intraventricular tumors as well as tumor-associated hydrocephalus. This technique has largely replaced pneumoencephalography, an older air-contrast imaging technique that provided limited diagnostic information and was poorly tolerated by patients because of associated headaches, nausea, and vomiting.

Skull Films

Although plain skull films are no longer routinely used in the diagnosis of brain tumors, tomograms of the sella turcica may be helpful in the diagnosis of pituitary tumors, craniopharyngiomas, and the so-called empty sella syndrome. Plain skull films also may be helpful in the diagnosis of bone (skull) metastases, but bone scans are generally superior in this regard.

Cerebral Angiography

In some cases, cerebral angiography may be important in delineating the vascular supply to a brain tumor before surgery.

Neuropsychological Testing

Neuropsychological testing can be very helpful in determining the extent of tumor-associated cognitive dysfunction and in providing baseline and pretreatment measures of cognitive functioning. It also may be helpful in assessing the efficacy of surgery, radiation therapy, and chemotherapy with respect to improvements in tumor-associated cognitive and neuropsychological dysfunction. It is also helpful in documenting postoperative and postradiation cognitive changes and monitoring the effectiveness of rehabilitative efforts with respect to them.

Lumbar Puncture

Lumbar puncture is now used less frequently than in the past in the diagnosis of brain tumors. Brain tumors may be associated with elevated CSF protein and increased intracranial pressure, but these findings are diagnostically nonspecific, and in the presence of the latter, herniation is a potential danger after a lumbar puncture. Therefore, before proceeding with a lumbar puncture in a patient with a brain tumor, increased intracranial pressure must be ruled out. With certain types of neoplastic diseases of the CNS, such as meningeal carcinomatosis and leukemia, however, lumbar puncture may play an important diagnostic role when other neurodiagnostic studies have been unrevealing.

Electroencephalography

Electroencephalograms in patients with brain tumors may show nonspecific electrical abnormalities, such as spikes and slow waves, either diffuse or focal and paroxysmal or continuous. Frequently, however, the electroencephalogram is normal in such patients. It is not a very specific or sensitive test and thus is not very helpful in differentiating brain tumors from other localized structural cerebral lesions.

Other Testing

Obtaining a chest radiograph is important in evaluating brain tumors because often they may be metastatic from primary lung neoplasms. Single-photon emission computed tomography (SPECT), positron emission tomography (PET), and brain electrical activity mapping (BEAM) are quantitative, computer-based techniques for evaluating various aspects of brain structure and metabolic and neurophysiological functioning. SPECT may have some utility in differentiating tumor recurrence from radiation necrosis in brain tumor patients who have received radiation therapy or in differentiating CNS lymphoma from toxoplasma encephalitis in AIDS patients (Ruiz et al. 1994). And PET scanning may improve diagnostic accuracy and help in the evaluation of the presence of residual or recurrent tumor tissue following initial treatments (Wong et al. 2002).

Magnetoencephalography (MEG) relies on measurement of magnetic fields to localize neuronal cells producing abnormal electrical activity. MEG is more precise than electroencephalography in localizing sources of abnormal electrical activity in the brain and has the potential additional advantage of being able to be used sequentially in assessing brain activity over time without radiation exposure.

TREATMENT OF PSYCHIATRIC AND BEHAVIORAL SYMPTOMS ASSOCIATED WITH CEREBRAL TUMORS

GENERAL CONSIDERATIONS

Psychiatric and behavioral symptoms may be completely relieved after removal of the cerebral tumor with which they are associated. When this does not happen, as is often the case, decreasing the size or interfering with the growth of the tumor through surgery, chemotherapy, or radiation therapy (alone, sequentially, or in combination) may significantly ameliorate the severity of associated behavioral symptoms. Improvement in cognitive and behavioral symptoms may be rapid and dramatic with treatments that diminish increased intracranial pressure or relieve hydrocephalus associated with brain tumors.

In cases in which neuropsychiatric or behavioral symptoms persist or worsen after optimal surgical and nonsurgical interventions, psychopharmacological, psychotherapeutic, and psychosocial interventions become a major treatment focus. The persistence of such psychiatric, behavioral, and neurocognitive symptoms should lead the neurosurgeon or neurologist to seek psychiatric consultation because these symptoms are distressing, cause functional impairment and disability, and have a very negative effect on the patient's overall quality of life (Weitzner 1999).

The interventions of the consulting psychiatrist—who works closely with the attending neurosurgeon—may significantly enhance the patient's level of functioning and overall quality of life (Fox 1998). Ameliorating the disabling dysphoria and anergia of severe depression, alleviating the distress caused by overwhelming anxiety, or simply providing consistent supportive contacts to fearful patients and their families may make an enormous difference to all concerned.

Although patients with cerebral tumors often have psychiatric and behavioral symptoms, only a portion of these are directly related to the tumor. Patients may also have persistent or recurrent symptoms of mood or anxiety disorders that were present premorbidly. Anxiety and depressive symptoms may arise de novo in any brain tumor patient, as a result of psychological reactions to the stress of the initial diagnosis of a brain tumor; concerns about how it will be treated; fears about the potential adverse effects of surgery, radiation therapy, and chemotherapy; and worries about long-term prognosis. Other psychiatric symptoms may emerge later in reaction to the difficulties of adjusting to functional disabilities or distressing life changes that may result from the tumor itself or from the side effects and complications of the various therapeutic interventions brought to bear on it.

PHARMACOLOGICAL MANAGEMENT OF PATIENTS WITH PRIMARY PSYCHIATRIC DISORDERS WHO DEVELOP BRAIN TUMORS

The psychopharmacological management of brain tumor patients with preexisting primary psychiatric illnesses should follow the same general therapeutic principles that apply to tumor-free patients with similar disorders. However, it is important for the psychiatrist to be cognizant of the potential need to make downward adjustments in medication dose and to use drugs that are less likely to cause delirium in patients with brain tumors, as a result of their increased susceptibility to many of the side effects of psychotropic medications. This is especially true of patients who are in the immediate postoperative period or are receiving chemotherapy or radiation therapy. Lithium, low-potency antipsychotic drugs, tertiary amine tricyclic antidepressants (TCAs), and antiparkinsonian agents all have significant dose-related deliriogenic potential when given individually, and this is even more true when they are given in combination or with other potentially deliriogenic agents. It may be necessary to substitute an atypical antipsychotic, carbamazepine, valproic acid, lamotrigine, oxcarbazepine, gabapentin, or a benzodiazepine, such as lorazepam or clonazepam, for lithium in patients with mania; a newer-generation heterocyclic or secondary amine TCA, a selective serotonin reuptake inhibitor (SSRI), or one of the newer, novel-structured antidepressants for tertiary amine TCAs in patients with depression; or one of the atypical antipsychotics for standard neuroleptics in patients with schizophrenia.

Another significant concern is the potential for precipitating seizures when using these drugs, especially in patients with brain tumors. Neuroleptics, antidepressants, and lithium all can lower seizure threshold to varying degrees. Although the available data are inconclusive, standard neuroleptics such as molindone and fluphenazine, and possibly haloperidol (Mendez et al. 1984), are among the older antipsychotic drugs that are believed to carry the smallest risk for seizures, whereas low-potency agents such as chlorpromazine and clozapine are associated with an increased frequency of seizures (Stoudemire et al. 1993). In general, the atypical antipsychotics are believed to have a lower likelihood of precipitating seizures and thus offer an important therapeutic advantage over the old-line antipsychotics. Among the antidepressants, maprotiline and bupropion appear to have the greatest seizure-inducing potential (Dubovsky 1992). It is unclear as to which antidepressants carry the smallest overall risk, but the SSRIs have been reported to have a low likelihood of precipitating seizures. In acutely manic patients with brain tumors, for whom lithium might otherwise be the drug of choice, carbamazepine, valproic acid, oxcarbazepine, lorazepam, clonazepam, and gabapentin—all of which have anticonvulsant properties—may be preferable alternatives.

The psychiatrist should also bear in mind that patients with brain tumors who have psychiatric disorders and are also taking anticonvulsants for a known seizure diathesis should be monitored carefully for the adequacy of anticonvulsant blood levels and should have their anticonvulsant dose increased or decreased as appropriate when psychotropic agents are given. Certain of these medications have epi-leptogenic effects, as well as the potential for decreasing or increasing anticonvulsant blood levels.

PSYCHOTHERAPEUTIC MANAGEMENT OF SYNDROMES ASSOCIATED WITH BRAIN TUMORS

Supportive psychotherapy geared to the patient's current overall functional status, psychosocial situation, interpersonal and family relationships, cognitive capacities, and emotional needs is a very important element in the treatment of any brain tumor patient. The often devastating psychological stress of initially receiving a brain tumor diagnosis and then having to undergo various invasive, painful, and potentially debilitating diagnostic studies and subsequent treatments for it can trigger both the recurrence of preexisting primary psychiatric disorders and the de novo appearance in the patient of reactive psychiatric symptoms resulting from the multiple stressors associated with the illness and its treatment. Likewise, the diagnosis and treatment of a brain tumor in a loved one is enormously stressful for families. Under any clinical scenario, supportive psychotherapy for patients and supportive psychoeducation and therapeutic interventions for their families are likely to be well received and very helpful for both and should play a major role in overall clinical management.

Ideally, supportive psychotherapy for both the patient and the family or significant others should focus primarily on concrete, reality-based cognitive and psychoeducational issues relating to diagnosis, treatment, and prognosis of the patient's brain tumor. Psychotherapeutic interactions with patients should be geared to the patient's cognitive capacities. Over time, the focus of psychotherapy often shifts to the effect of the illness on the patient's emotional and functional status, its effect on the family, the real and imagined challenges of coping with actual or anticipated functional disabilities, and the difficult processes of dealing with anticipatory grief related to potential losses and eventual death. Patients vary widely in their capacity to adjust to and cope with the potentially devastating consequences of brain tumors, and the success of their adjustment and adaptation greatly depends on the flexibility of their premorbid coping abilities. Some patients may appear to be little affected, whereas others may experience severe and even overwhelming symptoms of anxiety and depression. These latter patients may experience greater difficulty continuing to function optimally in their usual work and family roles and need more aggressive psychotherapeutic and psychopharmacological interventions.

Coping by brain tumor patients through the use of the defense mechanism of denial is common and may often be adaptive and effective in helping them to cope with their fears and anxieties, especially in the early stages of what may well turn out to be a life-threatening illness. On the other hand, maladaptive denial may result in the failure of patients and/or their families to comply with optimal treatment recommendations or deal appropriately and in a timely fashion with important legal, personal, family, and other reality-based issues and obligations that need to be addressed while the patient is still able. When denial is producing such maladaptive effects, the clinician may, in a sensitive and supportive manner, need to directly confront and encourage the patient and family to begin to address painful yet inevitable issues such as increasing disability, growing incapacity, and even impending death, and how to best deal with these issues, and then be available to them on a continuing basis as they begin to do so.

It should be kept in mind that psychodynamically focused, insight-oriented psychotherapy, which is usually used in primary psychiatric syndromes when psychodynamic factors are playing a major role and which generally requires intact higher-level cognitive and abstracting capacities, may be relatively contraindicated in psychiatrically ill brain tumor patients. Such patients may have a significant degree of neurocognitive impairment in addition to their psychiatric and behavioral symptoms as a result of the effects of the tumor

itself or of the various neurosurgical, chemotherapeutic, or radiotherapeutic interventions they may have undergone. When such cognitive impairment is present, psychodynamically oriented therapies are unlikely to be beneficial, and they also may cause substantial frustration and acute psychic distress as patients are confronted with psychological tasks and cognitive demands that they are unable to meet because of their brain dysfunction. In general, more concretely focused, "here-and-now" problem-solving psychotherapeutic approaches based on a cognitive-behavioral orientation with the psychiatrist assuming an active, supportive, and educational role in verbal interactions with the patient are likely to be most beneficial.

SOMATIC TREATMENT OF MENTAL DISORDERS DUE TO BRAIN TUMORS

The psychopharmacological treatment of organic mental symptoms and syndromes caused by cerebral tumors follows the same general principles as the drug treatment of phenomenologically similar symptoms due to primary psychiatric illnesses. In treating secondary psychiatric symptoms pharmacologically in patients with brain tumors, some important caveats must be borne in mind. Patients with psychiatric symptoms that are a direct consequence of a brain tumor frequently respond favorably to medications but will frequently tolerate them only in significantly lower doses. Thus, side-effect profiles of psychotropic drugs being considered for the treatment of brain tumor patients must be very carefully considered, especially with regard to sedative, extrapyramidal, deliriogenic, and epileptogenic effects and potential drug interactions.

DRUG TREATMENT OF PSYCHOTIC DISORDERS DUE TO BRAIN TUMORS

First-generation antipsychotic medications may be beneficial in treating the hallucinations, delusions, and thought content and process disturbances that may accompany tumor-associated psychotic syndromes. High-potency antipsychotics, which have fewer nonneurological side effects than do the low-potency antipsychotics, are generally preferable if one of the standard neuroleptics is to be used. However, the former more often cause extrapyramidal symptoms, which may be more severe and persistent in patients with brain tumors. In patients with "organic" psychotic disorders, the therapeutically effective dose of an antipsychotic is often lower than that required for the treatment of primary "functional" psychoses. Thus, as little as 1–5 mg, rather than 10–20 mg, of haloperidol per day (or equivalent doses with other antipsychotics) may be effective. The atypical antipsychotics have been reported to be effective in other psychotic syndromes associated with neurological disorders and have, as a result of their low side-effect profile, generally been well tolerated. Thus, they may well turn out to be the treatment of choice in brain tumor patients with psychotic symptoms. When initiating treatment with antipsychotics, one should "start low and go slowly." This is especially true in elderly patients, in whom effective antipsychotic doses may be lower than they are in younger patients.

Antiparkinsonian agents, such as benztropine, trihexyphenidyl, and orphenadrine, are effective in the treatment of extrapyramidal side effects resulting from the use of neuroleptics in patients with brain tumors. However, in such patients, these agents have a greater likelihood of causing or contributing to the occurrence of anticholinergic delirium when they are used in conjunction with low-potency neuroleptics and/or tertiary amine TCAs. Thus, their use generally should be avoided unless there is a clear-cut clinical indication, and the dose should be minimized when they are used. Diphenhydramine or amantadine for dystonic and parkinsonian symptoms and benzodiazepines or β-blockers for akathisia can be effective alternatives and have less potential for causing delirium.

TREATMENT OF MOOD DISORDERS DUE TO BRAIN TUMORS

Antidepressant medications are often effective in the treatment of depressive mood disorders in patients with brain tumors. Standard TCAs are useful, but currently the SSRIs, newer-generation heterocyclic antidepressants, or secondary amine TCAs are often used preferentially. The SSRIs are therapeutically effective and do not cause delirium, have a favorable side-effect profile, and, despite their relatively high cost, often may be effective in such patients. In recent years, methylphenidate has been shown to be effective (Masand et al. 1991) and to have a rapid onset of action (Woods et al. 1986) in patients with brain tumors. Because methylphenidate is generally well tolerated and does not lower the seizure threshold, its use as an antidepressant in brain tumor patients is increasing.

Monoamine oxidase inhibitors may be effective when other antidepressants are not. They do not ordinarily pose an undue risk in patients with brain tumors, but the clinician must bear in mind that the cognitive impairment that often occurs in such patients may interfere with their ability to maintain a tyramine-free diet.

If single antidepressant medication regimens are ineffective, various combinations may work. When pharmacological treatments have failed, electroconvulsive therapy or repetitive transcranial magnetic stimulation with appropriate precautions should be given serious consideration.

Mood disorders with manic features due to brain tumors, although relatively rare, generally respond to lithium in the usual therapeutic range of 0.8–1.2 mEq/L. For patients in whom seizures have been a part of the clinical picture, however, carbamazepine, valproate, oxcarbazepine, lorazepam, clonazepam, gabapentin, and—in cases in which drug therapy has been ineffective—electroconvulsive therapy may be preferable alternatives.

Newer treatment approaches, including vagal nerve stimulation and transcranial magnetic stimulation, have shown promise in early clinical trials with a variety of mood disorders, including depression, mania (Berman et al. 2000; Grisaru et al. 1998; Rush et al. 2000), and psychotic symptoms (Hoffman et al.

1999). Clarification of their future role in the treatment of brain tumor patients with depression and other neuropsychiatric syndromes awaits further research.

TREATMENT OF ANXIETY DISORDERS DUE TO BRAIN TUMORS

Anxiety symptoms caused either directly or indirectly by brain tumors should not be treated with neuroleptics unless psychotic features are present. The benzodiazepines are often effective and have the added benefit of possessing anticonvulsant properties. However, benzodiazepines may induce delirium in patients with organic brain disease, including brain tumors. This argues for the preferential use of short-acting agents in lower doses, especially in older patients. Other disadvantages of benzodiazepines include their abuse potential and their occasional propensity (especially with the varieties that have long half-lives) to cause seemingly paradoxical reactions, characterized by increased arousal and agitation. Buspirone, which is free of these potentially negative effects, should be considered an alternative to the benzodiazepines. Its main drawbacks are its delayed onset and only modest degree of anxiolytic action. Hydroxyzine, SSRIs, or low doses of tertiary amine TCAs, such as doxepin or amitriptyline, also may have beneficial anxiolytic effects in some patients. Finally, panic attacks associated with temporal lobe tumors may respond to carbamazepine, valproate, or primidone, as well as to the usual antidepressant and antianxiety drugs.

TREATMENT OF DELIRIUM ASSOCIATED WITH BRAIN TUMORS

Delirium in patients with brain tumors may be associated with a wide variety of psychiatric and behavioral symptoms. Hallucinations (especially visual) and delusions are common in delirious patients and often respond to symptomatic treatment with low doses of haloperidol, other high-potency neuroleptics, or one of the atypical antipsychotics while the underlying causes of the delirium are being sought and treated.

TREATMENT OF PERSONALITY CHANGES DUE TO BRAIN TUMORS

Mood lability may be associated with personality changes due to a brain tumor and may respond to lithium, carbamazepine, or other mood stabilizers. Some patients with frontal lobe syndromes associated with tumors may respond to carbamazepine, as do some patients with temporal lobe tumors who may present with associated interictal aggression and violent behavior. Patients with brain tumors who have impulse dyscontrol and rageful, explosive episodes, like patients with intermittent explosive disorders due to other medical and neurological conditions, may respond to empirical therapeutic trials of anticonvulsants, such as carbamazepine, valproic acid, or phenytoin; psychotropics, including lithium; high-potency neuroleptics; and stimulants or β-blockers.

COGNITIVE REHABILITATION

In addition to psychopharmacological and psychotherapeutic treatments, cognitive, occupational, and vocational rehabilitative interventions can be very helpful for patients whose tumors, or the treatments they have received for them, have produced behavioral, cognitive, or functional sequelae. Such sequelae can be identified and quantified by comparing preoperative with postoperative test results on the Halstead-Reitan Neuropsychological Test Battery or other comprehensive neuropsychological test batteries and various functional assessment tools. Serial testing at intervals during the patient's postoperative rehabilitation allows for objective documentation of neuropsychological and functional deficits and allows for objective monitoring of improvement or deterioration over time. Thus, in general, neuropsychological and functional assessments should be a standard part of the pretreatment evaluation and posttreatment follow-up of patients receiving treatment for brain tumors.

Cognitive, occupational, and vocational rehabilitative strategies can be developed that will seek to address deficits in intellectual, language, visuospatial, memory, and neurocognitive functioning, as well as vocational functioning and ability to carry out activities of daily living resulting from a brain tumor. In addition, behavioral techniques have been successfully applied to problematic behaviors resulting from insults to the brain. Such interventions may be used alone or in conjunction with other therapies. For a more detailed discussion of these various approaches, see "Cognitive Rehabilitation and Behavior Therapy for Patients With Neuropsychiatric Disorders," Chapter 18 of this book.

NEUROPSYCHIATRIC CONSEQUENCES OF TREATMENTS OF BRAIN TUMORS

Several psychiatric and behavioral symptoms, as well as neurocognitive deficits, may result from surgical, pharmacological, and radiation treatments of brain tumors and their complications. Unavoidable intraoperative injury to normal brain tissue in the vicinity of a brain tumor during the course of resection or debulking may result in the postoperative appearance of new or exacerbated behavioral or neurocognitive symptoms, depending on the location and connectivity of the tissues involved. The same is true of other perioperative and postoperative complications, such as infections and bleeding. Chemotherapy of brain tumors may cause transient delirium and neurocognitive dysfunction as well as other neurological complications, and the administration of steroids for secondary phenomena such as cerebral edema and increased intracranial pressure may result in the appearance of psychotic symptoms or manic, depressive, or mixed manic and depressive affective syndromes. Radiation therapy directed at brain tumors may result in immediate or delayed sequelae—neurocognitive, endocrine (in the form of late-onset hypothalamic-pituitary dysfunction) (Agha et al. 2005), and behavioral—

due to radiation-induced damage to white matter and other structures.

CONCLUSION

Brain tumors often are associated with, and frequently present, a broad range of psychiatric, behavioral, and neurocognitive symptoms. The differential diagnosis of any patient who has acute or progressive changes in behavior, personality, or cognitive function should include a brain tumor, especially if any focal neurological signs and symptoms are present. In addition to assessment of psychiatric and behavioral symptoms, a full neuropsychiatric evaluation should include physical, neurological, and mental status examinations (e.g., MMSE); appropriate brain imaging and other neurodiagnostic studies; and formal neuropsychological testing, particularly when there is any question of neurocognitive dysfunction on bedside testing with the MMSE.

The nature, frequency, and severity of psychiatric symptoms observed in patients with brain tumors depend on the combined effects of several clinical factors, including the type, location, size, rate of growth, connectivity of affected neurons, and malignancy of the tumor. In general, behavioral symptoms associated with smaller, slower-growing, less aggressive tumors are most likely to be misdiagnosed as psychiatric in origin, particularly when they occur in "silent" regions of the brain, which do not give rise to focal neurological signs or symptoms.

Although tumors of the frontal lobe, temporal lobe, and diencephalon appear to be most commonly associated with psychiatric and behavioral symptoms, the variation in symptoms that may occur with each of these types of tumors is exceedingly broad. In general, the relation between particular neuropsychiatric symptoms and specific anatomical locations of the brain tumors that are causing them is not very consistent.

Optimal treatment of tumor-associated psychiatric, neuropsychiatric, and neuropsychological dysfunctions should be multifaceted and is dependent on the coordinated interventions of a multidisciplinary treatment team. The psychopharmacological treatment of psychiatric and behavioral syndromes should follow the same general principles as those for corresponding primary psychiatric disorders. However, the choice of drugs and/or dosages may require modification because many of the psychotropic agents can induce seizures or delirium, and patients with brain tumors are more vulnerable to these and other side effects of psychotropic medications.

Adjunctive supportive psychotherapy for both the patient and the family is very important, as are psychosocial and psychoeducational interventions tailored to their specific needs. Such psychotherapeutic and psychosocial interventions must be carefully integrated with psychopharmacological, rehabiliative (neurocognitive, physical, occupational, vocational), and behavioral treatment approaches as clinically indicated. In turn, all of these must be coordinated with the neurosurgeon's ongoing treatment interventions to optimize the patient's overall medical and surgical management. With well-planned integration and coordination of these multiple complementary therapeutic approaches, both the quantity and the quality of the patient's life may be substantially enhanced.

RECOMMENDED READINGS

Cummings J: Clinical Neuropsychiatry. Orlando, FL, Grune & Stratton, 1985

Feinberg T, Frank M (eds): Behavioral Neurology and Neuropsychology. New York, McGraw-Hill, 1997

Jobe TH, Gaviria M: Clinical Neuropsychiatry. Oxford, UK, Blackwell Science, 1997

Kandel E, Schwartz J, Jessel T: Principles of Neural Science, 4th Edition. New York, McGraw-Hill, 2000

Lishman A, Malden MA: Organic Psychiatry: The Psychological Consequences of Cerebral Disorders, 3rd Edition. Oxford, UK, Blackwell Science, 1998

Mesulam M: Principles of Behavioral Neurology. Philadelphia, PA, FA Davis, 1986

Strub R, Black FW: Neurobehavioral Disorders: A Clinical Approach. Philadelphia, PA, FA Davis, 1988

REFERENCES

Agha A, Shenlock M, Brennan S, et al: Hypothalamic-pituitary dysfunction after irradiation of nonpituitary brain tumors in adults. J Clin Endocrinol Metab 90:6355–6360, 2005

Alexander GE, Crutcher MD: Functional architecture of basal ganglia circuits: neural substrates of parallel processing. Trends Neurosci 13:266–271, 1990

Allen IM: A clinical study of tumors involving the occipital lobe. Brain 53:196–243, 1930

Avery TL: A case of acromegaly and gigantism with depression. Br J Psychiatry 122:599–600, 1973

Bauer RM, Tobias B, Valenstein E: Amnesic disorders, in Clinical Neuropsychology, 3rd Edition. Edited by Heilman KM, Valenstein E. New York, Oxford University Press, 1993, pp 523–578

Belyi BI: Mental impairment in unilateral frontal tumors: role of the laterality of the lesion. Int J Neurosci 32:799–810, 1987

Benson DF: Aphasia, Alexia, and Agraphia. New York, Churchill Livingstone, 1979

Berman RM, Narasimhan M, Sanacora G, et al: A randomized clinical trial of repetitive transcranial magnetic stimulation in the treatment of major depression. Biol Psychiatry 47:332–337, 2000

Bhatia MS: Cotard's syndrome in parietal lobe tumor. Indian Pediatr 30:1019–1021, 1993

Bigler ED: Diagnostic Clinical Neuropsychology. Austin, University of Texas Press, 1984

Blackman M, Wheler GH: A case of mistaken identity: a fourth ventricular tumor presenting as school phobia in a 12 year old boy. Can J Psychiatry 32:584–587, 1987

Burkle FM, Lipowski ZJ: Colloid cyst of the third ventricle presenting as psychiatric disorder. Am J Psychiatry 135:373–374, 1978

Burns JM, Swerdlow RH: Right orbitofrontal tumor with pedophilia symptom and constructional apraxia sign. Arch Neurol 60:437–440, 2003

Butters N, Milotis P: Amnestic disorders, in Clinical Neuropsychology. Edited by Heilman KM, Valenstein E. New York, Oxford University Press, 1979, pp 403–439

Cairns H: Mental disorders with tumors of the pons. Folia Psychiatrica Neurologica Neurochirurgica 53:193–203, 1950

Cairns H, Mosberg WH: Colloid cysts of the third ventricle. Surg Gynecol Obstet 92:545–570, 1951

Cairns H, Oldfield RC, Pennybacker JB, et al: Akinetic mutism with an epidermoid cyst of the 3rd ventricle. Brain 64:273–290, 1941

Chipkevitch E: Brain tumors and anorexia nervosa syndrome. Brain Dev 16:175–179, 1994

Coffey RJ: Hypothalamic and basal forebrain germinoma presenting with amnesia and hyperphagia. Surg Neurol 31:228–233, 1989

Critchley M: Psychiatric symptoms and parietal disease: differential diagnosis. Proc R Soc Med 57:422–428, 1964

Cummings JL: Subcortical Dementia. New York, Oxford University Press, 1990

Cummings JL: Frontal-subcortical circuits and human behavior. Arch Neurol 50:873–880, 1993

Cummings JL, Mendez MF: Secondary mania with focal cerebrovascular lesions. Am J Psychiatry 141:1084–1087, 1984

Davison K, Bagley CR: Schizophrenia-like psychoses associated with organic disorders of the central nervous system: a review of the literature, in Current Problems in Neuropsychiatry: Schizophrenia, Epilepsy, the Temporal Lobe (British Journal of Psychiatry Special Publication No 4). Edited by Harrington RN. London, Headley Brothers, 1969, pp 126–130

Direkze M, Bayliss SG, Cutting JC: Primary tumours of the frontal lobe. Br J Clin Pract 25:207–213, 1971

Drubach DA, Kelly MP: Panic disorder associated with a right paralimbic lesion. Neuropsychiatry Neuropsychol Behav Neurol 2:282–289, 1989

Dubovsky SL: Psychopharmacological treatment in neuropsychiatry, in The American Psychiatric Press Textbook of Neuropsychiatry. Edited by Yudofsky SC, Hales RE. Washington, DC, American Psychiatric Press, 1992, pp 663–701

Dunn DW, Weisberg LA: Peduncular hallucinations caused by brainstem compression. Neurology 33:1360–1361, 1983

Filley CM, Kleinschmidt-DeMasters BK: Neurobehavioral presentations of brain neoplasms. West J Med 163:19–25, 1995

Fox S: Use of a quality of life instrument to improve assessment of brain tumor patients in an outpatient setting. J Neurosci Nurs 30:322–325, 1998

Galasko D, Kwo-On-Yuen PF, Thal L: Intracranial mass lesions associated with late-onset psychosis and depression. Psychiatr Clin North Am 11:151–166, 1988

Gamazo-Garran P, Soutullo CA, Ortuna F: Obsessive-compulsive disorder secondary to brain dysgerminoma in an adolescent boy: a positron emission tomography case report. J Child Adolesc Psychopharmacol 12:259–263, 2002

Gautier-Smith P: Parasagittal and Falx Meningiomas. London, Butterworth, 1970

Ghadirian AM, Gauthier S, Bertrand S: Anxiety attacks in a patient with a right temporal lobe meningioma. J Clin Psychiatry 47:270–271, 1986

Goldberg E: Varieties of perseverations: comparison of two taxonomies. J Clin Exp Neuropsychol 6:710–726, 1986

Greenberg DB, Brown GL: Mania resulting from brain stem tumor: single case study. J Nerv Ment Dis 173:434–436, 1985

Grisaru N, Chudakov B, Yaroslavsky Y, et al: Transcranial magnetic stimulation in mania: a controlled study. Am J Psychiatry 155:1608–1610, 1998

Gupta RK, Kumar R: Benign brain tumours and psychiatric morbidity: a 5-year retrospective data analysis. Aust N Z J Psychiatry 38:316–319, 2004

Gutmann DH, Grossman RI, Mollman JE: Personality changes associated with thalamic infiltration. J Neurooncol 8:263–267, 1990

Hahn CA, Dunn RH, Logue PE, et al: Prospective study of neuropsychologic testing and quality-of-life assessment of adults with primary malignant brain tumors. Int J Radiat Oncol Biol Phys 55:992–999, 2003

Heaton RK: Wisconsin Card Sorting Test. Odessa, FL, Psychological Assessment Resources, 1985

Hobbs GE: Brain tumours simulating psychiatric disorder. Can Med Assoc J 88:186–188, 1963

Hoffman RE, Boutros NN, Berman RM, et al: Transcranial magnetic stimulation of left temporoparietal cortex in three patients reporting hallucinated "voices." Biol Psychiatry 46:130–132, 1999

Hollister LE, Boutros N: Clinical use of CT and MR scans in psychiatric patients. J Psychiatry Neurosci 16:194–198, 1991

Jamieson RC, Wells CE: Manic psychosis in a patient with multiple metastatic brain tumors. J Clin Psychiatry 40:280–283, 1979

Jarquin-Valdivia AA: Psychiatric symptoms and brain tumors: a brief historical overview. Arch Neurol 61:1800–1804, 2004

Jones JB, Barklage NE: Conversion disorder: camouflage for brain lesions in two cases. Arch Intern Med 150:1343–1345, 1990

Jukich PJ, McCarthy BJ, Surawicz TS, et al: Trends in incidence of primary brain tumors in the United States, 1985–1994. Neuro-oncol 3:141–151, 2001

Kalayam B, Young RC, Tsuboyama GK: Mood disorders associated with acoustic neuromas. Int J Psychiatry Med 24:31–43, 1994

Kaplan CP, Miner ME: Anxiety and depression in elderly patients receiving treatment for cerebral tumours. Brain Inj 11:129–135, 1997

Keschner M, Bender MB, Strauss I: Mental symptoms in cases of tumor of the temporal lobe. Arch Neurol Psychiatry 35:572–596, 1936

Keschner M, Bender MB, Strauss I: Mental symptoms associated with brain tumor: a study of 530 verified cases. JAMA 110:714–718, 1938

Khouzam HR, Emery PE, Reaves B: Secondary mania in late life. J Am Geriatr Soc 42:85–87, 1994

Klotz M: Incidence of brain tumors in patients hospitalized for chronic mental disorders. Psychiatr Q 31:669–680, 1957

Ko SM, Kok LP: Cerebral tumours presenting with psychiatric symptoms. Singapore Med J 30:282–284, 1989

Kocher R, Linder M, Stula D: [Primary brain tumors in psychiatry.] Schweiz Arch Neurol Neurochir Psychiatr 135:217–227, 1984

Lampl Y, Barak Y, Achiron A, et al: Intracranial meningiomas: correlation of peritumoral edema and psychiatric disturbances. Psychiatry Res 58:177–180, 1995

Lezak MD: Neuropsychological Assessment, 3rd Edition. New York, Oxford University Press, 1995

Lin L, Lioa SC, Lee YJ, et al: Brain tumor presenting as anorexia nervosa in a 19-year-old man. J Formos Med Assoc 102:737–740, 2003

Lishman WA: Organic Psychiatry: The Psychological Consequences of Cerebral Disorder. New York, Oxford University Press, 1987

Madhusoodanan S, Danan D, Brenner R, et al: Brain tumor and psychiatric manifestations: a case report and brief review. Ann Clin Psychiatry 16:111–113, 2004

Mainio A, Hakko H, Niemela A, et al: The effect of brain tumour laterality on anxiety levels among neurosurgical patients. J Neurol Neurosurg Psychiatry 74:1278–1282, 2003

Malamud N: Psychiatric disorder with intracranial tumors of limbic system. Arch Neurol 17:113–123, 1967

Masand P, Murray GB, Pickett P: Psychostimulants in post-stroke depression. J Neuropsychiatry Clin Neurosci 3:23–27, 1991

Meadows JC: The anatomical basis of prosopagnosia. J Neurol Neurosurg Psychiatry 37:489–501, 1974

Mendez MF, Cummings JL, Benson DF: Epilepsy: psychiatric aspects and use of psychotropics. Psychosomatics 25:883–894, 1984

Minski L: The mental symptoms associated with 58 cases of cerebral tumor. J Neurol Psychopathol 13:330–343, 1933

Mulder DW, Daly D: Psychiatric symptoms associated with lesions of temporal lobe. JAMA 150:173–176, 1952

Nadvi SS, van Dellen JR: Transient peduncular hallucinations secondary to brain stem compression by a medulloblastoma. Surg Neurol 41:250–252, 1994

Nasrallah HA, McChesney CM: Psychopathology of corpus callosum tumors. Biol Psychiatry 16:663–669, 1981

Neuman E, Rancurel G, Lecrubier Y, et al: Schizophreniform catatonia in 6 cases secondary to hydrocephalus with subthalamic mesencephalic tumor associated with hypodopaminergia. Neuropsychobiology 34:76–81, 1996

Olney JW, Farber NB, Spitznagel E, et al: Increasing brain tumor rates: is there a link to aspartame? J Neuropathol Exp Neurol 55:1115–1123, 1996

Percy AK, Elveback LR, Okazaki H, et al: Neoplasms of the central nervous system: epidemiologic considerations. Neurology 22:40–48, 1972

Pincus JH, Tucker GJ: Behavioral Neurology, 2nd Edition. New York, Oxford University Press, 1978

Pollack L, Klein C, Rabey JM, et al: Posterior fossa lesions associated with neuropsychiatric symptomatology. Int J Neurosci 87:119–126, 1996

Pringle AM, Taylor R, Whittle IR: Anxiety and depression in patients with an intracranial neoplasm before and after tumor surgery. Br J Neurosurg 13:46–51, 1999

Radhakrishnan K, Bohnen NI, Kurland LT: Epidemiology of brain tumors, in Brain Tumors: A Comprehensive Text. Edited by Morantz RA, Walsh JW. New York, Marcel Dekker, 1994, pp 1–18

Reitan RM, Wolfson D: Neuroanatomy and Neuropathology for Neuropsychologists. Tucson, AZ, Neuropsychology Press, 1985, pp 167–192

Remington FB, Robert SL: Why patients with brain tumors come to a psychiatric hospital: a thirty-year survey. Am J Psychiatry 119:256–257, 1962

Roberts GW, Done DJ, Bruton C, et al: A "mock up" of schizophrenia: temporal lobe epilepsy and schizophrenia-like psychosis. Biol Psychiatry 28:127–143, 1990

Roberts JKA, Lishman WA: The use of CAT head scanner in clinical psychiatry. Br J Psychiatry 145:152–158, 1984

Ross E: Prosody and brain lateralization: fact vs. fancy or is it all just semantics? Arch Neurol 45:338–339, 1988

Ruiz A, Ganz WI, Donovan Post J, et al: Use of thallium-201 brain SPECT to differentiate cerebral lymphoma from toxoplasma encephalitis in AIDS patients. AJNR Am J Neuroradiol 15:1885–1894, 1994

Rush AJ, George MS, Sackheim HA, et al: Vagus nerve stimulation (VNS) for refractory depressions: a multicenter study. Biol Psychiatry 47:276–286, 2000

Russell RW, Pennybacker JB: Craniopharyngioma in the elderly. J Neurol Neurosurg Psychiatry 24:1–13, 1961

Salazar-Calderon Perriggo VH, Oommen KJ, Sobonya RE: Silent solitary right parietal chondroma resulting in secondary mania. Clin Neuropathol 12:325–329, 1993

Scheibel RS, Meyers CA, Levin VA: Cognitive dysfunction following surgery for intracerebral glioma: influence of histopathology, lesion location, and treatment. J Neurooncol 30:61–67, 1996

Schlesinger B: Mental changes in intracranial tumors and related problems. Confinia Neurologica 10:225–263, 1950

Selecki BR: Cerebral mid-line tumours involving the corpus callosum among mental hospital patients. Med J Aust 2:954–960, 1964

Selecki BR: Intracranial space-occupying lesions among patients admitted to mental hospitals. Med J Aust 1:383–390, 1965

Spreen O, Benton A, Fincham R: Auditory agnosia without aphasia. Arch Neurol 13:84–92, 1965

Starkstein SE, Boston JD, Robinson RG: Mechanisms of mania after brain injury: 12 case reports and review of the literature. J Nerv Ment Dis 176:87–100, 1988

Stoudemire A, Fogel BS, Gulley LR, et al: Psychopharmacology in the medical patient, in Psychiatric Care of the Medical Patient. Edited by Stoudemire A, Fogel BS. New York, Oxford University Press, 1993, pp 155–206

Strauss I, Keschner M: Mental symptoms in cases of tumor of the frontal lobe. Arch Neurol Psychiatry 33:986–1005, 1935

Strobos RRJ: Tumors of the temporal lobe. Neurology 3:752–760, 1953

Tanaghow A, Lewis J, Jones GH: Anterior tumour of the corpus callosum with atypical depression. Br J Psychiatry 155:854–856, 1989

Teuber HL: Unity and diversity of frontal lobe functions. Acta Neurobiol Exp 32:615–656, 1972

von Monakow C: Die Lokalisation im Grossheim und der Abbav der Funktion durch Kortikale Herde. Weisbaden, JF Bergmann, 1914

Warrington EK, Rabin P: Perceptual matching in patients with cerebral lesions. Neuropsychologia 8:475–487, 1970

Weitzner MA: Psychosocial and neuropsychiatric aspects of patients with primary brain tumors. Cancer Invest 17:285–291, 1999

Weitzner MA, Kanfer S, Booth-Jones M: Apathy and pituitary disease: it has nothing to do with depression. J Neuropsychiatry Clin Neurosci 17:159–166, 2005

Wellisch DK, Kaleita TA, Freeman D, et al: Predicting major depression in brain tumor patients. Psychooncology 11:230–238, 2002

White J, Cobb S: Psychological changes associated with giant pituitary neoplasms. Arch Neurol Psychiatry 74:383–396, 1955

Wilson G, Rupp C: Mental symptoms associated with extramedullary posterior fossa tumors. Trans Am Neurol Assoc 71:104–107, 1946

Wong TZ, van der Westhuizen GJ, Coleman RE: Positron emission tomography imaging of brain tumors. Neuroimaging Clin N Am 12:615–626, 2002

Woods SW, Tesar GE, Murray GB, et al: Psychostimulant treatment of depressive disorders secondary to medical illness. J Clin Psychiatry 47:12–15, 1986

10

NEUROPSYCHIATRIC ASPECTS OF HUMAN IMMUNODEFICIENCY VIRUS INFECTION OF THE CENTRAL NERVOUS SYSTEM

Francisco Fernandez, M.D.

Brian Giunta, M.D., M.S.

Jun Tan, M.D., Ph.D.

Human immunodeficiency virus (HIV) infection has become a major health and social issue of this era. Our aim is to outline the neuropathology and neurobehavioral symptomatology associated with HIV infection and delineate the challenging and perplexing range of possible neuropsychiatric complications that clinicians may encounter. We discuss treatment of the various neuropsychiatric entities in relation to the special characteristics and needs of this medically ill population.

CNS PATHOLOGY RESULTING DIRECTLY FROM HIV

Direct brain infection by HIV is now widely believed to be the likely cause of related cognitive and other neurobehavioral disorders (Janssen et al. 1991). The evidence for this theory includes detection of HIV-1 in the central nervous system (CNS) (Davis et al. 1992), direct HIV isolation from the brain and cerebrospinal fluid (CSF) (Chiodi et al. 1992), and electron microscopic findings of viral particles within infiltrating macrophages (Schindelmeiser and Gullotta 1991). Because the CNS in HIV infection can be regarded as a possible reservoir for the virus, antiviral drugs that can penetrate the blood-brain barrier and the blood-CSF barrier are clearly necessary. Gross examination of the brain indicates that the white matter, subcortical structures, and spinal cord are commonly involved in HIV-1-associated dementia (HAD), showing vacuolar myelopathy and multinucleated giant cells (Brew et al. 1988). Also, extensive atrophy is found. Because of long-term survival in the HIV-infected population, the epidemic is extending into older age brackets and is commonly characterized by pathology resembling that of Alzheimer's disease (AD). Several postmortem studies have revealed a significant incidence of AD-like pathology in the HIV-infected brain, including increased brain beta-amyloid (A-beta) deposition (Green et al. 2005), increased extracellular amyloid plaques (Achim et al. 2004), and CSF A-beta levels (Brew et al. 2005).

Although neurons are not the direct target of the virus (Weis et al. 1993), they sustain neurotoxic effects. Frequently involved subcortical gray matter structures include basal ganglia, thalamus, and temporolimbic structures. Wiley and colleagues (1991) applied sensitive quantitative methods to the histological analysis of cerebral cortex and found up to a 40% loss of cortical dendritic area. In this analysis, the severity of cortical damage was found to be correlated with level of HIV gp41 immunoreactivity (Masliah et al. 1992).

This CNS neuropathology often results in cognitive changes, from mild memory decline and cognitive slowing to a profound dementia (Everall et al. 1993). In addition, Price and colleagues noted in their series of findings that HIV-1 could be recovered mainly from brains of patients with the most severe form of dementia, in which multinucleated giant cell creation had occurred (Brew et al. 1988). However, dementia also has developed in individuals in whom the virus could not be recovered from the CNS, either directly or by hybridization methods.

Once the virus has entered the CNS, a complex cascade of events can occur to cause neural injury, which is thought to result in the various neurobehavioral syndromes (Lipton and Gendleman 1995). Lipton and Gendleman (1995) have detailed what is currently known about these events. First, in the process of binding to a $CD4^+$ receptor–containing cell, HIV gp120 irreversibly binds to a calcium channel and increases intracellular free calcium (Stefano et al. 1993). HIV gp120 also induces the cell to increase neurotoxin production (Lipton and Gendleman 1995) and may alter brain glucose metabolism, which could lead to brain dysfunction (Lipton and Gendleman 1995). Second, after the virus enters the cell and incorporates its genome into the host's genome, it can induce the infected macrophage to release more injurious compounds in the presence of other stimulators, such as other CNS infectious by-products and cytokines produced in response to infections by other immunologically active cells. Lipton and Gendleman (1995) described these compounds to include glutamate-like substances such as quinolinic acid; free radicals such as superoxide anions; other cytokines such as tumor necrosis factor (TNF)-α, interleukin-1-β, and interferon-γ; and eicosanoids such as arachidonic acid. Additionally, gp120 and certain fragment peptides are powerful activators of N-methyl-D-aspartate (NMDA) receptors of the CNS, the mechanism associated with neuroexcitotoxicity (Gemignani et al. 2000). These are all thought to cause neurocellular injury by several mechanisms, including increased intracellular calcium and increased concentrations of the toxic inorganic compound nitric oxide.

Apoptosis was proposed as an additional factor in the destruction of $CD4^+$ cells in HIV disease, for both lymphocytes and neural tissues. One protein thought to participate in this process is FAS (Lynch et al. 1995), and this genetically driven action has been shown to culminate in disruption of the cell's nucleus by activation of endonucleases (Silvestris et al. 1995). Certain immune factors, such as TNF-α, can trigger apoptosis (Talley et al. 1995).

In the case of HIV infection, several virus-related proteins can trigger apoptosis. Gp120 also has been reported to induce apoptosis (Maccarrone et al. 2000). TNF-α can be produced by HIV-related gp120 binding to macrophages, which may lead to this process (Sekigawa et al. 1995). Apoptosis also has been shown to be induced peripherally by the HIV-related Tat protein (Li et al. 1995). This cell-destroying mechanism can be inhibited, and knowledge of how to effect this inhibition can be applied to clinical AIDS treatment. Certain immunosuppressive compounds such as FK506 (Sekigawa et al. 1995) and glucocorticoids (Lu et al. 1995) have inhibited apoptosis, as have growth factors (Li et al. 1995), soluble CD4 (Maldarelli et al. 1995), N-acetylcysteine (Talley et al. 1995), and didanosine (preinfection only) (Corbeil and Richman 1995), but not zidovudine (Maldarelli et al. 1995). However, inhibiting apoptosis can present further difficulties because it has been shown that it can enhance viral production and lead to high levels of persistent viral infection (Antoni et al. 1995).

Additional work on the neuropathology of excitotoxins (Heyes et al. 1991, 1992; Lipton 1992; Lipton and Gendleman 1995; Walker et al. 1989), the role of NMDA receptor physiology and dysregulation (Lipton 1992; Lipton and Gendleman 1995), and the specific neurotoxicity of quinolinic acid, a metabolite of tryptophan (Lipton and Gendleman 1995), is also contributing to the explanation of how neuronal tissue is injured by remote metabolic effects of HIV infection. Quinolinic acid levels have been found to be highly correlated with levels of β_2-microglobulin and neopterin (Heyes et al. 1992) and with cognitive impairment (Heyes et al. 1991).

CNS NEUROPATHOLOGY DUE TO OPPORTUNISTIC INFECTIONS AND NEOPLASIA

When severe neurological disease, opportunistic infections, or malignancies arise, the patient's condition meets criteria for full-blown AIDS. This may occur at any time, although immune compromise is usually reflected by the clinical and laboratory markers—namely, fewer than 200 CD4$^+$ cells/mm^3. Additionally, syphilis and tuberculosis are increasingly found as coinfections in patients with AIDS. These disorders must be considered in the differential diagnosis of CNS infection. These infections and malignancies may contribute to severe neurological disorders or overwhelming dementia (Brew et al. 1988; Filley et al. 1988; Gonzales and David 1988; Ho et al. 1987; Petito 1988). Thus, it is important to investigate and treat aggressively the cause of the neurological problem in order to postpone mortality and to seek to restore normal neurobehavioral function. Bredesen and colleagues (1988) reviewed common CNS infections, as well as neoplasia and other infection- or treatment-induced complications. This range of CNS involvement is listed in Table 10–1 (Bredesen et al. 1988).

DIRECT ASSESSMENT OF CNS INJURY IN HIV DISEASE

NEUROIMAGING FINDINGS

Imaging, by both computed tomography (CT) and magnetic resonance imaging (MRI), has proved helpful in showing injury by the virus and other pathological processes in the brain (Dooneief et al. 1992; Flowers et al. 1990; Post et al. 1991). Aside from either method being able to show atrophy, as reflected by increased ventricular size and sulcal size, both can help to define pathological entities such as ring-enhancing lesions and some aspects of white matter involvement. MRI is superior to CT in showing areas of focal high-signal intensities in subcortical white and gray matter by the T2-weighted signal (Dooneief et al. 1992). T1 relaxation times have been examined and have not indicated structural differences between older HIV-infected patients and control subjects or temporal changes in these older patients as their disease progressed (Freund-Levi et al. 1989). MRI also has not proven useful in depicting structural correlates of neurologically asymptomatic HIV infection (Post et al. 1991). MRI, however, has disclosed neuro-

TABLE 10–1.   CNS conditions associated with AIDS and HIV infection

HIV-associated disorders

    HIV-1-associated cognitive/motor complex

        HIV-1-associated dementia

        HIV-1-associated minor cognitive/motor disorder

    HIV-1-associated myelopathy

Opportunistic viral infections

    Cytomegalovirus

    Herpes simplex virus, types 1 and 2

    Herpes varicella zoster virus

    Papovavirus (progressive multifocal leukoencephalopathy)

    Adenovirus type 2

Other opportunistic infections of the CNS

    Toxoplasma gondii

    Cryptococcus neoformans

    Candida albicans

    Aspergillus fumigatus

    Coccidioides immitis

    Mucormycosis

    Rhizopus species

    Acremonium alabamensis

    Histoplasma capsulatum

    Mycobacterium tuberculosis

    Mycobacterium avium-intracellulare

    Listeria monocytogenes

    Nocardia asteroides

Neoplasms

    Primary CNS lymphoma

    Metastatic lymphoma

    Metastatic Kaposi's sarcoma

Cerebrovascular pathology

    Infarction

    Hemorrhage

    Vasculitis

Adverse effects of treatments for HIV and AIDS-related disorders

Note.   AIDS = acquired immunodeficiency syndrome; CNS = central nervous system; HIV = human immunodeficiency virus.

Source.   Adapted from Bredesen DE, Levy RM, Rosenblum ML: "The Neurology of Human Immunodeficiency Virus Infection." *Quarterly Journal of Medicine* 68:665–677, 1988. Copyright 1988 Oxford University Press. Used with permission.

structural changes in medically symptomatic but neurologically asymptomatic HIV-positive patients. Jernigan et al. (1993) found volumetric reductions in cerebral gray and white matter in these patients.

Imaging reflecting functioning of the nervous system, such as positron emission tomography (PET) (Brunetti et al. 1989), single-photon emission computed tomography (SPECT) (Kuni et al. 1991; Sacktor et al. 1995), magnetic resonance spectroscopy (MRS) (Deicken et al. 1991), functional MRI (Navia and Gonzalez 1997), and regional cerebral blood flow (rCBF) (Schielke et al. 1990), has shown regional functional abnormalities in HIV infection. These imaging modalities have established themselves as sensitive to different aspects of functioning: PET reflects metabolism; SPECT, functional MRI, and rCBF reflect brain perfusion; and MRS reflects biochemical function and dysfunction.

CEREBROSPINAL FLUID FINDINGS

The CSF of HIV-infected patients who have fever with or without altered mental status or with complaints about mental functioning should be evaluated quickly for signs of opportunistic infection such as toxoplasmosis, cryptococcal infection, herpes simplex virus, varicella zoster virus, and cytomegalovirus so that anti-infective treatment can be initiated before CNS damage occurs (Buffet et al. 1991). Specific signs of HIV infection in CSF values include HIV virions, immunoglobulin G (IgG—in abnormally large quantities), HIV-specific antibody, mononuclear cells, neopterin, β_2-microglobulin, and oligoclonal bands (Brew et al. 1992; Buffet et al. 1991; Carrieri et al. 1992; Chiodi et al. 1992; Heyes et al. 1991; Larsson et al. 1991; Marshall et al. 1988; McArthur et al. 1992; Reboul et al. 1989; Shaskan et al. 1992; Tartaglione et al. 1991). The amount of intrathecal virus and antibody, however, has not been found to correlate with severity of neurological or cognitive symptomatology (Reboul et al. 1989). The concentration of CSF β_2-microglobulin is highly correlated with both dementia severity (Brew et al. 1992; McArthur et al. 1992) and level of systemic disease (asymptom-

atic seropositivity to fully developed AIDS). CSF β_2-microglobulin has shown some specificity in differentiating HAD from multiple sclerosis and other CNS disorders (Carrieri et al. 1992) with regard to absolute levels and CSF-to-serum ratios. Additionally, it can reflect positive symptomatic zidovudine therapy (Brew et al. 1992) (although the amount of virus in the CSF may not be reduced with treatment [Tartaglione et al. 1991]).

Analysis of neurotransmitter metabolites in CSF, specifically those of noradrenaline and dopamine, failed to detect significantly different levels of 3-methoxy-4-hydroxyphenylglycol (MHPG) between HIV-infected patients and noninfected, healthy volunteers (Larsson et al. 1991). However, CSF levels of homovanillic acid (HVA) were lower by almost half in HIV-infected patients than in noninfected volunteers and lowest in patients with AIDS; no direct relation was found between HVA levels and severity of dementia. The level of quinolinic acid, an excitotoxin and an NMDA receptor agonist (see earlier discussion in the section "CNS Pathology Resulting Directly From HIV"), is related to severity of dementia and clinical status (Heyes et al. 1991). In patients with early-stage disease, quinolinic acid levels were twice those of non-HIV-infected subjects, and more than 20 times normal levels were detected in patients with severe dementia or CNS AIDS involvement (opportunistic infection or CNS neoplasms) (Heyes et al. 1991). More recently, CSF quinolinic acid levels were found to correlate with regional brain atrophy as quantified by MRI, whereas CSF β_2-microglobulin levels were not (Heyes et al. 2001). The significance of these levels of an excitotoxin in the CNS continues to be investigated with regard to pathogenesis and pathophysiology of cognitive disorders.

NEUROBEHAVIORAL ASSESSMENT OF HIV INFECTION OF THE CNS

A revision of the American Academy of Neurology (AAN) criteria for HIV-1-associated cognitive/motor complex (Janssen et al. 1991) has been proposed (Antinori et al. 2007). The new criteria mainly recognized three neurocognitive disorders: asymptomatic neurocognitive impairment (ANI), minor neurocognitive disorder (MND) and HAD. ANI is a subclinical condition (*not* a formal disorder) that is characterized by significant cognitive decline in two or more domains of neuropsychological test performance but without significant decline in functional status. For a diagnosis of MND, there must be mild neurocognitive impairment in at least two domains of cognitive performance and, at most, a minor functional impairment in daily living, insufficient severity for a diagnosis of HAD, and no other known etiology for the symptoms. For HAD, there must be severe cognitive impairment in two or more domains, at least a moderate level of functional status impairment due to the cognitive symptoms, a lack of clouding of consciousness (i.e., delirium), and no support for another etiology accounting for these symptoms.

Dementia is an acquired intellectual impairment characterized by persistent deficits in multiple areas, including memory, language, cognition, visuospatial skills, personality, and emotional functioning (Cummings and Benson 1983). Until recently, HAD has been portrayed as a subcortical type of dementia affecting subcortical and frontostriatal brain processes (Brew et al. 1988). However, because other CNS cortical areas have been identified as being affected (Everall et al. 1991; Masliah et al. 1992; Navia et al. 1986; Wiley et al. 1991), a strict definition of HIV-related cognitive impairment as a subcortical disorder has been questioned (Poutiainen et al. 1991). Dementia's persistent cognitive impairment differentiates it from another common HIV-related mental disorder due to a general medical condition—delirium. The symptoms most frequently described and most closely associated with subcortical disorders such as Parkinson's disease and progressive supranuclear palsy, as well as multiple sclerosis, are found in HIV infection of the CNS. The description of HAD as a subcortical process suggests that neuropsychological tests that reflect

memory registration, storage, and retrieval; psychomotor speed; information processing rate; and fine motor function are important in a neuropsychological battery for assessment of HIV-related cognitive impairment (Butters et al. 1990). Other traditionally cortical syndromes, such as aphasia, agnosia, apraxia, and other sensory-perceptual functions, also can be present but usually not until later in the course of the disease and perhaps as a result of some focal opportunistic infection or neoplastic invasion of the CNS.

The earliest level of cognitive impairment is a subclinical cognitive inefficiency that can range in severity from a decrement in previous level of functioning in attention, speed of information processing, memory, abstraction, and fine motor skills to formal test-defined deficits in some of these domains. Disturbances in these functions may have no observable effects on activities of daily living (ADL) or on functional performance; thus, the new name—asymptomatic neurocognitive impairment. These changes occur in more than 20% of asymptomatic HIV-1-infected individuals (Wilkie et al. 1990), but the proportion of patients having these problems doubles with advanced disease (Heaton et al. 1995). More severe impairment interfering minimally with functional status is now defined as MND. Prevalence of MND is unknown, but estimates suggest that 20%–30% of asymptomatic HIV-1-infected individuals may meet formal AAN criteria for this disorder (Goodkin et al. 2001). Indications of MND may be mild and, as such, are frequently attributed to the systemic illness or a psychosocial reaction to HIV infection. However, even under the influence of an early organic process that affects cognition, many patients will be cognizant of their own mental and physical sluggishness and personality changes, and affective symptoms may occur concomitantly.

Fully developed HAD is commonly associated with significant declines in functional status. Table 10–2 shows signs and symptoms of both cognitive and psychiatric disturbances commonly encountered early in the course

TABLE 10–2.   Early signs and symptoms of HIV-related neurobehavioral impairment

Cognitive	Affective/behavioral
Memory impairment (especially with verbal, rote, or episodic)	Apathy
Concentration or attention disturbance	Depressed mood
Language comprehension problems	Anxiety
Conceptualization difficulties	Mild agitation
Problem-solving difficulties	Mild disinhibition
Visuospatial constructional deficits	Hallucinations or misperceptions
Motor slowing or impairment in coordination	
Mental tracking difficulties	
Mild frontal lobe–type symptoms	
Handwriting and fine motor control difficulties	

Note.   HIV = human immunodeficiency virus.
Source.   Adapted from Brew BJ, Sidtis JJ, Petito CK, et al.: "The Neurologic Complications of AIDS and Human Immunodeficiency Virus Infection," in *Advances in Contemporary Neurology.* Edited by Plum F. Philadelphia, PA, FA Davis, 1988, pp. 1–49.

of HAD (Brew et al. 1988), and Table 10–3 shows signs and symptoms of cognitive and psychiatric difficulties encountered late in the course of HAD (Brew et al. 1988). The course of HAD can steadily worsen, with the development of moderate to severe cognitive deficits, confusion, psychomotor slowing, and seizures. Patients may appear mute and catatonic. So-cially inappropriate behavior; psychosis; mania; marked motor abnormalities such as ataxia, spasticity, and hyperreflexia; and incontinence of bladder and bowel can occur.

Clinicians must, however, evaluate the patient's complaints—such as memory problems, mental slowing, and difficulty with attention and concentration—at any stage of the disease.

TABLE 10–3.   Late signs and symptoms of HIV-related neurobehavioral impairment

Cognitive	Affective/behavioral
Severe dementia affecting multiple cognitive areas	Severe behavioral disinhibition
Aphasia and/or mutism	Manic symptoms
Severe frontal lobe symptoms	Delusions
Severe psychomotor slowing	Severe hallucinations
Intense distractibility	Severe agitation
Disorientation	Paranoid ideation
	Severe depression with or without suicidality

Note.   HIV = human immunodeficiency virus.
Source.   Adapted from Brew BJ, Sidtis JJ, Petito CK, et al.: "The Neurologic Complications of AIDS and Human Immunodeficiency Virus Infection," in *Advances in Contemporary Neurology.* Edited by Plum F. Philadelphia, PA, FA Davis, 1988, pp. 1–49.

Dysphoria due to the seriousness of the illness or induced by medications or affective disturbances could theoretically cause cognitive difficulties (e.g., pseudodementia of depression) (Cummings and Benson 1983), but several studies (e.g., Syndulko et al. 1990) have reported that cognitive dysfunction is not correlated with mood disorder, and the level of cognitive impairment surpasses that expected from distraction due to affective causes.

The cardinal signs of HIV-related cognitive impairment include problems with verbal memory, difficulties with attention and concentration, slowing of information processing, slowed psychomotor speed, and in some cases, the nonverbal abilities of problem solving, visuospatial integration and construction, and nonverbal memory are impaired (Butters et al. 1990). Studies have shown that psychomotor tasks, such as the Digit Symbol and Block Design tests of the Wechsler Adult Intelligence Scale and the Trail Making Test Part B from the Halstead-Reitan Neuropsychological Test Battery, and memory tasks, such as the delayed Visual Reproduction subtest from the Wechsler Memory Scale and the delayed recall of the Rey-Osterrieth Complex Figure, were most affected in the early stages of cognitive impairment associated with HIV (Van Gorp et al. 1989). We and others have found that tasks detecting psychomotor and neuromotor disturbances in HIV-related neural dysfunction such as visuomotor reaction time (Dunlop et al. 1992; Nance et al. 1990) and fine motor dexterity as measured by pegboard activities are also sensitive measures for the early detection of impairment. Such motor speed tasks may be more vulnerable to the effects of HIV than is central processing speed. One investigation (Martin et al. 1992) implied that graphomotor and manual slowing may be a major component of impairment on psychomotor tasks. When a memory search or reaction time paradigm was used, speed of memory search in HIV-positive patients did not differ significantly from that in control subjects. This task did not test speed of movement but rather a cognitive reaction latency.

TABLE 10–4. HIV neuropsychological screening battery

Attention and memory

Wechsler Adult Intelligence Scale—Revised, Digit Span subtest

Rey Auditory-Verbal Learning Test

Language/speech and speed of cognitive production

Controlled Oral Word Association Test (from Benton Multilingual Aphasia Examination)

Executive/psychomotor

Symbol Digit Modalities Test

Trail Making Test, Parts A and B

Grooved Pegboard

Note. HIV = human immunodeficiency virus.
Source. Reproduced with permission of authors and publisher from Selnes OA, Jacobson L, Machado AM, Becker JT, Wesch J, Miller EN, Visscher B, and McArthur JC: "Normative Data for a Brief Neuropsychological Screening Battery." *Perceptual and Motor Skills* 73:539–550, 1991. © Perceptual and Motor Skills 1991.

Other areas of cognitive function that are assessed by neuropsychological batteries include aphasia, apraxia, and other complex language-associated functioning; verbal abstract reasoning and problem solving; and perceptual functioning of the different sensory modalities. If the patient's lack of stamina or other situation precludes an extensive battery, a comprehensive but briefer battery consisting of the tests listed in Table 10–4 (Selnes et al. 1991), or tests that address similar functions (Butters et al. 1990), can assess the critical areas of cognitive functioning to detect HIV involvement at an early stage.

Because early cognitive impairment may occur before the diagnosis of AIDS, a means of measuring cognitive functioning was needed to define cognitive disabilities at earlier stages of infection.

A scale that has been proposed to discriminate patients with HIV infection and dementia from patients with HIV infection but not dementia is the HIV Dementia Scale (HDS;

Power et al. 1995). It appears to be more sensitive than the Mini-Mental State Examination to the HIV-related subcortical effects of CNS infection. The HDS has been criticized because portions of the scale are difficult to administer by nonneurologically trained individuals. For example, it requires saccadic eye movement examination, for which no standardized scoring exists. However, even if this component is deleted, the HDS retains the ability to discriminate grossly among mild-moderate and moderate-severe dementia (Skolasky et al. 1998).

In the largest study of its kind to date, 267 HIV-positive individuals received comprehensive evaluations of neuropsychological functioning, medical status, and functional abilities, including laboratory measures of instrumental ADL (Heaton et al. 2004). A comparison of group test performance found that individuals classified as having abnormal neuropsychological functioning performed significantly worse on laboratory measures of daily functional abilities. The domains most strongly correlated with failure on the functional measures included abstraction and executive functioning, learning, attention and working memory, and verbal abilities. This suggests that neuropsychological impairment is related to functional deficits, further emphasizing the importance of objective cognitive assessment in addition to measures of cognitive complaints and other self-report measures.

TREATMENT OF HIV INFECTION OF THE CNS

PRIMARY THERAPY: ANTIVIRALS

For a detailed review of the primary and secondary salvage therapeutic strategies for the treatment of HIV/AIDS, the reader is referred to the federal guidelines for the use of antiretroviral therapies in adults and children (Panel on Antiretroviral Guidelines for Adults and Adolescents 2009). No specific guidelines exist for treating cognitive impairment and HAD. However, available studies suggest that the main thrust of treatment should be to produce virological suppression of both plasma and CNS compartments.

Zidovudine is a potent inhibitor of retrovirus replication in vitro and reduces morbidity by decreasing the number of serious complications in patients with AIDS as well as in asymptomatic patients (Fischl et al. 1987). Several studies also suggest zidovudine therapy attenuates the symptomatic course of the dementia and neurological disease in some patients (Arendt et al. 1991; Yarchoan et al. 1987). The compound penetrates the brain at a level at which one-half can be recovered from CSF (Wong et al. 1992). Therefore, findings such as those of Sidtis and colleagues (1993) that report improved cognitive functioning in patients who receive high levels of zidovudine—up to 2,000 mg/day—are consistent with this brain parenchymal bioavailability characteristic. Additionally, doses may need to be high to maintain therapeutic CNS levels of zidovudine because it is cleared from the brain through an active transport process (Wang and Sawchuk 1995; Wong et al. 1993). Clinicians should keep this finding in mind when calculating the maintenance dose of zidovudine in the patient with subjective complaints consistent with HIV-1-associated minor cognitive/motor disorder or HAD.

Human data regarding zidovudine indicate that with careful clinical monitoring and appropriate dose modification, it is a safe drug to use in neurologically impaired patients (Yarchoan et al. 1987). The principal toxicity of zidovudine is a decrease in the red blood cell, neutrophil, and, less commonly, platelet counts. Of these, neutrophil depression has proved to be the major limiting toxicity because anemia can be treated with transfusion. Most hematological side effects of zidovudine usually emerge after 6 weeks or more of therapy and, in many cases, require dose reduction or discontinuation. Typically, resuming treatment with zidovudine at a lower dose can be effective once hematopoietic toxicity has resolved. Minor side effects of zidovudine include myalgias, headache, insomnia, nausea, and depersonalization and derealization. Mania has been reported (Wright et al. 1989), and delirium also has been reported (Fernandez 1988). Macrocytosis is the only consistent laboratory index, excluding the previously described hematological changes. Concurrent treatment with acetaminophen may result in an increased frequency of neutropenia. Theoretically, drugs that are hepatically cleared and disturb the process of glucuronidation also have the potential to cause neutropenia. Thus, zidovudine should be used cautiously, with regular hematological monitoring. A single report exists of a patient who developed severe neurotoxicity and died (Hagler and Frame 1986); however, confirmatory studies of mortality risk from zidovudine are lacking.

Other antivirals such as zalcitabine (ddC) (Dickover et al. 1991; Neuzil 1994), didanosine (ddI) (Neuzil 1994), lamivudine (3TC) (van Leeuwen et al. 1995), and stavudine (d4T) (Murray et al. 1995; Neuzil 1994) are now being used in the control of HIV replication and, as such, may play a role in reducing the viral load available to the CNS via circulatory spread. These drugs, however, do not penetrate the blood-brain barrier as well as zidovudine. Additionally, the protease inhibitors that prevent maturation of HIV particles (Neuzil 1994) are also showing promise alone and in combination therapy with the reverse transcriptase agents (highly active antiretroviral therapy; HAART) (Greenlee and Rose 2000). Significant improvement in both cognitive (Tozzi et al. 1999) and motor (Sacktor et al. 2001) abilities on neuropsychological testing has been reported. Thus, antiviral therapy currently provides an important direct intervention for cognitive and emotional effects of HIV infection of the CNS.

What is not known is what particular combinations of antiretrovirals have the best penetration of the blood-brain barrier and provide the best parenchymal prophylaxis. Agents other than zidovudine theorized to do so include abacavir, nevirapine, and indinavir. Some advocate the use of these agents that are known to penetrate the brain better on the assumption that these might better treat HIV in-fection of the CNS (Cysique et al. 2004; Sacktor et al. 2001). However, this approach remains theoretical at this time.

ADJUNCTIVE THERAPY: ADDITIONAL BIOLOGICAL AND PHARMACOLOGICAL INTERVENTIONS

HIV-1 gp120 may be associated with neuronal cell injury by altering cellular calcium flux (Lipton 1991; Lipton and Gendleman 1995; Stefano et al. 1993). Lipton (1991) suggested that certain calcium channel blockers (e.g., flunarizine) were protective against gp120 toxicity in vitro. Nimodipine (30–60 mg orally 4–6 times daily) also was found to be protective and is being used to regulate neuron-injuring intracellular calcium increments (Dreyer et al. 1990). Verapamil and diltiazem were not as effective as nimodipine or did not help. In fact, in another study, verapamil enhanced HIV-1 replication in lymphoid cells (Harbison et al. 1991).

Microglia-associated chronic brain inflammation is the common final pathway in HAD. Galantamine is a potent allosteric potentiating ligand of nicotinic acetylcholine receptors (Samochocki et al. 2003; Santos et al. 2002) and cholinesterase inhibitors (Shytle et al. 2004). We showed that nicotine in the presence of galantamine synergistically attenuates HIV-1 gp120/interferon-γ–induced microglial activation, as evidenced by decreased TNF-α and nitric oxide releases (Giunta et al. 2004). This finding suggests a novel therapeutic combination to treat or prevent the onset of HAD through this modulation of the microglia inflammation mechanism.

Epigallocatechin gallate (EGCG), the major component of green tea, has been reported to have neuroprotective properties (Mandel et al. 2004). Most important, Kawai and colleagues (2003) reported that EGCG directly binds to the CD4 receptor and interferes with HIV-1 gp120 binding at the target cell surface. We have shown that EGCG treatment of primary neurons from normal mice reduced HAD-like neuronal injury mediated by interferon-γ and/or HIV-1 viral proteins gp120 and Tat, as evidenced by decreased lactate dehydrogenase release and increased ratio of Bcl-xL to Bax protein. In addition, primary neurons derived from Stat1-deficient mice were largely resistant to HAD-like neuronal damage. In accord with these findings, EGCG also attenuated HAD-like neuronal damage in mice (Giunta et al. 2006). Taken together, these data suggest that green tea–derived EGCG possibly represents a novel therapeutic approach for the prevention and treatment of HAD and its Alzheimer's-like pathology.

ADJUVANT THERAPY: PSYCHOPHARMACOLOGICAL ENHANCEMENT OF FUNCTION

Adjuvant therapy in the form of psychostimulant treatment (see also subsection "Depression in HIV Disease" later in this chapter) can help improve functioning in cognitive domains. Early data indicated that methylphenidate, when used to treat affective disorders in HIV-infected patients, significantly improved verbal rote memory and rate of cognitive tracking and mental set shifting (Fernandez et al. 1988a, 1988b). On average, this amounted to elevating associated scores on neuropsychological instruments into the normal range. Subsequent investigations (Angrist et al. 1991; White et al. 1992) have confirmed this effect. Possible support for the efficacy of psychostimulants may come from their enhancement of dopaminergic functioning in neural populations that subtend attention or concentration, memory retrieval, and speed of cognitive processing (Fernandez and Levy 1990).

MANIFESTATIONS OF SPECIFIC HIV-RELATED NEUROPSYCHIATRIC DISORDERS AND THEIR TREATMENT

The range of HIV-related neuropsychiatric disorders includes most of the major mental disorders listed in DSM-IV-TR (American Psychiatric Association 2000). The most common psychiatric effects are those "due to general medical conditions," such as delirium and psychosis (Fernandez et al. 1989b; Harris et al. 1991; Wolcott et al. 1985); dementia; mood disorder, including depression (Fernandez et al. 1995; Markowitz et al. 1994) and mania (McGowan et al. 1991); and stress syndromes such as anxiety disorders (Fernandez 1989).

DELIRIUM AND PSYCHOSIS IN HIV DISEASE

Delirium is the most prevalent and frequently undiagnosed; as many as 30% of hospitalized medical-surgical patients have an undetected delirium (Knights and Folstein 1977). In the post-HAART era, delirium is reported in 20% of patients (O'Dowd and McKegney 1990). The prompt detection of delirium is crucial because of potential reversibility and, thus, diminished morbidity and mortality.

Timely pharmacological intervention may help to suppress the delirium symptoms; however, in our study, complete reversal of delirium occurred in only 37% of the patients with AIDS (Fernandez et al. 1989b).

The atypical antipsychotic agents are entering the armamentarium to treat delirium. Risperidone (Singh et al. 1997) at various doses has been used with success to target psychotic symptoms. Olanzapine (Sockalingam et al. 2005) also may be used, but its affinity for the cytochrome P450 3A4 isoenzyme system may be problematic for patients taking specific protease inhibitors. Quetiapine, ziprasidone, aripiprazole, and paliperidone also may be tried, but there is little experience to date with these agents (Stolar et al. 2005).

The safety and efficacy of intravenous haloperidol treatment for delirium, either alone or in combination with lorazepam or additionally with hydromorphone for agitated patients with delirium, has been reported (Fernandez et al. 1989a). Neuroleptic malignant syndrome is perhaps the most ominous potential adverse effect (Breitbart et al. 1988); however, in our experience, this syndrome is rare in this population. The rarity of this complication may stem from the intravenous route of administration. The possible protective influence of lorazepam, when coadministered with haloperidol, against the extrapyramidal side effects of haloperidol must be delineated with further controlled trials.

Psychosis associated with HIV infection has been less frequently studied. The differential diagnosis of psychotic symptoms in an HIV seropositive patient includes delirium, late-stage HIV-associated dementia, and mania (which may be due to HIV infection itself); recurrence of premorbid psychotic illnesses; psychoactive substance intoxication; HAART medication toxicities (particularly with efavirenz) (Lowenhaupt et al. 2007); and general medical conditions manifesting with psychotic symptoms. The same atypical antipsychotic medications are effective in treating psychotic symptoms no matter what the etiology.

DEPRESSION IN HIV DISEASE

The prevalence of mood disorders in HIV-infected patients, especially during the asymptomatic stage, has been an issue of investigation since the first patients presented with these affective symptoms.

The relative risk of suicide is very high. Marzuk and colleagues (1988) found that the relative risk of suicide in men with AIDS living in New York City was 36.3 times that for men without an AIDS diagnosis and 66.2 times that of the general population. Although pharmacotherapy provides the most rapid intervention for remission of depression, specific guidelines for drug selection are conspicuously absent.

The low-anticholinergic tricyclic antidepressants (TCAs) may be useful for treating depression in HIV-infected patients because these drugs have less risk than do the highly anticholinergic TCAs of exacerbating cognitive deficits or causing a delirious process. The choice of a particular TCA should be guided by its specific action and side effects (Richelson 1988) in relation to the patient's depressive symptoms and concomitant medical condition (Fernandez and Levy 1991). The therapeutic dose of a TCA

may be much lower (10–75 mg) for an HIV-infected patient with neuropsychiatric impairment than for a noninfected person.

In general, all nontricyclic antidepressant agents are effective and lack significant anticholinergic, histaminergic, adrenergic, and cardiac side effects. However, most do inhibit the biochemical activity of drugs that metabolize the isoenzyme cytochrome P450 2D6 or 3A4. Citalopram (Currier et al. 2004), escitalopram, venlafaxine, and mirtazapine are the weakest 2D6 and 3A isoenzyme inhibitors (Greenblatt et al. 1998). Clinicians may use these agents with low affinity for the 2D6 and 3A isoenzyme system in HIV-related depression while carefully monitoring the coadministration of both prescribed and over-the-counter medications.

Bupropion has both noradrenergic and dopaminergic effects and has been used effectively in HIV/AIDS patients with depression (Maldonado et al. 2000). It has been associated with seizures and should be used cautiously in patients with neurological disease or avoided altogether (Maldonado et al. 2000).

Nefazodone is a serotonin receptor antagonist and serotonin reuptake inhibitor that works at the serotonin type 2 receptor site. It also is a minor noradrenergic reuptake inhibitor. Along with nefazodone's effectiveness in significant depressive illness, it appears not to potentiate the depressant effects of alcohol (Frewer and Lader 1993). Because of its affinity for cytochrome P450 and its propensity for hepatoxicity, nefazodone should be avoided in the treatment of depression in HIV/AIDS (Stolar et al. 2005).

The psychostimulants seem to be especially effective in HIV-infected patients who have cognitive impairment or depression and dementia (Fernandez and Levy 1991; Fernandez et al. 1988a, 1988b; Holmes et al. 1989). In HIV-infected patients without cognitive impairment, treatment with methylphenidate was associated with a remission of depressive symptoms that was statistically indistinguishable from that achieved with the TCA desipramine (Fernandez et al. 1995). For methylphenidate, the usual dosage is 5–20 mg taken on awakening in the morning, at midmorning, and again in early afternoon to avoid disturbing nighttime sleep (Fernandez et al. 1989a). Amelioration of secondary, subclinical depression in a double-blind clinical trial comparing methylphenidate and pemoline in the treatment of significant fatigue has been reported, with relatively few side effects (Breitbart et al. 2001).

Hypogonadism with associated changes in libido, diminished appetite, fatigue, and loss of lean body mass can be present in a significant number of men with HIV/AIDS and can present as depression. Hormone replacement therapy with testosterone has been reported to be effective in men (Rabkin et al. 2004) and women (Miller et al. 1998). Hormone replacement in neurobehaviorally impaired patients may be disinhibitory and may cause irritability, rage, and violent behavior; therefore, such therapy should be used with caution.

Depressed HIV-infected patients with psychotic symptoms or an organic mood disturbance, or for whom pharmacological treatment has failed, may benefit from electroconvulsive therapy (ECT). This modality may be tried after very careful review of its use in patients with complex medical illness (Weiner 1983); however, ECT may increase confusion in some encephalopathic HIV-infected patients (Schaerf et al. 1989).

MANIA IN HIV DISEASE

Acute mania with HIV disease may be the result of premorbid bipolar disorder; brain lesions from HIV, opportunistic infections, or AIDS-related neoplasms; or medications (McGowan et al. 1991; O'Dowd and McKegney 1988; Wright et al. 1989).

Treatment of mania in HIV-infected patients is similar to that in non-HIV-infected patients. Lithium has been found useful in the treatment of secondary mania due to zidovudine (O'Dowd and McKegney 1988). Close monitoring of levels and blood chemistry is essential for avoidance of toxicity in debilitated patients or those with the wasting syndrome. It is especially critical when infectious complica-

tions occur, such as with cryptosporidial infection or other causes of severe diarrhea, or with other severe fluid losses. Even when doses are used to maintain therapeutic serum concentrations of 0.5–1.0 mEq/L, patients with advanced disease cannot tolerate treatment with lithium.

Valproate also has been approved as a treatment for mania (McElroy et al. 1992). It may be tried cautiously in patients whose renal or electrolyte status makes lithium problematic. There is a single report of valproic acid decreasing intracellular concentration of glutathione and stimulating HIV (Melton et al. 1997). We have retrospectively evaluated our valproate-treated patients' medical records and have not found any increases in viral load to suggest that this is a clinically relevant concern.

At this time, no clinical reports are available on the efficacy of newer antiepileptic agents such as gabapentin, lamotrigine, and topiramate in HIV-related mania. Of these, lamotrigine is the only U.S. Food and Drug Administration–approved medication for maintenance therapy in bipolar affective disorder and therefore may be equally effective in HIV-related mania. It is safe to use in the context of HIV.

ANXIETY AND INSOMNIA IN HIV DISEASE

The stresses associated with treatment of HIV elicit anxiety (Fernandez 1989; Perry et al. 1992), especially for those predisposed to anxiety disorders. Anxiety disorders of any type often respond to supportive therapy, cognitive behavioral therapy, progressive muscular relaxation training, self-hypnosis, cognitive-imagery, and biofeedback without anxiolytic pharmacotherapy. Anxiolytic agents may help the patient to function better in all aspects of daily living.

However, the automatic use of benzodiazepines as anxiolytics is risky in cases of severe anxiety or restlessness because these compounds may further compromise the patient's coping capacity and may be disinhibiting.

But the anxiety and insomnia (ranging from mild to severe) that may result from treatment with zidovudine, efavirenz, or steroids, or be secondary to the effects of HIV on the CNS, may be helped with brief pharmacotherapy with short- to intermediate-acting benzodiazepines such as lorazepam and oxazepam (Fernandez 1988). Alprazolam for anxiety and triazolam and estazolam for insomnia should be avoided in patients receiving HAART because of their affinity for the cytochrome P450 3A4 subenzyme system. Chronic use of benzodiazepines may be warranted in some patients. If so, we advocate use of clonazepam tablets or wafers. If tolerance develops in these patients, 50–200 mg of trazodone at bedtime may be combined with or substituted for the benzodiazepine. Although the β-blocker propranolol is often useful for healthy individuals who are anxious or phobic, it has a propensity to result in hypotensive episodes, particularly in patients who may have undiagnosed HIV-related dysautonomia (Lin-Greenberger and Taneja-Uppal 1987). Antihistamines, such as hydroxyzine, have low efficacy for anxiolysis unless the anxiety is accompanied by specific respiratory problems.

Studies of the effectiveness of the non-benzodiazepine anxiolytic buspirone (Kastenholz and Crismon 1984) in HIV-infected patients indicate its value when the immediate attenuation of acute anxiety or phobias is not essential. Buspirone's anxiolytic effects lack excessive sedation or potential for dependence. It should be prescribed with caution for HIV-infected patients with CNS impairment, and its use should be monitored closely because buspirone-related dyskinesias (Strauss 1988) may be more easily elicited in HIV-infected patients than in noninfected, neurologically intact patients with anxiety. Cases of possible buspirone-related mania have been reported (McDaniel et al. 1990; Price and Bielefeld 1989).

Nonbenzodiazepines in use for insomnia include zolpidem, zaleplon, and eszopiclone (Sharma et al. 2005). Zolpidem is a nonbenzodiazepine sedative-hypnotic, and it is the most prescribed agent in HIV-related insomnia. Zolpidem is primarily a substrate of cytochrome P450 3A4. Clinically significant inter-actions may occur with concurrent use of cytochrome P450 3A4 inhibitors and inducers such as ritonavir, delavirdine, and nevirapine. Zaleplon is a short-acting nonbenzodiazepine sedative-hypnotic. Zaleplon is primarily metabolized by aldehyde oxidase to form 5-oxozaleplon. To a lesser extent, zaleplon is metabolized by the hepatic isoenzyme cytochrome P450 3A4, and all its metabolites are inactive. However, antiretroviral protease inhibitors may increase the levels of zaleplon. Although clinical data do not exist, and this interaction is not expected to require routine zaleplon dosage adjustment, one should remain vigilant for possible problems. Eszopiclone is a nonbenzodiazepine hypnotic agent that is a pyrrolopyrazine derivative of the cyclopyrrolone class. Eszopiclone is metabolized by cytochrome P450 3A4 and 2E1 via demethylation and oxidation. Inhibitors of cytochrome P450 3A4, like the protease inhibitors, will result in an increase in the levels of eszopiclone. Clinical experience with eszopiclone in patients with HIV-related insomnia is limited.

CONCLUSION

The neuropsychiatric complications of HIV infection and AIDS are a perplexing assortment of neurological, neurocognitive, and affective/behavioral effects that may arise at any time during the course of the illness. Thus, all neuropsychiatrists should maintain a high index of suspicion of even the most subtle of behavioral symptoms in previously asymptomatic persons because several means of investigation (e.g., electrophysiological, neuropsychological) have disclosed that neurological involvement may occur early in the course of the disease. As the AIDS epidemic continues, these symptoms may arise in individuals other than those in the initial high-risk categories, and a careful history of possible exposure must be included in any workup of unusual cognitive, neurological, or neuropsychiatric symptoms fitting the pattern described in this chapter. If the etiology is found to be HIV related, then prompt aggressive treatment of the conditions, perhaps with innovative measures, is warranted, to maintain as optimal a quality of life as can be promoted, for as long as possible.

RECOMMENDED READINGS

Fernandez F, Ruiz P (eds): Psychiatric Aspects of HIV/AIDS. Philadelphia, PA, Lippincott Williams & Wilkins, 2006

McArthur JC, Brew B, Nath A: Neurological complications of HIV infection. Lancet Neurol 4:543–555, 2005

REFERENCES

Achim CL, Masliah E, Schindelar J, et al: Immunophilin expression in the HIV-infected brain. J Neuroimmunol 157:126–132, 2004

American Psychiatric Association: Diagnostic and Statistical Manual of Mental Disorders, 4th Edition, Text Revision. Washington, DC, American Psychiatric Association, 2000

Angrist B, D'Hollosy M, Sanfilipo M, et al: Central nervous system stimulants as symptomatic treatments for AIDS-related neuropsychiatric impairment. J Clin Psychopharmacol 12:268–272, 1991

Antinori A, Arendt G, Becker JT, et al: Updated research nosology for HIV-associated neurocognitive disorders. Neurology 69:1789–1799, 2007

Antoni BA, Sabbatini P, Rabson AB, et al: Inhibition of apoptosis in human immunodeficiency virus–infected cells enhances virus production and facilitates persistent infection. J Virol 69:2384–2392, 1995

Arendt G, Hefter H, Buesher L, et al: Improvement of motor performance of HIV-positive patients under AZT therapy. Neurology 42:891–895, 1991

Bredesen DE, Levy RM, Rosenblum ML: The neurology of human immunodeficiency virus infection. Q J Med 68:665–677, 1988

Breitbart W, Marotta RF, Call P: AIDS and neuroleptic malignant syndrome. Lancet 2:1488–1489, 1988

Breitbart W, Rosenfeld B, Kaim M, et al: A randomized, double-blind, placebo controlled trial of psychostimulants for the treatment of fatigue in ambulatory patients with human immunodeficiency virus disease. Arch Intern Med 161:411–420, 2001

Brew BJ, Sidtis JJ, Petito CK, et al: The neurologic complications of AIDS and human immunodeficiency virus infection, in Advances in Contemporary Neurology. Edited by Plum F. Philadelphia, PA, FA Davis, 1988, pp 1–49

Brew BJ, Bhalla RB, Paul M, et al: Cerebrospinal fluid β2 microglobulin in patients infected with AIDS dementia complex: an expanded series including response to zidovudine treatment. AIDS 6:461–465, 1992

Brew BJ, Pemberton L, Blennow K, et al: CSF amyloid beta42 and tau levels correlate with AIDS dementia complex. Neurology 65:1490–1492, 2005

Brunetti A, Berg G, Di Chiro G, et al: Reversal of brain metabolic abnormalities following treatment of AIDS dementia complex with 3'-azido-2',3'-dideoxythymidine (AZT, zidovudine): a PET-FDG study. J Nucl Med 30:581–590, 1989

Buffet R, Agut H, Chieze F, et al: Virological markers in the cerebrospinal fluid from HIV-1 infected individuals. AIDS 5:1419–1424, 1991

Butters N, Grant I, Haxby J, et al: Assessment of AIDS-related cognitive changes: recommendations of the NIMH workshop on neuropsychological assessment approaches. J Clin Exp Neuropsychol 12:963–978, 1990

Carrieri PB, Indaco A, Maiorino A, et al: Cerebrospinal fluid beta-2-microglobulin in multiple sclerosis and AIDS dementia complex. Neurol Res 14:282–283, 1992

Chiodi F, Keys B, Albert J, et al: Human immunodeficiency virus type 1 is present in the cerebrospinal fluid of a majority of infected individuals. J Clin Microbiol 30:1768–1771, 1992

Corbeil J, Richman DD: Productive infection and subsequent interaction of CD4-gp120 at the cellular membrane is required for HIV-induced apoptosis of CD4+ T cells. J Gen Virol 76 (pt 3): 681–690, 1995

Cummings JL, Benson DF: Dementia: A Clinical Approach. Boston, MA, Butterworths, 1983

Currier MB, Molina G, Kato M: Citalopram treatment of major depressive disorder in Hispanic HIV and AIDS patients: a prospective study. Psychosomatics 45:210–216, 2004

Cysique LA, Maruff P, Brew BJ: Antiretroviral therapy in HIV infection: are neurologically active drugs important? Arch Neurol 61:1699–1704, 2004

Davis LE, Hjelle BL, Miller VE, et al: Early viral brain invasion in iatrogenic human immunodeficiency virus infection. Neurology 42:1736–1739, 1992

Deicken RF, Hubesch B, Jensen PC, et al: Alterations in brain phosphate metabolite concentrations in patients with human immunodeficiency virus infection. Arch Neurol 48:203–209, 1991

Dickover RE, Donovan RM, Goldstein E, et al: Decreases in unintegrated HIV DNA are associated with antiretroviral therapy in AIDS patients. J Acquir Immune Defic Syndr 5:31–36, 1991

Dooneief G, Bello J, Todak G, et al: A prospective controlled study of magnetic resonance imaging of the brain in gay men and parenteral drug users with human immunodeficiency virus infection. Arch Neurol 49:38–43, 1992

Dreyer EB, Kaiser PK, Offermann JT, et al: HIV-1 coat protein neurotoxicity prevented by calcium channel antagonists. Science 248:364–367, 1990

Dunlop O, Bjørklund RA, Abedelnoor M, et al: Five different tests of reaction time evaluated in HIV seropositive men. Acta Neurol Scand 8:260–266, 1992

Everall I, Luthert PJ, Lantos PL: Neuronal loss in the frontal cortex in HIV infection. Lancet 337:1119–1121, 1991

Everall I, Luthert PJ, Lantos PL: A review of neuronal damage in human immunodeficiency virus infection: its assessment, possible mechanism and relationship to dementia. J Neuropathol Exp Neurol 52:561–566, 1993

Fernandez F: Psychiatric complications in HIV-related illnesses, in American Psychiatric Association AIDS Primer. Washington, DC, American Psychiatric Press, 1988

Fernandez F: Anxiety and the neuropsychiatry of AIDS. J Clin Psychiatry 50(suppl):9–14, 1989

Fernandez F, Levy JK: Adjuvant treatment of HIV dementia with psychostimulants, in Behavioral Aspects of AIDS and Other Sexually Transmitted Diseases. Edited by Ostrow D. New York, Plenum, 1990, pp 279–286

Fernandez F, Levy JK: Psychopharmacotherapy of psychiatric syndromes in asymptomatic and symptomatic HIV infection. Psychiatr Med 9:377–393, 1991

Fernandez F, Adams F, Levy JK, et al: Cognitive impairment due to AIDS-related complex and its response to psychostimulants. Psychosomatics 29:38–46, 1988a

Fernandez F, Levy JK, Galizzi H: Response of HIV-related depression to psychostimulants: case reports. Hosp Community Psychiatry 39:628–631, 1988b

Fernandez F, Holmes VF, Levy JK, et al: Consultation-liaison psychiatry and HIV-related disorders. Hosp Community Psychiatry 40:146–153, 1989a

Fernandez F, Levy JK, Mansell PWA: Management of delirium in terminally ill AIDS patients. Int J Psychiatry Med 19:165–172, 1989b

Fernandez F, Levy JK, Sampley HR, et al: Effects of methylphenidate in HIV-related depression: a comparative trial with desipramine. Int J Psychiatry Med 25:53–67, 1995

Filley CM, Franklin GM, Heaton RK, et al: White matter dementia: clinical disorders and implications. Neuropsychiatry Neuropsychol Behav Neurol 1:239–254, 1988

Fischl MA, Richman DD, Grieco MH, et al: The efficacy of azidothymidine (AZT) in the treatment of patients with AIDS and AIDS-related complex: a double-blind, placebo-controlled study. N Engl J Med 317:185–191, 1987

Flowers CH, Mafee MF, Crowell R, et al: Encephalopathy in AIDS patients: evaluation with MR imaging. AJNR Am J Neuroradiol 11:1235–1245, 1990

Freund-Levi Y, Saaf J, Wahlund L-O, et al: Ultra low field brain MRI in HIV transfusion infected patients. Magn Reson Imaging 7:225–230, 1989

Frewer LJ, Lader M: The effects of nefazodone, imipramine, and placebo, alone and combined with alcohol, in normal subjects. Int Clin Psychopharmacol 8:13–20, 1993

Gemignani A, Paudice P, Pittaluga A, et al: The HIV-1 coat protein gp120 and some of its fragments potently activate native cerebral NMDA receptors mediating neuropeptide release. Eur J Neurosci 12:2839–2846, 2000

Giunta B, Ehrhart J, Townsend K, et al: Galantamine and nicotine have a synergistic effect on inhibition of microglial activation induced by HIV-1 gp120. Brain Res Bull 64:165–170, 2004

Giunta B, Obregon D, Hou H, et al: Green tea derived EGCG modulates AIDS dementia-like neuronal damage via inhibition of STAT1 activation. Brain Res 1123:216–225, 2006

Gonzales MF, David RL: Neuropathology of acquired immunodeficiency syndrome. Neuropathol Appl Neurobiol 14:345–363, 1988

Goodkin K, Baldewicz TT, Wilkie FL, et al: Cognitive-motor impairment and disorder in HIV-1 infection. Psychiatr Ann 31:37–44, 2001

Green DA, Masliah E, Vinters HV, et al: Brain deposition of beta-amyloid is a common pathologic feature in HIV positive patients. AIDS 19:407–411, 2005

Greenblatt DJ, VonMolke LL, Harmatz JS, et al: Drug interactions with newer antidepressants: role of human cytochromes P450. J Clin Psychiatry 59 (suppl 15):19–27, 1998

Greenlee JE, Rose JW: Controversies in neurological infectious diseases. Semin Neurol 20:375–386, 2000

Hagler DN, Frame PT: Azidothymidine neurotoxicity. Lancet 2:1392–1393, 1986

Harbison MA, Kim S, Gillis JM, et al: Effect of the calcium channel blocker verapamil on human immunodeficiency virus type 1 replication in lymphoid cells. J Infect Dis 164:43–60, 1991

Harris MJ, Jeste DV, Gleghorn A, et al: New-onset psychosis in HIV-infected patients. J Clin Psychiatry 52:369–376, 1991

Heaton RK, Grant I, Butters N, et al: The HNRC 500: neuropsychology of HIV infection at different disease stages. J Int Neuropsychol Soc 1:231–251, 1995

Heaton RK, Marcotte TD, Rivera Mindt M, et al: The impact of HIV-associated neuropsychological impairment on everyday functioning. J Int Neuropsychol Soc 10:317–331, 2004

Heyes MP, Brew BJ, Martin A, et al: Quinolinic acid in cerebrospinal fluid and serum in HIV-1 infection: relationship to clinical neurological status. Ann Neurol 29:202–209, 1991

Heyes MP, Brew BJ, Saito K, et al: Inter-relationships between quinolinic acid, neuroactive kynurenines, neopterin and β2-microglobulin in cerebrospinal fluid and HIV-1-infected patients. J Neuroimmunol 40:71–80, 1992

Heyes MP, Ellis RJ, Ryan L, et al: Elevated cerebrospinal fluid quinolinic acid levels are associated with region-specific cerebral volume loss in HIV infection. Brain 124 (pt 5):1033–1042, 2001

Ho DD, Pomerantz RJ, Kaplan JC: Pathogenesis of infection with human immunodeficiency virus. N Engl J Med 317:278–286, 1987

Holmes VF, Fernandez F, Levy JK: Psychostimulant response in AIDS-related complex patients. J Clin Psychiatry 50:5–8, 1989

Janssen RS, Cornblath DR, Epstein LG, and the Working Group of the American Academy of Neurology AIDS Task Force: Nomenclature and research case definitions for neurologic manifestations of human immunodeficiency virus–type 1 (HIV-1) infection. Neurology 41:778–785, 1991

Jernigan TL, Archibald S, Hesselink JR, et al: Magnetic resonance imaging morphometric analysis of cerebral volume loss in human immunodeficiency virus: the HNRC group. Arch Neurol 50:250–255, 1993

Kastenholz KV, Crismon ML: Buspirone, a novel nonbenzodiazepine anxiolytic. Clin Pharmacol Ther 3:600–607, 1984

Kawai K, Tsuno NH, Kitayama J, et al: Epigallocatechin gallate, the main component of tea polyphenol, binds to CD4 and interferes with gp120 binding. J Allergy Clin Immunol 112:951–957, 2003

Knights EB, Folstein MF: Unsuspected emotional and cognitive disturbance in medical patients. Ann Intern Med 87:723–724, 1977

Kuni CC, Phame FS, Meier MJ, et al: Quantitative I-123-IMP brain SPECT and neuropsychological testing in AIDS dementia. Clin Nucl Med 16:174–177, 1991

Larsson M, Hagbreg L, Forsman A, et al: Cerebrospinal fluid catecholamine metabolites in HIV-infected patients. J Neurosci Res 28:406–409, 1991

Li CJ, Friedman DJ, Wang C, et al: Induction of apoptosis in uninfected lymphocytes by HIV-1 Tat protein. Science 268:429–431, 1995

Lin-Greenberger A, Taneja-Uppal N: Dysautonomia and infection with the human immunodeficiency virus (letter). Ann Intern Med 106:167, 1987

Lipton SA: Calcium channel antagonists and human immunodeficiency virus coat protein-mediated neuronal injury. Ann Neurol 30:110–114, 1991

Lipton SA: Models of neuronal injury in AIDS: another role for the NMDA receptor. Trends Neurosci 15:75–79, 1992

Lipton SA, Gendleman HE: Dementia associated with the acquired immunodeficiency syndrome. N Engl J Med 332:934–940, 1995

Lowenhaupt EA, Matson K, Qureishi B, et al: Psychosis in a 12-year-old HIV-positive girl with an increased serum concentration of efavirenz. Clin Infect Dis 45:e128–130, 2007

Lu W, Salerno-Goncalves R, Yuan J, et al: Glucocorticoids rescue CD4+ T lymphocytes from activation-induced apoptosis triggered by HIV-1: implications for pathogenesis and therapy. AIDS 9:35–42, 1995

Lynch DH, Ramsdell F, Alderson MR: Fas and FasL in the homeostatic regulation of immune responses. Immunol Today 16:569–574, 1995

Maccarrone M, Bari M, Corasaniti MT, et al: HIV-1 coat glycoprotein gp 120 induces apoptosis in rat brain neocortex by deranging the arachidonate cascade in favor of prostanoids. J Neurochem 75:196–203, 2000

Maldarelli F, Sato H, Berthold E, et al: Rapid induction of apoptosis by cell-to-cell transmission of human immunodeficiency virus type 1. J Virol 69:6457–6465, 1995

Maldonado JL, Fernandez F, Levy JK: Acquired immunodeficiency syndrome, in Psychiatric Management of Neurological Disease. Edited by Lauterbach EC. Washington, DC, American Psychiatric Press, 2000, pp 271–295

Mandel S, Weinreb O, Amit T, et al: Cell signaling pathways in the neuroprotective actions of the green tea polyphenol (-)-epigallocatechin-3-gallate: implications for neurodegenerative diseases. J Neurochem 88:1555–1569, 2004 [published erratum in: J Neurochem 89:527, 2004]

Markowitz JC, Rabkin JG, Perry SW: Treating depression in HIV-positive patients. AIDS 8:403–412, 1994

Marshall DW, Brey RL, Cahill WT, et al: Spectrum of cerebrospinal fluid findings in various stages of human immunodeficiency virus infection. Arch Neurol 45:954–958, 1988

Martin EM, Robertson LC, Sorensen DJ, et al: Speed of memory scanning is not affected in early HIV-1 infection (abstract). J Clin Exp Neuropsychol 14:102, 1992

Marzuk PM, Tierney H, Tardiff K, et al: Increased risk of suicide in persons with AIDS. JAMA 259:1333–1337, 1988

Masliah E, Achim CL, Ge N, et al: Spectrum of human immunodeficiency virus–associated neocortical damage. Ann Neurol 32:321–329, 1992

McArthur JC, Nance-Sproson TE, Griffin DE, et al: The diagnostic utility of elevation in cerebral spinal fluid β2-microglobulin in HIV-1 dementia. Neurology 42:1707–1712, 1992

McDaniel SJ, Niran PT, Magnuson JV: Possible induction of mania by buspirone. Am J Psychiatry 147:125–126, 1990

McElroy SL, Keck PE, Pope HG, et al: Valproate in the treatment of bipolar disorder: literature review and clinical guidelines. J Clin Psychopharmacol 12 (suppl 1):42S–52S, 1992

McGowan I, Potter M, George RJD, et al: HIV encephalopathy presenting as hypomania. Genitourin Med 67:420–424, 1991

Melton ST, Kirkwood CK, Ghanemi SN: Pharmacotherapy of HIV dementia. Ann Pharmacother 31:457–473, 1997

Miller K, Corcoran C, Armstrong C, et al: Transdermal testosterone administration in women with acquired immunodeficiency syndrome wasting: a pilot study. J Clin Endocrinol Metab 83:2717–2725, 1998

Nance M, Pirozzolo FJ, Levy JK, et al: Simple and choice reaction time in HIV-seronegative, HIV-seropositive and AIDS patients. Abstracts of the 6th International Conference on AIDS, Vol 2. San Francisco, CA, June 22, 1990, p 173

Navia BA, Gonzalez RG: Functional imaging of the AIDS dementia complex and the metabolic pathology of the HIV-1-infected brain. Neuroimaging Clin North Am 7:431–445, 1997

Navia BA, Cho E-S, Petito CK, et al: The AIDS dementia complex, II: neuropathology. Ann Neurol 19:525–535, 1986

Neuzil KM: Pharmacologic therapy for human immunodeficiency virus infection: a review. Am J Med Sci 307:368–373, 1994

O'Dowd MA, McKegney FP: Manic syndrome associated with zidovudine. JAMA 260:3587–3588, 1988

O'Dowd MA, McKegney FP: AIDS patients compared to others seen in psychiatric consultation. Gen Hosp Psychiatry 12:50–55, 1990

Panel on Antiretroviral Guidelines for Adults and Adolescents. Guidelines for the use of antiretroviral agents in HIV-1-infected adults and adolescents. Washington, DC, U.S. Department of Health and Human Services. December 1, 2009. Available at: http://www.aidsinfo.nih.gov/ContentFiles/AdultandAdolescentGL.pdf. Accessed February 24, 2010.

Perry S, Fishman B, Jacobsberg L, et al: Relationships over 1 year between lymphocyte subsets and psychosocial variables among adults with infection by human immunodeficiency virus. Arch Gen Psychiatry 49:396–401, 1992

Petito CK: Review of central nervous system pathology in human immunodeficiency virus infection. Ann Neurol 23(suppl):S54–S57, 1988

Post MJD, Berger JR, Quencer RM: Asymptomatic and neurologically symptomatic HIV-seropositive individuals: prospective evaluation with cranial MR imaging. Radiology 178:131–139, 1991

Poutiainen E, Haltia M, Elovaara I, et al: Dementia associated with human immunodeficiency virus: subcortical or cortical? Acta Psychiatr Scand 83:297–301, 1991

Power C, Selnes OA, Grim JA, et al: HIV Dementia Scale: a rapid screening test. J Acquir Immune Defic Syndr Hum Retrovirol 8:273–278, 1995

Price WA, Bielefeld M: Buspirone induced mania. J Clin Psychopharmacol 9:150–151, 1989

Rabkin JG, Wagner JG, McElhiney MC, et al: Testosterone versus fluoxetine for depression and fatigue in HIV/AIDS patients: a placebo controlled trial. J Clin Psychopharmacol 24:379–385, 2004

Reboul J, Schuller E, Pialoux G, et al: Immunoglobulins and complement components in 37 patients infected by HIV-1 virus: comparison of general (systemic) and intrathecal immunity. J Neurol Sci 89:243–252, 1989

Richelson E: Synaptic pharmacology of antidepressants: an update. McLean Hospital Journal 13:67–88, 1988

Sacktor N, Prohovnik I, Van Heertum RL, et al: Cerebral single-photon emission computed tomography abnormalities in human immunodeficiency virus type 1–infected gay men without cognitive impairment. Arch Neurol 52:607–611, 1995

Sacktor N, Tarwater PM, Skolasky RL, et al: CSF antiretroviral drug penetrance and the treatment of HIV-associated psychomotor slowing. Neurology 57:542–544, 2001

Samochocki M, Hoffle A, Fehrenbacher A, et al: Galantamine is an allosterically potentiating ligand of neuronal nicotinic but not of muscarinic acetylcholine receptors. J Pharmacol Exp Ther 305:1024–1036, 2003

Santos MD, Alkondon M, Pereira EF, et al: The nicotinic allosteric potentiating ligand galantamine facilitates synaptic transmission in the mammalian central nervous system. Mol Pharmacol 61:1222–1234, 2002

Schaerf FW, Miller RS, Lipsey JR, et al: ECT for major depression in four patients infected with human immunodeficiency virus. Am J Psychiatry 146:782–784, 1989

Schielke E, Tatsch K, Pfister HW, et al: Reduced cerebral blood flow in early stages of human immunodeficiency virus infection. Arch Neurol 47:1342–1345, 1990

Schindelmeiser J, Gullotta F: HIV-p24-antigen-bearing macrophages are only present in brains of HIV-seropositive patients with AIDS-encephalopathy. Clin Neuropathol 10:109–111, 1991

Sekigawa I, Koshino K, Hishikawa T, et al: Inhibitory effect of the immunosuppressant FK506 on apoptotic cell death induced by HIV-1-gp120. J Clin Immunol 15:312–317, 1995

Selnes OA, Jacobson L, Machado AM, et al: Normative data for a brief neuropsychological screening battery. Percept Mot Skills 73:539–550, 1991

Sharma SM, McDaniel JS, Sheehan NL: General principles of pharmacotherapy for the patient with HIV infection, in HIV and Psychiatry: A Training and Resource Manual. Edited by Citron K, Brouillete MJ, Beckett A. Cambridge, UK, Cambridge University Press, 2005, pp 56–87

Shaskan EG, Brew BJ, Rosenblum M, et al: Increased neopterin levels in brains of patients with human immunodeficiency virus type 1 infection. J Neurochem 59:1541–1546, 1992

Shytle RD, Mori T, Townsend K, et al: Cholinergic modulation of microglial activation by alpha 7 nicotinic receptors. J Neurochem 89:337–343, 2004

Sidtis JJ, Gatsonis C, Price RW, et al: Zidovudine treatment of the AIDS dementia complex: results of a placebo-controlled trial: AIDS Clinical Trials Group. Ann Neurol 33:343–349, 1993

Silvestris F, Ribatti D, Nico B, et al: Apoptosi, o morte cellulare programmata: meccanismi regolatori e fisiopatologia [Apoptosis or programmed cell death: regulatory and pathophysiological mechanisms]. Ann Ital Med Int 10:7–13, 1995

Singh AN, Golledge H, Catalan J: Treatment of HIV related psychotic disorders with risperidone a series of 21 cases. J Psychosom Res 42:489–493, 1997

Skolasky RL, Esposito DR, Selnes OA, et al: Modified HIV Dementia Scale: accurate staging of HIV-associated dementia: neuroscience of HIV infection (abstract). J Neurovirol 4(suppl):366, 1998

Sockalingam S, Parekh N, Bogoch II, et al: Delirium in the postoperative cardiac patient: a review. J Card Surg 20:560–567, 2005

Stefano GB, Smith EM, Cadet P, et al: HIV gp120 alteration of DAMA and IL-1 alpha induced chemotaxic responses in human and invertebrate immunocytes. J Neuroimmunol 43:177–184, 1993

Stolar A, Catalano G, Hakala SM, et al: Mood disorders and psychosis in HIV, in HIV and Psychiatry: A Training and Resource Manual. Edited by Citron K, Brouillete MJ, Beckett A. Cambridge, UK, Cambridge University Press, 2005, pp 88–109

Strauss A: Oral dyskinesia associated with buspirone use in an elderly woman. J Clin Psychiatry 49:322–323, 1988

Syndulko K, Singer E, Fahychandon B, et al: Relationship of self-rated depression and neuropsychological changes in HIV-1 neurological dysfunction (abstract). J Clin Exp Neuropsychol 12:72, 1990

Talley AK, Dewhurst S, Perry SW, et al: Tumor necrosis factor alpha-induced apoptosis in human neuronal cells: protection by the antioxidant *N*-acetylcysteine and the genes *bcl-2* and *crmA*. Mol Cell Biol 15:2359–2366, 1995

Tartaglione TA, Collier AC, Coombs RW, et al: Acquired immunodeficiency syndrome, cerebrospinal fluid findings in patients before and during long-term oral zidovudine therapy. Arch Neurol 48:695–699, 1991

Tozzi V, Balestra P, Galgani S, et al: Positive and sustained effects of highly active antiretroviral therapy on HIV-1 associated neurocognitive impairment. AIDS 13:1889–1897, 1999

Van Gorp WG, Miller E, Satz P, et al: Neuropsychological performance in HIV-1 immunocompromised patients (abstract). J Clin Exp Neuropsychol 11:35, 1989

van Leeuwen R, Katlama C, Kitchen V, et al: Evaluation of safety and efficacy of 3TC (Lamivudine) in patients with asymptomatic or mildly symptomatic human immunodeficiency virus infection: a phase I/II study. J Infect Dis 171:1166–1171, 1995

Walker DG, Itagaki J, Berry K, et al: Examination of brains of AIDS cases for human immunodeficiency virus and human cytomegalovirus nucleic acids. J Neurol Neurosurg Psychiatry 52:583–590, 1989

Wang Y, Sawchuk RJ: Zidovudine transport in the rabbit brain during intravenous and intracerebroventricular infusion. J Pharm Sci 84:871–876, 1995

Weiner RD: ECT in the physically ill. J Psychiatr Treat Eval 5:457–462, 1983

Weis S, Haug H, Budka H: Neuronal damage in the cerebral cortex of AIDS brains: a morphometric study. Acta Neuropathol (Berl) 85:185–189, 1993

White JC, Christensen JF, Singer CM: Methylphenidate as a treatment for depression in acquired immunodeficiency syndrome: an n-of-1 trial. J Clin Psychiatry 53:153–156, 1992

Wiley CA, Masliah E, Morey M, et al: Neocortical damage during HIV infection. Ann Neurol 29:651–657, 1991

Wilkie FL, Eisdorfer C, Morgan R, et al: Cognition in early human immunodeficiency virus infection. Arch Neurol 47:433–440, 1990

Wolcott DL, Fawzy FI, Pasnau RO: Acquired immune deficiency syndrome (AIDS) and consultation-liaison psychiatry. Gen Hosp Psychiatry 7:280–293, 1985

Wong SL, Wang Y, Sawchuk RJ: Analysis of zidovudine distribution to specific regions in rabbit brain using microdialysis. Pharm Res 9:332–338, 1992

Wong SL, Van Bell K, Sawchuk RJ: Distributional transport kinetics of zidovudine between plasma and brain extracellular fluid/cerebrospinal fluid in the rabbit: investigation of the inhibitory effect of probenecid utilizing microdialysis. J Pharmacol Exp Ther 264:899–909, 1993

Wright JM, Sachdev PS, Perkins RJ, et al: Zidovudine related mania. Med J Aust 150:339–341, 1989

Yarchoan R, Berg G, Brouwers P, et al: Response of human immunodeficiency virus associated neurological disease to 3'-azido-3'-deoxythymidine. Lancet 1:132–135, 1987

11

NEUROPSYCHIATRIC ASPECTS OF ETHANOL AND OTHER CHEMICAL DEPENDENCIES

Eric J. Nestler, M.D., Ph.D.
David W. Self, Ph.D.

Drug addiction continues to exact enormous human and financial costs on society, at a time when the available treatments remain inadequately effective for most people. Given that advances in treating other medical disorders have resulted directly from research of the molecular and cellular pathophysiology of the disease process, an improved understanding of the basic neurobiology of addiction should likewise translate into more efficacious treatments.

Our knowledge of the basic neurobiology of drug addiction is leading psychiatric neuroscience in establishing the biological basis of a complex and clinically important behavioral abnormality. This is because many features of drug addiction in people can be reproduced in laboratory animals, in which findings are directly referable back to the clinical situation. Earlier work on drug reinforcement mechanisms, and more recently developed animal models that target the addiction process and drug craving, has made it possible to identify regions of the brain that play important roles in distinct behavioral features of addiction. These neural substrates are now the focus of extensive research on the molecular and cellular alterations that underlie these behavioral changes.

In this chapter we provide an overview of recent progress made in our understanding of the neurobiological basis of drug addiction. After providing brief definitions of commonly used terminology, we summarize the anatomi-

This work was supported by grants from the National Institute on Drug Abuse.

cal and neurochemical substrates that mediate the reinforcing effects of short-term drug exposure. We then describe how repeated drug exposure can induce gradually developing, progressive alterations in molecular and cellular signaling pathways, and how these neuroadaptive changes may ultimately contribute to addictive behavior.

DEFINITION OF TERMS

From a pharmacological perspective, drug addiction can be defined by processes such as tolerance, sensitization, dependence, and withdrawal. *Tolerance* refers to a progressive weakening of a given drug effect after repeated exposure, which may contribute to an escalation of drug intake as the addiction process proceeds. *Sensitization*, or *reverse tolerance*, refers to the opposite circumstance, whereby repeated administration of the same drug dose elicits an even stronger effect; sensitization to certain "incentive motivational" effects of drugs is believed to contribute to high relapse rates seen in addicted individuals. Thus, both tolerance and sensitization to different aspects of drug action can occur simultaneously. *Dependence* is defined as the need for continued drug exposure to avoid a withdrawal syndrome, which is characterized by physical or motivational disturbances when the drug is withdrawn. Presumably, the processes of tolerance, sensitization, dependence, and withdrawal are each caused by molecular and cellular adaptations in specific brain regions in response to repeated drug exposure. It is important to emphasize that these phenomena are not associated uniquely with drugs of abuse, as many clinically used medications that are not addicting (e.g., clonidine, propranolol, most antidepressants) can produce similar phenomena. Rather, the manifestation of tolerance, sensitization, dependence, and withdrawal specifically in brain regions that regulate motivation is believed to underlie addiction-related changes in behavior.

Drugs of abuse are unique in terms of their reinforcing properties. A drug is defined as a reinforcer if the probability of a drug-seeking response is increased and maintained by pairing drug exposure with the response. Initially, most abused drugs function as positive reinforcers, presumably because they produce a positive affective state (e.g., euphoria). Such rapid and powerful associations between a drug reinforcer and a drug-seeking response probably reflect the drug's ability to usurp preexisting brain reinforcement mechanisms, which normally mediate the reinforcing effects of natural rewards such as food, sex, and social interaction.

Long-term exposure to reinforcing drugs can lead to drug addiction, which is characterized by an escalation in both the frequency and the amount of drug use and by intense drug craving during withdrawal despite grave adverse consequences. In the context of long-term drug use, a drug may serve not only as a positive reinforcer, but also as a negative reinforcer by alleviating the negative consequences of drug withdrawal. The persistence of drug craving and drug seeking (relapse) despite prolonged periods of abstinence suggests that long-lasting adaptations have occurred in the neural substrates that mediate acute drug reinforcement.

Addictive disorders are often defined clinically as a state of "psychological dependence"—for example, in DSM-IV-TR (American Psychiatric Association 2000). However, it is important to emphasize that in more precise pharmacological terms, we do not yet know the relative contributions of neurobiological changes that underlie tolerance, sensitization, or dependence/withdrawal to the compulsive drug-seeking behavior that is the clinical hallmark of an addictive disorder. It is possible that drug craving and relapse involve dependence-related dysphoria associated with drug withdrawal. Such factors are likely to be important during the relatively early phases of abstinence. However, a major question remains regarding the types of adaptations that underlie particularly long-lived aspects of addiction—for example, the increased risk of relapse that many addicts show even after years of abstinence. As stated above, such persistent drug craving may involve adaptations that underlie sensitization to the incentive motivational properties of drugs, drug-associated (conditioned) stimuli, and stressful

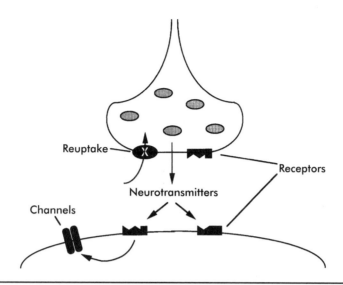

FIGURE 11–1. A classic working model of synaptic transmission.

In classic terms, synaptic transmission was conceived as the release of neurotransmitter from a nerve terminal, the binding of the neurotransmitter to specific receptor sites on target neurons, and the resulting alterations in the conductances of specific ion channels. The action of the neurotransmitter is then terminated by its reuptake into the nerve terminal or by enzymatic degradation (not shown).

events. In other words, sensitization to these various stimuli would increase their ability to "reinstate"—or "prime"—drug seeking despite prolonged abstinence. Identification of long-lasting adaptations that underlie these persisting behavioral changes is paramount to the ultimate development of truly effective treatments.

THE SYNAPSE AS THE IMMEDIATE TARGET OF DRUGS OF ABUSE

The initial actions of drugs of abuse on the brain can be understood at the level of synaptic transmission. Figure 11–1 depicts a classic view of a synapse, in which a presynaptic nerve terminal, in response to a nerve impulse along its axon, releases a neurotransmitter that acts on a postsynaptic receptor to elicit changes in neuronal excitability of the postsynaptic neuron. The activity of the neurotransmitter is then turned off by its reuptake into the nerve terminal, or by enzymatic degradation (for review, see Nestler et al. 2001).

All drugs of abuse initially affect the brain by influencing the amount of a neurotransmitter present at the synapse or by interacting with specific neurotransmitter receptors. Table 11–1 lists examples of such acute pharmacological actions of some commonly used drugs of abuse. The fact that drugs of abuse initially influence different neurotransmitter and receptor systems in the brain explains the very different actions produced by these drugs acutely. For example, the presence of high levels of opioid receptors in the brain stem and spinal cord explains why opiates can exert such profound effects on respiration, level of consciousness, and nociception. In contrast, the importance of noradrenergic mechanisms in the regulation of cardiac function explains why cocaine can exert potent cardiotoxic effects.

In contrast to the many disparate acute actions of drugs of abuse, the drugs do appear to exert some common behavioral effects: as discussed above, they are all positively reinforcing after short-term exposure and cause a similar behavioral syndrome (addiction) after long-term exposure. This suggests that there are

TABLE 11–1.   Examples of acute pharmacological actions of drugs of abuse

Drug	Action
Amphetamine	Stimulates monoamine release
Cannabinoids	Agonists at CB_1 cannabinoid receptors[a]
Cocaine	Inhibits monoamine reuptake transporters
Ethanol	Facilitates $GABA_A$ receptor function and inhibits NMDA glutamate receptor function[b]
Hallucinogens	Partial agonists at $5\text{-}HT_{2A}$ serotonin receptors
Nicotine	Agonist at nicotinic acetylcholine receptors
Opiates	Agonists at μ, δ, and κ opioid receptors[c]
Phencyclidine (PCP)	Antagonist at NMDA glutamate receptors

Note. $GABA_A$ = γ-aminobutyric acid type A; NMDA = *N*-methyl-D-aspartate; $5\text{-}HT_{2A}$ = 5-hydroxytryptamine (serotonin) type 2A.
[a]The endogenous ligand(s) for these receptors have not yet been definitively identified; one candidate is anandamide.
[b]The mechanism by which ethanol produces these effects has not been established. In addition, ethanol affects many other neurotransmitter systems in brain.
[c]Activity at μ and δ receptors is thought to mediate the reinforcing actions of opiates.

certain regions of the brain where the distinct acute pharmacological actions of these drugs converge at the level of a common reinforcement substrate. That is, in certain regions of the brain, which are discussed below, the activation of opioid receptors (by opiates), the inhibition of monoamine reuptake (by cocaine), or the facilitation of γ-aminobutyric acid (GABA)–ergic and inhibition of *N*-methyl-D-aspartate (NMDA) glutamatergic neurotransmission (by ethanol) would appear to elicit some common neurobiological responses that mediate their reinforcing properties.

MOLECULAR AND CELLULAR ADAPTATIONS AS THE LONG-TERM CONSEQUENCES OF DRUGS OF ABUSE

The acute pharmacological actions of a drug of abuse per se do not explain the long-term effects of repeated drug exposure. To understand such long-term effects, it is necessary to move beyond the classic view of a synapse, such as that shown in Figure 11–1. We now know that neurotransmitter-receptor activation does more to influence a target neuron than simply regulate its ion channels and immediate electrical properties: virtually every process in a neuron can be affected by neurotransmitter-receptor activation (Hyman et al. 2006; Nestler et al. 2001) (Figure 11–2). Such effects are mediated by modulating the functional activity of proteins that are already present in the neuron or by regulating the actual amount of the proteins. Most neurotransmitters and receptors produce these diverse effects through biochemical cascades of intracellular messengers, which involve G proteins (guanosine triphosphate–binding membrane proteins that couple extracellular receptors to intracellular effector proteins), and the subsequent regulation of second messengers (such as cyclic adenosine monophosphate [cAMP], calcium, phosphatidylinositol, or nitric oxide) and protein phosphorylation (see Nestler et al. 2001). Protein phosphorylation is a process whereby phosphate groups are added to proteins by protein kinases or are removed from proteins by protein phosphatases. Addition or removal of phosphate groups dramatically alters protein function and leads to the myriad biological responses in question.

Neurotransmitter receptors function presynaptically to regulate the synthesis and storage of neurotransmitter via phosphorylation of synthetic enzymes and transporter proteins. In addition, altered phosphorylation of synaptic vesicle–associated proteins can modulate the release of neurotransmitters from presynaptic nerve terminals. Postsynaptically, altered phosphorylation of receptors and ion channels can modify the ability of neurotransmitters to regulate the physiological responses to the same or different neurotransmitter stimuli. Neurotransmitter-mediated phosphorylation of cytoskeletal proteins can produce structural and morphological changes in target neurons. Finally, altered phosphorylation of nuclear or ribosomal proteins can alter gene transcription and protein synthesis and hence the total amounts of these various types of proteins in the target neurons. Given the gradual development of drug addiction in most people and the persistence of drug craving for long periods after cessation of drug exposure, it is likely that repeated drug exposure causes altered patterns of gene expression and protein synthesis that underlie some of these long-term actions of drugs of abuse on the nervous system (Chao and Nestler 2004; Hyman et al. 2006; Nestler 1992).

Neurotransmitter regulation of G proteins and second messenger–dependent protein phosphorylation is a small part of a neuron's intracellular regulatory machinery (see Figure 11–2) (Nestler et al. 2001). Neurons also express high levels of protein tyrosine kinases (e.g., Trk proteins) that mediate the actions of neurotrophins and other growth factors. Growth factors play an important role in neuronal development, but more recently they have been shown to exert powerful effects on fully differentiated adult neurons. This implies that the traditional distinction between neurotransmitters and growth factors is becoming increasingly arbitrary. In addition, neurons contain high levels of protein kinases that are not regulated directly by extracellular signals but are influenced by those signals indirectly via "cross-talk" among various intracellular pathways. Thus, each neurotransmitter-receptor system can interact with others via

secondary, tertiary, etc., effects on various intracellular signaling pathways, all of which will contribute to the myriad effects of the original neurotransmitter stimulus.

This means that despite the initial actions of a drug of abuse on the activity of a neurotransmitter or receptor system, the many actions of drugs of abuse on brain function are achieved ultimately through the complex network of intracellular messenger pathways that mediate physiological responses to neurotransmitter-receptor interactions. Moreover, repeated exposure to drugs of abuse would be expected to produce molecular and cellular adaptations as a result of repeated perturbation of these intracellular pathways. These adaptations may be responsible for tolerance, sensitization, dependence, withdrawal, and, ultimately, the addiction process.

ADAPTATIONS IN THE MESOLIMBIC DOPAMINE SYSTEM AFTER LONG-TERM DRUG EXPOSURE

A substantial body of literature has established the mesolimbic dopamine system as a major neural substrate for the reinforcing effects of opiates, psychostimulants, ethanol, nicotine, and cannabinoids in animals (see Dworkin and Smith 1993; Ikemoto and Wise 2004; Koob et al. 1998; Kuhar et al. 1991; Olds 1982). This system consists of dopaminergic neurons in the ventral tegmental area (VTA) of the midbrain and their target neurons in forebrain regions such as the nucleus accumbens (NAc) and other ventral striatal regions. Long-lasting adaptations within these brain reward regions are believed to cause key motivational symptoms of drug addiction, which include an escalation of drug intake (tolerance), increased drug craving (sensitization), and withdrawal-induced dysphoria (dependence). Indeed, studies over the past two decades have found that long-term drug exposure produces adaptations at the molecular and cellular levels in VTA dopamine neurons, and in their target neurons in the NAc, that may underlie motivational

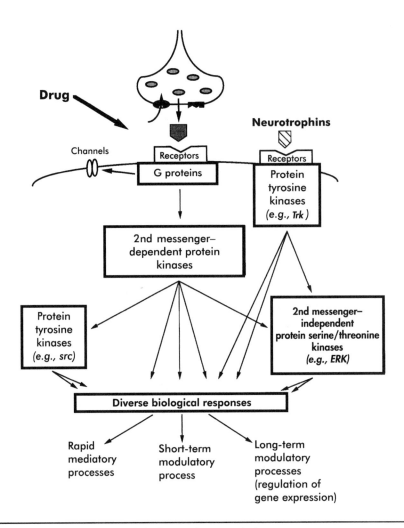

FIGURE 11–2.   A working model of synaptic transmission.

Studies in basic neuroscience have provided a much more complex view of synaptic transmission than that shown in Figure 11–1. These studies focused on the involvement of intracellular messenger systems involving coupling factors (termed G proteins), second messengers (e.g., cyclic adenosine monophosphate [cAMP], calcium, nitric oxide, and the metabolites of phosphatidylinositol), and protein phosphorylation (involving the phosphorylation of phosphoproteins by protein kinases and their dephosphorylation by protein phosphatases) in mediating multiple actions of neurotransmitters on their target neurons. Second messenger–dependent protein kinases (e.g., those activated by cAMP or calcium) are classified as protein serine/threonine kinases, because they phosphorylate substrate proteins on serine or threonine residues. Each second messenger–dependent protein kinase phosphorylates a specific array of substrate proteins (which can be considered third messengers) and thereby leads to multiple biological responses of the neurotransmitter. Brain also contains many important intracellular regulatory pathways in addition to those regulated directly by G proteins and second messengers. This includes numerous protein serine/threonine kinases (e.g., the extracellular signal–regulated kinases [ERKs] or mitogen-activated protein [MAP] kinases), as well as numerous protein tyrosine kinases (which phosphorylate substrate proteins on tyrosine residues), some of which reside in the receptors for neurotrophins and most other growth factors (e.g., the trk proteins), and others that are not associated with growth factor receptors (e.g., src kinase). Each of these various protein kinases is highly regulated by extracellular stimuli. The second messenger–dependent protein kinases are regulated by receptor–G protein–second messenger pathways as mentioned above. The receptor-associated protein tyrosine kinases are activated on growth factor binding to the receptor. The second messenger–independent protein serine/threonine

---

FIGURE 11–2. A working model of synaptic transmission (*continued*).

kinases and the protein tyrosine kinases that are not receptor associated seem to be regulated indirectly via the second messenger–dependent and growth factor–dependent pathways as depicted in the figure. The brain also contains numerous types of protein serine/threonine and protein tyrosine phosphatases, not shown in the figure, which are also subject to regulation by extracellular and intracellular stimuli. Thus, the binding of neurotransmitter to its receptor extracellularly results in numerous short-term and long-term biological responses through the complex regulation of multiple intracellular regulatory pathways and the phosphorylation or dephosphorylation of numerous substrate proteins.

aspects of tolerance, sensitization, and dependence associated with drug addiction (e.g., see Hyman et al. 2006; Kalivas et al. 2005; Nestler 2001; Self 2004; Self and Nestler 1998; Shaham et al. 2003; White and Kalivas 1998; M.E. Wolf 1998). The results from these studies provide the basis for specific hypotheses that will guide future investigations to test, more directly, the role of specific adaptations in mediating drug craving in addicted subjects.

The ability of various drugs of abuse to produce similar types of changes in drug-taking and drug-seeking behavior after repeated administration raises the possibility that these drugs also produce similar types of molecular and cellular adaptations in specific brain regions. Support for this possibility comes from behavioral data, which show that long-term exposure to stimulants, opiates, or ethanol can cross-sensitize the animal to the effects of the other drugs (e.g., see Kelley 2004; Stewart 2003; Vezina 2004). As demonstrated below, there is also now considerable biochemical evidence that different drugs of abuse can produce similar molecular adaptations in the VTA–NAc pathway after long-term administration. These adaptations may be part of a common general mechanism of drug addiction and craving (Figure 11–3) (Nestler 2005).

REGULATION OF DOPAMINE IN THE VENTRAL TEGMENTAL AREA– NUCLEUS ACCUMBENS PATHWAY

A widely held view is that repeated exposure to a drug of abuse may produce some of its behavioral effects (e.g., drug craving or locomotor sensitization) by facilitating drug-induced dopamine release in the NAc. This possibility is best established for stimulants and opiates, which can result in augmented synaptic levels of dopamine as measured by in vivo microdialysis, under some experimental conditions. However, the large body of literature on this subject is inconsistent and confusing overall, given that these drugs have been reported to both increase and decrease synaptic levels of dopamine depending on the drug-treatment regimen employed and the time of withdrawal studied (for references, see Kalivas 2004; Robinson and Berridge 2003; Self and Nestler 1995; Spanagel and Weiss 1999; White and Kalivas 1998; M.E. Wolf 1998). Although altered regulation of dopamine release in the NAc or other brain regions is one likely mechanism underlying aspects of long-term drug exposure, its precise role remains uncertain.

It also has been difficult to identify the precise molecular targets of drugs of abuse that mediate the altered synaptic levels of dopamine observed. Long-term exposure to cocaine upregulates dopamine reuptake transporter proteins specifically in the mesolimbic dopamine system during late phases of withdrawal from the drug (Pilotte 1997). By increasing dopamine reuptake at the synapse, this molecular change would be expected to reduce synaptic levels of dopamine in the VTA–NAc pathway. Long-term exposure to opiates, cocaine, amphetamine, or ethanol has been shown to increase levels of tyrosine hydroxylase in the VTA but to reduce the total amount and phosphorylation state (and hence the enzymatic activity) of the enzyme in the NAc during early phases of withdrawal (Nestler 1992; Ortiz et al. 1995; Schmidt et al. 2001). Decreases in tyrosine hydroxylase activity in the NAc and increases in presynaptic dopa-

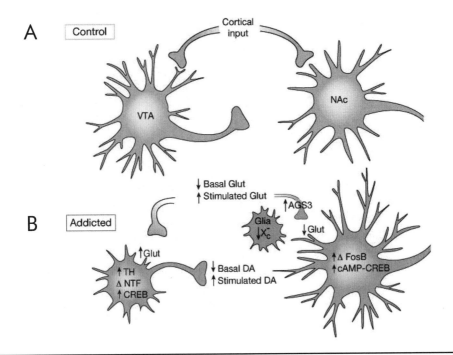

FIGURE 11–3. Schematic summary of some common, chronic actions of drugs of abuse on the ventral tegmental area (VTA)–nucleus accumbens (NAc) circuit.

Panel A (Control) shows a VTA neuron innervating an NAc neuron, and glutamatergic inputs to the VTA and NAc neurons, under normal conditions. *Panel B* (Addicted) illustrates several adaptations that occur after chronic drug administration. In the VTA, drug exposure induces tyrosine hydroxylase (TH) and increases α-amino-3-hydroxy-5-methylisoxazole-4–propionic acid (AMPA) glutamatergic responses (Glut), possibly via induction of GluR1 (an AMPA glutamate receptor subunit) and altered trafficking of AMPA receptors. There is also evidence that VTA dopamine neurons decrease in size, an effect demonstrated thus far with chronic opiates only, but presumed for other drugs of abuse due to common associated biochemical adaptations (e.g., reduced levels of neurofilament proteins). Induction of cyclic adenosine monophosphate (cAMP) response element binding protein (CREB) activity and alterations in neurotrophic factor (NTF) signaling may partly mediate these various effects. In the NAc, all drugs of abuse induce the transcription factor ΔFosB, which may then mediate some of the shared aspects of addiction via regulation of numerous target genes. Several, but not all, drugs of abuse also induce CREB activity in this region, which may be mediated via upregulation of the cAMP pathway. Several additional changes have been found for stimulant exposure; it is not yet known whether they generalize to other drugs. Stimulants decrease AMPA glutamatergic responses in NAc neurons, possibly mediated via induction of GluR2 or repression of several postsynaptic density proteins (e.g., PSD95, Homer-1). These changes in postsynaptic glutamate responses are associated with complex changes in glutamatergic innervation of the NAc, including reduced glutamatergic transmission at baseline and in response to normal rewards, but enhanced transmission in response to cocaine and associated cues, effects mediated in part via upregulation of AGS3 (activator of G protein signaling) in cortical neurons and downregulation of the cystine-glutamate transporter (system X_c^-) in glia. Stimulants and nicotine also induce dendritic outgrowth of NAc neurons, although opiates are reported to produce the opposite action. The net effect of this complex dysregulation in glutamate function and synaptic structure is not yet known.

Source. Reprinted from Nestler EJ: "Is There a Common Molecular Pathway for Addiction?" *Nature Neuroscience* 8:1445–1449, 2005. Used with permission.

mine reuptake could contribute to the reductions in basal extracellular dopamine levels and anhedonia seen during withdrawal (see Koob et al. 2004).

REGULATION OF OPIOID AND DOPAMINE RECEPTORS IN THE VENTRAL TEGMENTAL AREA AND NUCLEUS ACCUMBENS

It also has been proposed that altered levels of various opioid, dopamine, or other neurotransmitter receptors in the mesolimbic dopamine system could mediate some of the long-term effects of drugs of abuse on this neural pathway. The literature on this subject, although vast, is unsatisfying. In general, it has been difficult to establish altered levels of opioid receptors in the VTA and NAc or any other brain regions in response to long-term opiate treatment, although μ and κ receptors are reported to be upregulated by long-term cocaine treatment (Unterwald et al. 1994). There have also been numerous reports of stimulant regulation of dopamine receptors in specific brain regions. Although conflicting data exist, most studies have found reductions in D_1 and D_2 receptors in the NAc in early withdrawal from self-administration or bingelike administration of cocaine. An in vivo positron emission tomography study in rats found reductions in D_1 receptor binding that were mainly attributable to a reduced receptor affinity (Tsukada et al. 1996). In contrast, long-term self-administration or bingelike administration of cocaine is associated with a reduction in D_1 and D_2 receptor numbers in the NAc and with a reduction in maximal D_1-stimulated adenylyl cyclase activity (De Montis et al. 1998; Maggos et al. 1998; Moore et al. 1998), consistent with receptor downregulation. These findings in laboratory animals are consistent with observations in human cocaine and methamphetamine addicts, in whom decreases in D_2 receptor binding have been documented by brain imaging (Volkow et al. 1999).

The various changes seen at the receptor level cannot, however, explain consistent effects of stimulants on dopamine receptor function, which have been well documented in recent years. Electrophysiological studies have shown that long-term exposure to cocaine or other stimulants causes transient subsensitivity of D_2-like autoreceptors in the VTA as well as longer-lasting supersensitivity to the effects of D_1-like receptor activation in the NAc at later withdrawal times (see White and Kalivas 1998; M. Wolf 1998). These changes in dopamine receptor function in both the VTA and the NAc are not accompanied by corresponding changes in dopamine receptor levels, which suggests that they are mediated via adaptations in postreceptor, intracellular signaling pathways.

ROLE OF GLUTAMATERGIC SYSTEMS IN LONG-TERM DRUG ACTION

Adaptations in glutamatergic systems have gained significant attention because of their prominent interactions with central dopamine function and their reported role in locomotor sensitization (see Kalivas 2004; White and Kalivas 1998; M.E. Wolf 1998). Specifically, glutamate receptor antagonists can block the development of locomotor sensitization to stimulants and opiates as well as the electrophysiological perturbations in mesolimbic dopamine function that accompany repeated stimulant exposure. Repeated stimulant exposure has been shown to increase the electrophysiological responsiveness of VTA dopamine neurons to glutamate and to decrease the responsiveness of NAc neurons to glutamate (White et al. 1995). These observations are consistent with the ability of drug exposure to induce a long-term potentiation-like effect in the VTA, and a long-term depression-like effect in the NAc, with respect to synaptic responses to glutamate (Thomas and Malenka 2003).

Supersensitivity of VTA dopamine neurons to glutamate could be mediated via upregulation of specific glutamate receptor subunits in this region, specifically GluR1 (an α-amino-3-hydroxy-5-methylisoxale-4–propionic acid [AMPA] glutamate receptor subunit), which has been seen after long-term administration of cocaine, opiates, or ethanol (Carlezon and Nestler 2002). Thus, mimicking drug-induced increases in GluR1 in the VTA, by use of viral-mediated gene transfer, causes sensitized responses to drugs of abuse. Altered levels of glutamate receptor subunits in the NAc are more variable, with different changes observed in early and late withdrawal (Churchill et al. 1999; Kelz et al. 1999; W. Lu and Wolf 1999). Changes in postsynaptic glutamate responses in the NAc could also be mediated by altered AMPA receptor trafficking or by adaptations in the neurons' postsynaptic densities, including reduced levels of PSD95 (postsynaptic density-95) and Homer or increased levels of F-actin, all of which help anchor AMPA receptors at the synapse (Kalivas et al. 2005; Yao et al. 2004).

In addition, chronic administration of stimulants is reported to alter glutamatergic innervation of the NAc by decreasing levels of the cystine-glutamate transporter in glial cells in this brain region (Kalivas 2004). This transporter normally promotes release of glutamate from prefrontal cortical glutamatergic nerve terminals. These findings highlight the complexity of drug-induced adaptations in glutamate function in the brain's reward circuitry (see Figure 11–3) and would suggest a profound dysfunction in cortical control over the NAc, which could in turn relate to the impulsive and compulsive features of drug addiction (Kalivas et al. 2005). A critical question remains as to whether dysfunctional cortical-NAc glutamatergic transmission in addiction involves a decrease in basal function, an increase in stimulated function, or both, and how these changes contribute to a loss of control over drug use.

REGULATION OF G PROTEINS AND cAMP PATHWAY IN THE VENTRAL TEGMENTAL AREA AND NUCLEUS ACCUMBENS

Repeated cocaine treatment produces transient decreases in the level of inhibitory G protein subunits, Gi and Go, that couple to D_2 autoreceptors in the VTA (Nestler 1992; Striplin and Kalivas 1992). The level of these G proteins in the VTA is negatively correlated with the initial level of locomotor activation produced by cocaine (Striplin and Kalivas 1992). In addition, pertussis toxin injected directly into the VTA, which functionally inactivates these G proteins, increases the locomotor activating effects of cocaine and thereby mimics locomotor sensitization. Together, these findings support the possibility that reduced levels of Gi and Go could account for the D_2 receptor subsensitivity observed electrophysiologically after long-term cocaine exposure and may play a role in some of the long-term effects of cocaine on mesolimbic dopamine function.

Repeated cocaine treatment also decreases levels of Gi and Go in the NAc (Nestler 1992; Striplin and Kalivas 1993) and increases levels of adenylyl cyclase and of cAMP-dependent protein kinase in this brain region (Terwilliger et al. 1991). Together, these changes would be expected to result in a concerted upregulation in the functional activity of the cAMP pathway. Because D_1 receptors are generally thought to produce their effects via activation of the cAMP pathway, these molecular adaptations could account for D_1 receptor supersensitivity observed during later withdrawal times. Long-term exposure to morphine, cocaine, heroin, or ethanol—but not to several drugs without reinforcing properties—produces similar changes in G proteins and the cAMP pathway (Ortiz et al. 1995; Self et al. 1995; Terwilliger et al. 1991). Although the long-term effects of morphine and ethanol on the electrophysiological state of NAc neurons have not yet been investigated, the biochemical findings suggest that an upregulated cAMP pathway may be part of a common mechanism of altered NAc function associated with the drug-treated state (see Figure 11–3). A critical question regarding these neuroadaptations is whether they contribute to changes in drug self-administration habits and to drug craving and relapse during abstinence.

We tested the former possibility by artificially upregulating the cAMP pathway in the

NAc of animals during drug self-administration tests (Self et al. 1994, 1998). In these studies, escalation of drug self-administration is produced by inactivation of inhibitory G proteins with pertussis toxin or by sustained protein kinase A activity after microinfusion of a membrane-permeable cAMP analogue into the NAc. Artificially mimicking the drug-induced neuroadaptations by sustained downregulation of inhibitory G proteins or by sustained increases in protein kinase A activity produces increases in drug self-administration. This effect is usually interpreted as a reduction in drug reward, with animals compensating by increasing their drug intake. These findings suggest that neuroadaptations in the NAc–cAMP pathway caused by repeated drug use may represent an intracellular mechanism of tolerance to the rewarding effects of drugs, which leads to escalating drug intake during drug self-administration. One possible mechanism for such tolerance may involve protein kinase A–mediated phosphorylation, desensitization, and downregulation of D_1 receptors (see Sibley et al. 1998). On the other hand, activation of the cAMP pathway in the NAc was shown to produce an enhancement of conditioned reinforcement produced by cues associated with food reward (Kelley and Holahan 1997) and to facilitate the ability of D_2 receptors to trigger cocaine seeking (Self 2004). This suggests that upregulation of the cAMP pathway in the NAc may potentiate the incentive motivational effects of reward-associated cues, and possibly their ability to elicit craving. Although further work is needed, these studies suggest that upregulation of cAMP–protein kinase A signaling in the NAc can produce both tolerance and sensitization-like effects associated with addiction. Interestingly, upregulation of the cAMP–protein kinase A pathway has been shown to be a shared adaptation to chronic exposure to drugs of abuse in several regions of the central and peripheral nervous systems (e.g., Bonci and Williams 1997; Jolas et al. 2000; Nestler 2001) and remains one of the best-established molecular mechanisms of long-term adaptations to abused drugs (Nestler 2004).

EVIDENCE FOR STRUCTURAL CHANGES IN THE VENTRAL TEGMENTAL AREA–NUCLEUS ACCUMBENS PATHWAY

Although changes in levels of signal transduction proteins could mediate some of the long-term actions of drugs of abuse, they are unlikely to be responsible for the extremely long-lived adaptations that characterize an addicted state. One hypothesis is that adaptations in signaling pathways may cause longer-lasting structural changes in neurons (Bolaños and Nestler 2004). Several examples of such changes have been documented in recent years.

Long-term administration of morphine, for example, has been shown to decrease the size of VTA dopamine neurons as well as the caliber of their proximal processes (Sklair-Tavron et al. 1996). This is depicted in Figure 11–3. Morphine also causes a reduction in axoplasmic transport from the VTA to the NAc (see Nestler 1992). These findings may be related to the observation that long-term morphine use decreases levels of neurofilament proteins in this brain region, an effect also seen after long-term cocaine or ethanol exposure (Beitner-Johnson et al. 1992; Nestler 1992; Ortiz et al. 1995). The observed decrease in axonal transport rates could decrease the amount of tyrosine hydroxylase transported from dopamine cell bodies in the VTA to nerve terminals in the NAc. At a constant rate of tyrosine hydroxylase synthesis, this would tend to lead to the buildup of tyrosine hydroxylase observed in the VTA (as described in the earlier section on dopamine regulation in the VTA–NAc pathway) and to decreased levels of enzyme in the NAc. Such decreased levels of tyrosine hydroxylase, along with its reduced phosphorylation, have been reported (Nestler 1992; Schmidt et al. 2001; Self et al. 1995). Decreases in tyrosine hydroxylase in the NAc could explain the short-term reductions (also described earlier) in levels of basal and stimulated dopamine release during early phases of drug withdrawal.

Long-term morphine, cocaine, or ethanol treatment also increases levels of glial fibrillary acidic protein, specifically in the VTA (Beitner-Johnson et al. 1993; Ortiz et al. 1995). Drug-induced decreases in neurofilament proteins and increases in glial filament proteins in the VTA are reminiscent of neural insult or injury (see Figure 11–3). Such findings raise the possibility that perturbations in neurotrophic factor signaling are involved in long-term drug action. Indeed, direct infusion of any of several neurotrophic factors into the VTA has been shown to oppose the ability of long-term drug exposure to produce some of its characteristic biochemical and morphological changes in the VTA (Berhow et al. 1995; Messer et al. 2000; Sklair-Tavron et al. 1996). Such infusions of neurotrophic factors also potently modify behavioral responses to drug exposure (Bolaños and Nestler 2004; Horger et al. 1999; L. Lu et al. 2004; Pierce and Bari 2001). Of particular interest are the abnormal biochemical and behavioral responses to drugs of abuse in mice lacking brain-derived neurotrophic factor or glial cell line–derived neurotrophic factor and the alterations in certain neurotrophic factor signaling proteins after long-term drug exposure (Bolaños et al. 2003; He et al. 2005; Horger et al. 1999; Messer et al. 2000; D.H. Wolf et al. 1999). Together, these results indicate not only that exogenous neurotrophic factors can modify responses to drugs of abuse, but also that endogenous neurotrophic factor pathways are involved in mediating some of the long-term effects of drug exposure on the brain.

Drugs of abuse also cause structural changes in the medium spiny neurons of the NAc. Long-term administration of cocaine, amphetamine, or nicotine increases the dendritic arborizations of these neurons as well as the density of their terminal dendritic spines (Robinson and Kolb 1997). Similar changes have been found for pyramidal neurons in the prefrontal cortex. In contrast, long-term morphine administration causes the opposite changes in dendritic structure in the NAc (Robinson and Kolb 2004). Because alterations in dendritic spines are implicated in controlling

the efficacy of synaptic transmission in other regions of brain, the observed drug-induced changes in the NAc represent an attractive mechanism by which long-term drug exposure might produce very long-lived changes in NAc function and, hence, motivational processes.

MOLECULAR MECHANISMS UNDERLYING DRUG-INDUCED ADAPTATIONS IN THE NUCLEUS ACCUMBENS

The precise mechanisms by which long-term drug treatment alters levels of specific proteins in the VTA–NAc pathway are still unknown, but there are now many studies that show that gene expression can be regulated by drug exposure (see Chao and Nestler 2004; Nestler 1992). Such studies have focused on the role played by two families of transcription factors (shown in Figure 11–4): cAMP response element binding protein (CREB) and CREB-like proteins and the products of certain immediate early genes (IEGs), such as the Fos and Jun family proteins (see Nestler 2001). Fos and Jun proteins form heterodimeric complexes that bind to specific DNA sequences referred to as activator protein 1 (AP-1) sites to regulate transcription of a target gene. Most genes likely contain numerous response elements for these and many other transcription factors, suggesting that complex interactions and multiple mechanisms control the expression of a given gene.

Short-term administration of cocaine or amphetamine increases the expression of several Fos and Jun family members and increases AP-1 binding activity in the NAc and dorsal striatum (for references, see McClung et al. 2004). One possible mechanism of cocaine action is that the drug induces c-Fos via dopamine activation of D_1 receptors and the subsequent activation of the cAMP pathway. These drugs also induce Egr1 (also known as Zif268) in these brain regions. Egr1 is a transcription factor that binds to a distinct response element but is regulated as an IEG product in a fashion similar to

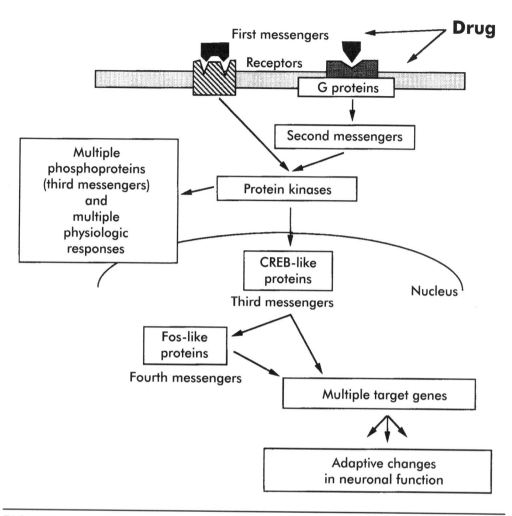

FIGURE 11–4. Schematic illustration of the hypothetical role played by gene expression in drug addiction.

According to this scheme, an initial extracellular effect of a drug of abuse would trigger changes in multiple intracellular messenger pathways in target neurons. Changes in the intracellular messengers would result in numerous physiologic responses to the drug (as shown in Figure 11–2), including alterations in gene expression. The latter types of alterations would occur through the regulation of many classes of nuclear, DNA-binding proteins termed transcription factors, such as cyclic adenosine monophosphate (cAMP) response element binding protein (CREB) and Fos. CREB exemplifies a transcription factor that is regulated by extracellular agents primarily through changes in its degree of phosphorylation. Fos exemplifies a transcription factor that is expressed at very low levels under basal conditions and is regulated by extracellular agents primarily through induction of its expression (in some cases via CREB). Both types of transcription factors would then result in altered levels of expression of specific target proteins that underlie the adaptive changes in brain function associated with addiction.

Fos- and Jun-like proteins (O'Donovan et al. 1999). Other drugs of abuse also induce these various IEGs in the NAc and dorsal striatum.

The ability to induce c-Fos and the other IEG products in the NAc is attenuated on re-peated cocaine treatment, whereas the increased AP-1 binding activity persists for weeks after drug treatment ceases (Daunais and McGinty 1994; Hope et al. 1994). We now know that this persistent AP-1 binding activity

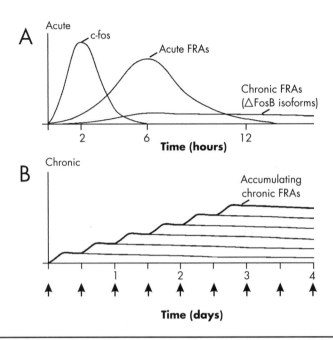

FIGURE 11–5. Scheme for the gradual accumulation of ΔFosB (also called chronic Fos-related antigens [FRAs]) versus the rapid and transient induction of acute FRAs in the brain.

Panel A. Several waves of FRAs are induced in neurons by many acute stimuli. c-Fos is induced rapidly and degrades within several hours of the acute stimulus, whereas other "acute FRAs" (e.g., FosB, FRA-1, and FRA-2) are induced somewhat later and persist somewhat longer than c-Fos. The chronic FRAs are phosphorylated isoforms of ΔFosB; they, too, are induced (although at low levels) after a single acute stimulus but persist in the brain for long periods (with a half-life longer than 1 week). In a complex with Jun-like proteins, these waves of FRAs form activator protein 1 (AP-1)–binding complexes with shifting composition over time. *Panel B.* With repeated (e.g., twice daily) stimulation, each acute stimulus induces a low level of ΔFosB. This is indicated by the lower set of overlapping lines, which indicates ΔFosB induced by each acute stimulus. The result is a gradual increase in the total levels of ΔFosB with repeated stimuli during a course of long-term treatment. This is indicated by the increasing stepped line in the graph. The increasing levels of ΔFosB with repeated stimulation would result in the gradual induction of significant levels of a long-lasting AP-1 complex, which could underlie persisting forms of neural plasticity in the brain.

Source. Adapted from Hope BT, Nye HE, Kelz MB, et al:. "Induction of a Long-Lasting AP-1 Complex Composed of Altered Fos-Like Proteins in Brain by Chronic Cocaine and Other Chronic Treatments. *Neuron* 13:1235–1244, © +1994, with permission from Elsevier.

is caused by the long-lived expression of biochemically modified isoforms of ΔFosB, a member of the Fos family of transcription factors. ΔFosB persists in the brain for a long time due to its extraordinary stability mediated in part by its phosphorylation by casein kinase II. Thus, it could represent a type of sustained molecular switch that contributes to prolonged aspects of cocaine addiction (Figure 11–5). Similar induction of ΔFosB is seen after long-term (but not after short-term) administration of

opiates, nicotine, alcohol, cannabinoids, and phencyclidine (see McClung et al. 2004). Studies of transgenic mice in which ΔFosB, or an antagonist of ΔFosB, can be induced in adult animals selectively within the NAc and dorsal striatum demonstrate that ΔFosB expression increases an animal's sensitivity to the rewarding and locomotor-activating effects of cocaine and may increase the motivation to pursue cocaine reward as well (Colby et al. 2003; Kelz et al. 1999; Peakman et al. 2003). ΔFosB causes this behavioral phenotype via the regulation of numerous target genes, which are just now beginning to be identified and characterized (McClung and Nestler 2003). Interestingly, some of these target genes have been related to the decreased glutamate sensitivity and increased dendritic spine densities of NAc neurons observed after chronic drug exposure (see McClung et al. 2004).

Because long-term cocaine and morphine treatments upregulate the cAMP pathway in the NAc, the CREB family of transcription factors is also likely influenced by these drugs. Indeed, long-term drug treatments regulate CREB phosphorylation and functional activity in this brain region (see Cole et al. 1995; Shaw-Lutchman et al. 2003). By use of virus-mediated gene transfer, it has been shown that increases in CREB levels in the NAc decrease an animal's sensitivity to the rewarding effects of cocaine and of morphine, whereas inactivation of CREB has the opposite effect (Barrot et al. 2002; Carlezon et al. 1998). The effects of CREB are mediated in part by the opioid peptide dynorphin, which is increased by CREB and decreased on inactivation of CREB. Dynorphin acts on κ opioid receptors within the NAc and VTA to produce aversive effects by reducing dopamine release from presynaptic terminals. Thus, activation of CREB, and the resulting induction of dynorphin, in response to long-term drug exposure would appear to represent a mechanism of tolerance to drug reward as well as dysphoria during drug withdrawal (dependence) (Carlezon et al. 2005).

Current research is focused on identifying additional target genes for CREB and for ΔFosB and on identifying additional transcriptional control mechanisms that mediate the long-term actions of drugs of abuse on the mesolimbic dopamine system (McClung and Nestler 2003).

CONCLUSION

The availability of animal models that accurately reproduce important features of drug addiction in humans has made it possible to identify specific regions in the brain that play an important role in addictive disorders. Whereas the locus coeruleus plays an important role in physical dependence on opiates, it is the mesolimbic dopamine system as well as regions of the prefrontal cortex and amygdala that appears to be integrally involved in drug-seeking behavior, the essential clinical feature of drug addiction. Basic neurobiological investigations are now providing an increasingly complete understanding of the adaptations at the molecular and cellular levels that occur in these various brain regions and are responsible for behavioral features of drug addiction. Work to date has focused on adaptations in intracellular messenger pathways, particularly G proteins and the cAMP pathway, although many other types of adaptations will also prove to be involved. As the pathophysiological mechanisms underlying drug addiction become increasingly understood, it will be possible to develop more efficacious pharmacotherapies for the treatment of addictive disorders. Parallel studies, not covered in this chapter, of different inbred animal strains and of individual differences among large outbred populations promise to yield information concerning the specific proteins that underlie inherent differences in an individual's responsiveness to drugs of abuse. This work will lead eventually to the identification of specific genes and environmental factors that control individual variations in the susceptibility to drug addiction. Ultimately, this work could lead to the development of specific interventions that prevent drug addiction in particularly vulnerable individuals.

RECOMMENDED READINGS

Goldstein A: Addiction: From Biology to Drug Policy, 2nd Edition. New York, Oxford University Press, 2001

Hyman SE, Malenka RC: Addiction and the brain: the neurobiology of compulsion and its persistence. Nature Rev Neurosci 2:695–703, 2001

Kalivas PW, Volkow N, Seamans J: Unmanageable motivation in addiction: a pathology in prefrontal-accumbens glutamate transmission. Neuron 45:647–650, 2005

Koob GF, Sanna PP, Bloom FE: Neuroscience of addiction. Neuron 21:467–476, 1998

Nestler EJ: Molecular basis of neural plasticity underlying addiction. Nature Rev Neurosci 2:119–128, 2001

Nestler EJ, Malenka RC: The addicted brain. Sci Am 290:78–85, 2004

Robinson TE, Kolb B: Structural plasticity associated with exposure to drugs of abuse. Neuropharmacology 47 (suppl 1):33–46, 2004

REFERENCES

American Psychiatric Association: Diagnostic and Statistical Manual of Mental Disorders, 4th Edition, Text Revision. Washington, DC, American Psychiatric Association, 2000

Barrot M, Olivier JDA, Perrotti LI: CREB activity in the nucleus accumbens shell controls gating of behavioral responses to emotional stimuli. Proc Natl Acad Sci U S A 99:11435–11440, 2002

Beitner-Johnson D, Guitart X, Nestler EJ: Neurofilament proteins and the mesolimbic dopamine system: common regulation by chronic morphine and chronic cocaine in the rat ventral tegmental area. J Neurosci 12:2165–2176, 1992

Beitner-Johnson D, Guitart X, Nestler EJ: Glial fibrillary acidic protein and the mesolimbic dopamine system: regulation by chronic morphine and Lewis-Fischer strain differences in the rat ventral tegmental area. J Neurochem 61:1766–1773, 1993

Berhow MT, Russell DS, Terwilliger RZ, et al: Influence of neurotrophic factors on morphine- and cocaine-induced biochemical changes in the mesolimbic dopamine system. Neuroscience 68:969–979, 1995

Bolaños CA, Nestler EJ: Neurotrophic mechanisms in drug addiction. Neuromolecular Med 5:69–83, 2004

Bolaños CA, Perrotti LI, Edwards S, et al: Viral-mediated expression of phospholipase Cγ in distinct regions of the ventral tegmental area differentially modulates mood-related behaviors. J Neurosci 23:7569–7576, 2003

Bonci A, Williams JT: Increased probability of GABA release during withdrawal from morphine. J Neurosci 17:796–803, 1997

Carlezon WA Jr, Nestler EJ: Elevated levels of GluR1 in the midbrain: a trigger for sensitization to drugs of abuse? Trends Neurosci 25:610–615, 2002

Carlezon WA Jr, Thome J, Olson VG, et al: Regulation of cocaine reward by CREB. Science 282:2272–2275, 1998

Carlezon WA Jr, Duman RS, Nestler EJ: The many faces of CREB. Trends Neurosci 28:436–445, 2005

Chao J, Nestler EJ: Molecular neurobiology of drug addiction. Annu Rev Med 55:113–132, 2004

Churchill L, Swanson CJ, Urbina M, et al: Repeated cocaine alters glutamate receptor subunit levels in the nucleus accumbens and ventral tegmental area of rats that develop behavioral sensitization. J Neurochem 72:2397–2403, 1999

Colby CR, Whisler K, Steffen C, et al: FosB enhances incentive for cocaine. J Neurosci 23:2488–2493, 2003

Cole RL, Konradi C, Douglass J, et al: Neuronal adaptation to amphetamine and dopamine: molecular mechanisms of prodynorphin gene regulation in rat striatum. Neuron 14:813–823, 1995

Daunais JB, McGinty JF: Acute and chronic cocaine administration differentially alters striatal opioid and nuclear transcription factor mRNAs. Synapse 18:35–46, 1994

De Montis MG, Co C, Dworking SI, et al: Modifications of dopamine D1 receptor complex in rats self-administering cocaine. Eur J Pharmacol 362:9–15, 1998

Dworkin SI, Smith JE: Opiates/opioids and reinforcement, in Biological Basis of Substance Abuse. Edited by Korenman SG, Barchas JD. New York, Oxford University Press, 1993, pp 327–338

He DY, McGough NN, Ravindranathan A, et al: Glial cell line-derived neurotrophic factor mediates the desirable actions of the anti-addiction drug ibogaine against alcohol consumption. J Neurosci 25:619–628, 2005

Hope BT, Nye HE, Kelz MB, et al: Induction of a long-lasting AP1 complex composed of altered Fos-like proteins in brain by chronic cocaine and other chronic treatments. Neuron 13:1235–1244, 1994

Horger BA, Iyasere CA, Berhow MT, et al: Enhancement of locomotor activity and conditioned reward to cocaine by brain-derived neurotrophic factor. J Neurosci 19:4110–4122, 1999

Hyman SE, Malenka RC, Nestler EJ: Neural mechanisms of addiction: the role of reward-related learning and memory. Annu Rev Neurosci 29:565–598, 2006

Ikemoto S, Wise RA: Mapping of chemical trigger zones for reward. Neuropharmacology 47 (suppl 1):190–201, 2004

Jolas T, Nestler EJ, Aghajanian GK: Chronic morphine increases GABA tone on serotonergic neurons of the dorsal raphe nucleus: association with an upregulation of the cyclic AMP pathway. Neuroscience 95:433–443, 2000

Kalivas PW: Glutamate systems in cocaine addiction. Curr Opin Pharmacol 4:23–29, 2004

Kalivas PW, Volkow N, Seamans J: Unmanageable motivation in addiction: a pathology in prefrontal-accumbens glutamate transmission. Neuron 45:647–650, 2005

Kelley AE: Memory and addiction: shared neural circuitry and molecular mechanisms. Neuron 44:161–179, 2004

Kelley AE, Holahan MR: Enhanced reward-related responding following cholera toxin infusion into the nucleus accumbens. Synapse 26:46–54, 1997

Kelz MB, Chen JS, Carlezon WA, et al: Expression of the transcription factor deltaFosB in the brain controls sensitivity to cocaine. Nature 401:272–276, 1999

Koob GF, Sanna PP, Bloom FE: Neuroscience of addiction. Neuron 21:467–476, 1998

Koob GF, Ahmed SH, Boutrel B, et al: Neurobiological mechanisms in the transition from drug use to drug dependence. Neurosci Biobehav Rev 27:739–749, 2004

Kuhar MJ, Ritz MC, Boja JW: The dopamine hypothesis of the reinforcing properties of cocaine. Trends Neurosci 14:299–302, 1991

Lu L, Dempsey J, Liu SY, et al: A single infusion of brain-derived neurotrophic factor into the ventral tegmental area induces long-lasting potentiation of cocaine seeking after withdrawal. J Neurosci 24:1604–1611, 2004

Lu W, Wolf ME: Repeated amphetamine administration alters AMPA receptor subunit expression in rat nucleus accumbens and medial prefrontal cortex. Synapse 32:119–131, 1999

Maggos CE, Tsukada H, Kakiuchi T, et al: Sustained withdrawal allows normalization of in vivo [^{11}C]N-methylspiperone dopamine D2 receptor binding after chronic binge cocaine: a positron emission tomography study in rats. Neuropsychopharmacology 19:146–153, 1998

McClung CA, Nestler EJ: Regulation of gene expression and cocaine reward by CREB and FosB. Nat Neurosci 11:1208–1215, 2003

McClung CA, Ulery PG, Perrotti LI, et al: FosB: A molecular switch for long-term adaptation. Brain Res Mol Brain Res 132:146–154, 2004

Messer CJ, Eisch AJ, Carlezon WA Jr, et al: Role of GDNF in biochemical and behavioral adaptations to drugs of abuse. Neuron 26:247–257, 2000

Moore RJ, Vinsant SL, Nader MA, et al: Effect of cocaine self-administration on striatal dopamine D1 receptors in rhesus monkeys. Synapse 28:1–9, 1998

Nestler EJ: Molecular basis of long-term plasticity underlying addiction. Nat Rev Neurosci 2:119–128, 2001

Nestler EJ: Historical review: molecular and cellular mechanisms of opiate and cocaine addiction. Trends Pharmacol Sci 25:210–218, 2004

Nestler EJ: Is there a common molecular pathway for addiction? Nat Neurosci 8:1445–1449, 2005

Nestler EJ, Aghajanian GK: Molecular and cellular basis of addiction. Science 278:58–63, 1997

Nestler EJ, Hyman SE, Malenka RC: Molecular Neuropharmacology: A Foundation for Clinical Neuroscience. New York, McGraw-Hill, 2001

O'Donovan KJ, Tourtellotte WG, Millbrandt J, et al: The EGR family of transcription-regulatory factors: progress at the interface of molecular and systems neuroscience. Trends Neurosci 22:167–173, 1999

Olds ME: Reinforcing effects of morphine in the nucleus accumbens. Brain Res 237:429–440, 1982

Ortiz J, Fitzgerald LW, Charlton M, et al: Biochemical actions of chronic ethanol exposure in the mesolimbic dopamine system. Synapse 21:289–298, 1995

Peakman MC, Colby C, Perrotti LI, et al: Inducible, brain region specific expression of a dominant negative mutant of c-Jun in transgenic mice decreases sensitivity to cocaine. Brain Res 970:73–86, 2003

Pierce RC, Bari AA: The role of neurotrophic factors in psychostimulant-induced behavioral and neuronal plasticity. Rev Neurosci 12:95–110, 2001

Pilotte NS: Neurochemistry of cocaine withdrawal. Curr Opin Neurol 10:534–538, 1997

Robinson TE, Berridge KC: Addiction. Annu Rev Psychol 54:25–53, 2003

Robinson TE, Kolb B: Persistent structural modifications in nucleus accumbens and prefrontal neurons produced by previous experience with amphetamine. J Neurosci 17:8491–8497, 1997

Robinson TE, Kolb B: Structural plasticity associated with exposure to drugs of abuse. Neuropharmacology 47 (suppl 1):33–46, 2004

Schmidt EF, Sutton MA, Schad CA, et al: Extinction training regulates tyrosine hydroxylase during withdrawal from cocaine self-administration (rapid communication). J Neurosci 21 (RC137):1–5, 2001

Self DW: Regulation of drug-taking and -seeking behaviors by neuroadaptations in the mesolimbic dopamine system. Neuropharmacology 47:242–255, 2004

Self DW, Nestler EJ: Molecular mechanisms of drug reinforcement and addiction. Annu Rev Neurosci 18:463–495, 1995

Self DW, Nestler EJ: Relapse to drug seeking: neural and molecular mechanisms. Drug Alcohol Depend 51:49–60, 1998

Self DW, Terwilliger RZ, Nestler EJ, et al: Inactivation of Gi and Go proteins in nucleus accumbens reduces both cocaine and heroin reinforcement. J Neurosci 14:6239–6247, 1994

Self DW, McClenahan AW, Beitner-Johnson D, et al: Biochemical adaptations in the mesolimbic dopamine system in response to heroin self-administration. Synapse 21:312–318, 1995

Self DW, Genova LM, Hope BT, et al: Involvement of cAMP-dependent protein kinase in the nucleus accumbens in cocaine self-administration and relapse of cocaine-seeking behavior. J Neurosci 18:1848–1859, 1998

Shaham Y, Shalev U, Lu L, et al: The reinstatement model of drug relapse: history, methodology and major findings. Psychopharmacology 168:3–20, 2003

Shaw-Lutchman SZ, Impey S, Storm D, et al: Regulation of CRE-mediated transcription in mouse brain by amphetamine. Synapse 48:10–17, 2003

Sibley DR, Ventura AL, Jiang D, et al: Regulation of the D1 receptor through cAMP-mediated pathways. Adv Pharmacol 42:447–450, 1998

Sklair-Tavron L, Shi W-X, Lane SB, et al: Chronic morphine induces visible changes in the morphology of mesolimbic dopamine neurons. Proc Natl Acad Sci U S A 93:11202–11207, 1996

Spanagel R, Weiss F: The dopamine hypothesis of reward: past and current status. Trends Neurosci 22:521–527, 1999

Stewart J: Stress and relapse to drug seeking: studies in laboratory animals shed light on mechanisms and sources of long-term vulnerability. Am J Addict 12:1–17, 2003

Striplin CD, Kalivas PW: Correlation between behavioral sensitization to cocaine and G protein ADP-ribosylation in the ventral tegmental area. Brain Res 579:181–186, 1992

Striplin CD, Kalivas PW: Robustness of G protein changes in cocaine sensitization shown with immunoblotting. Synapse 14:10–15, 1993

Terwilliger RZ, Beitner-Johnson D, Sevarino KA, et al: A general roll for adaptations in G-proteins and the cyclic AMP system in mediating the chronic actions of morphine and cocaine on neuronal function. Brain Res 548:100–110, 1991

Thomas MJ, Malenka RC: Synaptic plasticity in the mesolimbic dopamine system. Philos Trans R Soc Lond B Biol Sci 358:815–819, 2003

Tsukada H, Kreuter J, Maggos CE, et al: Effects of binge pattern cocaine administration on dopamine D1 and D2 receptors in the rat brain: an in vivo study using positron emission tomography. J Neurosci 16:7670–7677, 1996

Unterwald EM, Cox BM, Creek MJ, et al: Chronic repeated cocaine administration alters basal and opioid-regulated adenylyl cyclase activity. Synapse 15:33–38, 1993

Vezina P: Sensitization of midbrain dopamine neuron reactivity and the self-administration of psychomotor stimulant drugs. Neurosci Biobehav Rev 27:827–839, 2004

Volkow ND, Fowler JS, Wang GJ: Imaging studies on the role of dopamine in cocaine reinforcement and addiction in humans. J Psychopharmacol 13:337–345, 1999

White FJ, Kalivas PW: Neuroadaptations involved in amphetamine and cocaine addiction. Drug Alcohol Depend 51:141–153, 1998

White FJ, Hu X-T, Zhang X-F, et al: Repeated administration of cocaine or amphetamine alters neuronal responses to glutamate in the mesoaccumbens dopamine system. J Pharmacol Exp Ther 273:445–454, 1995

Wolf DH, Numan S, Nestler EJ, et al: Regulation of phospholipase Cgamma in the mesolimbic dopamine system by chronic morphine administration. J Neurochem 73:1520–1528, 1999

Wolf ME: The role of excitatory amino acids in behavioral sensitization to psychomotor stimulants. Prog Neurobiol 54:679–720, 1998

Yao WD, Gainetdinvo RR, Arbuckle MI, et al: Identification of PSD-95 as a regulator of dopamine-mediated synaptic and behavioral plasticity. Neuron 41:625–638, 2004

12

NEUROPSYCHIATRIC ASPECTS OF DEMENTIAS ASSOCIATED WITH MOTOR DYSFUNCTION

Alan J. Lerner, M.D.

David Riley, M.D.

The degenerative dementias associated with motor system dysfunction are diverse disorders that present a particular challenge to the clinician. Depending on where the primary pathology occurs in the motor system (basal ganglia, cerebellum, or motor neuron), symptoms can include abnormal movements, incoordination, or weakness in addition to the neuropsychiatric features. In this chapter, we review Huntington's disease (HD), Parkinson's disease (PD), progressive supranuclear palsy (PSP), and other conditions in which movement or motor disorders are cardinal clinical features. In contrast, in primary degenerative dementias such as Alzheimer's disease (AD) and frontotemporal dementia (FTD), motor signs are relatively incidental and usually become prominent only in later stages of the disease.

As degenerative disorders, the dementias included in this chapter are characterized by gradual loss of function caused by progressive loss of neurons in specific regions of the brain associated with pathological hallmarks that are characteristic of the individual diseases. The specific etiologies of these diseases are often unknown, and clinical features frequently overlap among different conditions, making a clear nosology difficult.

As the genetic basis of these conditions is being elucidated, a firmer basis has developed for deciphering the variability in clinical and neuropsychiatric symptoms. Despite these impressive, concerted advances in knowledge, specific biological interventions are limited in effectiveness.

The combination of motor, cognitive, and behavioral abnormalities is particularly stressful for patients, family members, and professional caregivers because of the multifaceted impairment in quality of life. Medications available to treat the motor symptoms for some of these conditions may aggravate the cognitive and behavioral dysfunction. Motor impairments themselves create special difficulties in neuropsychiatric and neuropsychological testing of the cognitive and psychiatric dysfunction.

The classification of the dementias included in this chapter and their nosological relations to those considered by Apostolova and Cummings in Chapter 13 of this volume are controversial. Ideally, classification depends on proper understanding of essential clinical and biological features. However, our understanding of the relations between brain changes, aging, and behavioral alterations in these disorders is limited. One approach was the development of the concept of cortical and subcortical dementia (Albert et al. 1974; McHugh and Folstein 1975). AD and Pick's disease (see section "Frontotemporal Dementia" later in this chapter) are thought to represent cortical dementias in which the predominant pathology is neocortical and the clinical symptoms such as aphasia, apraxia, and agnosia supposedly reflect cortical pathology. Subcortical dementias show prominent deficits in processing speed, memory dysfunction, and affective changes. However, dementias cannot be easily classified into these two large categories, since there is overlap in site of pathology and symptomatology (Apaydin et al. 2002; Brown and Marsden 1988; Cummings 1990; Mayeux et al. 1983; Whitehouse 1986).

HUNTINGTON'S DISEASE

HD is an autosomal dominant progressive neuropsychiatric disorder with peak period of onset in the fourth and fifth decades. Chorea—defined as brief, random, nonstereotyped, purposeless movements—is usually considered the first sign of the disease. However, the clinical presentation is variable, and cognitive and psychiatric manifestations are often evident before the movement disorder (S.E. Folstein 1989). Depression, irritability, and impulsive or erratic behavior are the most common psychiatric symptoms. Memory and concentration difficulties are early cognitive symptoms (S.E. Folstein 1989; Martin and Gusella 1986).

EPIDEMIOLOGY

Point prevalence among Caucasians is 5–7 cases per 100,000. The prevalence in European populations is relatively uniform, although there are isolated populations with much higher or lower rates (e.g., Spain, Finland) (Harper 1992).

Early onset is associated with paternal transmission and has a more rapid course. In adult-onset cases, death usually occurs after 16–20 years. The rate of decline may be slower in patients with onset after the fifth decade of life.

ETIOLOGY

Genetic linkage analysis, based on a Venezuelan population with a very high prevalence of the disease, identified the HD gene locus at the distal end of the short arm of chromosome 4 (Gusella et al. 1983). The mutant gene consists of an expanded trinucleotide cytosine-adenine-guanine (CAG) repeat sequence longer than a normal gene. Normal alleles have a range of 9 to 30 CAG repeats, whereas HD patients have from 40 to at least 121 repeats (Albin and Tagle 1995; Huntington's Disease Collaborative Research Group 1993; Monckton and Caskey 1995). Patients with repeat lengths between 36 and 39 may or may not become symptomatic.

The isolation of the gene has permitted some accounting for the apparent allelic heterogeneity of the disease, with family, race, and gender variation in age at onset (Farrer and Conneally 1985; S.E. Folstein et al. 1987). Although age at onset is related to the number of gene repeats, environmental factors contribute as much as 38% of the variability in this important aspect of the disease (Wexler et al. 2004).

DIAGNOSIS AND CLINICAL FEATURES

The key step in clinical diagnosis is to consider HD among the diagnostic possibilities, since laboratory diagnosis requires only confirmation of the expanded CAG repeats. The classic clinical syndrome of HD consists of typical clinical findings in the setting of a positive family history consistent with autosomal dominant inheritance. Clinical diagnosis may become problematic if patients present with other movement disorders, if they present with psychiatric rather than cognitive dysfunction, and if the family history is incomplete or misleading (e.g., mistaken paternity). In the 3%–9% of cases in which onset occurs before or during adolescence, the so-called Westphal variant, parkinsonism, myoclonus, or dystonia may be the predominant movements.

The differential diagnosis of HD includes PD, Sydenham's chorea, ataxias, cerebrovascular disease, systemic lupus erythematosus, schizophrenia, mood disorder, thyroid disease, acanthocytosis, drug-induced chorea, and alcoholism.

Nearly half of HD patients initially present with emotional or cognitive symptoms. These symptoms are diverse and include depression, irritability, hallucinations, and apathy. Motor symptoms, if present, may be mild and may be attributed to another disorder. However, when the patient has a positive family history, HD is a very likely explanation of these symptoms.

With direct genetic testing, the clinical and ethical issues involved in preclinical testing for HD have been widely discussed. These issues must be explored on an individual basis and may be aided by employing an experienced genetic counselor.

NEUROBIOLOGY

The most obvious gross pathology in HD occurs in the basal ganglia. The striatum is consistently affected, with degeneration beginning in the medial caudate nucleus and proceeding laterally to the putamen and occasionally to the globus pallidus.

The gene product of the HD gene is a protein called huntingtin. In unaffected individuals, it is a cytosolic protein, but in HD it is transported to the cell nucleus. The mechanism by which its abnormal transport and de-

position in intraneuronal inclusions relate to molecular pathophysiology is currently unknown. The actual mechanisms of cell destruction in the caudate nucleus are also unclear. One theory focuses on abnormal posttranslation cleavage products that disturb cellular metabolism and function (Albin and Tagle 1995). A second model proposes an excitotoxic basis for HD involving the glutamate/N-methyl-D-aspartate (NDMA) receptor.

γ-Aminobutyric acid (GABA), the most abundant neurotransmitter of the spiny output neurons, and acetylcholine, the principal neurotransmitter of type I aspiny interneurons, are especially reduced (Martin and Gusella 1986). The alterations in absolute neurotransmitter concentrations and relative balance among different systems may account for some of the symptoms of HD.

Rich interconnections are found between the striatum and the prefrontal and parietal cortices. There are five distinct parallel corticostriatal circuits subserving distinct neurobehavioral functions, including eye movements, motor behavior, emotion, and cognitive functions. Except for the motor circuit involving the putamen, the others are caudate nucleus–frontal circuits. Interestingly, lesions at any of the segments of the circuit produce similar functional consequences.

Major inputs to the striatum include limbic structures, the primary motor cortex, and motor association areas. These sources may account for the co-occurrence of movement abnormalities and behavioral symptoms, and for the influence of emotional states on motor symptoms.

The degree of atrophy of the caudate nucleus correlates with cognitive dysfunction, including intelligence, memory, and visuospatial deficits. Atrophy of the caudate nucleus is generally more consistently correlated than measures of frontal atrophy, with executive functions typically considered to be evidence of prefrontal cortical pathology. Similar associations between functional impairments and caudate nucleus pathology have been reported with positron emission tomography (PET)

(Bamford et al. 1989; M. Morris 1995; Starkstein et al 1988).

MOTOR ABNORMALITIES

HD was formerly known as Huntington's chorea, emphasizing the prominence of chorea, characterized by involuntary sudden, jerky movements of the limbs, face, or trunk, unpredictable in timing or distribution. Patients can generally suppress chorea for only short periods. Parkinsonism or dystonia, in the absence of chorea, is common in juvenile-onset (Westphal variant) cases.

Motor abnormalities change over the course of the disease. Early motor abnormalities include brief, irregular, jerky movements along with slower, writhing movements, often occurring in conjunction with the initiation of action. Irregular flexion-extension of individual fingers and ulnar deviation of the hands while walking are also common. Later, movements become almost constant, with severe grimacing, nodding, head bobbing, and a "dancing" gait. In late disease, chorea may decrease and dystonia and an akinetic-rigid syndrome may supervene, especially in those with drug-induced parkinsonism (Feigin et al. 1995; Furtado and Suchowersky 1995).

Chorea may be misdiagnosed as nervousness, mannerisms, or intentional movements early in the course of the disease. Abnormalities in voluntary movements are helpful in the diagnosis because they are present in HD even in the absence of chorea. Patients have abnormalities in initiation and inhibition of eye movements (saccades, fixation, and smooth pursuit), coordination of limb movements, and articulation (Furtado and Suchowersky 1995; Leigh et al. 1983). Although nonspecific, these abnormalities correlate better with intellectual impairment, memory disorder, and capacity for activities of daily living than does the chorea severity.

COGNITIVE ABNORMALITIES

Cognitive deficits usually appear early in the course of HD and are progressive (M. Morris 1995). Very early in the disease, intelligence may be normal, and detailed neuropsychological testing is helpful. Although cognitive deficits can occur very early, it is questionable whether neuropsychological deficits appear before other clinical signs of the disease, but they can contribute to early disability (Giordani et al. 1995; Mayeux et al. 1986a; Strauss and Brandt 1990). When the deficits are severe, a brief mental status test is sufficient.

Memory deficits are the best-characterized neuropsychological feature of the disease. Early studies (Brandt and Butters 1986) suggested that HD was characterized by major deficits in the encoding or storage of new information. However, deficits in retrieval of memories and the acquisition of procedural memory appear to be even more pronounced (S.E. Folstein et al. 1990).

Mendez (1994) found that for any given level of dementia, the pattern of failure is different in HD and AD. At mild levels of dementia (scores of 20–24 on the Mini-Mental State Examination [MMSE; M.F. Folstein et al. 1975]), HD patients are more impaired in the serial subtraction of 7 from 100, whereas AD patients are more likely to have errors in recall.

The cognitive deficits of HD also include difficulties in sustained concentration and visuospatial skills. HD patients may have difficulty identifying or using their position in space relative to some fixed point, unlike in AD, where the deficit is mainly in the perception of extrapersonal space.

Executive dysfunction (problems with planning, organizing, and mental flexibility) is also affected early in HD. Examples of such tasks are those requiring keeping track of several things at once, discovering rules, or frequently changing mental sets (Bylsma et al. 1990; Starkstein et al. 1988; Wexler 1979).

Language, with the exception of verbal fluency and prosody, is relatively preserved in HD (Furtado and Suchowersky 1995; Mendez 1994; M. Morris 1995). Patients may answer questions with single words or short phrases, punctuated by pauses and silences. There may be deficits in the ability to understand prosodic elements of speech, which may contribute to the impairments in interpersonal relationships. Problems in writing often correlate with verbal difficulties.

PSYCHIATRIC ABNORMALITIES

Psychiatric symptoms are common in HD and are often the first signs of the disorder. Estimates of the proportion of patients who first present with psychiatric symptoms range from 24% to 79%, and the prevalence of psychiatric disorders in HD patients ranges from 35% to 73% (Cummings 1995; Mendez 1994).

Shiwach and Norbury (1994) found no increase in schizophrenia, depression, psychiatric episodes, or behavior disorders in asymptomatic HD heterozygotes compared with their mutation-free siblings. The number of CAG repeats did not correlate with psychiatric symptoms or onset symptoms in two studies in which this variable was included (Claes et al. 1995; Zappacosta et al. 1996).

Studies suggest that affective disorders and intermittent explosive disorders are the most prevalent psychiatric conditions in HD (S.E. Folstein 1989; S.E. Folstein et al. 1990). Unipolar depression is common, but mania can also be seen in conjunction with HD. A markedly elevated risk of suicide is found in persons with HD, with the period of greatest risk in the 50s and 60s (Cummings 1995; Mendez 1994).

Irritability, often precipitated by previously innocuous stimuli or events and anxiety, is common in HD. Approximately 30% of patients are reported to show altered sexual behavior, including sexual aggression, promiscuity, exhibitionism, voyeurism, and pedophilia (Cummings 1995; Mendez 1994). Whereas early HD may be accompanied by irritability, anxiety, aggression, and antisocial behavior, the middle stages often contain depression, psychosis, or mania. Later on in the disease, apathy and abulia are common psychiatric manifestations.

TREATMENT

Tetrabenazine has been approved in the United States for treatment of chorea and is marketed under the trade name Xenazine. It acts by depleting neurotransmitters. Tetrabenazine can increase the risk of depression and suicidal thoughts and behavior (suicidality) in patients with HD, and given the frequency of depression in HD, its use must be carefully monitored.

Neuroleptics have long been used for suppressing chorea. Treatment is not always effective, and use of dopamine blockade brings with it risk of tardive dyskinesia, worsening depression, and cognitive effects. Amantadine has been tried for chorea treatment with mixed results. Because the impairment of voluntary movement persists, reducing chorea generally does not improve disability.

Tricyclic antidepressants or lithium can be effective in the treatment of affective symptoms. Improvement may be greater for the somatic-vegetative aspects of the syndrome than for the subjective elements of depression. The lessened responsiveness of helplessness-hopelessness to pharmacotherapy is understandable. Although rarely used, monoamine oxidase inhibitors and electroconvulsive therapy may be helpful (Ranen et al. 1994).

Manic symptoms may respond to neuroleptics and carbamazepine more than to lithium (Mendez 1994). Irritability and aggressive outbursts respond to both environmental changes and neuroleptics. Irritability can be decreased by a reduction in environmental complexity and the institution of unchanging routines.

Social support along with case management can be very important in the adaptation of the family to the diagnosis of HD and the management of the illness within the family (Shoulson 1982). Referral to the Huntington's Disease Society is helpful to provide educational materials and needed psychological support.

PARKINSON'S DISEASE

In 1817, James Parkinson described a new disorder he referred to as *the shaking palsy*, now referred to as *Parkinson's disease*. The cardinal neurological features include tremor, muscle rigidity, bradykinesia, and postural instability.

When these features occur in another identified entity, the term *parkinsonism* or *secondary parkinsonism* is used. Neuropsychiatric symptoms, particularly dementia and depression, are frequently associated with PD or parkinsonism.

EPIDEMIOLOGY AND ETIOLOGY

PD affects perhaps 1 million individuals in North America and shows dramatic age-related increases in prevalence. The prevalence of PD is approximately 150 per 100,000, increasing after age 65 to nearly 1,100 per 100,000 (Kessler 1972).

Genetic causes of PD are now thought to be involved in 10%–20% of cases, beginning with discovery of mutations in α-synuclein (Lucking et al. 2000). Other genes, including *Parkin, LRRK2,* and the glucocerebrosidase gene, appear to account for far more cases of PD among the general population (Lucking et al. 2000).

Parkinsonism has also been associated with use of a meperidine analogue (Langston et al. 1983), invigorating searches for environmental risks. There are positive associations between the risk for PD and rural living and drinking well water, possibly mediated by pesticide exposure. A negative association between the risk for PD and smoking has been established in numerous studies.

Dementia probably occurs in 20%–40% of patients and depression occurs in up to 50% of patients (Ebmeier et al. 1990). Mayeux (1990) found that the cumulative incidence of dementia in PD may be as high as 60% by age 88. Family histories of dementia, depression, and severe motor disability increase dementia risk (Aarsland et al. 1996; Marder et al. 1995). The decline in mental status scores on the MMSE is similar to that observed in AD (Aarsland et al. 2004).

NEUROBIOLOGY

The neuronal loss in PD is accompanied by the formation of Lewy bodies—hyaline inclusion bodies. Lewy bodies occur in brain stem nuclei, particularly the substantia nigra and locus coeruleus (Jellinger 1986). Occurrence of Lewy bodies in the neocortex has led to the recognition of dementia with Lewy bodies (DLB). Braak and colleagues (2003) showed the sequential pathology of PD beginning in lower brain stem structures (an asymptomatic stage), followed by the substantia nigra (onset of motor manifestations of PD), and ultimately into other cerebral structures, including cortex. Although a rigid sequence of pathological evolution does not always explain clinical variability of PD, the consistent distribution of PD lesions provides a framework for understanding the numerous nonmotor manifestations of PD, including dementia.

The loss of dopaminergic cells in the substantia nigra relates most directly to the motor abnormalities, particularly the akinesia and rigidity. Dementia in PD is most clearly associated with the finding of cortical Lewy body disease, consisting of neuronal degeneration and Lewy body formation in surviving neurons.

In depressed PD patients, metabolic imaging shows bilateral decreases in regional cerebral blood flow in anteromedial frontal and cingulate cortex, overlapping with areas shown to be affected in primary depression (Ring et al. 1994). Mayeux et al. (1984, 1988) associated raphe pathology with depression.

MOTOR SYMPTOMS

The most disabling motor features of PD are bradykinesia and rigidity. The patient has difficulty initiating movements, and when movement is started, it is executed slowly. Poverty of associated movements (such as blinking or arm swing when walking) is characteristic. Lack of facial expression reflects akinesia of facial musculature. Rigidity can affect all muscle groups—proximal and distal, agonist and antagonist. Tremor is the presenting feature in most cases and is relatively slow (3–7 Hz), often occurs distally, and occurs most often at rest. It increases with distraction and may be prominent during walking. All of these motor manifestations typically occur asymmetrically in PD.

Postural changes are a late development in PD and take two forms. One is a characteristic flexion at the neck, waist, elbows, and knees. The other, postural instability or disequilibrium, can lead to falls and serious injury. Early occurrence of postural instability should raise suspicion of PSP, multiple system atrophy (MSA), or another akinetic-rigid syndrome. Treatment may improve tremor, rigidity, and akinesia but rarely has any effect on postural instability or dementia.

PD is frequently associated with development of restless legs syndrome, which responds to levodopa, dopamine agonists, or benzodiazepines.

COGNITIVE IMPAIRMENTS

Cognitive impairment may complicate PD at any time during its course, from preceding motor manifestations to occurring decades later.

Visuospatial impairment, including impairments in spatial capacities, facial recognition, body schema, pursuit tracking, spatial attention, visual analysis, and judgments concerning position in space, is common in PD (Levin 1990). Constructional praxis is affected in PD, perhaps partly because of problems with spatial attention.

The communication difficulties of PD are mostly due to hypophonia and dysarthria. Language impairments can also occur and include reduced verbal fluency and naming difficulties (Matison et al. 1982).

Executive and attentional abnormalities can be attributed to frontal lobe dysfunction. These deficits include difficulties in sequencing voluntary motor activities, difficulties in maintaining and switching set, and abnormalities in selective attention (Freedman 1990).

The relations between the cognitive impairments in PD and the motor symptoms are complex. Poor performance on cognitive tests is not purely related to motor abnormalities. For example, visuospatial deficits continue to be detectable when tasks with limited roles for eye movements (e.g., tachistoscopy) are used. However, the presence of akinetic-rigid motor deficit makes comparisons with dementias such as AD or HD difficult to interpret.

PSYCHIATRIC ABNORMALITIES

Premorbid Personality

In the 1940s, patients who appeared to suppress anger and to be quite perfectionistic ("masked personality") were claimed to be at risk for PD (Sands 1942). Later studies did not bear this out, but the notion of a common premorbid personality in PD patients persists.

Psychiatric Disturbances

Affective disorder is the most common psychiatric disturbance in PD, with estimated incidence from 20% to 90% (Mayeux et al. 1986b). Depression does not always correlate with duration of disease, degree of disability, or response to medications (Troster et al. 1995). There is a higher frequency of depression in early-onset cases (Kostic et al. 1994).

Anxiety such as fear of falling (a real risk in advanced PD) is common. Sleep is frequently affected in PD, but this disturbance is frequently multifactorial, with medications, motor and nonmotor symptoms, and age playing as large a role as depression and anxiety.

Psychosis

Psychosis may occur in PD in the absence of medication effects, but medications trigger the vast majority of episodes of psychosis in PD. Dementia is the most important risk factor for psychosis, and age and visual impairment also contribute to risk. All of the antiparkinsonian medications have been implicated in the occurrence of hallucinations in PD. Of these, anticholinergic drugs, such as trihexyphenidyl, are the most notorious causes of delirium with psychotic features. Levodopa is the antiparkinsonian agent least likely to provoke hallucinations and delusions and is the preferred agent for management of PD symptoms and signs in psychotic patients.

Dementia

The occurrence of dementia in Parkinson's disease presents a diagnostic and therapeutic challenge, and the diagnosis may change over time as the patient's full clinical picture develops.

In a study of rivastigmine, moderate improvements occurred, but treated patients had higher rates of nausea, vomiting, and tremor (Emre et al. 2004).

TREATMENT OF MOTOR DYSFUNCTION

Six drugs or drug classes are currently available for treating motor dysfunction, and surgery is being used increasingly. Medication classes include levodopa, which may be given with inhibitors of its breakdown such as monoamine oxidase–B (MAO-B) inhibitors and catechol O-methyltransferase (COMT) inhibitors, dopamine agonists, amantadine, and anticholinergic agents. As PD progresses, treatment with levodopa is often complicated by dose-related fluctuations and dyskinesias, particularly in younger patients. Use of extended-release levodopa and MAO-B and COMT inhibitors can help with this symptom. Other agents helping treat motor fluctuations are selegiline and subcutaneous apomorphine (Bowron 2004). Selegiline may cause the unusual side effect of transvestic fetishism, which resolved when selegiline was discontinued (Riley 2002).

Dopamine agonists are associated with cognitive side effects, postural hypotension, and peripheral edema. Dopamine agonists may cause sedation, including sleep attacks while driving, and compulsive behaviors related to gambling, sexual activity, and eating.

Behavioral treatment begins with a careful assessment of the medical aspects and the functional effects of the illness on the patient and family. Nursing and social work assessments are important in providing a baseline for following the course of the illness, and follow-up care to modify the treatment plan is essential. Early planning, both financial and legal, is helpful to minimize the difficulty of gaining access to and financing home care, day care, or institutional care.

Interventions such as individual psychotherapy can help with depression early in the illness. Physical and occupational therapy may be very helpful, and a home safety evaluation may prevent falls.

Biological Treatment of Dementia in PD

Most important is prevention of so-called excess disability, which is frequently a result of intercurrent illnesses, psychological stress, or iatrogenic disease such as that due to overuse of medication.

Treatment of depression in PD parallels that of non-PD depression. Virtually all antidepressants may aggravate tremor, with the notable exception of mirtazapine, which may improve tremor or dyskinesias. While helping motor disabilities, antidepressants or other medications with significant anticholinergic potential can aggravate dementia or orthostatic hypotension.

Antipsychotics may worsen either motor symptoms or dementia, or both. Cholinesterase inhibitors may provide relief from psychosis in milder cases and spare patients from antipsychotic therapy. However, treatment with dopamine receptor blockers is often necessary. Fortunately, small doses of these agents are often sufficient to control PD-related hallucinosis. The atypical neuroleptics that produce little if any exacerbation of parkinsonism are quetiapine and clozapine (Motsinger et al. 2003; Parsa and Bastani 1998). Other atypical antipsychotics that were thought to cause few extrapyramidal side effects, such as risperidone, olanzapine, and aripiprazole, have been disappointments in this regard. Atypical antipsychotics have relatively high anticholinergic potential and can cause lethargy and conceivably affect cognition. Sleep disturbances are common with psychotic disorders, and the primary focus should be placed on sleep hygiene.

Although cholinesterase inhibitors occasionally lead to worsening of parkinsonism, they are usually well tolerated and may produce measurable levels of cognitive enhancement that equal or surpass their effectiveness in AD (Emre et al. 2004). The role of memantine in treating PD-related dementia is unclear, but no contraindication to its use is apparent.

Surgical Treatment

Patients whose motor manifestations prove to be difficult to control with medication, or who develop intolerable side effects, may benefit from stereotactic surgery. The surgical treatment of choice is deep brain stimulation (DBS) targeting the subthalamic nucleus, which has supplanted destructive internal pallidotomy. DBS surgery often leads to more consistent control of PD symptoms and may allow for medication reduction, sometimes ameliorating cognitive dysfunction. Rarely, electrode implantation results in irreversible cognitive deterioration; worsened cognitive outcomes are more common in older patients and in those with preexisting dementia. A decrease in verbal fluency, particularly with left subthalamic nucleus stimulation, has been reported. Changes in personality and acute depression also have been reported (Hugdahl and Wester 2000; Schmand et al. 2000). Some patients may experience improved cognitive scores secondary to surgery itself, such as improvements in cognitive flexibility (Witt et al. 2004). In most patients, surgery is well tolerated from a cognitive standpoint, and cognitive complications are typically transient.

DEMENTIA WITH LEWY BODIES

DLB is an increasingly recognized and studied form of dementia, accounting for about 20% of cases. DLB occurs as the sole pathology but is often (approximately 50% of the time) mixed with AD pathology. Compared with AD patients, DLB patients show no difference in age at onset, age at death, or duration of disease (Z. Walker et al. 2000). Rest tremor was more common in PD than in DLB, whereas myoclonus was more common in DLB. The frequency of rigidity, bradykinesia, dystonia, and gaze palsies did not differ (Louis et al. 1997). Response to levodopa is much more predictable in PD than in DLB.

CLINICAL DIAGNOSIS

Diagnostic criteria for DLB include the presence of two of three cardinal features: hallucinations (especially visual), spontaneous parkinsonism, and daily fluctuations in cognition.

The clinical criteria have been criticized as being of low sensitivity (Hohl et al. 2000). An autopsy study using international consensus criteria found that the 1996 criteria (McKeith et al. 1996) were both sensitive and specific; false-negative DLB cases tended to lack hallucinations and spontaneous parkinsonism (McKeith et al. 2000).

To improve the diagnostic sensitivity, the diagnostic criteria have been revised (McKeith et al. 2006). Dementia is now obligatory for diagnosis of possible or probable DLB, with frequent occurrence of supportive features recognized, including rapid eye movement sleep behavior disorder, repeated falls and syncope, autonomic dysfunction, nonvisual hallucinations, delusions, depression, reduced occipital regional cerebral blood flow, abnormally low uptake of ^{123}I-metaiodobenzylguanidine (MIBG) on myocardial scintigraphy, and prominent slow-wave activity on electroencephalograms along with transient sharp waves in the temporal lobe.

One clinical feature of DLB is fluctuating consciousness. Ferman and colleagues (2004) identified four features of cognitive fluctuations: daytime drowsiness, sleep during the daytime of 2 hours or more, prolonged staring into space, and episodic disorganized speech. At least three of these features were present in 63% of their DLB patients but in only 12% of the AD patients (M.P. Walker et al. 2000).

NEUROBIOLOGY

Genetic forms of DLB exist, including autosomal dominant forms, and patients with these forms of DLB may respond well to levodopa therapy. Autopsy studies have shown that about half of DLB patients have similar numbers of neuritic plaques to AD but fewer neurofibrillary tangles (NFTs) (Samuel et al. 1997a). Samuel et al. (1997b) found neocortical neuritic plaque burden and NFT counts in entorhinal cortex and loss of choline acetyltransferase correlated with dementia severity, but neocortical NFTs and synaptophysin were not correlated with dementia. Sabbagh et al. (1999) found that reductions in synaptophysin and choline acetyltransferase did not correlate with dementia severity in DLB as in AD.

NEUROIMAGING

Neuroimaging is not helpful in diagnosing DLB. Frontal lobe atrophy may be prominent in DLB but is nonspecific. Attempts are being made to use other forms of neuroimaging to differentiate these conditions. Functional neuroimaging also has not proved to be specific in diagnosing DLB.

TREATMENT

Patients with DLB need to be watched carefully when neuroleptics are administered because they may develop neuroleptic malignant syndrome and related phenomena. DLB patients may respond as well as or better than AD patients to cholinesterase inhibitors (Fergusson and Howard 2000). No large controlled trials of memantine have been done yet to support a recommendation for its use in DLB.

PROGRESSIVE SUPRANUCLEAR PALSY

Progressive supranuclear palsy (also known as Steele-Richardson-Olszewski syndrome) is a progressive disorder with eye movement abnormalities, parkinsonism, and dementia. It may present with deficient downward gaze, which causes trouble walking down stairs. The prevalence of PSP is estimated at 1.4 per 100,000. Median age at onset of symptoms is approximately 63, and median survival is 6–10 years (Golbe et al. 1988).

DIAGNOSIS

In PSP, there is often parkinsonism without tremor, with early disequilibrium and eye movement abnormalities, including decreased saccadic velocity (Leigh and Riley 2000). With disease progression, pursuit eye movements are also impaired. Testing of reflex eye movements with passive head turning shows relative preservation of vertical eye movements (hence supranuclear, because the oculocephalic

reflexes determine the integrity of the lower motor neuron pathways for up and down gaze). Lack of vertical eye movement abnormalities is the largest obstacle to correct antemortem diagnosis of PSP (Litvan et al. 1997, 1999).

Many patients with PSP have no noticeable dementia or it is often not severe early in the course. There can be forgetfulness, slowing of thought processes, emotional or personality changes, and impaired ability to manipulate knowledge in the relative absence of aphasia, apraxia, or agnosia (Albert et al. 1974). There may be deficits in visual scanning and search as well as verbal fluency, digit span, verbal memory, and logical memory.

Patients usually have symmetrical extensor rigidity of the neck and face; bradykinetic, less rigid extremities; and a parkinsonian gait. The postural instability is coupled with a tendency toward retropulsion. Other signs include axial dystonia, bradyphrenia, perseveration, forced grasping, and utilization behaviors. Pseudobulbar palsy may be observed in the later stages.

NEUROPSYCHIATRIC MANIFESTATIONS

PSP patients often have disturbances of sleep and depression and, occasionally, a schizophreniform psychosis. Patients with PSP also show memory loss, slowness of thought processes, changes in personality with apathy or depression, irritability, inappropriate crying or laughing, and obsessive-compulsive behaviors (Destee et al. 1990).

Apathy is particularly prominent and should be differentiated from concomitant depression. Levy et al. (1998) found that apathy correlated with lower cognitive function but not with depression. There is particular impairment in sequential movement tasks and in tasks requiring shifting of concepts, monitoring of the frequency of stimuli, or rapid retrieval of verbal information (Grafman et al. 1990). These symptoms are thought to be a reflection of frontal lobe impairment resulting from pathology in orbitofrontal-cortical circuits. Apraxia may be prominent in cases with prominent cerebral cortical involvement (Bergeron et al. 1997).

DIAGNOSTIC IMAGING

Neuroimaging shows early atrophy of midbrain structures with later atrophy of the pons and frontotemporal regions (Savoiardo et al. 1989). Fluorodeoxyglucose PET studies show marked frontal and temporal hypometabolism. The loss of striatal dopamine receptors, as demonstrated by PET scanning, during life may explain the poor therapeutic efficacy of dopamine agonist therapy in PSP.

NEUROBIOLOGY

Neuropathological findings include neuronal loss associated with gliosis and NFTs, most marked in the substantia nigra, basal forebrain, subthalamic nucleus, pallidum, and superior colliculus. The tangles in PSP are straight filaments. Additional areas involved to a lesser extent include the locus coeruleus, striatum, and a variety of upper brain stem and midbrain structures (Agid et al. 1986). Standardized criteria for the neuropathological diagnosis of PSP have been proposed and should widen our understanding of the clinical spectrum of PSP (Litvan et al. 1996).

Mutations in the tau gene on chromosome 17 are responsible for most clinical cases of PSP. In PSP, only the four-repeat tau isoform aggregating into straight filaments is found.

The neurochemistry of PSP is characterized by massive dopamine depletion in the striatum and reduced density of dopamine type 2 receptors in striatum (Pierot et al. 1988). There is also widespread reduction in choline acetyltransferase levels in frontal cortex, basal forebrain, and basal ganglia (Whitehouse et al. 1988).

TREATMENT

No treatment has been found to be effective in relieving the motor or cognitive deficiencies in PSP. Levodopa treatment is generally not successful, correlating with the loss of postsynaptic striatal dopamine receptors, and may worsen cognitive function. Poor responses with frequent dose-limiting side effects often occur with dopamine agonists.

CORTICAL–BASAL GANGLIONIC DEGENERATION

Cortical–basal ganglionic degeneration (CBD) presents with asymmetric basal ganglia (akinesia, rigidity, dystonia) and cerebral cortical (apraxia, cortical sensory loss, alien limb) manifestations (Riley et al. 1990). The alien limb is seen with parietal, medial frontal, and corpus callosum pathology. Dementia is a variable but may be the presenting symptom (Lang 2003). The neuropsychological profile shows prominent executive dysfunction, explicit memory deficits without retention difficulties, and asymmetric apraxias (Pillon et al. 1995). Other neuropsychiatric abnormalities include depression, apathy or disinhibition, aberrant motor behaviors, and delusions (Litvan et al. 1998). Oculomotor involvement similar to that in PSP may occur, particularly in advanced cases. Survival ranges from 2.5 to 12 years, with a median of about 8 years.

CBD pathology shows abundant ballooned, achromatic neurons and focal cortical atrophy predominating in medial frontal and parietal lobes, plus degeneration of the substantia nigra. Astrocytic plaques are also seen in neocortex. CBD neuronal tau pathology shows wispy, fine-threaded tau inclusions (Dickson 1999).

Magnetic resonance imaging (MRI) may show asymmetric atrophy in the frontal and parietal lobes contralateral to the dominantly affected limbs (Soliveri et al. 1999). Dopamine binding is reduced asymmetrically in CBD (Frisoni et al. 1995).

Treatment of CBD is limited, with only a minority of patients responding to levodopa preparations given for parkinsonism. Myoclonus may respond to benzodiazepines, particularly clonazepam. No specific treatment for the dementia is available, but it may not be cholinergic in nature, suggesting that cholinesterase inhibitors are of limited value. Depression is common in CBD, but few data exist on treatment response (Kampoliti et al. 1998; Litvan et al. 1998).

FRONTOTEMPORAL DEMENTIA

The frontotemporal dementias constitute a heterogeneous group of conditions, often with prominent early behavioral disinhibitory symptoms. There are a confusing number of phenotypes, subsuming Pick's disease, semantic aphasia, hereditary dysphasic dementia (J.C. Morris et al. 1984), progressive aphasias (fluent and nonfluent), PSP, and CBD. Neuropsychiatric symptoms include Klüver-Bucy syndrome or social withdrawal, depression, and a schizophrenia-like illness in middle adulthood. Patients may develop parkinsonism and occasionally amyotrophy (Josephs et al. 2006).

The FTDs have been linked to mutations in the tau protein gene and progranulin and to TDP-43. Although consensus diagnostic criteria have been proposed, the incidence of these conditions has varied widely in different regions, possibly because of differences in case identification.

MULTIPLE SYSTEM ATROPHY

Multiple system atrophy is a disease concept that unifies striatonigral degeneration, Shy-Drager syndrome, and sporadic olivopontocerebellar atrophy. Consensus diagnostic criteria require that patients show evidence of orthostatic hypotension or urinary incontinence in combination with either levodopa-unresponsive parkinsonism or cerebellar dysfunction, but partial syndromes may present clinically. Cognitive dysfunction was considered so unusual that dementia is considered an exclusionary criterion for diagnosis (Gilman et al. 1998). However, autopsy-proven cases of MSA have been associated with dementia (Schlossmacher et al. 2004). Neuropsychiatric studies report subtle deficits in frontal lobe function, verbal fluency, and verbal memory (Burk et al. 2006; Robbins et al. 1992).

FRIEDREICH'S ATAXIA

Friedreich's ataxia is an autosomal recessive disorder presenting with a slowly progressive ataxia, areflexia, pes cavus, and scoliosis. Mental changes are present in about a quarter of cases but have not been well characterized. There may be generalized decline or specific nonverbal intellectual impairments. Psychiatric disorders, including schizophrenia-like psychoses and depression, can occur. Personality abnormalities may be marked and are associated with juvenile delinquency and irritability.

SPINOCEREBELLAR ATAXIAS

Spinocerebellar ataxia (SCA) classification has been revolutionized by the discovery of gene loci, with more than 25 loci described. The molecular pathogenesis may involve excess polyglutamine repeats, channelopathies, or gene expression disorders but remains unknown in most cases.

The ataxic disorders may not be accompanied by intellectual changes until late in the illness. In a study by Skre (1974), dementia was found in one-third of autosomal dominant cases and in more than one-half of those with autosomal recessive cerebellar disease. There may be apathy and psychomotor retardation and occasionally depression or schizophrenia-like psychosis.

Cognitive and behavior changes may be particularly prominent or presenting features of SCA-17, which can also have an HD-like phenotype (Bruni et al. 2004; Rolfs et al. 2003). SCA-1 can have prominent executive dysfunction, whereas mild verbal memory deficits can be seen in SCA-1, SCA-2, and SCA-3 (Burk et al. 2003). With disease progression, about one-third of patients with SCA-2 develop dementia, and dementia may occur in SCA-12 (Geschwind 1999; O'Hearn et al. 2001; Storey et al. 1999).

Cerebellar ataxia itself is generally considered resistant to medications. Brief trials of many agents have been attempted, usually with minimal effect.

MOTOR NEURON DISEASE WITH DEMENTIA

Loss of strength with diminished muscle mass (amyotrophy) and dementia may be seen in motor neuron disease, also known as *amyotrophic lateral sclerosis* (ALS). Motor neuron disease is also increasingly associated with FTD, especially the behavioral subtype. This is consistent with the observation of personality changes; hallucinations; and impairments in judgment, memory, abstract thinking, calculations, and anomia in ALS cases. A loss of neurons occurs in layers 2 and 3 of the cortical mantle, particularly in the frontal and temporal regions.

Western New Guinea, the Kii Peninsula of Japan, and the island of Guam have a high incidence of ALS, often associated with parkinsonism and dementia. On Guam, 10% of adult deaths in the native Chamorro population result from ALS, and 7% are attributed to the Parkinson-dementia complex. Although various toxins have been implicated in its etiology, the exact cause of this symptom complex is unknown.

THALAMIC DEGENERATION

Thalamic degeneration may be isolated or seen in association with MSA. Abnormal movements include tremor, choreoathetosis, and occasionally myoclonus. Alterations in sleep may be observed, such as in the prion-related disorder of fatal familial insomnia (Gambetti et al. 1995). Ataxia, paraparesis, blindness, spasticity, optic atrophy, nystagmus, and dysarthria also may be present. Depression may be prominent, and there may be apathy with personality changes and hypersomnolence. Memory and calculations are poor, and patients may have incomprehensible spontaneous verbal output. Executive functions may be impaired early in the course. Severe gliosis and neuronal loss occur in the thalamus and also in limbic projection nuclei.

Fatal familial insomnia is associated with mutations of the prion protein gene. Fatal familial insomnia preferentially involves limbic thalamocortical circuits, correlating with the prominent sleep and autonomic disturbance, sympathetic hyperactivity, and flattening of circadian rhythms (Cortelli et al. 1999).

WILSON'S DISEASE

Wilson's disease, also called hepatolenticular degeneration, affects the basal ganglia in association with abnormalities in liver function. It is autosomally recessive due to a mutation causing a defect in copper metabolism, in a defective P-type adenosine triphosphatase (Cuthbert 1995; Petrukhin and Gilliam 1994). This leads to excessive copper deposition in the liver, corneas, and basal ganglia. Onset is usually in the second or third decade with dystonia, parkinsonism, or cerebellar ataxia. Patients also may have dysarthria, dysphagia, hypophonia, or seizures. Chronic hepatitis or hemolytic anemia may be detected. Kayser-Fleischer rings consist of brown or green discolorations near the limbus of the cornea and are seen in nearly all patients with neurological signs. Imaging shows ventricular enlargement and cortical atrophy and MRI shows abnormal signal in the lenticular nuclei, caudate nuclei, thalamus, dentate nuclei, and brain stem. The diagnosis may be established by slit-lamp examination of the cornea, laboratory studies reporting a serum ceruloplasmin level less than 20 mg/dL, a 24-hour copper excretion of more than 100 mg, or a liver biopsy showing increased hepatic copper concentration.

Wilson's disease may present with affective and behavior changes including schizophrenia-like changes, depression, or manic-depressive states. Sexual preoccupation and reduced sexual inhibitions are common. Aggressive and self-destructive or antisocial acts may also occur. Intellectual deterioration is relatively mild in the early symptomatic stages (Akil and Brewer 1995).

Treatment of Wilson's disease consists of establishing and maintaining a negative copper balance. Induction is performed with either zinc or tetrathiomolybdate, and maintenance requires zinc or a copper-chelating agent such as trientine (trien) (Brewer 2005). D-Penicillamine has fallen out of favor because of multiple severe toxicities and the potential for severe worsening with initiation of therapy. Maintaining a copper-deficient diet also may be helpful. Patients with advanced disease may require liver transplantation. Neurological symptoms, including the dementia syndrome, improve with long-term therapy. Levodopa may be of some benefit in reversing neurological symptoms not improved by chelation or negative copper balance.

CALCIFICATION OF THE BASAL GANGLIA (FAHR'S DISEASE)

Calcification of the basal ganglia is a rare disorder, occasionally inherited in an autosomal dominant fashion (Geschwind et al. 1999). Patients may present in early adulthood with a schizophrenia-like psychosis or mood disorder or may present later in life with an extrapyramidal syndrome, dementia, and mood changes. Apathy, poor judgment, and impaired memory are usually prominent, and language function is often spared. Computed tomography (CT) scans show extensive calcification of the basal ganglia and periventricular white matter. Choreoathetosis, cerebellar ataxia, and dystonia also may be seen. Psychosis may respond to lithium.

Minor degrees of calcification are not pathological. Dystrophic calcification occurs in pediatric acquired immunodeficiency syndrome, Aicardi-Goutières syndrome, trisomy 21, Kearns-Sayre syndrome, tumors (e.g., astrocytomas) or vascular lesions, and hypoparathyroidism. The pathogenesis of basal ganglia calcification is unknown (Baba et al. 2005).

PANTOTHENATE KINASE–ASSOCIATED NEURODEGENERATION

Pantothenate kinase–associated neurodegeneration (PKAN) is also referred to as neurodegeneration with brain iron accumulation type 1 (NBIA-1; Arawaka et al. 1998). PKAN is a rare progressive autosomal recessive disease of childhood and adolescence characterized by stiffness of gait, distal wasting, dysarthria, and occasionally dementia. PKAN is part of the group of infantile neuraxonal dystrophies, of which it may be an allelic variant.

Olive or golden brown discoloration of the medial segment of the globus pallidus is seen. There may also be widespread α-synuclein–positive Lewy bodies and axonal swellings. Some patients may have lipid abnormalities, acanthocytosis, and pigmentary retinal degeneration (Arawaka et al. 1998; Halliday 1995; Newell et al. 1999). There may be dopamine deficiency in substantia nigra and striatum with relatively preserved limbic system dopamine concentrations (Jankovic et al. 1985).

CT shows mild atrophy with caudate nucleus atrophy. MRI scans may show the so-called eye of the tiger sign, a result of bilateral hyperintensity of the rostral globus pallidus. There may be loss of T2-weighted signal in the substantia nigra pars reticularis, red nucleus, pulvinar, and globus pallidus resulting from iron accumulation.

Dystonia may respond to pallidotomy or thalamotomy, and dopa-responsive parkinsonism has been described (Justesen et al. 1999). No specific treatment for the dementia is available.

NORMAL-PRESSURE HYDROCEPHALUS

Normal-pressure hydrocephalus (NPH) is a syndrome composed of the triad of dementia, gait disturbance, and urinary incontinence. It may be associated with a history of meningitis, intracranial bleeding, or head injury. A wide-based gait with slow steps and difficulty initiating locomotion are characteristic. Usually, no changes occur in motor strength or tone.

The diagnosis requires symptom recognition and neuroimaging showing an enlarged ventricle disproportionate to cerebral atrophy. MRI scanning may show transependymal fluid flux. Difficulties in diagnosis arise in determining whether hydrocephalus is congenital or secondary to cerebral atrophy. It may be difficult to determine if dementia in suspected

NPH is not due to other causes. In series in which shunted patients also underwent brain biopsy, the prevalence of AD ranged from 31% to 50% (Savolainen et al. 1999).

Dementia of NPH presents primarily with attentional difficulties in the early stages. Frontal dysfunction, including apathy, lethargy, mental slowing, and perseveration, is very common. Up to 50% of patients have some memory dysfunction. Language is typically spared early in the course, although late-stage patients may have an akinetic-mutism syndrome. Occasional patients may present with psychosis as an initial symptom. The motor deficits of hydrocephalic patients may be similar to those seen in PD or other basal ganglia disorders.

High-volume lumbar puncture (up to 50 mL) and cerebrospinal fluid (CSF) pressure measurement and analysis is commonly recommended but has low sensitivity. Transient improvement in gait, urinary incontinence, or neuropsychological functioning may help predict surgical treatment response. Use of external lumbar drainage (up to 500 mL over several days) and CSF outflow resistance testing may confirm the diagnosis.

CSF shunting may help up to 70% of patients (Bergsneider et al. 2005; Verrees and Selman 2004). The best cognitive results occur in patients whose cognitive disturbances are relatively mild and who have early onset of urinary incontinence and gait disturbance. Memory may improve more than frontostriatal dysfunction after shunting (Iddon et al. 1999). Use of programmable pressure valves reduces the complication rate of postshunting hematomas while ensuring optimal shunting in a given patient. Late shunt failure, as a result of mechanical failure or obstruction, may present as worsening clinical status (Williams et al. 1998).

RECOMMENDED READINGS

Huntington's Disease

Hague SM, Klaffke S, Bandmann O: Neurodegenerative disorders: Parkinson's disease and Huntington's disease. J Neurol Neurosurg Psychiatry 76:1058–1063, 2005

Landles C, Bates GP: Huntingtin and the molecular pathogenesis of Huntington's disease. Fourth in molecular medicine review series. EMBO Rep 5:958–963, 2004

Parkinson's Disease

Jankovic J: An update on the treatment of Parkinson's disease. Mt Sinai J Med 73:682–689, 2006

Savitt JM, Dawson VL, Dawson TM: Diagnosis and treatment of Parkinson disease: molecules to medicine. J Clin Invest 116:1744–1754, 2006

Dementia With Lewy Bodies

Lippa CF, Duda JE, Grossman M, et al: DLB and PDD boundary issues: diagnosis, treatment, molecular pathology, and biomarkers. Neurology 68:812–819, 2007

McKeith IG, Rowan E, Askew K, et al: More severe functional impairment in dementia with Lewy bodies than Alzheimer disease is related to extrapyramidal motor dysfunction. Am J Geriatr Psychiatry 14:582–588, 2006

Mosimann UP, Rowan EN, Partington CE, et al: Characteristics of visual hallucinations in Parkinson disease dementia and dementia with Lewy bodies. Am J Geriatr Psychiatry 14:153–160, 2006

Weisman D, McKeith I: Dementia with Lewy bodies. Semin Neurol 27:42–47, 2007

Progressive Supranuclear Palsy

Rampello L, Butta V, Raffaele R, et al: Progressive supranuclear palsy: a systematic review. Neurobiol Dis 20:179–186, 2005

Cortical–Basal Ganglionic Degeneration

Sha S, Hou C, Viskontas IV, et al: Are frontotemporal lobar degeneration, progressive supranuclear palsy and corticobasal degeneration distinct diseases? Nat Clin Pract Neurol 2:658–665, 2006

Frontotemporal Dementia

Boxer AL, Miller BL: Clinical features of frontotemporal dementia. Alzheimer Dis Assoc Disord 19 (suppl 1):S3–S6, 2005

Multiple System Atrophy

Bak TH, Rogers TT, Crawford LM, et al: Cognitive bedside assessment in atypical parkinsonian syndromes. J Neurol Neurosurg Psychiatry 76:420–422, 2005

Singer W, Opfer-Gehrking TL, McPhee BR, et al: Acetylcholinesterase inhibition: a novel approach in the treatment of neurogenic orthostatic hypotension. J Neurol Neurosurg Psychiatry 74:1294–1298, 2003

Friedreich's Ataxia and Spinocerebellar Ataxia

Geschwind DH: Focusing attention on cognitive impairment in spinocerebellar ataxia. Arch Neurol 56:20–22, 1999

Motor Neuron Disease With Dementia

Ringholz GM, Greene SR: The relationship between amyotrophic lateral sclerosis and frontotemporal dementia. Curr Neurol Neurosci Rep 6:387–392, 2006

Thalamic Degeneration

Montagna P, Gambetti P, Cortelli P, et al: Familial and sporadic fatal insomnia. Lancet Neurol 2:167–176. 2003

Wilson's Disease

Ala A, Walker AP, Ashkan K, et al: Wilson's disease. Lancet 369:397–408, 2007

Fahr's Disease

Geschwind DH, Loginov M, Stern JM: Identification of a locus on chromosome 14Q for idiopathic basal ganglia calcification (Fahr disease). Am J Hum Genet 65:764–772, 1999

Schmidt U, Mursch K, Halatsch ME: Symmetrical intracerebral and intracerebellar calcification ("Fahr's disease"). Funct Neurol 20:15, 2005

Pantothenate Kinase–Associated Neurodegeneration

Gregory A, Hayflick SJ: Neurodegeneration with brain iron accumulation. Folia Neuropathol 43:286–296, 2005

Nemeth AH: The genetics of primary dystonias and related disorders. Brain 125 (pt 4):695–721, 2002

Normal-Pressure Hydrocephalus

McGirt MJ, Woodworth G, Coon AL, et al: Diagnosis, treatment, and analysis of long-term outcomes in idiopathic normal-pressure hydrocephalus. Neurosurgery 57:699–705, 2005

Relkin N, Marmarou A, Klinge P, et al: Diagnosing idiopathic normal-pressure hydrocephalus. Neurosurgery 57 (3 suppl):S4–S16, 2005

REFERENCES

Aarsland D, Tandberg E, Larson JP, et al: Frequency of dementia in Parkinson's disease. Arch Neurol 53:538–542, 1996

Aarsland D, Andersen K, Larsen JP, et al: The rate of cognitive decline in Parkinson disease. Arch Neurol 61:1906–1911, 2004

Agid Y, Javoy-Agid F, Ruberg M, et al: Progressive supranuclear palsy: anatomoclinical and biochemical considerations, in Parkinson's Disease (Advances in Neurology Series, Vol 45). Edited by Yahr MD, Bergmann KJ. New York, Raven, 1986, pp 191–206

Akil M, Brewer GJ: Psychiatric and behavioral abnormalities in Wilson's disease, in Behavioral Neurology of Movement Disorders (Advances in Neurology Series, Vol 46). Edited by Weiner WS, Lang AE. New York, Raven, 1995, pp 171–178

Albert ML, Feldman RG, Willis AL: The "subcortical dementia" of progressive supranuclear palsy. J Neurol Neurosurg Psychiatry 37:121–130, 1974

Albin RL, Tagle DA: Genetics and molecular biology of Huntington's disease. Trends Neurosci 18:11–14, 1995

Apaydin H, Ahlskog JE, Parisi JE, et al: Parkinson disease neuropathology: later-developing dementia and loss of the levodopa response. Arch Neurol 59:102–112, 2002

Arawaka S, Saito Y, Murayama S, et al: Lewy body in neurodegeneration with brain iron accumulation type 1 is immunoreactive for alpha-synuclein. Neurology 51:887–889, 1998

Baba Y, Broderick DF, Uitri RJ, et al: Heredofamilial brain calcinosis syndrome. Mayo Clin Proc 80:641–651, 2005

Bamford K, Caine E, Kido D, et al: Clinical-pathologic correlation in Huntington's disease: a neuropsychological and computed tomography study. Neurology 39:796–801, 1989

Bergeron C, Pollanen MS, Weyer L, et al: Cortical degeneration in progressive supranuclear palsy: a comparison with cortical-basal ganglionic degeneration. J Neuropathol Exp Neurol 56:726–734, 1997

Bergsneider M, Black PM, Klinge P, et al: Surgical management of idiopathic normal-pressure hydrocephalus. Neurosurgery 57 (3 suppl):S29–S39, 2005

Bowron A: Practical considerations in the use of apomorphine injectable. Neurology 62 (suppl 4):S32–S36, 2004

Braak H, Del Tredici K, Rub U, et al: Staging of brain pathology related to sporadic Parkinson's disease. Neurobiol Aging 24:197–211, 2003

Brandt J, Butters N: The neuropsychology of Huntington's disease. Trends Neurosci 9:118–120, 1986

Brewer GJ: Neurologically presenting Wilson's disease: epidemiology, pathophysiology and treatment. CNS Drugs 19:185–192, 2005

Brown RE, Marsden CD: "Subcortical dementia": the neuropsychological evidence. Neuroscience 25:363–387, 1988

Bruni AC, Takahashi-Fujigasaki J, Maltecca F, et al: Behavioral disorder, dementia, ataxia, and rigidity in a large family with TATA box-binding protein mutation. Arch Neurol 61:1314–1320, 2004

Burk K, Globas C, Bosch S, et al: Cognitive deficits in spinocerebellar ataxia type 1, 2, and 3. J Neurol 250:207–211, 2003

Burk K, Daum I, Rub U: Cognitive function in multiple system atrophy of the cerebellar type. Mov Disord 21:772–776, 2006

Bylsma FW, Brandt J, Strauss ME: Aspects of procedural memory are differentially impaired in Huntington's disease. Arch Clin Neuropsychol 5:287–297, 1990

Claes S, Van Zand K, Legius K, et al: Correlations between triplet repeat expansion and clinical features in Huntington's disease. Arch Neurol 52:749–753, 1995

Cortelli P, Gambetti P, Montagna P, et al: Fatal familial insomnia: clinical features and molecular genetics. J Sleep Res 8 (suppl 1):23–29, 1999

Cummings JL (ed): Subcortical Dementia. New York, Oxford University Press, 1990

Cummings JL: Behavioral and psychiatric symptoms associated with Huntington's disease, in Behavioral Neurology of Movement Disorders (Advances in Neurology Series, Vol 65). Edited by Weiner WJ, Lang AE. New York, Raven, 1995, pp 179–186

Cuthbert JA: Wilson's disease: a new gene and an animal model for an old disease. J Investig Med 43:323–326, 1995

Destee A, Gray F, Parent M, et al: Obsessive-compulsive behavior and progressive supranuclear palsy. Rev Neurol 146:12–18, 1990

Dickson DW: Neuropathologic differentiation of progressive supranuclear palsy and corticobasal degeneration. J Neurol 246 (suppl 2):6–15, 1999

Ebmeier KP, Calder SA, Craford JR, et al: Clinical features predicting dementia in idiopathic Parkinson's disease: a followup study. Neurology 40:1222–1224, 1990

Emre M, Aarsland D, Albanese A, et al: Rivastigmine for dementia associated with Parkinson's disease. N Engl J Med 351:2509–2518, 2004

Farrer LA, Conneally PM: A genetic model for age at onset in Huntington's disease. Am J Hum Genet 37:350–357, 1985

Feigin A, Kieburtz K, Bordwell K, et al: Functional decline in Huntington's disease. Mov Disord 10:211–214, 1995

Fergusson E, Howard R: Donepezil for the treatment of psychosis in dementia with Lewy bodies. Int J Geriatr Psychiatry 15:280–281, 2000

Ferman TJ, Smith GE, Boeve BF, et al: DLB fluctuations: specific features that reliably differentiate DLB from AD and normal aging. Neurology 62:181–187, 2004

Folstein MF, Folstein SE, McHugh PR: Mini-Mental State: a practical method for grading the cognitive state of patients for the clinician. J Psychiatr Res 12:189–198, 1975

Folstein SE: Huntington's Disease: A Disorder of Families. Baltimore, MD, Johns Hopkins University Press, 1989

Folstein SE, Chase GA, Wahl WE, et al: Huntington's disease in Maryland: clinical aspects of racial variation. Am J Hum Genet 41:168–179, 1987

Folstein SE, Brandt J, Folstein MF: Huntington's disease, in Subcortical Dementia. Edited by Cummings JL. New York, Oxford University Press, 1990, pp 87–107

Freedman M: Parkinson's disease, in Subcortical Dementia. Edited by Cummings JL. New York, Oxford University Press, 1990, pp 108–122

Frisoni GB, Pizzolato G, Zanetti O, et al: Corticobasal degeneration: neuropsychological assessment and dopamine D_2 receptor SPECT analysis. Eur Neurol 35:50–54, 1995

Furtado S, Suchowersky O: Huntington's disease: recent advances in diagnosis and management. Can J Neurol Sci 22:5–12, 1995

Gambetti P, Parchi P, Petersen RB, et al: Fatal familial insomnia and familial Creutzfeldt-Jakob disease: clinical, pathological and molecular features. Brain Pathol 5:43–51, 1995

Geschwind DH: Focusing attention on cognitive impairment in spinocerebellar ataxia. Arch Neurol 56:20–22, 1999

Geschwind DH, Loginov M, Stern JM: Identification of a locus on chromosome 14Q for idiopathic basal ganglia calcification (Fahr disease). Am J Hum Genet 65:764–772, 1999

Gilman S, Low PA, Quinn N, et al: Consensus statement on the diagnosis of multiple system atrophy. J Auton Nerv Syst 74:189–192, 1998

Giordani B, Berent S, Boivin MJ, et al: Longitudinal neuropsychological and genetic linkage analysis of persons at risk for Huntington's disease. Arch Neurol 52:59–64, 1995

Golbe LI, Davis PH, Schoenberg BS, et al: Prevalence and natural history of progressive supranuclear palsy. Neurology 38:1031–1034, 1988

Grafman J, Litvan I, Gomez C, et al: Frontal lobe function in progressive supranuclear palsy. Arch Neurol 47:553–558, 1990

Gusella J, Wexler NS, Conneally PM, et al: A polymorphic DNA marker genetically linked to Huntington's disease. Nature 306:234–238, 1983

Halliday W: The nosology of Hallervorden-Spatz disease. J Neurol Sci 134(suppl):84–91, 1995

Harper PS: The epidemiology of Huntington's disease. Hum Genet 89:365–376, 1992

Hohl U, Tiraboschi P, Hansen LA, et al: Diagnostic accuracy of dementia with Lewy bodies. Arch Neurol 57:347–351, 2000

Hugdahl K, Wester K: Neurocognitive correlates of stereotactic thalamotomy and thalamic stimulation in parkinsonian patients. Brain Cogn 42:231–252, 2000

Huntington's Disease Collaborative Research Group: A novel gene containing a trinucleotide repeat that is expanded and unstable on Huntington's disease chromosomes. Cell 72:971–983, 1993

Iddon JL, Pickard JD, Cross JJ, et al: Specific patterns of cognitive impairment in patients with idiopathic normal pressure hydrocephalus and Alzheimer's disease: a pilot study. J Neurol Neurosurg Psychiatry 67:723–732, 1999

Jankovic J, Kirkpatrick JB, Blomquist KA, et al: Late-onset Hallervorden-Spatz disease presenting as familial parkinsonism. Neurology 35:227–234, 1985

Jellinger K: Overview of morphological changes in Parkinson's disease, in Parkinson's Disease (Advances in Neurology Series, Vol 45). Edited by Yahr MD, Bergmann KJ. New York, Raven, 1986, pp 1–18

Josephs KA, Parisi JE, Knopman DS, et al: Clinically undetected motor neuron disease in pathologically proven frontotemporal lobar degeneration with motor neuron disease. Arch Neurol 63:506–512, 2006

Justesen CR, Penn RD, Kroin JS, et al: Stereotactic pallidotomy in a child with Hallervorden-Spatz disease: case report. J Neurosurg 90:551–554, 1999

Kampoliti K, Goetz CG, Boeve BF, et al: Clinical presentation and pharmacological therapy in corticobasal degeneration. Arch Neurol 55:957–961, 1998

Kessler H: Epidemiological studies of Parkinson's disease, III: a community based study. Am J Epidemiol 96:242–254, 1972

Kostic VS, Filipovic SR, Lecic D, et al: Effect of age at onset on frequency of depression in Parkinson's disease. J Neurol Neurosurg Psychiatry 57:1265–1267, 1994

Lang AE: Corticobasal degeneration: selected developments. Mov Disord 18 (suppl 6):S51–S56, 2003

Langston JW, Ballard P, Tetrud JW, et al: Chronic parkinsonism in humans due to a product of meperidine-analog synthesis. Science 219:979–980, 1983

Leigh RJ, Riley DE: Eye movements in parkinsonism: it's saccadic speed that counts. Neurology 54:1018–1019, 2000

Leigh RJ, Newman SA, Folstein SE, et al: Abnormal ocular motor control in Huntington's disease. Neurology 33:1268–1275, 1983

Levin BE: Spatial cognition in Parkinson's disease. Alzheimer Dis Assoc Disord 4:161–170, 1990

Levy ML, Cummings JL, Fairbanks LA, et al: Apathy is not depression. J Neuropsychiatry Clin Neurosci 10:314–319, 1998

Litvan I, Hauw JJ, Bartko JJ, et al: Validity and reliability of the preliminary NINDS neuropathologic criteria for progressive supranuclear palsy and related disorders. J Neuropathol Exp Neurol 55:97–105, 1996

Litvan I, Campbell G, Mangone CA, et al: Which clinical features differentiate progressive supranuclear palsy (Steele-Richardson-Olszewski syndrome) from related disorders? A clinicopathological study. Brain 120:65–74, 1997

Litvan I, Cummings JL, Mega M: Neuropsychiatric features of corticobasal degeneration. J Neurol Neurosurg Psychiatry 65:717–721, 1998

Litvan I, Grimes DA, Lang AE, et al: Clinical features differentiating patients with postmortem confirmed progressive supranuclear palsy and corticobasal degeneration. J Neurol 246 (suppl 2): 1–5, 1999

Louis ED, Klatka LA, Liu Y, et al: Comparison of extrapyramidal features in 31 pathologically confirmed cases of diffuse Lewy body disease and 34 pathologically confirmed cases of Parkinson's disease. Neurology 48:376–380, 1997

Lucking CB, Durr A, Bonifati V, et al: Association between early onset Parkinson's disease and mutations in the Parkin gene. N Engl J Med 342:1560–1567, 2000

Marder K, Tang MX, Cote L, et al: The frequency and associated risk factors for dementia in patients with Parkinson's disease. Arch Neurol 52:695–701, 1995

Martin JB, Gusella JF: Huntington's disease: pathogenesis and management. N Engl J Med 20:1267–1276, 1986

Matison R, Mayeux R, Rosen J, et al: "Tip of the tongue" phenomenon in Parkinson's disease. Neurology 32:567–570, 1982

Mayeux R: Dementia in extrapyramidal disorders. Curr Opin Neurol Neurosurg 3:98–102, 1990

Mayeux R, Stern Y, Rosen J, et al: Is "subcortical dementia" a recognizable clinical entity? Ann Neurol 14:278–283, 1983

Mayeux R, Stern Y, Cote L, et al: Altered serotonin metabolism in depressed patients with Parkinson's disease. Neurology 34:642–646, 1984

Mayeux R, Stern Y, Herman A, et al: Correlates of early disability in Huntington's disease. Ann Neurol 20:727–731, 1986a

Mayeux R, Stern Y, Williams JBW, et al: Clinical and biochemical features of depression in Parkinson's disease. Am J Psychiatry 143:756–759, 1986b

Mayeux R, Stern Y, Sano M, et al: The relationship of serotonin to depression in Parkinson's disease. Mov Disord 3:236–244, 1988

McHugh PR, Folstein ME: Psychiatric syndromes in Huntington's disease: a clinical and phenomenologic study, in Psychiatric Aspects of Neurologic Disease. Edited by Benson DF, Blumer D. New York, Grune & Stratton, 1975, pp 267–285

McKeith IG, Galasko D, Kosaka K, et al: Consensus guidelines for the clinical and pathological diagnosis of dementia with Lewy bodies (DLB): report of the Consortium on DLB International Workshop. Neurology 47:1113–1124, 1996

McKeith IG, Ballard CG, Perry RH, et al: Prospective validation of consensus criteria for the diagnosis of dementia with Lewy bodies. Neurology 54:1050–1058, 2000

McKeith IG, Dickson DW, Lowe J, et al: Diagnosis and management of dementia with Lewy bodies: third report of the DLB Consortium. Neurology 65:1863–1872, 2006

Mendez MF: Huntington's disease: update and review of neuropsychiatric aspects. Int J Psychiatry Med 24:189–208, 1994

Monckton DG, Caskey CT: Unstable triplet repeat diseases. Circulation 91:513–520, 1995

Morris JC, Cole M, Banker BQ, et al: Hereditary dysphasic dementia and the Pick-Alzheimer spectrum. Ann Neurol 16:455–466, 1984

Morris M: Dementia and cognitive changes in Huntington's disease, in Behavioral Neurology of Movement Disorders (Advances in Neurology Series, Vol 65). Edited by Weiner WS, Lang AE. New York, Raven, 1995, pp 187–200

Motsinger CD, Perron GA, Lacy TJ: Use of atypical antipsychotic drugs in patients with dementia. Am Fam Physician 67:2335–2340, 2003

Newell KL, Boyer P, Gomez-Tortosa E, et al: Alpha-synuclein immunoreactivity is present in axonal swellings in neuroaxonal dystrophy and acute traumatic brain injury. J Neuropathol Exp Neurol 58:1263–1268, 1999

O'Hearn E, Holmes SE, Calvert PC, et al: SCA-12: tremor with cerebellar and cortical atrophy is associated with a CAG repeat expansion. Neurology 56:299–303, 2001

Parsa MA, Bastani B: Quetiapine (Seroquel) in the treatment of psychosis in patients with Parkinson's disease. J Neuropsychiatry Clin Neurosci 10:216–219, 1998

Petrukhin K, Gilliam TC: Genetic disorders of copper metabolism. Curr Opin Pediatr 6:698–701, 1994

Pierot L, Desnos C, Blin J, et al: D1 and D2-type dopamine receptors in patients with Parkinson's disease and progressive supranuclear palsy. J Neurol Sci 86:291–306, 1988

Pillon B, Blin J, Vidailhet M, et al: The neuropsychological pattern of corticobasal degeneration: comparison with progressive supranuclear palsy and Alzheimer's disease. Neurology 45:1477–1483, 1995

Ranen NG, Peyser CE, Folstein SE: ECT as a treatment for depression in Huntington's disease. J Neuropsychiatry Clin Neurosci 6:154–159, 1994

Riley DE: Reversible transvestic fetishism in a man with Parkinson's disease treated with selegiline. Clin Neuropharmacol 25:234–237, 2002

Riley DE, Lang AE, Lewis A, et al: Cortical-basal ganglionic degeneration. Neurology 40:1203–1212, 1990

Ring HA, Bench CJ, Trimble MR, et al: Depression in Parkinson's disease: a positron emission study. Br J Psychiatry 165:333–339, 1994

Robbins TW, James M, Lange KW, et al: Cognitive performance in multiple system atrophy. Brain 115:271–291, 1992

Rolfs A, Koeppen AH, Bauer I, et al: Clinical features and neuropathology of autosomal dominant spinocerebellar ataxia (SCA17). Ann Neurol 54:367–375, 2003

Sabbagh MN, Corey-Bloom J, Tiraboschi P, et al: Neurochemical markers do not correlate with cognitive decline in the Lewy body variant of Alzheimer disease. Arch Neurol 45:1458–1461, 1999

Samuel W, Alford M, Hofstetter CR, et al: Dementia with Lewy bodies versus pure Alzheimer disease: differences in cognition, neuropathology, cholinergic dysfunction, and synapse density. J Neuropathol Exp Neurol 56:499–508, 1997a

Samuel W, Crowder R, Hofstetter CR, et al: Neuritic plaques in the Lewy body variant of Alzheimer disease lack paired helical filaments. Neurosci Lett 223:73–76, 1997b

Sands IR: The type of personality susceptible to Parkinson disease. J Mt Sinai Hosp N Y 9:792–794, 1942

Savoiardo M, Strada L, Girotti F, et al: MR imaging in progressive supranuclear palsy and Shy-Drager syndrome. J Comput Assist Tomogr 13:555–560, 1989

Savolainen S, Paljarvi L, Vapalahti M: Prevalence of Alzheimer's disease in patients investigated for presumed normal pressure hydrocephalus: a clinical and neuropathological study. Acta Neurochir (Wien) 141:849–853, 1999

Schlossmacher MG, Hamann C, Cole AG, et al: Case records of the Massachusetts General Hospital: weekly clinicopathological exercises. Case 27-2004: a 79-year-old woman with disturbances in gait, cognition, and autonomic function. N Engl J Med 351:912–922, 2004

Schmand B, de Bie RM, Koning-Haanstra M, et al: Unilateral pallidotomy in PD: a controlled study of cognitive and behavioral effects. The Netherlands Pallidotomy Study (NEPAS) group. Neurology 54:1058–1064, 2000

Shiwach RS, Norbury CG: A controlled psychiatric study of individuals at risk for Huntington's disease. Br J Psychiatry 165:500–505, 1994

Shoulson I: Care of patients and families with Huntington's disease, in Movement Disorders. Edited by Marsden CD, Fahn S. London, Butterworths International Medical Reviews, 1982, pp 277–290

Skre H: Spino-cerebellar ataxia in western Norway. Clin Genet 6:265–288, 1974

Soliveri P, Monza D, Paridi D, et al: Cognitive and magnetic resonance imaging aspects of corticobasal degeneration and progressive supranuclear palsy. Neurology 53:502–507, 1999

Starkstein SE, Brandt J, Folstein S, et al: Neuropsychologic and neuropathologic correlates in Huntington's disease. J Neurol Neurosurg Psychiatry 51:1259–1263, 1988

Storey E, Forrest SM, Shaw JH, et al: Spinocerebellar ataxia type 2: clinical features of a pedigree displaying prominent frontal-executive dysfunction. Arch Neurol 56:43–50, 1999

Strauss ME, Brandt J: Are there neuropsychologic manifestations of the gene for Huntington's disease in asymptomatic, at-risk individuals? Arch Neurol 47:905–908, 1990

Troster AI, Stalp LD, Paolo AM, et al: Neuropsychological impairment in Parkinson's disease with and without depression. Arch Neurol 52:1164–1169, 1995

Verrees M, Selman WR: Management of normal pressure hydrocephalus. Am Fam Physician 70:1071–1078, 2004

Walker MP, Ayre GA, Cummings JL, et al: Quantifying fluctuation in dementia with Lewy bodies, Alzheimer's disease, and vascular dementia. Neurology 54:1616–1625, 2000

Walker Z, Allen RL, Shergill S, et al: Three years survival in patients with a clinical diagnosis of dementia with Lewy bodies. Int J Geriatr Psychiatry 15:267–273, 2000

Wexler NS: Perceptual, motor, cognitive, and emotional characteristics of persons at risk for Huntington's disease, in Huntington's Disease (Advances in Neurology Series, Vol 23). Edited by Chase TN, Wexler NS, Barbeau A. New York, Raven, 1979, pp 257–271

Wexler NS, Lorimer J, Porter J, et al: Venezuelan kindreds reveal that genetic and environmental factors modulate Huntington's disease age of onset. Proc Natl Acad Sci USA 101:3498–3503, 2004

Whitehouse PJ: The concept of subcortical and cortical dementia: another look. Ann Neurol 19:1–6, 1986

Whitehouse PJ, Martino AM, Marcus KA, et al: Reductions in acetylcholine and nicotine binding in several degenerative diseases. Arch Neurol 45:722–724, 1988

Williams MA, Razumovsky AY, Hanley DF: Evaluation of shunt function in patients who are never better, or better than worse after shunt surgery for NPH. Acta Neurochir (Wien) 71:368–370, 1998

Witt K, Pulkowski U, Herzog J, et al: Deep brain stimulation of the subthalamic nucleus improves cognitive flexibility but impairs response inhibition in Parkinson disease. Arch Neurol 61:697–700, 2004

Zappacosta B, Monza D, Meoni C, et al: Psychiatric symptoms do not correlate with cognitive decline, motor symptoms, or CAG repeat length in Huntington's disease. Arch Neurol 53:493–497, 1996

13

NEUROPSYCHIATRIC ASPECTS OF ALZHEIMER'S DISEASE AND OTHER DEMENTING ILLNESSES

Liana G. Apostolova, M.D.

Jeffrey L. Cummings, M.D.

The dementias are a large group of neuropsychiatric disorders that preferentially affect the elderly. Their socioeconomic significance is on a steady rise as the number of elderly persons continues to increase. The most common dementia—Alzheimer's disease (AD)—accounts for 60%–70% of all dementias in older individuals. More than 90% of all patients with AD are 65 years or older. The second most common dementia—dementia with Lewy bodies (DLB)—accounts for 15%–20% of the newly diagnosed cases, and vascular dementia (VaD) for another 5%–10% (Corey-Bloom 2004). DLB and VaD also occur in seniors. Before age

65 years, frontotemporal dementia (FTD) is as common as AD; it accounts for 5%–9% of all newly diagnosed dementia cases (Graff-Radford and Woodruff 2004).

DIAGNOSTIC CRITERIA

DSM-IV-TR (American Psychiatric Association 2000) defines *dementia* as an acquired cognitive syndrome of sufficient severity to result in functional decline. The diagnosis requires the following two conditions to be met: impairments of memory and at least one additional cognitive domain, and functional decline

This project was supported by a grant from the National Institute on Aging for the UCLA Alzheimer's Disease Research Center (P50 16570), the Kassel Parkinson's Disease Foundation, and the Sidell-Kagan Foundation.

resulting in impaired activities of daily living, vocational abilities, or social interactions. As these criteria are broad and nonspecific, dementia experts have developed more refined research criteria for each of the major dementia syndromes (Tables 13–1, 13–3, 13–4, and 13–5) (Dubois et al. 2007; McKeith et al. 2005; Neary et al. 1998; Roman et al. 1993).

THE PRODROMAL DEMENTIA STAGES

AD and many other neurodegenerative disorders have a long latent stage of steady, relentless pathology spread. Once a critical threshold of pathology is reached, symptoms evolve. While it is still challenging to define diagnostic criteria for the presymptomatic stages, recent progress suggests that AD can be identified, diagnosed, and potentially treated in the predementia stage. Dubois et al. have proposed a set of criteria that can be applied to label underlying AD in subjects with only mild memory decline (Dubois et al. 2007). The criteria recognize the importance of disease-specific biomarkers such low cerebrospinal fluid (CSF) amyloid beta protein (Aβ) concentration or hippocampal atrophy. This approach moves the field closer to the concept of very early AD and away from the previously widely accepted but rather nonspecific research concept of mild cognitive impairment (MCI). MCI was diagnosed in patients with cognitive decline greater than expected for chronological age but no impairment of activities of daily living (Petersen et al. 2001). It is very important to establish cognitive decline in the elderly; however, MCI as a diagnostic construct does not adequately specify the underlying disease process. Although most MCI subjects who came to autopsy demonstrated AD-type changes, up to 30% of MCI subjects show other pathologic substrates (Jicha et al. 2006).

In addition to cognitive impairment, the predementia stages of AD present a host of behavioral and personality changes (Apostolova and Cummings 2008). Administration of the Neuropsychiatric Inventory (NPI) (Cummings et al. 1994) to the caregivers of MCI subjects elicited evidence of one or more neuropsychiatric symptoms in 43%–59% (Apostolova and Cummings 2008). The most commonly reported symptoms were dysphoria, apathy, irritability and anxiety, whereas hallucinations, delusions, euphoria, abnormal motor behavior, and disinhibition were relatively uncommon (Figure 13–1). Neuropsychiatric symptoms have been shown to correlate with more severe cognitive and functional impairment in MCI (Apostolova and Cummings 2008).

ALZHEIMER'S DISEASE

AD (Table 13–1) is the most common cause of cognitive decline among the elderly. It frequently follows a prodromal stage during which amyloid pathology is already accumulating but has not reached the threshold for interfering with activities of daily living (Dubois et al. 2007). As the disease progresses, the initially isolated memory deficits evolve into more multidimensional cognitive decline with disturbance in language, visuospatial skills, and executive and social functioning. Early in the disease course, the patients have deficient verbal and visual encoding, impaired delayed recall, concrete thinking, and mild anomia (Pasquier 1999). They may have trouble operating a vehicle and managing their finances. Patients may have deficient emotional processing manifested in difficulty with interpretation of facial expression and speech prosody (Cummings 2003). As the disease progresses, they develop transcortical sensory aphasia with relatively preserved syntax and phonological abilities (Pasquier 1999). Their judgment and ability to perform instrumental activities of daily living decline. Neurovegetative disturbances such as appetite loss and sleep-wake cycle disruption are common (Cummings 2003). As patients continue to deteriorate, they progressively lose the ability to perform the more basic activities of daily living, such as dressing, eating, toileting, and finally communicating and ambulating. They typically succumb to the complications of immobilization (Kukull et al. 1994).

TABLE 13–1.   Diagnostic criteria for Alzheimer's disease (AD)

Definite AD	Probable AD
Sporadic late-onset AD: Both a diagnosis of probable AD **and** histopathologic evidence of AD should be present Autosomal dominant AD: Both clinical **and** genetic evidence for autosomal dominant AD should be present	*Core criterion:* Early significant episodic memory impairment • With gradual and progressive course over more than 6 months • With objective evidence of impaired episodic memory on neuropsychological testing that does not normalize with cueing or recognition testing • Concomitant impairments of other cognitive domains are possible *Supportive features (one or more required):* • Evidence of medial temporal lobe atrophy (hippocampus, amygdala, entorhinal atrophy) • Positive cerebrospinal fluid biomarkers such as low $A\beta$ (amyloid beta protein), increased total tau or phosphorylated tau individually or in combination • Functional neuroimaging suggestive of AD pathology (bilateral temporoparietal hypometabolism/ hypoperfusion or positive amyloid ligand imaging [using PIB or FDDNP]) • Proven AD autosomal dominant mutation in the immediate family *Exclusion criteria:* • Sudden onset of cognitive decline or early occurrence of gait or behavioral disturbances or seizures • Clinical features: focal neurological signs or early extrapyramidal signs • Other disorders severe enough to account for the clinical manifestation such as non-AD dementia, major depression, cerebrovascular disease, toxic/metabolic abnormalities

Source.   Dubois et al. 2007.

NEUROPSYCHIATRIC FEATURES OF AD

Aside from cognitive decline, AD patients display a host of personality and behavior changes. Some behaviors are more stage specific than others (Figure 13–2).

Early in the disease course, AD patients show apathy, depressed mood, anxiety, and irritability (Lyketsos et al. 2000; Mega et al. 1996). Depression in AD is associated with decreased quality of life, functional impairment, increased aggression, and increased institutionalization as well as caregiver burden and caregiver depression (Cummings 2003; Lyketsos and Olin 2002). Depression in AD has been linked to more precipitous cognitive decline (Heun et al. 2003).

Apathy in AD is a complex syndrome consisting of loss of interest, motivation, volition, enjoyment, spontaneity, and emotional behavior. It is the most common neuropsychiatric symptom in AD, affecting 42% of the patients with mild, 80% with moderate, and 92% with advanced AD (Mega et al. 1996). It may occur up to 3 years prior to diagnosis (Jost and Grossberg 1996). Apathy and the associated executive dysfunction (Boyle et al. 2003; McPherson et al. 2002) result in inefficient social and environmental interaction, decreased engagement in day-to-day activities and personal care, and worse quality of life (Boyle et

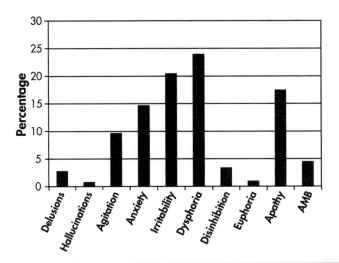

FIGURE 13–1.   Frequency of neuropsychiatric symptoms in mild cognitive impairment.

AMB = aberrant motor behavior.

Source.   Data from Baquero et al. 2004; Geda et al. 2004; Hwang et al. 2004; Lyketsos et al. 2002.

al. 2003; Freels et al. 1992). Apathy most likely results from disruption of the anterior cingulate and dorsolateral prefrontal circuits (Apostolova et al. 2007a; Mega and Cummings 1994).

Anxiety is another early feature of AD. It can present with apprehension and inner feelings of nervousness and autonomic signs such as tachycardia, perspiration, dry mouth, or chest tightness. Relative to nondemented elderly persons, in whom the prevalence of anxiety is 5.8% (Lyketsos et al. 2002), and to persons with MCI, in whom it is 11%–39% (Apostolova and Cummings 2008), the frequency of anxiety in persons with AD dementia averages 48% (Mega et al. 1996).

Irritability increases from the cognitively normal elderly population, where it is seen in 4.6%, to MCI and to AD, where it occurs in 29% and 42% of the patients, respectively (Lyketsos et al. 2002).

As AD progresses, its behavioral profile expands. Some behaviors that are only rarely encountered in the premorbid amnestic MCI or in the mild AD stages, such as disinhibition, abnormal motor behaviors, hallucinations, and delusions ensue (Piccininni et al. 2005). In advanced AD, agitation, aggression, irritability,

and violent behaviors may be prominent and prompt nursing home placement.

Disinhibition may manifest with impulsivity, tactlessness, loss of empathy, and violation of social boundaries. It results from dysfunction in the frontosubcortical circuits (Cummings 1993).

Aberrant motor behaviors include a variety of manifestations, such as fidgetiness, pacing, and/or inability to stay still. The prevalence of these behaviors exponentially increases with disease progression (Lyketsos et al. 2000; Mega et al. 1996).

Psychotic symptoms such as delusions and hallucinations are common features of AD and several other neurodegenerative disorders. They can result in patient distress, caregiver dissatisfaction, and early residential placement (Steele et al. 1990). The delusions are rarely as bizarre as in some primary psychiatric disorders such as schizophrenia. Common delusional themes are paranoia, theft, and infidelity. Content-specific delusions and misidentification syndromes (Table 13–2) occur mostly later in the disease course (Devanand et al. 1997).

Hallucinations in AD are typically in the visual modality and tend to resolve with time (Marin et al. 1997). Both hallucinations and

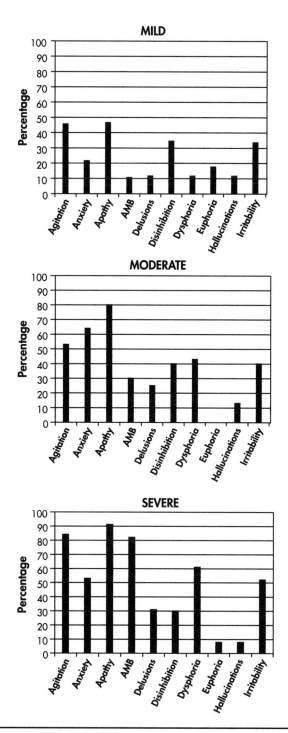

FIGURE 13–2.   Frequency of neuropsychiatric symptoms in mild, moderate, and severe Alzheimer's disease.

AMB = aberrant motor behavior.

Source.   Data from Mega et al. 1996.

TABLE 13–2.   Delusional misidentification syndromes

Capgras syndrome	Others (usually close relatives) have been replaced by impostors
Doppelganger/Heautoscopy	One has a double
Fregoli syndrome	Strangers are replaced by familiar people
Intermetamorphosis	Two people exchange their appearance
Autoscopy	One perceives one's own body as a double
Foley's syndrome	Delusion that one's image in the mirror is that of another person
Reduplicative paramnesia	One believes a physical location (e.g., home) has been duplicated
Reduplication for time	Delusion that the chronological time is duplicated and one exists in two time points

delusions correlate with poor insight (Migliorelli et al. 1995) and faster cognitive and functional decline (J. Rosen and Zubenko 1991).

Other disturbing behaviors are wandering, occurring in as many as 43% of AD patients, and disturbed diurnal sleep, occurring in 56% (Jost and Grossberg 1996).

PATHOLOGY OF AD

AD is a neurodegenerative disorder that results from accumulation of Aβ and tau protein. Aβ is a segment of the amyloid precursor protein (APP) that is liberated by the joint action of two proteases—the β- and the γ-secretase. In healthy individuals, these two enzymes are responsible for only a small fraction of the APP cleavage, while the majority is accomplished by a third protease—the α-secretase, which splits the large APP molecule in the midst of the Aβ sequence and prevents the formation of the potentially toxic 39– to 43–amino acid long Aβ protein (Mesulam 2000). Aβ polymerizes, producing first oligomeres and later polymers that clump together and form several types of amyloid inclusions. The diffuse and neuritic plaques deposit extracellularly. *Vascular amyloid* is the term for Aβ accumulation within the walls of cortical blood vessels (Duyckaerts and Dickson 2003).

Tau is a structural protein of the microtubular transport system and plays a role in microtubule stabilization. Tau's affinity for microtubules is closely regulated by phosphorylation/dephosphorylation. AD tau is hyperphosphorylated, whereby its function is severely compromised. Tau forms intracellular neurofibrillary tangles and dendritic inclusions in the form of neuropil threads and dystrophic neurites (Duyckaerts and Dickson 2003).

GENETICS OF AD

Sporadic AD (e.g., late-onset AD) generally occurs after age 65. Its mode of inheritance is governed by the synergistic action of a constellation of genes further modified by epigenetic influences. The risk for and the age at onset of AD are modified by the *APOE* gene on chromosome 19. The *APOE* gene encodes a 299–amino acid glycoprotein functioning as cholesterol transporter. *APOE*E4*, one of its three alleles, promotes Aβ aggregation (Esler et al. 2002) and suppresses neural plasticity (Nathan et al. 2002). It has been shown to accelerate disease onset in a dose-dependent fashion (Khachaturian et al. 2004). The *APOE*E4* effect is modified by race, being stronger in Caucasians than African Americans (Evans et al. 2003), and inversely by advancing age (Blacker et al. 1997). Epigenetic influences such as mental and physical exercise, high educational level, and a healthy diet rich in polyunsaturated as opposed to saturated fats (Luchsinger et al. 2007) offer protection from AD.

When AD presents before age 65 years (early-onset AD; EOAD), consideration should be given to three autosomal dominant mutations—the APP gene mutation on chromosome 21, the presenilin-1 gene mutation on chromosome 14, and the presenilin-2 gene mutation on chromosome 1. Autosomal dominant EOAD is known for its atypical clinical features, which may include aphasia, dysarthria, myoclonus, seizures, paraplegia, or dystonia (Binetti et al. 2003; Miklossy et al. 2003; Rippon et al. 2003).

Some of EOAD's atypical neuropsychiatric symptoms are emotional lability, obsessive-compulsive behavior (Rippon et al. 2003), an FTD type of presentation, or hyperoral, hyperphagic, and hypersexual behavior resembling Klüver-Bucy syndrome (Tang-Wai et al. 2002).

NEUROIMAGING IN AD

The American Academy of Neurology currently recommends a noncontrast structural image—either computed tomography or magnetic resonance imaging (MRI)—as part of the initial evaluation for cognitive impairment. MRI has several advantages—most notably, better resolution. The classical structural changes of AD are global cerebral atrophy with mesial temporal and parietal predilection. Hippocampal volume loss is evident not only in the predementia stage of MCI (Apostolova et al. 2006) but also in the presymptomatic (i.e., pre-MCI) stages of AD (Apostolova et al. 2009a). Gray matter atrophy can now be visualized easily with computational anatomy techniques. It is most pronounced in the association cortices, while primary cortices are relatively spared (Apostolova and Thompson 2008; Apostolova et al. 2007b).

Functional neuroimaging techniques such as single-photon emission computed tomography and positron emission tomography add another dimension to the workup. They provide an estimate of neuronal function rather than cerebral structure and reveal early hypoperfusion/hypometabolic changes in lateral temporal and parietal distribution and in the posterior cingulate (Apostolova et al. 2009b). Later in the disease, global hypoperfusion/hypometabolism is the rule, with relative sparing of the basal ganglia and the primary sensorimotor and visual cortices (Silverman 2004).

THERAPY FOR AD

The acetylcholinesterase inhibitors (AChEIs) donepezil (Doody 2003), galantamine (Raskind 2003), and rivastigmine (Farlow 2003) were the first class of pharmaceuticals approved by the U.S. Food and Drug Administration (FDA) for treatment of AD. Their effect is mediated by increased availability of acetylcholine in the synaptic cleft. These three agents have modest cognitive, functional, and behavioral effects and a safe side-effect profile.

Memantine is approved for treatment of moderate to severe AD. Memantine is a weak N-methyl-D-aspartate (NMDA) receptor blocker and as such prevents the deleterious effects of continuous toxic low levels of glutamate while allowing the physiologically advantageous large glutamate surge to exert its required cognitive effect. More recently, memantine was shown to stimulate long-term potentiation and ameliorate tau hyperphosphorylation (Li et al. 2004; Voisin et al. 2004).

The symptomatic therapies described above have a modest effect. The need for disease-modifying therapy has long been recognized. AD immunotherapy has recently received significant interest, and several promising passive and active immunization approaches are currently being studied. The enthusiasm for AD immunotherapy followed the successful development of anti-Aβ monoclonal antibodies, which were first shown to inhibit Aβ aggregation and later to promote dissolution of Aβ deposits and inhibit Aβ cytotoxicity in vitro (Solomon et al. 1996, 1997). The first attempt for active anti-Aβ vaccination in humans was, however, prematurely halted because 6% of the patients developed meningoencephalitis (Orgogozo et al. 2003). Resources are currently invested in other immunotherapy approaches, such as passive immunization or the use of Aβ fragments or plasmid DNA encoding Aβ (Manea et al. 2004; Schiltz et al. 2004).

Passive immunization techniques are under intense investigation following reports that passive delivery of mid-domain or amino-terminal Aβ antibodies successfully decreased plaque burden in APP mice (Bard et al. 2003;

Cribbs et al. 2003). Passive immunization may be safer, as it is unlikely to elicit a T-cell autoimmune reaction. Other benefits are the short life of the antibodies and the opportunity to quickly clear them via plasmapheresis in the event of severe side effects.

Another focus for pharmaceutical development is Aβ production and aggregation. Several β- and γ-secretase inhibitors are currently being tested. Various peptide or nonpeptide inhibitors of Aβ polymerization are likewise being explored (Boyle et al. 2003; Wolfe 2002).

The presence of activated microglia in AD brains led to several clinical trials of anti-inflammatory agents. Nevertheless, the trials of prednisone (Aisen 2000; Aisen et al. 2000), diclofenac (Scharf et al. 1999), rofecoxib, and naproxen (Aisen et al. 2003) were all negative (Weggen et al. 2003).

Until recently, however, standard therapy in AD was 2,000 IU of vitamin E, because its administration to AD patients in a large placebo-controlled trial had resulted in functional benefit (Sano et al. 1997). However, its more recent association with increased frequency of cardiac events and death (Miller et al. 2005) has resulted in more cautious prescribing patterns among dementia specialists and geriatricians (lower doses: 400–800 IU) and avoidance of this vitamin's use in patients with heart disease. Curcumin, a nutraceutical compound and an ingredient in curry spice, has been demonstrated to decrease Aβ deposition both in vitro and in transgenic mice (Lim et al. 2001; Ono et al. 2004), but it has proven difficult to test in human subjects because of its low bioavailability and thus low concentrations in the central nervous system in one recent trial (Ringman et al. 2008). Newer formulations of curcumin are currently being tested.

Several inhibitors of tau hyperphosphorylation are being investigated (Iqbal et al. 2002). Candidate agents include lithium (Bhat et al. 2004), valproate (Loy and Tariot 2002), memantine, (Li et al. 2004), and methylene blue derivatives.

MANAGEMENT OF NEUROPSYCHIATRIC DISTURBANCES IN AD

Treatment of the neuropsychiatric manifestations of AD remains rather empiric to date. No agents for the behavioral aspects of AD have been approved by the FDA. Depressive mood may respond to selective serotonin reuptake inhibitors (SSRIs) such as citalopram, sertraline, and escitalopram. In depression with psychotic symptoms or for treatment of psychosis in AD, the newer-generation antipsychotics such as risperidone, quetiapine, olanzapine, aripiprazole, and ziprasidone are typically helpful. Anxiety is best approached with SSRIs rather than benzodiazepines. The atypical antipsychotics may be useful in refractory cases. Agitation, irritability, and aggression, when mild, are best treated with behavioral modifications such as structure, gentle reassurance, and redirection. The educational and emotional support of caregivers in the management of these challenging behaviors is of utmost importance. When absolutely necessary, one should once again consider the atypical antipsychotics or the SSRIs.

When prescribing atypical antipsychotics, physicians should take into consideration the FDA warning of the associated increased risk for stroke in elderly persons with dementia—which emerged after post hoc data analyses of randomized, placebo-controlled trials of risperidone and olanzapine—and the increased risk of death associated with all antipsychotics, typical and atypical. This risk is highest for patients with risk factors for stroke, such as hypertension, diabetes, and atrial fibrillation (Bullock 2005; Sink et al. 2005).

DEMENTIA WITH LEWY BODIES

DLB accounts for 15%–20% of all late-onset dementias and is the second most prevalent dementing disorder of the elderly (Corey-Bloom 2004). The most recent diagnostic criteria (McKeith et al. 2005) are listed in Table 13–3.

TABLE 13–3. Diagnostic criteria for dementia with Lewy bodies (DLB)

Central feature

Progressive cognitive decline interfering with activities of daily living (with prominent decline in attention, executive function, or visuospatial performance)

Core features

Cognitive fluctuations

Recurrent visual hallucinations

Spontaneous features of parkinsonism (bradykinesia, rigidity, gait disturbance)

Suggestive features

Repeated falls

Severe autonomic dysfunction (orthostatic hypotension, urinary incontinence)

Transient loss of consciousness

Neuroleptic sensitivity

Systematized delusions

Hallucinations in other modalities

Depression

Relative preservation of medial temporal lobe structures on CT/MRI

Generalized hypometabolism/hypoperfusion with reduced occipital activity

Low uptake on myocardial scintigraphy

Prominent slow-wave activity on electroencephalographic examination with transient sharp waves in the temporal lobes

Source.   McKeith et al. 2005.

Cognitive decline in DLB is somewhat different than that observed in AD. Memory impairment is less severe in DLB, but attention and visuospatial and visuoperceptual functions can be severely affected early in the disease course. Cognitive fluctuations in AD are minor; in DLB they are profound, resulting in significant variability in cognitive performance, fluctuating alertness, and frank episodes of delirium. Cognitive fluctuations could be short-lived, lasting a few minutes, or persist for several days. Fluctuations are described in as many as 50%–75% of DLB patients (McKeith et al. 2004).

DLB is closely related to Parkinson's disease dementia; it is arbitrarily accepted to diagnose Parkinson's disease dementia if motor symptoms precede cognitive decline by more than 12 months and DLB if they occur within a year of each other. The extrapyramidal symptoms (EPS) observed in DLB—bradykinesia, rigidity, resting tremor, and gait disturbance—are typically symmetric. EPS are one of the initial presenting symptoms of DLB in 25%–50% and develop later in the disease course in up to 100% of the patients (McKeith et al. 2004).

Distinguishing DLB from AD and VaD may be challenging. Early falls and presyncopal/syncopal episodes are characteristic of DLB. DLB features prominent sleep disorders, most notably rapid eye movement sleep behavior disorder (RBD). RBD bears a positive predictive value of 92% for DLB (Boeve et al. 2001) and can precede the onset of EPS, cognitive decline, and fluctuations and visual hallucinations (VH) in up to 80% of DLB patients. (Ferman et al. 2002).

A characteristic but ominous clinical symptom in DLB is the unusual sensitivity of DLB patients to neuroleptic medications. Adverse EPS have been reported in 81% of DLB versus 19% of AD patients. The reactions included sedation, confusion, severe parkinsonism with extreme rigidity and immobility, and neuroleptic malignant syndrome. The mortality hazard ratio is 2.3 (McKeith et al. 1992). Thus, neuroleptic use is contraindicated in DLB.

NEUROPSYCHIATRIC FEATURES OF DLB

Up to 98% of all DLB patients experience at least one psychiatric symptom during the course of their illness. Multiple simultaneous psychiatric symptoms are almost universal (Ballard et al. 1996). At disease onset, neuropsychiatric features are much more common in DLB than in AD (Simard et al. 2000) (Figure 13–3).

As many as 65% of pathologically proven DLB but only 25% of AD patients experience VH at disease onset. In mild dementia (Mini-Mental State Examination score of 20 or higher), 93% of patients experiencing VH had

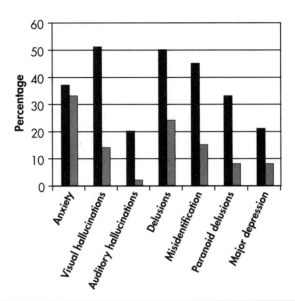

FIGURE 13–3. Prevalence of some neuropsychiatric features at disease onset in dementia with Lewy bodies (*dark shading*) and Alzheimer's disease (*light shading*).

Source. Data from Simard et al. 2000.

DLB pathology (Ballard et al. 1999). VH consist of complex, detailed, brightly colored 3D images of people and animals. Less frequent are hallucinations of inanimate objects (Aarsland et al. 2001; Ballard et al. 1996, 1997). Most VH are of normal size, complete, and animated, and half are associated with auditory hallucinations (AH). Multiple VH or VH associated with AH are exceedingly rare in AD, whereas both are relatively common in DLB (Ballard et al. 1997). VH tend to worsen in the evening (Ballard et al. 1997; McKeith et al. 1996), reflecting the impact of solitude, inactivity, and poor lighting. Patients are rarely disturbed by their VH, although the occasional patient may feel fear, amusement, or anger (McKeith et al. 1992, 1996). The reported frequency of AH in DLB (19%–25%) is much greater than that observed in AD (4%–6%) (Ballard et al 1999; Simard et al. 2000), but remission rates are similar (Ballard et al. 1996, 2001). Olfactory hallucinations are reported in 7%–12% of DLB patients and tactile in up to 3% (Aarsland et al. 2001; Ballard et al. 1996; Simard et al. 2000).

Delusions are common in DLB, with a prevalence of 50% compared with 30% in AD (Simard et al. 2000). The most common themes are delusional misidentification (see Table 13–2), followed by paranoid beliefs (theft, conspiracy, harassment, abandonment, infidelity) and phantom boarder syndrome. Of the delusional misidentifications, mistaking TV images for real occurs in 19%, followed by Capgras syndrome in 10%, mistaking one's mirror image for another person in 9.5%, and reduplicative paramnesia in 2.4% (Ballard et al. 1996).

Depression is more common in DLB than in AD (Ballard et al. 1999), although the symptomatology seems not to differ (Samuels et al. 2004). The depressed cognitively impaired patient has a 16 times higher likelihood to have DLB than AD pathology (Papka et al. 1998). Major depression per DSM-III-R criteria (American Psychiatric Association 1987) was observed in 33% of the patients with DLB (McKeith et al. 1992).

Anxiety disorder per DSM-IV-TR criteria is rare in DLB, whereas feeling anxious is very common (Ballard et al. 1996). Up to 84% of DLB patients appear or feel anxious (Rockwell et al. 2000). Among three studies using the NPI, two found anxiety as one of the most prominent neuropsychiatric features (Del Ser et al. 2000; Hirono et al. 1999; McKeith 2000).

Very few studies have assessed the full neuropsychiatric spectrum in DLB. Among the three NPI studies, apathy emerged as the most common psychopathology. Agitation, aberrant motor behavior, and aggression were also significant in DLB, while euphoria and disinhibition rarely were reported (Del Ser et al. 2000; Hirono et al. 1999; McKeith 2000).

Neuropsychiatric remission occurs less frequently in DLB than in AD or VaD patients (28%, 63%, and 33%, respectively), largely because of persistent VH.

PATHOLOGY OF DLB

The major pathological finding in DLB is the Lewy body (LB). Its major component—α-synuclein—is a natively unfolded 140–amino acid polypeptide. α-Synuclein functions as a modulator of synaptic transmission and synaptic vesicle transport. It also plays a role in neuronal plasticity (Jellinger 2003; Spillantini 2003).

LBs are frequently seen in the amygdala and brain stem nuclei of DLB, PD, and AD patients, and occasionally in cognitively intact elderly persons. Cortical LBs, however, are seen in temporal, insular, and cingulate cortices in dementia patients with DLB, Parkinson's disease dementia, and sometimes AD (Jellinger 2003).

NEUROIMAGING IN DLB

DLB patients manifest brain atrophy in a similar pattern to that observed in AD but with lesser severity (Burton et al. 2002; Harvey et al. 1999; Hashimoto et al. 1998).

Functional imaging has demonstrated temporoparietal and occipital involvement in DLB. Occipital involvement helps differentiate DLB from AD (Lobotesis et al. 2001; Minoshima et al. 2001).

The most distinctive and useful imaging modality to date is dopamine transporter imaging, which shows impaired dopamine transporter function in DLB and normal function in AD (O'Brien et al. 2004).

THERAPY FOR DLB

Similar to AD, DLB is characterized by cholinergic deficits. Two randomized, placebo-controlled rivastigmine trials showed cognitive improvement specifically in vigilance, working memory, episodic memory, attention, and executive function (McKeith et al. 2000; Wesnes et al. 2002).

The noncognitive symptoms in DLB also tend to respond favorably to AChEI therapy. Most responsive to AChEI therapy are hallucinations, paranoid delusions, daytime somnolence, apathy, aggression, and agitation (Simard and van Reekum 2004). Most importantly, neuroleptic use is contraindicated in DLB because of the extreme risk of severe side effects such as neuroleptic malignant syndrome and death. Neuroleptic malignant syndrome is only rarely reported with atypical antipsychotics (McKeith et al. 1995). Extreme caution in instituting atypical antipsychotic therapy in DLB is advised. Treatment should begin with very low doses under close supervision for cognitive or extrapyramidal side effects (Swanberg and Cummings 2002).

FRONTOTEMPORAL DEMENTIA

FTD (Table 13–4) is a group of disorders that, as the name implies, result from focal atrophy of the frontal and/or temporal lobes, with characteristic behavioral and neuropsychological features. The three subtypes of FTD are frontal variant FTD (fvFTD), primary progressive aphasia (PPA), and semantic dementia (SD). Onset around age 70 is typical for SD, whereas PPA and fvFTD tend to occur in younger persons.

FRONTAL VARIANT FTD

FvFTD, the most common subtype, is characterized by insidious early personal conduct and personality changes. Patients are frequently socially inappropriate, tactless and disinhibited, or aloof and socially isolated. FvFTD patients readily disobey socially accepted

TABLE 13–4.   Diagnostic criteria for frontotemporal dementia (FTD)

Frontal variant FTD (fvFTD)

Insidious onset and gradual progression

Early decline in interpersonal conduct

Early decline in personal conduct

Emotional blunting

Loss of insight

Decline in personal hygiene and grooming

Mental rigidity and inflexibility

Distractibility and impersistence

Hyperorality and dietary changes

Preparations and/or stereotyped behavior

Utilization behavior

Neuroimaging evidence of predominant frontal and temporal lobe involvement

Primary progressive aphasia

Insidious onset and gradual progression

Dysfluent speech output with at least one of the following: agrammatism, phonemic paraphasias, anomia

Supportive features: stuttering, apraxia of speech, impaired repetition, alexia, agraphia, early preservation of single word comprehension, late mutism, early preservation of social skills, late behavioral changes similar to fvFTD

Neuroimaging evidence of predominant superior temporal, inferior frontal, and insular involvement

Semantic dementia

Insidious onset and gradual progression

Progressive fluent empty spontaneous speech

Loss of semantic word knowledge with impaired naming and single word comprehension

Semantic paraphasias

Supportive features: pressured speech, idiosyncratic word substitution, surface dyslexia and dysgraphia

Neuroimaging evidence of predominant anterior temporal lobe involvement

Source.   Modified from Neary et al. 1998.

norms and boundaries, becoming self-centered and lacking empathy and insight. Some develop hyperorality, including compulsive

consumption of the same food item (especially sweets) or consumption of nonedible items (Bathgate et al. 2001).

Despite the paucity of cognitive complaints, detailed neuropsychological evaluation reveals impairment of frontal-executive abilities such as abstract thinking, decision making, planning, sequencing, and set shifting, and diminished free verbal recall with characteristic sparing of visual memory (Hodges and Miller 2001).

PRIMARY PROGRESSIVE APHASIA

PPA is characterized by early prominent language impairment, with dysfluent, effortful, and agrammatic language output in the context of preserved language comprehension until late in the disease course. Anomia and phonemic paraphasic errors are pronounced. Yet the behavioral disturbances are mild and PPD patients are typically socially competent until late in the disease.

SEMANTIC DEMENTIA

SD presents with characteristic language impairment resulting from semantic knowledge loss (i.e., loss of conceptual knowledge and word meaning). The language output in SD, while being fluent, well articulated, and grammatically correct, shows impoverished content and semantic supraordinate paraphasias (such as naming a lion an "animal" or a flower a "plant"). Further semantic loss leads to frequent substitutions of "it" or "thing" for many nouns, to the point that the message the patients try to convey is completely lost. Impaired comprehension for both spoken and written language is also characteristic. Unlike PPA subjects, SD patients show frontally mediated behavioral abnormalities similar to those seen in FTD (Bozeat et al. 2000; Hodges and Miller 2001).

NEUROPSYCHIATRIC FEATURES OF FTD

Figure 13–4 shows the frequency of neuropsychiatric symptoms in FTD assessed with the NPI. Relative to AD, FTD patients have signif-

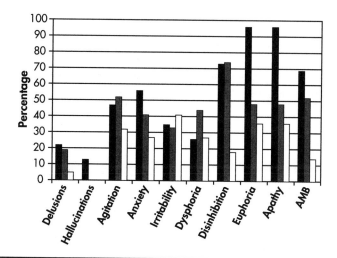

FIGURE 13–4.   Comparison of the frequency of neuropsychiatric symptoms in frontal variant FTD (*black*), temporal variant FTD (*gray*), and Alzheimer's disease (*white*).

AMB = aberrant motor behavior; FTD = frontotemporal dementia.

Source.   Liu et al. 2004.

icantly more apathy, euphoria, disinhibition, and abnormal motor behavior. In addition, fvFTD patients show other behavioral features such as emotional lability, profound emotional coldness, loss of social comportment, and loss of empathy. Obsessive-compulsive behavior, in its simple form (lip smacking, hand clapping, counting) or its complex form (hoarding, repeating a fixed route, having a strict routine, hyperorality, food craving, eating the same food item every day, or complex ritualistic behaviors), is present in 24% of FTD patients at presentation and in 47% two years after diagnosis (Bathgate et al. 2001; Mendez and Perryman 2002).

PATHOLOGY OF FTD

Pathologically, FTD is divided into tau-positive and tau-negative forms. Pick's disease is characterized by striking frontotemporal atrophy, with underlying intraneuronal argyrophylic spherical tau inclusions (i.e., Pick bodies), striking neuronal loss, and swollen neurons (i.e., Pick's cells) (Lantos and Cairns 2001). Some hereditary FTD forms show tau inclusions in neurons and glia, neuronal loss, and vacuolation

of the superficial cortical layers (Ghetti et al. 2003; Lantos and Cairns 2001).

Several tau-negative forms of FTD have been described. One is pathologically defined as dementia lacking distinctive histopathology (DLDH), in which neuronal loss, gliosis, and microvacuolation are the sole pathological features. Nevertheless, when biochemical analyses were conducted, substantial reductions in the soluble brain tau content in both gray and white matter were found (Zhukareva et al. 2003). The tau-negative ubiquitin-positive FTD is frequently a familial disorder and may present as FTD, as amyotrophic lateral sclerosis (ALS), or as a combination of the two (Lantos and Cairns 2001).

GENETICS OF FTD

Forty percent of FTD patients have a positive family history. Such kinships have allowed the identifications of multiple pathogenic mutations of the tau gene on chromosome 17. These mutations are all autosomal dominant and have high penetrance but also significant phenotypic variability (Ghetti et al. 2003; Hodges and Miller 2001). FTD with DLDH pathology has been linked to chromosome 3, and the ubiquitin positive–tau negative FTD-ALS forms have revealed causative mutations on chromosomes 9 and 17 (Lowe and Rossor 2003). The responsible gene on chromosome 17 was recently recognized as the progranulin gene (Gijselinck et al. 2008).

NEUROIMAGING IN FTD

The neuroimaging profiles of the three subtypes of FTD are distinct (Gorno-Tempini et al. 2004; H.J. Rosen et al. 2002). The behavioral variant of FTD has predominant frontal and to a lesser extent temporal atrophy, usually more significant on the right. PPA is associated with left inferior frontal, left insular, and left superior temporal involvement. SD is associated with atrophy of the left anterior temporal pole and gray matter loss in temporal, parietal, and frontal lobes. Functional imaging shows frontotemporal changes.

THERAPY FOR FTD

Presently, no effective therapy for FTD is available. SSRIs have been tested in open-label fashion. They provide symptomatic relief from compulsive behaviors, depression, disinhibition, and carbohydrate craving, and reduce caregiver burden (Moretti et al. 2003; Swartz et al. 1997). Selegiline, a monoamine oxidase B inhibitor, may influence behavior and improve executive performance (Moretti et al. 2002).

VASCULAR DEMENTIA

VaD (Table 13–5) is the third leading cause of dementia in the elderly population, with an incidence of 6–12 per 1,000 persons over age 70 years (Corey-Bloom 2004). VaD is a highly heterogeneous dementia syndrome that can result from small or large vessel arteriosclerotic disease, cardiac embolism, vasospasm, hypoperfusion, hematological/rheological disturbances, or hypoxic ischemic injury. Currently the following VaD syndromes are recognized: multi-infarct dementia, single strategically placed infarct, lacunar state, and poststroke cognitive deterioration (Bowler

2002; Korczyn 2002). Common risk factors for VaD are cerebrovascular atherosclerosis, hypertension, hyperlipidemia, hyperhomocysteinemia, diabetes mellitus, and smoking (Bowler 2002; Korczyn 2002).

The cognitive deficits in VaD are frequently those of psychomotor slowing and executive dysfunction. Difficulty with spontaneous retrieval of previously learned information, as well as declines in attention, processing speed, and set shifting, are readily observed (Schmidtke and Hull 2002). Cortical (aphasia) and subcortical (dysarthria) language deficits may be present. Confrontation naming is frequently impaired. Visuospatial difficulties may result either from parietal or frontal lobe involvement, and these impairments are associated with deficiencies in planning and executive functioning (McPherson and Cummings 1996).

The neurological examination is an important step in the evaluation of VaD patients, as it frequently reveals abnormalities. Focal or generalized upper motor neuron signs (weakness, spasticity, hyperreflexia, extensor plantar reflex), extrapyramidal findings (bradykinesia, rigidity, lower-body parkinsonism), and gait apraxia are common (Chui 2001).

NEUROPSYCHIATRIC FEATURES OF VaD

A large epidemiological study of community-dwelling elderly persons with VaD used the NPI to assess the frequency and severity of individual neuropsychiatric symptoms. The most common were depression and aggressive behaviors, followed by apathy, irritability, and anxiety. Less frequent were delusions, hallucinations, disinhibition, and abnormal motor behaviors, and the least common was euphoria (Lyketsos et al. 2000) (Figure 13–5). Relative to AD, VaD has more severe depression, agitation, and apathy (Aharon-Peretz et al. 2000).

PATHOLOGY OF VaD

The pathological findings in VaD are heterogeneous (Jellinger 2002). Multi-infarct dementia typically has underlying infarcts in the terri-

---

TABLE 13–5.   Diagnostic criteria for vascular dementia (VaD)

Probable VaD

Cognitive decline in two or more cognitive domains interfering with activities of daily living

Absence of delirium, aphasia, or sensorimotor impairment that would preclude administration of neuropsychological tests

Absence of another medical or psychiatric disorder that can cause cognitive decline

Focal neurological signs consistent with stroke

Neuroimaging evidence of extensive cerebrovascular disease

Onset of dementia within 3 months of a documented stroke

Abrupt onset, stepwise deterioration, and/or fluctuating course

Supporting features

Early gait disturbance

History of unsteadiness and frequent falls

Early urinary problems not explained by genitourinary condition

Pseudobulbal palsy

Neuropsychiatric manifestations such as mood changes, abulia, depression, emotional incontinence

Psychomotor retardation or executive dysfunction

Possible VaD

Dementia otherwise meeting criteria for probable VaD but without neuroimaging confirmation of definite cerebrovascular disease

Dementia otherwise meeting criteria for probable VaD but without a clear temporal relationship with a stroke event

Dementia otherwise meeting criteria for probable VaD but with subtle onset and gradual course of cognitive decline

---

Source.   Adapted from Roman et al. 1993.

---

tory of the middle cerebral artery and the watershed regions. Microangiopathic changes and lacunar infarcts are commonly seen in the basal ganglia, periventricular white matter, or cortical and subcortical areas. They can lead to strategic infarct dementia syndrome in the case of thalamic, mesial temporal lobe, posterior cerebral artery territory, or basal forebrain strokes; to Binswanger's disease in the case of confluent lacunes and/or cystic infarcts in periventricular or hemispheric white matter; or to multilacunar state in the case of basal ganglia and brain stem lacunar infarcts. Hypoperfusion VaD is characterized by multiple watershed cortical and subcortical microinfarcts and is most commonly due to tight stenosis of the internal carotid or middle cerebral arteries. Postischemic encephalopathy is characterized by cortical laminar necrosis and hippocampal and cerebellar ischemia and is most commonly due to cardiorespiratory collapse.

NEUROIMAGING IN VaD

Chronic VaD lesions are best visualized on T2 and fluid-attenuated inverse recovery (FLAIR) MRI sequences as hyperintense lesions. Acutely, infarcts are most easily appreciated on diffusion-weighted imaging as hyperintense and on apparent diffusion coefficient maps as hypointense lesions. Functional imaging shows deficits in the areas corresponding with the stroke location.

THERAPY FOR VaD

The most important therapy in VaD is stroke prevention. Smoking cessation and tight control of hypertension, hyperlipidemia, diabetes

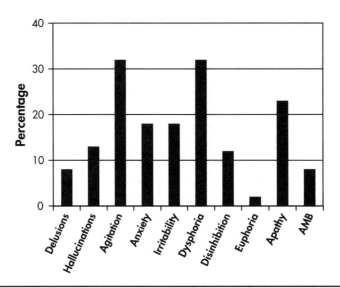

FIGURE 13–5.   Frequency of neuropsychiatric symptoms in vascular dementia.

AMB = aberrant motor behavior.

Source.   Adapted from Lyketsos et al. 2000.

mellitus are imperative. Aspirin should be used for routine prophylaxis. Physical, occupational, and speech therapy may be beneficial for the functional recovery of many patients.

In VaD, cognitive, behavioral, and functional scales showed improvement in AChEI trials (Erkinjuntti et al. 2004). Depression may respond to antidepressant therapy (Alexopoulos et al. 1997a, 1997b; Starkstein and Robinson 1994). Pseudobulbar palsy may improve with antidepressant therapy or a combination of dextromethorphan and quinidine. Atypical antipsychotics are best avoided or used only with greatest caution in this patient population, as they have been shown to increase the risk of stroke and death in elderly dementia patients with vascular risk factors (Bullock 2005; Sink et al. 2005).

CREUTZFELDT-JAKOB DISEASE

Prion disorders are a rare subgroup of the neurodegenerative diseases caused by infectious agents with proteinlike properties. Creutzfeldt-Jakob Disease (CJD), the most common prion disorder, characteristically pre-

sents with rapid cognitive decline. In its sporadic form, CJD presents mostly in the seventh decade of life (range 45–75 years) (Collinge and Palmer 1996), while the familial forms and new variant CJD (nvCJD) tend to present at a younger age.

The classic CJD presentation is that of rapidly progressing cognitive decline, with ataxia, multifocal myoclonic jerks, and startle myoclonus. Other features may include weakness, neuropathy, chorea, hallucinations, visual field cuts, language disturbance, and seizures. A third of the patients have prodromal fatigue, headache, insomnia, malaise, or depression. Once myoclonus appears, electroencephalographic recording typically shows periodic paroxysmal triphasic or sharp wave discharges against a slow background. CSF exam may show nonspecific abnormalities such as increased protein (Collinge and Palmer 1996). A sensitive but not specific CSF laboratory finding is the presence of protein 14-3-3 (Collinge and Palmer 1996; Mastrianni and Roos 2000). To date the only definitive means for establishing the diagnosis of CJD is brain biopsy or postmortem examination of the brain. Several promising diagnostic techniques under development rely on immunostaining for the causative variant of the prion protein (PrP^{Sc}) in tonsillar, olfactory mucosal, or muscle tissue (Collinge and Palmer 1996; Glatzel et al. 2005; Mastrianni and Roos 2000).

Iatrogenic CJD has been reported from inoculation of prion protein via blood transfusions, inadequately sterilized surgical equipment or depth electrodes, dural grafts, corneal implants, and human pituitary–derived growth hormone. In these cases, ataxia may be the predominant presentation following severe cerebellar involvement (Collinge and Palmer 1996; Mastrianni and Roos 2000).

The first reports of nvCJD came in 1995 from the United Kingdom. These cases represented interspecies (cow-to-human) transmission of bovine spongiform encephalopathy via alimentary intake of beef or beef products. Most commonly affected were children and adolescents (average age at onset = 26.3 years). nvCJD manifests with early prominent anxiety, depression and apathy, rapidly progressive ataxia, dementia, chorea, or myoclonus. Dysesthesias may be present. Average survival time is 14 months (Collinge and Palmer 1996; Ironside and Bell 1996).

Familial CJD accounts for about 15% of the CJD cases and is caused by point mutations, insertions, or deletions in the prion gene on chromosome 20. It tends to present a decade earlier than the sporadic variant and has a longer course (Collinge and Palmer 1996; Mastrianni and Roos 2000).

NEUROPSYCHIATRIC FEATURES OF CJD

Apathy, depression, sleep disorders, anorexia (Ajax and Rodnitzky 1998), and/or voracious appetite (personal observation) can occur. Hallucinations can occur in some (Mastrianni and Roos 2000). Prominent early neuropsychiatric changes are a classic feature in nvCJD (Collinge and Palmer 1996).

PATHOLOGY OF CJD

PrP^{Sc} is a protease-resistant, β-pleated isoform of the normal nonpathogenic membrane-bound PrP protein. Disease progression is thought to occur by template-directed refolding, whereas PrP^{Sc} serves as a template for misfolding of the nonpathogenic PrP protein to PrP^{Sc} within the cells. The most striking microscopic abnormality in sporadic CJD is the pancortical vacuolation commonly referred to as *spongiosis*. The vacuoles are axonal and dendritic swellings with accumulation of membranous material. Neuronal vacuolation may occasionally be present. Vacuoles can be seen in the cerebellum, white matter, basal ganglia, and brain stem. Reactive gliosis is present, but inflammatory cells are characteristically absent. Spongiosis is commonly found in the occipital, inferior temporal, and parietal cortex. Prion amyloid plaques rarely seen in sporadic and familial CJD are typical of nvCJD and iatrogenic CJD (Ajax and Rodnitzky 1998; Ironside and Bell 1996). Immunostaining of PrP^{Sc} is a sensitive technique allowing for definitive diagnosis of CJD and is extremely useful for questionable cases with very mild spongiform change; even the normal-appearing tissue without vacuolation stains positive in affected cases (Ironside and Bell 1996).

NEUROIMAGING IN CJD

MRI in CJD can show very specific abnormalities and aid the correct diagnosis. Increased T2, FLAIR, and diffusion signal intensity in the basal ganglia or the cortical ribbon are thought to be pathognomonic in patients with rapidly progressive cognitive decline (Hirose et al. 1998; Matoba et al. 2001; Milton et al. 1991; Yee et al. 1999; Zeidler et al. 2000).

THERAPY OF CJD

As definitive therapy for CJD is not yet available, only secondary prevention through transmission interception is possible.

CONCLUSION

The dementias are a prominent group of neurological disorders occurring mainly in the elderly. The full assessment of the patient with cognitive decline includes a thorough history of the current illness with particular attention to activities of daily living as well as social, family, and medication history. Alcohol and drug abuse and sexually transmitted diseases (e.g., syphilis, AIDS) need to be excluded in the appropriate patients. A detailed neuropsychiatric assessment of personality changes, mood disorders, and psychotic symptoms can help in the differential diagnosis. Such changes are sometimes present years before the onset of the cognitive decline. Genetic tests may be considered in young patients with a family history of dementia.

RECOMMENDED READINGS

Apostolova LG, Cummings JL: Neuropsychiatric features of dementia with Lewy bodies, in Dementia With Lewy Bodies and Parkinson's Disease. Edited by O'Brien J, McKeith I, Ames D, et al. Oxford, UK, Taylor and Francis, 2006, pp 73–94

Ballard C, Waite J, Birks J: Atypical antipsychotics for aggression and psychosis in Alzheimer's disease. Cochrane Database of Systematic Reviews. Wiley, 2006, pp 1–108

Craig D, Mirakhur A, Hart DJ, et al: A cross-sectional study of neuropsychiatric symptoms in 435 patients with Alzheimer's disease. Am J Geriatr Psychiatry 13:460–468, 2005

Lyketsos CG, Lopez O, Jones B, et al: Prevalence of neuropsychiatric symptoms in dementia and mild cognitive impairment: results from the cardiovascular health study. JAMA 288:1475–1483, 2002

McKeith IG, Dickson DW, Lowe J, et al: Diagnosis and management of dementia with Lewy bodies: third report of the DLB Consortium. Neurology 65:1863–1872, 2005

Sink KM, Holden KF, Yaffe K: Pharmacological treatment of neuropsychiatric symptoms of dementia: a review of the evidence. JAMA 293:596–608, 2005

REFERENCES

Aarsland D, Ballard C, Larsen JP, et al: A comparative study of psychiatric symptoms in dementia with Lewy bodies and Parkinson's disease with and without dementia. Int J Geriatr Psychiatry 16:528–536, 2001

Aharon-Peretz J, Kliot D, Tomer R: Behavioral differences between white matter lacunar dementia and Alzheimer's disease: a comparison on the neuropsychiatric inventory. Dement Geriatr Cogn Disord 11:294–298, 2000

Aisen PS: Anti-inflammatory therapy for Alzheimer's disease: implications of the prednisone trial. Acta Neurol Scand Suppl 176:85–89, 2000

Aisen PS, Davis KL, Berg JD, et al: A randomized controlled trial of prednisone in Alzheimer's disease. Alzheimer's Disease Cooperative Study. Neurology 54:588–593, 2000

Aisen PS, Schafer KA, Grundman M, et al: Effects of rofecoxib or naproxen vs placebo on Alzheimer disease progression: a randomized controlled trial. JAMA 289:2819–2826, 2003

Ajax T, Rodnitzky R: Creutzfeldt-Jacob disease. Home Healthcare Consultant 5:8–16, 1998

Alexopoulos GS, Meyers BS, Young RC, et al: Clinically defined vascular depression. Am J Psychiatry 154:562–565, 1997a

Alexopoulos GS, Meyers BS, Young RC, et al: "Vascular depression" hypothesis. Arch Gen Psychiatry 54:915–922, 1997b

American Psychiatric Association: Diagnostic and Statistical Manual of Mental Disorders, 3rd Edition, Revised. Washington, DC, American Psychiatric Association, 1987

American Psychiatric Association: Diagnostic and Statistical Manual of Mental Disorders, 4th Edition, Text Revision. Washington, DC, American Psychiatric Association, 2000

Apostolova LG, Cummings JL: Neuropsychiatric manifestations in mild cognitive impairment: a systematic review of the literature. Dement Geriatr Cogn Disord 25:115–126, 2008

Apostolova LG, Thompson PM: Mapping progressive brain structural changes in early Alzheimer's disease and mild cognitive impairment. Neuropsychologia 46:1597–612, 2008

Apostolova LG, Dutton RA, Dinov ID, et al: Conversion of mild cognitive impairment to Alzheimer disease predicted by hippocampal atrophy maps. Arch Neurol 63:693–699, 2006

Apostolova LG, Akopyan GG, Partiali N, et al: Structural correlates of apathy in Alzheimer's disease. Dement Geriatr Cogn Disord 24:91–97, 2007a

Apostolova LG, Steiner CA, Akopyan GG, et al: Three-dimensional gray matter atrophy mapping in mild cognitive impairment and mild Alzheimer disease. Arch Neurol 64:1489–1495, 2007b

Apostolova LG, Mosconi L, Thompson PM, et al: Subregional hippocampal atrophy predicts future decline to Alzheimer's dementia in cognitively normal subjects. Neurobiol Aging (in press). doi: 10.1016/j.neurobiolaging.2008.08.008, 2009a

Apostolova LG, Thompson PM, Rogers SA, et al: Surface feature-guided mapping of cerebral metabolic changes in cognitively normal and mildly impaired elderly [Epub ahead of print]. Mol Imaging Biol 2009b Jul 28

Ballard C, Lowery K, Harrison R, et al: Noncognitive symptoms in Lewy body dementia, in Dementia With Lewy Bodies. Edited by Perry R, McKeith I, Perry E. Cambridge, UK, Cambridge University Press, 1996, pp 67–84

Ballard C, McKeith I, Harrison R, et al: A detailed phenomenological comparison of complex visual hallucinations in dementia with Lewy bodies and Alzheimer's disease. Int Psychogeriatr 9:381–388, 1997

Ballard C, Holmes C, McKeith I, et al: Psychiatric morbidity in dementia with Lewy bodies: a prospective clinical and neuropathological comparative study with Alzheimer's disease. Am J Psychiatry 156:1039–1045, 1999

Ballard CG, O'Brien JT, Swann AG, et al: The natural history of psychosis and depression in dementia with Lewy bodies and Alzheimer's disease: persistence and new cases over 1 year of follow-up. J Clin Psychiatry 62:46–49, 2001

Baquero M, Blasco R, Campos-Garcia A, et al: [Descriptive study of behavioural disorders in mild cognitive impairment] (Spanish). Rev Neurol 38:323–326, 2004

Bard F, Barbour R, Cannon C, et al: Epitope and isotype specificities of antibodies to beta-amyloid peptide for protection against Alzheimer's disease-like neuropathology. Proc Natl Acad Sci U S A 100:2023–2028, 2003

Bathgate D, Snowden JS, Varma A, et al: Behaviour in frontotemporal dementia, Alzheimer's disease and vascular dementia. Acta Neurol Scand 103:367–378, 2001

Bhat RV, Budd Haeberlein SL, Avila J: Glycogen synthase kinase 3: a drug target for CNS therapies. J Neurochem 89:1313–1317, 2004

Binetti G, Signorini S, Squitti R, et al: Atypical dementia associated with a novel presenilin-2 mutation. Ann Neurol 54:832–836, 2003

Blacker D, Haines JL, Rodes L, et al: ApoE-4 and age at onset of Alzheimer's disease: the NIMH genetics initiative. Neurology 48:139–147, 1997

Boeve BF, Silber MH, Ferman TJ, et al: Association of REM sleep behavior disorder and neurodegenerative disease may reflect an underlying synucleinopathy. Mov Disord 16:622–630, 2001

Bowler JV: The concept of vascular cognitive impairment. J Neurol Sci 203-204:11–15, 2002

Boyle PA, Malloy PF, Salloway S, et al: Executive dysfunction and apathy predict functional impairment in Alzheimer disease. Am J Geriatr Psychiatry 11:214–221, 2003

Bozeat S, Gregory CA, Ralph MA, et al: Which neuropsychiatric and behavioural features distinguish frontal and temporal variants of frontotemporal dementia from Alzheimer's disease? J Neurol Neurosurg Psychiatry 69:178–186, 2000

Bullock R: Treatment of behavioural and psychiatric symptoms in dementia: implications of recent safety warnings. Curr Med Res Opin 21:1–10, 2005

Burton EJ, Karas G, Paling SM, et al: Patterns of cerebral atrophy in dementia with Lewy bodies using voxel-based morphometry. Neuroimage 17:618–630, 2002

Chui H: Dementia attributable to subcortical ischemic vascular disease. Neurologist 7:208–219, 2001

Collinge J, Palmer M: Human prion diseases, in Prion Diseases. Edited by Collinge J, Palmer M. New York, Oxford University Press, 1996, pp 18–56

Corey-Bloom J: Alzheimer's disease. Continuum Lifelong Learning Neurol 10:29–57 2004

Cribbs DH, Ghochikyan A, Vasilevko V, et al: Adjuvant-dependent modulation of Th1 and Th2 responses to immunization with beta-amyloid. Int Immunol 15:505–514, 2003

Cummings JL: Frontal-subcortical circuits and human behavior. Arch Neurol 50:873–880, 1993

Cummings JL: Alzheimer's disease, in The Neuropsychiatry of Alzheimer's Disease and Related Dementias. Edited by Cummings JL. London, Martin Dunitz, 2003, pp 57–116

Cummings JL, Mega M, Gray K, et al: The Neuropsychiatric Inventory: comprehensive assessment of psychopathology in dementia. Neurology 44:2308–2314, 1994

Del Ser T, McKeith I, Anand R, et al: Dementia with Lewy bodies: findings from an international multicentre study. Int J Geriatr Psychiatry 15:1034–1045, 2000

Devanand DP, Jacobs DM, Tang MX, et al: The course of psychopathologic features in mild to moderate Alzheimer disease. Arch Gen Psychiatry 54:257–263, 1997

Doody RS: Update on Alzheimer drugs: donepezil. Neurologist 9:225–229, 2003

Dubois B, Feldman HH, Jacova C, et al: Research criteria for the diagnosis of Alzheimer's disease: revising the NINCDS-ADRDA criteria. Lancet Neurol 6:734–746, 2007

Duyckaerts C, Dickson DW: Neuropathology of Alzheimer's disease, in Neurodegeneration: The Molecular Pathology of Dementia and Movement Disorders. Edited by Dickson DW. Basel, Switzerland, ISN Neuropath Press, 2003, pp 47–65

Erkinjuntti T, Roman G, Gauthier S: Treatment of vascular dementia: evidence from clinical trials with cholinesterase inhibitors. J Neurol Sci 226:63–66, 2004

Esler WP, Marshall JR, Stimson ER, et al: Apolipoprotein E affects amyloid formation but not amyloid growth in vitro: mechanistic implications for apoE4 enhanced amyloid burden and risk for Alzheimer's disease. Amyloid 9:1–12, 2002

Evans DA, Bennett DA, Wilson RS, et al: Incidence of Alzheimer disease in a biracial urban community: relation to apolipoprotein E allele status. Arch Neurol 60:185–189, 2003

Farlow M: Update on rivastigmine. Neurologist 9:230–234, 2003

Ferman TJ, Boeve BF, Smith GE, et al: Dementia with Lewy bodies may present as dementia and REM sleep behavior disorder without parkinsonism or hallucinations. J Int Neuropsychol Soc 8:907–914, 2002

Freels S, Cohen D, Eisdorfer C, et al: Functional status and clinical findings in patients with Alzheimer's disease. J Gerontol 47:M177–M182, 1992

Geda YE, Smith GE, Knopman DS, et al: De novo genesis of neuropsychiatric symptoms in mild cognitive impairment (MCI). Int Psychogeriatr 16:51–60, 2004

Ghetti B, Hutton ML, Wszolek ZK: Frontotemporal dementia and parkinsonism linked to chromosome 17 associated with tau gene mutations, in Neurodegeneration: The Molecular Pathology of Dementia and Movement Disorders. Edited by Dickson DW. Basel, Switzerland, ISN Neuropath Press, 2003, pp 86–102

Gijselinck I, Van Broeckhoven C, Cruts M: Granulin mutations associated with frontotemporal lobar degeneration and related disorders: an update. Hum Mutat 29:1373–86, 2008

Glatzel M, Stoeck K, Seeger H, et al: Human prion diseases: molecular and clinical aspects. Arch Neurol 62:545–552, 2005

Gorno-Tempini ML, Dronkers NF, Rankin KP, et al: Cognition and anatomy in three variants of primary progressive aphasia. Ann Neurol 55:335–346, 2004

Graff-Radford N, Woodruff B: Frontotemporal dementia. Continuum Lifetime Learning Neurol 10:58–80, 2004

Harvey GT, Hughes J, McKeith IG, et al: Magnetic resonance imaging differences between dementia with Lewy bodies and Alzheimer's disease: a pilot study. Psychol Med 29:181–187, 1999

Hashimoto M, Kitagaki H, Imamura T, et al: Medial temporal and whole-brain atrophy in dementia with Lewy bodies: a volumetric MRI study. Neurology 51:357–362, 1998

Heun R, Kockler M, Ptok U: Lifetime symptoms of depression in Alzheimer's disease. Eur Psychiatry 18:63–69, 2003

Hirono N, Mori E, Tanimukai S, et al: Distinctive neurobehavioral features among neurodegenerative dementias. J Neuropsychiatry Clin Neurosci 11:498–503, 1999

Hirose Y, Mokuno K, Abe Y, et al: [A case of clinically diagnosed Creutzfeldt-Jakob disease with serial MRI diffusion weighted images] (Japanese). Rinsho Shinkeigaku 38:779–782, 1998

Hodges JR, Miller B: The neuropsychology of frontal variant frontotemporal dementia and semantic dementia: introduction to the special topic papers, part II. Neurocase 7:113–121, 2001

Hwang TJ, Masterman DL, Ortiz F, et al: Mild cognitive impairment is associated with characteristic neuropsychiatric symptoms. Alzheimer Dis Assoc Disord 18:17–21, 2004

Iqbal K, Alonso Adel C, El-Akkad E, et al: Pharmacological targets to inhibit Alzheimer neurofibrillary degeneration. J Neural Transm Suppl (62):309–319, 2002

Ironside J, Bell J: Pathology of prion diseases, in Prion Diseases. Edited by Collinge J, Palmer M. Oxford University Press, 1996, pp 57–88

Jellinger KA: The pathology of ischemic-vascular dementia: an update. J Neurol Sci 203-204:153–157, 2002

Jellinger KA: Neuropathological spectrum of synucleinopathies. Mov Disord 18 (suppl 6):S2–S12, 2003

Jicha GA, Parisi JE, Dickson DW, et al: Neuropathologic outcome of mild cognitive impairment following progression to clinical dementia. Arch Neurol 63:674–681, 2006

Jost BC, Grossberg GT: The evolution of psychiatric symptoms in Alzheimer's disease: a natural history study [see comment]. J Am Geriatr Soc 44:1078–1081, 1996

Khachaturian AS, Corcoran CD, Mayer LS, et al: Apolipoprotein E epsilon4 count affects age at onset of Alzheimer disease, but not lifetime susceptibility: the Cache County Study. Arch Gen Psychiatry 61:518–524, 2004

Korczyn AD: The complex nosological concept of vascular dementia. J Neurol Sci 203-204:3–6, 2002

Kukull WA, Brenner DE, Speck CE, et al: Causes of death associated with Alzheimer disease: variation by level of cognitive impairment before death. J Am Geriatr Soc 42:723–726, 1994

Lantos PL, Cairns NJ: Neuropathology, in Early Onset Dementia. Edited by Hodges JR. New York, Oxford University Press, 2001, pp 227–262

Li L, Sengupta A, Haque N, et al: Memantine inhibits and reverses the Alzheimer type abnormal hyperphosphorylation of tau and associated neurodegeneration. FEBS Lett 566:261–269, 2004

Lim GP, Chu T, Yang F, et al: The curry spice curcumin reduces oxidative damage and amyloid pathology in an Alzheimer transgenic mouse. J Neurosci 21:8370–8377, 2001

Liu W, Miller BL, Kramer JH, et al: Behavioral disorders in the frontal and temporal variants of frontotemporal dementia. Neurology 62:742–748, 2004

Lobotesis K, Fenwick JD, Phipps A, et al: Occipital hypoperfusion on SPECT in dementia with Lewy bodies but not AD. Neurology 56:643–649, 2001

Lowe J, Rossor M: Frontotemporal lobar degeneration, in Neurodegeneration: The Molecular Pathology of Dementia and Movement Disorders. Edited by Dickson DW. Basel, Switzerland, ISN Neuropath Press, 2003, pp 342–348

Loy R, Tariot PN: Neuroprotective properties of valproate: potential benefit for AD and tauopathies. J Mol Neurosci 19:303–307, 2002

Luchsinger JA, Noble JM, Scarmeas N: Diet and Alzheimer's disease. Curr Neurol Neurosci Rep 7:366–72, 2007

Lyketsos CG, Olin J: Depression in Alzheimer's disease: overview and treatment. Biol Psychiatry 52:243–252, 2002

Lyketsos CG, Steinberg M, Tschanz JT, et al: Mental and behavioral disturbances in dementia: findings from the Cache County Study on Memory in Aging. Am J Psychiatry 157:708–714, 2000

Lyketsos CG, Lopez O, Jones B, et al: Prevalence of neuropsychiatric symptoms in dementia and mild cognitive impairment: results from the cardiovascular health study. JAMA 288:1475–1483, 2002

Manea M, Mezo G, Hudecz F, et al: Polypeptide conjugates comprising a beta-amyloid plaque-specific epitope as new vaccine structures against Alzheimer's disease. Biopolymers 76:503–511, 2004

Marin DB, Green CR, Schmeidler J, et al: Noncognitive disturbances in Alzheimer's disease: frequency, longitudinal course, and relationship to cognitive symptoms. J Am Geriatr Soc 45:1331–1338, 1997

Mastrianni JA, Roos RP: The prion diseases. Semin Neurol 20:337–352, 2000

Matoba M, Tonami H, Miyaji H, et al: Creutzfeldt-Jakob disease: serial changes on diffusion-weighted MRI. J Comput Assist Tomogr 25:274–277, 2001

McKeith IG: Spectrum of Parkinson's disease, Parkinson's dementia, and Lewy body dementia. Neurol Clin 18:865–902, 2000

McKeith IG, Perry RH, Fairbairn AF, et al: Operational criteria for senile dementia of Lewy body type (SDLT). Psychol Med 22:911–922, 1992

McKeith IG, Ballard CG, Harrison RW: Neuroleptic sensitivity to risperidone in Lewy body dementia. Lancet 346:699, 1995

McKeith IG, Galasko D, Kosaka K, et al: Consensus guidelines for the clinical and pathologic diagnosis of dementia with Lewy bodies (DLB): report of the Consortium on DLB International Workshop. Neurology 47:1113–1124, 1996

McKeith I, Del Ser T, Spano P, et al: Efficacy of rivastigmine in dementia with Lewy bodies: a randomised, double-blind, placebo-controlled international study [see comment]. Lancet 356:2031–2036, 2000

McKeith I, Mintzer J, Aarsland D, et al: Dementia with Lewy bodies. Lancet Neurol 3:19–28, 2004

McKeith IG, Dickson DW, Lowe J, et al: Diagnosis and management of dementia with Lewy bodies: third report of the DLB Consortium. Neurology 65:1863–1872, 2005

McPherson SE, Cummings JL: Neuropsychological aspects of vascular dementia. Brain Cogn 31:269–282, 1996

McPherson S, Fairbanks L, Tiken S, et al: Apathy and executive function in Alzheimer's disease. J Int Neuropsychol Soc 8:373–381, 2002

Mega MS, Cummings JL: Frontal-subcortical circuits and neuropsychiatric disorders. J Neuropsychiatry Clin Neurosci 6:358–370, 1994

Mega MS, Cummings JL, Fiorello T, et al: The spectrum of behavioral changes in Alzheimer's disease. Neurology 46:130–135, 1996

Mendez MF, Perryman KM: Neuropsychiatric features of frontotemporal dementia: evaluation of consensus criteria and review. J Neuropsychiatry Clin Neurosci 14:424–429, 2002

Mesulam MM: Aging, Alzheimer's disease and dementia, in Principles of Behavioral and Cognitive Neurology. Edited by Mesulam MM. Oxford, UK, Oxford University Press, 2000, pp 439–510

Migliorelli R, Teson A, Sabe L, et al: Prevalence and correlates of dysthymia and major depression among patients with Alzheimer's disease [see comment]. Am J Psychiatry 152:37–44, 1995

Miklossy J, Taddei K, Suva D, et al: Two novel presenilin-1 mutations (Y256S and Q222H) are associated with early onset Alzheimer's disease. Neurobiol Aging 24:655–662, 2003

Miller ER 3rd, Pastor-Barriuso R, Dalal D, et al: Meta-analysis: high-dosage vitamin E supplementation may increase all-cause mortality. Ann Intern Med 142:37–46, 2005

Milton WJ, Atlas SW, Lavi E, et al: Magnetic resonance imaging of Creutzfeldt-Jacob disease. Ann Neurol 29:438–440, 1991

Minoshima S, Foster NL, Sima AA, et al: Alzheimer's disease versus dementia with Lewy bodies: cerebral metabolic distinction with autopsy confirmation. Ann Neurol 50:358–365, 2001

Moretti R, Torre P, Antonello RM, et al: Effects of selegiline on fronto-temporal dementia: a neuropsychological evaluation. Int J Geriatr Psychiatry 17:391–392, 2002

Moretti R, Torre P, Antonello RM, et al: Frontotemporal dementia: paroxetine as a possible treatment of behavior symptoms: a randomized, controlled, open 14-month study. Eur Neurol 49:13–19, 2003

Nathan BP, Jiang Y, Wong GK, et al: Apolipoprotein E4 inhibits, and apolipoprotein E3 promotes neurite outgrowth in cultured adult mouse cortical neurons through the low-density lipoprotein receptor-related protein. Brain Res 928:96–105, 2002

Neary D, Snowden JS, Gustafson L, et al: Frontotemporal lobar degeneration: a consensus on clinical diagnostic criteria. Neurology 51:1546–1554, 1998

O'Brien JT, Colloby S, Fenwick J, et al: Dopamine transporter loss visualized with FP-CIT SPECT in the differential diagnosis of dementia with Lewy bodies. Arch Neurol 61:919–925, 2004

Ono K, Hasegawa K, Naiki H, et al: Curcumin has potent anti-amyloidogenic effects for Alzheimer's beta-amyloid fibrils in vitro. J Neurosci Res 75:742–750, 2004

Orgogozo JM, Gilman S, Dartigues JF, et al: Subacute meningoencephalitis in a subset of patients with AD after Abeta42 immunization. Neurology 61:46–54, 2003

Papka M, Rubio A, Schiffer RB, et al: Lewy body disease: can we diagnose it? J Neuropsychiatry Clin Neurosci 10:405–412, 1998

Pasquier F: Early diagnosis of dementia: neuropsychology. J Neurol 246:6–15, 1999

Petersen RC, Doody R, Kurz A, et al: Current concepts in mild cognitive impairment. Arch Neurol 58:1985–1992, 2001

Piccininni M, Di Carlo A, Baldereschi M, et al: Behavioral and psychological symptoms in Alzheimer's disease: frequency and relationship with duration and severity of the disease. Dement Geriatr Cogn Disord 19:276–281, 2005

Raskind MA: Update on Alzheimer drugs: galantamine. Neurologist 9:225–229, 2003

Ringman JM, Cole GM, Teng E, et al: Oral curcumin for the treatment of mild-to-moderate Alzheimer's disease: tolerability and clinical and biomarker efficacy results of a placebo-controlled 24-week study. Alzheimers Dement 4 (suppl 2):T774, 2008

Rippon GA, Crook R, Baker M, et al: Presenilin 1 mutation in an African American family presenting with atypical Alzheimer dementia. Arch Neurol 60:884–888, 2003

Rockwell E, Choure J, Galasko D, et al: Psychopathology at initial diagnosis in dementia with Lewy bodies versus Alzheimer disease: comparison of matched groups with autopsy-confirmed diagnoses. Int J Geriatr Psychiatry 15:819–823, 2000

Roman GC, Tatemichi TK, Erkinjuntti T, et al: Vascular dementia: diagnostic criteria for research studies. Report of the NINDS-AIREN International Workshop. Neurology 43:250–260, 1993

Rosen HJ, Gorno-Tempini ML, Goldman WP, et al: Patterns of brain atrophy in frontotemporal dementia and semantic dementia. Neurology 58:198–208, 2002

Rosen J, Zubenko GS: Emergence of psychosis and depression in the longitudinal evaluation of Alzheimer's disease. Biol Psychiatry 29:224–232, 1991

Samuels SC, Brickman AM, Burd JA, et al: Depression in autopsy-confirmed dementia with Lewy bodies and Alzheimer's disease. Mt Sinai J Med 71:55–62, 2004

Sano M, Ernesto C, Thomas RG, et al: A controlled trial of selegiline, alpha-tocopherol, or both as treatment for Alzheimer's disease. The Alzheimer's Disease Cooperative Study. N Engl J Med 336:1216–1222, 1997

Scharf S, Mander A, Ugoni A, et al: A double-blind, placebo-controlled trial of diclofenac/misoprostol in Alzheimer's disease. Neurology 53:197–201, 1999

Schiltz JG, Salzer U, Mohajeri MH, et al: Antibodies from a DNA peptide vaccination decrease the brain amyloid burden in a mouse model of Alzheimer's disease. J Mol Med 82:706–714, 2004

Schmidtke K, Hull M: Neuropsychological differentiation of small vessel disease, Alzheimer's disease and mixed dementia. J Neurol Sci 203-204:17–22, 2002

Silverman DH: Brain 18F-FDG PET in the diagnosis of neurodegenerative dementias: comparison with perfusion SPECT and with clinical evaluations lacking nuclear imaging. J Nucl Med 45:594–607, 2004

Simard M, van Reekum R: The acetylcholinesterase inhibitors for treatment of cognitive and behavioral symptoms in dementia with Lewy bodies. J Neuropsychiatry Clin Neurosci 16:409–425, 2004

Simard M, van Reekum R, Cohen T: A review of the cognitive and behavioral symptoms in dementia with Lewy bodies. J Neuropsychiatry Clin Neurosci 12:425–450, 2000

Sink KM, Holden KF, Yaffe K: Pharmacological treatment of neuropsychiatric symptoms of dementia: a review of the evidence. JAMA 293:596–608, 2005

Solomon B, Koppel R, Hanan E, et al: Monoclonal antibodies inhibit in vitro fibrillar aggregation of the Alzheimer beta-amyloid peptide. Proc Natl Acad Sci USA 93:452–455, 1996

Solomon B, Koppel R, Frankel D, et al: Disaggregation of Alzheimer beta-amyloid by site-directed mAb. Proc Natl Acad Sci USA 94:4109–4112, 1997

Spillantini MG: Introduction to synucleinopathies, in Neurodegeneration: The Molecular Pathology of Dementia and Movement Disorders. Edited by Dickson DW. Basel, Switzerland, ISN Neuropath Press, 2003, pp 156–158

Starkstein S, Robinson R: Neuropsychiatric aspects of stroke, in The American Psychiatric Press Textbook of Geriatric Neuropsychiatry. Edited by Coffey C, Cummings J. Washington, DC, American Psychiatric Press, 1994, pp 457–475

Steele C, Rovner B, Chase GA, et al: Psychiatric symptoms and nursing home placement of patients with Alzheimer's disease. Am J Psychiatry 147:1049–1051, 1990

Swanberg MM, Cummings JL: Benefit-risk considerations in the treatment of dementia with Lewy bodies. Drug Saf 25:511–523, 2002

Swartz JR, Miller BL, Lesser IM, et al: Frontotemporal dementia: treatment response to serotonin selective reuptake inhibitors. J Clin Psychiatry 58:212–216, 1997

Tang-Wai D, Lewis P, Boeve B, et al: Familial frontotemporal dementia associated with a novel presenilin-1 mutation. Dement Geriatr Cogn Disord 14:13–21, 2002

Voisin T, Reynish E, Portet F, et al: What are the treatment options for patients with severe Alzheimer's disease? CNS Drugs 18:575–583, 2004

Weggen S, Eriksen JL, Sagi SA, et al: Evidence that nonsteroidal anti-inflammatory drugs decrease amyloid beta 42 production by direct modulation of gamma-secretase activity. J Biol Chem 278:31831–31837, 2003

Wesnes K, McKeith I, Ferrara R, et al: Effects of rivastigmine on cognitive function in dementia with Lewy bodies: a randomized placebo-controlled international study using the cognitive drug research computerised assessment system. Dement Geriatr Cogn Disord 13:183–192, 2002

Wolfe MS: Therapeutic strategies for Alzheimer's disease. Nat Rev Drug Discov 1:859–866, 2002

Yee AS, Simon JH, Anderson CA, et al: Diffusion-weighted MRI of right-hemisphere dysfunction in Creutzfeldt-Jakob disease. Neurology 52:1514–1515, 1999

Zeidler M, Sellar RJ, Collie DA, et al: The pulvinar sign on magnetic resonance imaging in variant Creutzfeldt-Jakob disease. Lancet 355:1412–1418, 2000

Zhukareva V, Sundarraj S, Mann D, et al: Selective reduction of soluble tau proteins in sporadic and familial frontotemporal dementias: an international follow-up study. Acta Neuropathol (Berl) 105:469–476, 2003

14

NEUROPSYCHIATRIC ASPECTS OF SCHIZOPHRENIA

Carol A. Tamminga, M.D.

Mujeeb U. Shad, M.D.

Subroto Ghose, M.D., Ph.D.

We know that schizophrenia is a psychiatric illness with well-established diagnostic criteria, clear signs and symptoms, and variably effective symptomatic treatments (Andreasen et al. 1995; Carpenter and Buchanan 1994). However, not enough of the pieces of this puzzle have yet been manifested to arrange with any certainty the areas of sure knowledge into a complete disease picture. In this chapter, we examine the pieces of knowledge we possess today that define the biology of schizophrenia and how we can view these pieces to rationally increase our understanding of the illness.

CLINICAL CHARACTERISTICS OF SCHIZOPHRENIA

Schizophrenia-like conditions have been known for millennia. Not until the mid-twentieth century were broadly effective pharmacological

treatments available and modern disease formulations applied to the condition.

DIAGNOSIS

Throughout history, the identification of psychosis has always been straightforward because of its distinctive cognitive symptoms. DSM-IV-TR (American Psychiatric Association 2000) details clear diagnostic criteria accepted throughout North America and the worldwide scientific community. The use of these criteria has led to the consistent and reliable diagnosis of schizophrenia. The DSM-IV-TR criteria and the tenth revision of the *International Statistical Classification of Diseases and Related Health Problems* (ICD-10; World Health Organization 1992) criteria are the world's two major diagnostic systems for schizophrenia; with the current editions, they have reconciled their major differences. These structured diagnostic criteria have led to the examination and identification of schizophrenia around the world and to the observation that the incidence and the symptomatic expression are similar between countries and across cultures (Sartorius 1974).

Although the schizophrenia phenotype has been traditionally defined by chronic psychosis and functional deterioration, the boundary of the phenotype now is often viewed as broader than the schizophrenia diagnosis itself. Schizophrenia may well be the tip of an iceberg of schizophrenia-related diagnoses, augmented by the related personality disorders (Tsuang et al. 2000).

SYMPTOMATOLOGY

In the International Pilot Study of Schizophrenia conducted by the World Health Organization (Sartorius 1974), symptoms were rated in schizophrenic persons in seven different countries. The symptoms were noted to be similar in all countries.

Although DSM-IV-TR clearly identifies a syndrome, investigators remain unsure that schizophrenia is a unitary illness with a single etiology and pathophysiology as opposed to a group of syndromes or a collection of interrelated conditions (Carpenter and Buchanan 1994). Therefore, various attempts have been made to delineate testable subtypes of the illness on the basis of clinical characteristics, which then can be evaluated for distinguishing brain characteristics (Carpenter et al. 1993). In several investigations of large populations of schizophrenic patients, the symptom presentations have been analyzed for the clustering of symptoms into symptomatic subgroups. These analyses have consistently identified three distinct symptom domains in schizophrenia: 1) psychosis domain: hallucinations, delusions, and paranoia; 2) cognitive deficit domain: thought disorder; and 3) negative symptom domain: anhedonia, social withdrawal, and thought poverty (Andreasen et al. 1995; Arndt et al. 1991; Barnes and Liddle 1990; Carpenter and Buchanan 1989; Kay and Sevy 1990; Lenzenweger et al. 1991; Liddle 1987).

Cognitive deficits are core symptoms of schizophrenia. Schizophrenic patients as a group perform poorly on most neuropsychological tests compared with healthy subjects. Abnormalities in abstraction, problem solving, and other executive functions have been particularly noted in individuals with schizophrenia (Goldberg et al. 1987). Specific neuropsychological deficits are broad; they include memory, executive function, and motor performance (Braff et al. 1991; Gold et al. 1992; Goldberg et al. 1990; Gruzelier et al. 1988; R.C. Gur et al. 1991; Liddle and Morris 1991). No cognitive domains are entirely spared, and deficits in performance are highly intercorrelated (Sullivan et al. 1994).

Similarly, persons with schizophrenia consistently perform poorly on tasks that require sustained attention or vigilance (Nuechterlein et al. 1992). Other studies document deficits in memory, including explicit memory and verbal memory (Gold et al. 1994; Saykin et al. 1991). Working memory, which permits task-relevant information to be kept active for brief periods, has received much attention in the schizophrenia literature. Individuals with schizophrenia have difficulties maintaining working memory (Goldman-Rakic 1994; Park and Holzman 1992). Deficits may explain some of the serious disorganization and functional deterioration observed in the schizophrenia spectrum. This is because the ability to hold information "online" is critical for organizing future thoughts and actions in the context of the recent past (Goldman-Rakic 1994).

When clinical symptoms (i.e., psychosis, cognitive deficits, and negative symptoms) are related to imaging findings, specific brain areas are found to be differentially involved in symptom manifestations in schizophrenia. Whether these regionally specific changes are a cause or an effect of the disorder is not known, but they do suggest the presence of distinct neuroanatomical substrates, possibly distinct cerebral systems, for the different symptom clusters. One importance of this distinction lies in its therapeutic implications. Is there one treatment for schizophrenia? Or are there several treatments for symptom-specific domains of the illness?

This question remains open, and its answer is being aggressively pursued in ongoing research.

COURSE

The diagnosis of schizophrenia usually implies a lifelong course of psychotic illness. Occasionally, the illness is of fast onset and episodic, with symptoms first occurring in late teenage and early adult years and with satisfactory recovery between episodes. However, more often other patterns of illness occur, characterized by an insidious onset, a partial recovery, or a remarkable lack of recovery between episodes (Bleuler 1978; Ciompi and Müller 1976). In most schizophrenic patients, a profound deterioration in mental and social functioning occurs within the first few years of the illness. After the initial deteriorating years, the further course of illness settles at a low, but flat, plateau. That the disease course is generally flat in its middle years distinguishes schizophrenia from traditional neurodegenerative disorders in which the course is progressively downhill (such as Parkinson's disease or Alzheimer's dementia) and from traditional neurodevelopmental disorders (such as mental retardation) in which the course is steady and low from the beginning of life.

RISK FACTORS IN SCHIZOPHRENIA

Although the etiology of schizophrenia is not known, genetic and environmental factors have been associated with a propensity toward the illness. Each risk factor alone is believed to confer a small risk, yet when they occur together, these risks may be multiplicative (Barr et al. 1990; Kendell and Kemp 1989; O'Callaghan et al. 1991). Moreover, these risk factors suggest the importance of early life events in the onset of an illness whose florid symptoms appear later in life.

GENETICS

The evidence is currently clear and consistent across many methodologically sound studies that schizophrenia aggregates in families. Twin studies have been pivotal in identifying the familial factor as a genetic rather than an environmental risk (Gottesman and Shields 1982; Kety 1987). The monozygotic twin of a person with schizophrenia has a 31%–78% chance of contracting the illness, compared with a 0%–28% chance for a dizygotic twin. The heritability is estimated to be approximately 80% (Cardno and Gottesman 2000), with a complex mode of transmission (Gottesman and Shields 1967; McGue and Gottesman 1989). Detailed studies of linked regions and other studies have identified several candidate genes (see reviews by Harrison and Weinberger 2005; Owen et al. 2005), and here we briefly review the genes for which strong evidence and biological plausibility exist.

Dystrobrevin Binding Protein-1 (DTNBP1 or Dysbindin)

Dysbindin is a promising candidate gene implicated in schizophrenia. Associations between dysbindin and schizophrenia have been shown in several studies (Funke et al. 2004; Kirov et al. 2004; Numakawa et al. 2004; Schwab et al. 2003; Straub et al. 2002; Williams et al. 2004) although not in all (Morris et al. 2003; Van Den Bogaert et al. 2003). Dysbindin is a component of the dystrophin glycoprotein complex believed to play a role in stabilization of the postsynaptic membrane, cytoskeletal rearrangement (Adams et al. 2000; Grady et al. 2000), and signal transduction (Grady et al. 1999). A possible functional role of dysbindin in schizophrenia is supported by the finding of decreased messenger RNA (mRNA) and protein in human postmortem brain tissue from schizophrenic donors (Talbot et al. 2004; C.S. Weickert et al. 2004).

Neuregulin-1 (NRG1)

Neuregulin is believed to be a susceptibility gene for schizophrenia (Corvin et al. 2004; Stefansson et al. 2002, 2003; Tang et al. 2004; Williams et al. 2003; Yang et al. 2003; Zhao et al. 2004), although negative findings also have been reported (Iwata et al. 2004; Thiselton et al. 2004). Three studies (Stefansson et al. 2002, 2003; Williams et al. 2003), however, find an association between a specific core haplotype in *NRG1* and schizophrenia. Neuregulin is a large gene with 4 different isoforms that give rise to at least 15 different peptides (Harrison and Law 2006). Neuregulin peptides are involved in a host of physiological processes including neuronal migration, axon guidance, synaptogenesis, glial differentiation, myelination, neurotransmission, and synaptic plasticity.

D–Amino Acid Oxidase Activator and D–Amino Acid Oxidase

Association mapping in the linkage region on 13q22–34 found two genes—*G72* (also called D–amino acid oxidase activator [*DAOA*]) and *G30*—to be associated with schizophrenia in two populations (Chumakov et al. 2002). *DAOA* enhances activity of D–amino acid oxidase (DAO), an enzyme that is involved in the metabolism of D-serine, a potent activator of the *N*-methyl-D-aspartate (NMDA) glutamate receptor. Subsequent studies supported *DAOA* and DAO as important to the genetics of schizophrenia (Addington et al. 2004; Ma et al. 2006; Schumacher et al. 2004; Wang et al. 2004; Zou et al. 2005).

Regulator of G-Protein Signaling-4 (*RGS4*)

RGS4 is a gene that maps to 1q21–22, a region implicated in linkage studies. Associations were found with four single-nucleotide polymorphisms (SNPs) of varying haplotypes in *RGS4* in three different populations of subjects (Chowdari et al. 2002), and decreased expression levels of this gene in human postmortem microarray studies suggest candidacy of this gene in the susceptibility to schizophrenia (Mirnics et al. 2001). RGS proteins are a family of about 30 proteins that are guanosine triphosphatase–activating proteins serving to negatively regulate G protein–coupled receptors. *RGS4* is abundantly expressed in the brain and can regulate multiple G protein–coupled receptors, including dopaminergic and metabotropic glutamate receptors.

Catechol *O*-Methyltransferase (*COMT*)

COMT maps to 22q11, the deletion of which produces velocardiofacial syndrome, a disease associated with a high incidence of psychosis. COMT is an enzyme involved in monoamine metabolism and a functional polymorphism at codon 108/158. A G-to-A substitution converts valine (Val) to methionine (Met), which influences *COMT* activity. Numerous association studies examining the *COMT* Val/Met polymorphism in schizophrenia have been inconsistent, and a meta-analysis reported no association (Glatt et al. 2003). This polymorphism does influences prefrontal cortical and hippocampal function (de Frias et al. 2004; Egan et al. 2001; Goldberg et al. 2003; Joober et al. 2002; Malhotra et al. 2002) and the clinical response of persons with schizophrenia to antipsychotic medication (Bertolino et al. 2004; T.W. Weickert et al. 2004). Haplotypes carrying the Val158Met SNP show strong associations with schizophrenia (Chen et al. 2004; Sanders 2005; Shifman et al. 2002), perhaps suggesting that *COMT* may be a candidate gene, but not because of the Val158Met SNP.

Disrupted-in-Schizophrenia-1 and -2 (*DISC1* and *DISC2*)

A balanced translocation in chromosomes 1 and 11 (1;11) (q42.1;q14.3) linked to the major mental disorders—schizophrenia, depression, and mania—was found to disrupt two genes: *DISC1* and *DISC2* (St Clair et al. 1990). Linkage analysis and association studies implicate *DISC1* in schizophrenia (Ekelund et al. 2001, 2004). Positive associations have been found in several later studies (Callicott et al. 2005; Hennah et al. 2003; Hodgkinson et al. 2004; Zhang et al. 2006). *DISC1* interacts with components of the cytoskeletal system such as NudE-like and the centromere proteins to impair neurite growth and development of the cerebral cortex (Kamiya et al. 2005).

Metabotropic Glutamate Receptor-3 (*GRM3*)

Single-nucleotide polymorphisms in *GRM3* have been implicated in schizophrenia (Egan et al. 2004; Fujii et al. 2003; Marti et al. 2002), one of which has been determined to influence prefrontal- and hippocampal-dependent tasks in both control and schizophrenic volunteers.

Effects of Risk Genes

Understanding the effects of risk genes will undoubtedly be complex. Even though several risk genes have been implicated, the precise variations in the genes are inconsistent, and until specific mutations are identified, it will be difficult to determine the biological effect of each risk gene. Another level of complexity to factor in is the interaction between risk genes as well as the interaction between the risk genes and environmental factors.

ENVIRONMENTAL FACTORS

The role of environmental factors in the development of schizophrenia is evident from the fact that monozygotic twins have less than 100% concordance rates of schizophrenia. The neurodevelopmental hypothesis of schizophrenia suggests that a disruption of brain development underlies the later emergence of psychosis during adulthood. Brain development occurs well into the third decade of life, and environmental influences can have an effect at any time from the early prenatal to the late adolescent period.

Pre- and Perinatal Factors

Pre- and perinatal factors include in utero stress such as exposure to toxins, nutritional deficiencies and severe maternal duress, and obstetrical complications. Infections have been postulated to be responsible for the association between winter births and schizophrenia. Offspring of mothers who had influenza during the second trimester had a twofold risk of developing schizophrenia (Mednick et al. 1988; O'Callaghan et al. 1991). Famine (Susser et al. 1996), significant maternal stress (Huttunen

and Niskanen 1978), or living through catastrophes (Van Os and Selten 1998) is associated with an increased risk of schizophrenia. In a meta-analysis, factors associated with schizophrenia were found to be related to certain complications of pregnancy, abnormal fetal growth and development, and hypoxic delivery complications (Cannon et al. 2002).

Childhood and Adolescent Factors

Social stress has been postulated to be a factor in the development of schizophrenia (Bebbington et al. 1993; Hirsch et al. 1996). Substantial evidence indicates that childhood neglect and abuse are risk factors for schizophrenia (for review, see Read et al. 2005; Whitfield et al. 2005). Adverse socioeconomic conditions (Wicks et al. 2005) and migration (Cantor-Graae and Selten 2005; Hutchinson et al. 1996; Sugarman et al. 1994) are also associated with the risk of developing psychosis.

Stimulants and cannabis are psychotomimetics. The association between cannabis use and psychosis is well established (Andreasson et al. 1987; Arseneault et al. 2002; Fergusson et al. 2003; Hall and Degenhardt 2000; van Os et al. 2002; Weiser et al. 2002; Zammit et al. 2002). Particular susceptibility of adolescents with genetic makeup (described in the next section) has been suggested (Caspi et al. 2005). It is important to put these risk factors in perspective. Although there is an association with the factors mentioned earlier, most individuals who experience these early adversities do not develop schizophrenia, perhaps suggesting the importance of genetic predisposition.

GENE-ENVIRONMENT INTERACTIONS

Both genetic and environmental factors are associated with schizophrenia. A currently accepted construct to understand schizophrenia entails a genetic vulnerability with environmental determinants of disease. In schizophrenia, specific evidence is accumulating to support gene-environment interactions. For example, adolescent cannabis use in individuals with the COMT Val/Val genotype greatly increased risk for developing schizophrenia spectrum disorders in later life (Caspi et al. 2005). Another example shows that among adoptees at high genetic risk for schizophrenia, those raised in dysfunctional adoptive families are more likely to develop schizophrenia or schizophrenia-spectrum disorders (Tienari and Wynne 1994; Wahlberg et al. 1997). Complex interactions between genetic and environmental factors are likely to occur, contributing to the etiology of schizophrenia. Investigators argue that an important impediment in understanding the neurobiology of schizophrenia is disease heterogeneity. Attempts are being made to define more homogeneous phenotypes of schizophrenia in persons with the illness and in family members ("intermediate phenotypes") to test these genetically.

ENDOPHENOTYPES

The features most often used to develop phenotypes in the illness are neurocognitive characteristics, eye movements (Avila et al. 2002; Ross et al. 2002; Sweeney et al. 1998), prepulse inhibition (Braff and Geyer 1990; Swerdlow and Geyer 1998), evoked potentials (R. Freedman 2003), and in vivo brain imaging features (reviewed in Gottesman and Gould 2003). These are spontaneous behaviors of the brain occurring in response to external cues that have a known neural anatomy and hence may be more direct reflections of neural pathology (Tregellas et al. 2004).

Smooth pursuit is the use of slow eye movement to track a small moving object. To carry out this function, the ocular motor system processes the motion of the target image on the retina and then generates a combination of fast (i.e., saccadic) and slow (i.e., smooth pursuit) eye movements to capture the image quickly on the fovea (Lisberger et al. 1987). Abnormalities in smooth-pursuit and saccadic eye movements have been extensively reported in schizophrenia (Holzman et al. 1984). The ability of some probands (60%–70%) with

schizophrenia to follow a smooth pendulum movement with their eyes is deficient. Instead of describing smooth movements following a pendulum stimulus, some show jerky and irregular (delayed and catch-up movements) tracking patterns. Also, antisaccadic eye movements (those directed away from a stimulus) are abnormal in persons with the illness (Thaker et al. 1989, 2000).

Neurophysiological studies have identified abnormalities in information processing that often can be elicited in the absence of a behavioral response. P300 evoked potential response is a reliable positive change in potential occurring about 300 ms after a task-relevant stimulus or an unexpected stimulus. P300 has increased latency and decreased amplitude in persons with schizophrenia. Although these electroencephalographic measures may vary with changes in symptoms, the P300 amplitude is consistently small in schizophrenia, even during relative remission of psychotic symptoms (Blackwood et al. 1991; Pfefferbaum et al. 1984).

Measures of sensory gating are obtained by examining a process called prepulse inhibition. Prepulse inhibition is a normal phenomenon evident across all sensory modalities, in which a small initial ("pre") stimulus decreases the electrophysiological response to a second, higher-intensity stimulus. In schizophrenia, many probands show abnormal prepulse inhibition, as do unaffected family members. The neural systems influencing both oculomotor movements and prepulse inhibition have been well described in animals and are believed to be highly conserved in humans (Swerdlow et al. 1994, 1999). P50 is an electrophysiological measure produced when two equal auditory stimuli are presented 500 ms apart and their evoked potential is measured. Healthy persons show a reduced response in amplitude to the second signal, whereas persons with schizophrenia (estimated at 80%) show less or no suppression. Detection of endophenotypes will help identify candidate genes and allow rational selection of molecular targets for further investigation.

HISTOLOGICAL AND NEUROCHEMICAL FEATURES OF SCHIZOPHRENIA

MAGNETIC RESONANCE IMAGING OF IN VIVO BRAIN STRUCTURE

Initial magnetic resonance imaging (MRI) studies detected a reduction in overall brain size, an increase in ventricular size, and variable cortical wasting in schizophrenia (Shelton and Weinberger 1987). The studies confirmed and extended older literature describing the examination of schizophrenic patients with computed axial tomography (CAT), which showed the ventricular enlargement with the cruder CAT technique (Johnstone et al. 1976). More recent MRI studies demonstrate a volume decrease in the medial temporal cortical structures, hippocampus, amygdala, and parahippocampal gyrus with some consistency, especially in the studies with dense sampling (Barta et al. 1990; Bogerts et al. 1990; Breier et al. 1992; Kuperberg et al. 2003; Lawrie et al. 2002; Suddath et al. 1990). Newer analytic techniques allowing shape analysis of the hippocampus have identified striking regional shape differences in the hippocampus in schizophrenia (Csernansky et al. 1998). Not only has the volume of the superior temporal gyrus been reported to be reduced in schizophrenia, but the magnitude of the reduction has been correlated with the presence of hallucinations (Menon et al. 1995; Shenton et al. 1992) and with electrophysiological changes in the patients (McCarley et al. 1993). Other studies have found increases in sulcal size, decreases in gray matter volume, and altered gyral patterns (Giuliani et al. 2005; Niznikiewicz et al. 2000; Pearlson and Marsh 1993); increases in white matter volume (Breier et al. 1992); and reductions in thalamic volume (Andreasen et al. 1994; Csernansky et al. 2004). Although positive MRI data can identify a brain area for further study, negative results do not rule out areas as pathologic. It is important to follow up the identification of structural abnormalities with functional, pharmacological, or electrophysiological techniques.

MICROSCOPIC ANALYSIS OF POSTMORTEM CENTRAL NERVOUS SYSTEM TISSUE

It is widely accepted that no obvious, currently identifiable neuropathological lesion is present in schizophrenia as occurs in Parkinson's disease or Alzheimer's dementia. Certainly a more subtle pathology must be the expectation.

A significant number of modern postmortem studies of pathology in tissue of schizophrenic persons have now been published (Bogerts 1993; Harrison 1999). The changes that have most consistently been found suggest a common localization for a neural defect in the illness (i.e., in the prefrontal and limbic cortex) but not necessarily a common neuropathological feature. The primary limbic structures in brain (namely, hippocampus, cingulate cortex, anterior thalamus, and mamillary bodies) and their intimately associated cortical areas (entorhinal cortex) often have been found to have pathological abnormalities in cell size (Jeste and Lohr 1989), cell number (Falkai and Bogerts 1986), area (Suddath et al. 1989), neuronal organization (Scheibel and Kovelman 1981), and gross structure (Colter et al. 1987).

The neocortex (especially frontal cortex) has been studied more recently, with varying reports of cell or tissue loss (Goldman-Rakic 1995; Heckers et al. 1991; Pakkenberg 1987; Rosenthal and Bigelow 1972). The thalamus, because of its pivotal position in relation to afferent sensory information and as a station in the cortical-subcortical circuits, has been the occasional object of study, with inconsistent but not negative results (Lesch and Bogerts 1984; Pakkenberg 1990; Treff and Hempel 1958).

Although these postmortem findings are highly provocative and interesting, replication and extension studies are critical to confirm the initial results obtained and reported with low subject numbers and specialized technical procedures. Although it is necessary to report early on these findings to inform the field, further replication is certainly necessary. These kinds of postmortem results are compelling in schizophrenia because their presence is theoretically consistent with the cognitive changes of the illness.

BIOCHEMICAL STUDIES IN SCHIZOPHRENIA

The compelling impetus to study biochemical measures in schizophrenia derived from the early pharmacological observation that blockade of dopamine receptors in the brain reduces psychotic symptoms in schizophrenia (Carlsson and Lindquist 1963). The hypothesis derived from this observation—namely, that dysfunction of the CNS dopaminergic system either in whole or in part accounts for psychosis in schizophrenia—has been explored in all body fluids and in various conditions of rest and stimulation over the last half-century (Davis et al. 1991; Elkashef et al. 1995) with little real support. Work comparing individual D_2-family receptors (D_2, D_3, and D_4) in tissue from neuroleptic-free schizophrenic persons with caudate nucleus or putamen tissue from healthy control subjects showed no differences in density of the D_2-family subtypes in striatum (Lahti et al. 1995a; Reynolds and Mason 1995). More recent imaging studies, however, showed higher occupancy of D_2 receptors by dopamine in patients with schizophrenia (Abi-Dargham et al. 2000) and changes in dopamine release in acute illness phases (Laruelle et al. 1999), suggesting that a defect exists in the release of dopamine in the disease.

Other transmitter systems have more recently drawn interest as well, including serotonergic systems (Reynolds 1983; van Praag 1983), peptidergic (Nemeroff et al. 1983; Widerlöv et al. 1982), and most recently glutamatergic systems (reviewed in Tamminga 1998). Because of its ubiquitous and prominent location in the CNS, and because the antiglutamatergic drugs phencyclidine (PCP) and ketamine cause a schizophrenic-like reaction in humans, the glutamate system has become a focus of study. Alterations in the composition of the NMDA-sensitive glutamate receptor in

prefrontal cortex and hippocampus have been reported (Gao et al. 2000; Meador-Woodruff and Healy 2000). Most studies have focused on the mesial temporal lobe, and many have reported abnormalities in α-amino-3-hydroxy-5-methylisoxazole-4–propionic acid (AMPA), kainate, and NMDA receptor expression at the mRNA, protein, and ligand-binding level. Studies in the prefrontal cortex have been inconsistent, although AMPA abnormalities probably exist (Dracheva et al. 2005; Scarr et al. 2005). Other brain regions, such as the thalamus, show abnormal ionotropic receptor expression (Ibrahim et al. 2000). The group II metabotropic glutamate (mGluR2 and 3) receptors are implicated in animal (Moghaddam and Adams 1998) and human (Krystal et al. 2005) studies of schizophrenia. An endogenous agonist of mGluR3, N-acetylaspartylglutamate (Coyle 1997; Neale et al. 2000), and its metabolic enzyme (Ghose et al. 2004; Tsai et al. 1995) are abnormally expressed in the schizophrenic brain. It is also interesting to note that mGluR3 may be a risk gene for schizophrenia (Egan et al. 2004).

Akbarian and colleagues (1995) and Volk et al. (2000) reported decreased expression of glutamic acid decarboxylase (GAD) mRNA in prefrontal cortex of schizophrenic persons without significant cell loss. Evidence of γ-aminobutyric acid (GABA)–ergic involvement is found in reduced expression of presynaptic markers in subpopulations of interneurons in the frontal cortex and the hippocampal formation (Benes and Berretta 2001; Lewis et al. 2004). GABAergic neurons can be defined by the presence of one of three calcium-binding proteins—namely, parvalbumin, calretinin, and calbindin. The most characteristic morphological types of neurons that express parvalbumin are the large basket and chandelier cells (Lewis and Lund 1990). Decreased 67-kDa glutamic acid decarboxylase (GAD 67) and GABA transporter subtype 1 (GAT1) are found in the parvalbumin-expressing prefrontal interneurons (Lewis et al. 2005).

Serotonin was hypothesized to be central to the pathophysiology of schizophrenia because of the psychotomimetic actions of serotonergic drugs, such as lysergic acid diethylamide (LSD) (D.X. Freedman 1975). More recently, the affinity of newer antipsychotic drugs for serotonergic receptors has raised further speculation over the role of this neurotransmitter system in the pathophysiology of the illness. Further, drugs without any dopamine receptor affinity, but with only serotonin type 2A ($5\text{-}HT_{2A}$) receptor antagonism, do behave as antipsychotic drugs in animal models and show antipsychotic activity in humans (de Paulis 2001). The serotonin system has diverse receptors and functions, and it is not surprising that this aspect is not yet fully explored.

Clinically, it is well known that schizophrenic patients have a much higher incidence of cigarette smoking (Hughes et al. 1986). The upregulation in nicotinic receptors (Benwell et al. 1988; Wonnacott 1990) seen in "normal" smokers is not seen in schizophrenia. On the contrary, decreased levels of nicotinic and muscarinic receptors are reported in the hippocampus, frontal cortex, thalamus, and striatum in schizophrenia (Hyde and Crook 2001). In addition, cholinergic neurotransmission is known to be integral to cognition and memory, functions disrupted in schizophrenia. These findings suggest cholinergic dysfunction in schizophrenia.

In summary, molecular abnormalities are found in several anatomical regions and in several neurotransmitter systems in the neuropathology of schizophrenia. Abnormalities in molecular targets should be examined in terms of pathways (not only neurotransmitter pathways) affecting circuit function. Additionally, identification of primary pathology from epiphenomena is essential. For example, neurotransmitter systems are dynamic, and disruption of one system would lead to compensatory mechanisms in other relevant pathways. Universal cautions in reviewing any schizophrenia neuropathological studies include careful attention to the possible confounds of tissue artifacts, long-term neuroleptic treatment, lifelong altered mental state, and relevant demographic factors. Converging data from in vivo human studies, postmortem human studies, and animal model studies would provide clues to the primary pathology.

FUNCTIONAL STUDIES IN SCHIZOPHRENIA WITH IN VIVO IMAGING TECHNIQUES

The advances made in neuroimaging technology now allow us to study neurochemical and physiological changes in the living human brain. Functional BOLD (blood oxygen level dependent) MRI indirectly measures changes in regional cerebral blood flow (rCBF), which reflects regional brain activity.

FUNCTIONAL IMAGING

rCBF studies have identified frontal cortex blood flow abnormalities associated with impaired task performance (e.g., the Wisconsin Card Sorting Test) (reviewed in Holcomb et al. 1989). A meta-analysis suggested that hypofrontality at rest is found in schizophrenia (Hill et al. 2004). Although the potential confound exists of antipsychotic drug action reducing prefrontal cortex perfusion and activation, most studies where this is examined do find prefrontal reductions independent of drug. Studies have certainly confirmed frontal cortex alterations in schizophrenia with variable, complex, and still incompletely understood characteristics.

Fluorodeoxyglucose positron emission tomography (FDG PET) in young, medication-free, floridly psychotic schizophrenic individuals (Tamminga et al. 1992) reveal reduced metabolism in schizophrenia in limbic structures (anterior cingulate and hippocampal cortices) (Figure 14–1). Within the schizophrenic group, primary negative-symptom patients showed the additional abnormalities of reduced metabolism in frontal and parietal cortices and thalamus compared with the non-negative-symptom group. Both of these findings (limbic changes overall in schizophrenia and frontal cortex reductions in negative symptoms) are consistent with considerable other literature in their regional localization (Andreasen et al. 1992; Tamminga et al. 1992).

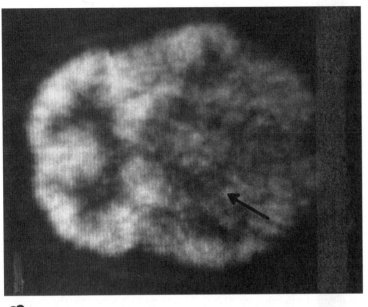

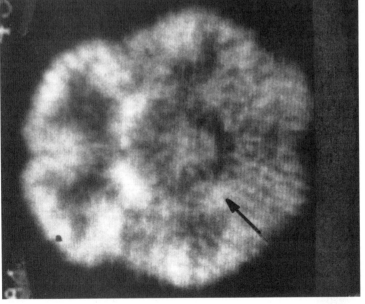

FIGURE 14–1.   Positron emission tomography images with fluorodeoxyglucose.

Both images are at the same axial level and show, among other areas, the medial temporal structures. *Panel A.* Image from a healthy control subject; the general area of parahippocampal gyrus/hippocampus is indicated by the *arrow.* *Panel B.* The schizophrenic individual has a remarkable reduction in glucose metabolism in the medial temporal structures (*arrow*). This reduction in parahippocampal gyrus metabolism is representative of differences in the entire schizophrenic group.

Liddle and colleagues (1992) studied the correlation between well-delineated symptom clusters in schizophrenia (negative symptoms, hallucinations or delusions, and disorganization) and rCBF. Negative symptoms were negatively associated with rCBF in left frontal cortex and left parietal areas. Hallucinations and delusions were positively associated with flow in the left parahippocampal gyrus and the left ventral striatum. Disorganization was associated with flow in anterior cingulate cortex and mediodorsal thalamus. This study showed that brain areas are differently involved in symptom manifestations in schizophrenia, perhaps as either a cause or an effect of the disorder. Silbersweig et al. (1995) scanned hallucinating schizophrenic persons to show involvement of specific brain regions with psychosis.

Other studies also have found evidence for limbic abnormalities in schizophrenia both at rest (Taylor et al. 1999) and with cognitive challenge (Artiges et al. 2000; Heckers et al. 1998; Spence et al. 1997). Heckers et al. (1998) found reduced hippocampal activation in schizophrenic subjects during a memory retrieval task. These limbic region abnormalities are probably the result of a dysfunctional network of regions and not a series of separate lesions.

Imaging during pharmacological manipulation of the NMDA-sensitive glutamate receptor system identifies specific brain regions that correlate with the severity of psychosis. PCP, an NMDA antagonist, can induce a psychotic state in nonschizophrenic persons characterized by many of the signs and symptoms often found in schizophrenia. Moreover, PCP (Luby et al. 1959) and ketamine (Lahti et al. 1995b) can both selectively exacerbate a patient's psychotic symptoms in schizophrenia. Ketamine alters rCBF in hippocampal and anterior cingulate cortices. Ketamine stimulates positive, not negative, symptoms in schizophrenia, and its action is not blocked by dopamine receptor antagonism (Lahti et al. 1995b). This action of ketamine would be most parsimoniously explained by assuming that the drug stimulates a brain system that is already active in mediating (possibly even in originating) the psychosis.

We used $H_2{}^{15}O$ and PET to study the localization and time course of ketamine action in brain by measuring rCBF (Figure 14–2). Schizophrenic subjects who were taking a dose of ketamine active in exacerbating psychosis (0.3 mg/kg) showed increased rCBF in the anterior cingulate gyrus and decreased rCBF in hippocampus and lingual gyrus (Lahti et al. 1995a), each with different time course patterns, suggesting that each area of brain has its own sensitivity to ketamine. Questions of how this ketamine-induced psychosis stimulation might be related to schizophrenia still need to be answered.

Abnormal functional connections between brain regions have been suggested as the cause of abnormal rCBF patterns seen in schizophrenia (Frith et al. 1995; Weinberger et al. 1992). In studies of verbal fluency (Spence et al. 2000) and semantic processing (Jennings et al. 1998), a network analysis identified a functional disconnection between the anterior cingulate and prefrontal regions of schizophrenic subjects. Frontal lobe functional connectivity was abnormal in the schizophrenic subjects, even though they had significantly activated the regions and their behavior on the tasks was not impaired. These findings suggest that the abnormalities seen in the frontal lobes of schizophrenic persons may be a problem of integration across regions as well as a specific regional abnormality.

NEURORECEPTOR IMAGING

Neuroreceptor single-photon emission computed tomography (SPECT) and PET imaging allows the direct assessments of receptor density and indirect estimations of neurotransmitter release in the living brain. Human brain imaging ligand studies suggested abnormalities in D_1 receptor density in the frontal cortex of persons with schizophrenia (Karlsson et al. 2002), leading to speculation that an agonist at the D_1 receptor may be therapeutic in treating cognitive dysfunctions in schizophrenia (Goldman-Rakic et al. 2004). Imaging studies with D_2 receptor ligands reported increases in D_2-family receptors in neuroleptic-naive and neuroleptic-free schizophrenia (Wong et al.

SPM, $P<0.01$, $n=5$, 6 minutes

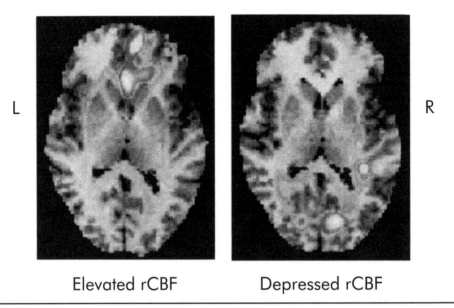

L   R

Elevated rCBF   Depressed rCBF

FIGURE 14-2. Regional cerebral blood flow (rCBF) localization of ketamine action in schizophrenic brain.

See Appendix for color version. rCBF increases occurred in anterior cingulate gyrus, extending to medial frontal areas (*left scan*); rCBF decreases are apparent in the hippocampus and lingual gyrus (*right scan*). The areas indicating significant flow change are plotted onto a magnetic resonance imaging template for ease of localization. SPM = statistical parametric mapping.

Source. Images contributed by Dr. Henry Holcomb and Dr. Adrienne Lahti.

1986), but subsequent studies did not replicate this finding (Farde et al. 1990; Hietala et al. 1991; Martinot et al. 1990, 1991).

More recently, Laruelle et al. (1996) measured dopamine release into the synapse by using SPECT or PET imaging with low-affinity dopamine receptor ligands. They reported that persons with schizophrenia had an increased release of dopamine in the striatum in response to amphetamine challenge (Abi-Dargham et al. 1998; Laruelle et al. 1999). This increase in dopaminergic tone in the striatum appears, at least in part, to be under glutamatergic regulation (Kegeles et al. 2000; Smith et al. 1998).

CLINICAL THERAPEUTICS IN SCHIZOPHRENIA

Advances in clinical therapeutics in schizophrenia have all been empirical, not theoretical, and rarely rational. Chlorpromazine was first tested in schizophrenic patients because of its known sedative properties as a preanesthetic agent (Delay and Deniker 1952). Its selective antipsychotic activity was immediately noted, and this became the springboard for hypotheses of altered dopaminergic transmission in schizophrenia.

The conventional antipsychotics (butyrophenones, phenothiazines, and thioxanthenes) with potent antidopaminergic activity were used successfully to treat psychosis for 50 years, albeit with acute and chronic motor side effects. These drugs have vastly improved the lives of those afflicted with schizophrenia; however, these patients still endure considerable residual symptom burden and lifelong psychosocial impairments. In 1990, newer drugs were introduced with higher antiserotonergic potency accompanying the dopamine receptor blockade. These drugs were less likely to cause motor side effects and dysphoria but had their own serious side effects. The metabolic syndrome (weight gain, hyperlipidemia, diabetes, hypertension) is a side effect of concern with many of the new antipsychotics. Clozapine remains the only antipsychotic with demonstrably greater antipsychotic efficacy; the mechanism of its better effect is still not known. In recent years, the concept of partial agonism at the D_2 receptors has added a novel and interesting perspective to the pharmacotherapy for schizophrenia (Carlsson et al. 2001). The efficacy of the first D_2 partial agonist, aripiprazole, has been established in preclinical trials, resulting in its approval by the U.S. Food and Drug Administration for the treatment of schizophrenia.

Existing treatments of schizophrenia generally have been unsuccessful in treating cognitive deficits in schizophrenia. There is controversy over whether second-generation antipsychotics improve cognition more than classic antipsychotics do (Green et al. 2002; Meltzer and McGurk 1999; Meltzer and Sumiyoshi 2003). The MATRICS (measurement and treatment research to improve cognition in schizophrenia) program was developed to identify potential molecular targets to treat cognitive deficits in schizophrenia (Geyer and Tamminga 2004). The molecular targets identified as having the greatest promise to improve cognition include the D_1 receptor (Goldman-Rakic et al. 2004), α_7 nicotinic receptor (Martin et al. 2004), muscarinic receptor (Friedman 2004), 5-HT$_{1A}$ and 5-HT$_{2A}$ receptors (Roth et al. 2004), noradrenergic receptors (Arnsten 2004), and the NMDA receptor (Coyle and Tsai 2004). The metabotropic glutamate receptors mGluR2, 3, and 5 modulate NMDA receptor function and also may provide a means to enhance cognition (Moghaddam 2004). Agonists of these receptors are being evaluated as new adjunctive drug treatments, and not as alternatives to current antipsychotics, in schizophrenia. Thus, they will be tested in volunteers whose positive symptoms are optimally treated and stable. For example, we are currently testing atomoxetine, a norepinephrine reuptake inhibitor that increases norepinephrine and dopamine levels in the frontal cortex, and M_1 muscarinic agonists (N-desmethyl clozapine, a derivative of clozapine with M_1 agonist properties).

INTEGRATIVE BASIC BRAIN MECHANISMS IMPORTANT TO UNDERSTANDING CEREBRAL FUNCTION

Systems neuroscience, the study of the function of neural circuits, is concerned with the functional organization and processing of information in cellular networks, thereby linking molecular and cellular biology to behaviors such as cognitive, motivational, perceptual, and motor processes. In schizophrenia, specific neural networks may underlie each of the symptom domains. The degree of dysfunction in neural systems may vary, and predominantly affected systems may have a greater effect on the clinical presentation. The notion is that abnormal networks, not just an abnormal protein, are found in schizophrenia. This neural system–based approach provides a plausible and scientifically sound framework in which to conceptualize the pathophysiology of schizophrenia.

CORTICAL-SUBCORTICAL CIRCUITS

Alexander and DeLong (Alexander and Crutcher 1990; Alexander et al. 1986; DeLong 1990) described multiple parallel segregated neural circuits that connect specific areas of the frontal cortex reciprocally with specific regions of the basal ganglia and thalamus. Parallel, segregated neuronal tracts project from specific areas in the frontal cortex to homologous target areas of basal ganglia, organized somatotopically and by functional system (for example, motor, oculomotor, limbic, prefrontal). Both within the basal ganglia and within the thalamus, the somatotopic organization is preserved.

This same feedback system mechanism was postulated to also be operative in other frontal functions (memory, attention, and other aspects of cognition) (Alexander et al. 1986). Schizophrenia, by extrapolation, could hypothetically result from abnormal regulation of aspects of frontal cortical function. Findings from human imaging and postmortem studies in schizophrenia provide a basis for us to speculate on the neural circuits that may underlie symptom domains described earlier (Figure 14–3).

SYMPTOM CLUSTER CIRCUITS

Psychosis Neural Circuit

Significant association between regional cerebral glucose metabolic rate in the limbic cortex (anterior cingulate cortex plus hippocampus) and the magnitude of positive symptoms was seen in medication-free schizophrenic volunteers (Tamminga et al. 1992). These studies allow us to speculate that the limbic cortex is associated with the positive symptoms of the illness, whereas the prefrontal cortex may support negative and cognitive symptoms. The anterior cingulate cortex and adjacent medial prefrontal cortex correlate with induction of positive symptoms with the NMDA antagonist ketamine (Lahti et al. 1995a). PET scanning in hallucinating schizophrenic persons is associated with activations in the medial prefrontal cortex, left superior temporal gyrus, right medial temporal gyrus, left hippocampus/parahippocampal region, thalamus, putamen, and cingulate (Copolov et al. 2003; Silbersweig et al. 1995). These studies provide clues to the anatomical structures that may be involved in a "psychosis neural circuit." Limbic regions, in particular, are frequently implicated in these in vivo studies. We postulate that a core pathology in the hippocampus affects other brain regions (e.g., the anterior cingulate cortex and medial prefrontal cortex) in the network. The proposed psychosis circuit consists of the anterior hippocampus, anterior cingulate, medial prefrontal cortex (Brodmann area 32), thalamus, ventral pallidum, striatum, and substantia nigra/ventral tegmental area (see Figure 14–3).

Negative Affect Neural Circuit

Brain activation patterns associated with negative symptoms show hypoactivation of the frontal lobe (Andreasen et al. 1992, 1994;

Schroeder et al. 1994; Volkow et al. 1987; Wolkin et al. 1992). Decreased rCBF is seen in both the prefrontal and the parietal cortices of schizophrenic persons experiencing negative symptoms (Friston 1992; Liddle et al. 1992; Tamminga et al. 1992). The dorsolateral prefrontal cortex and parietal cortex have dense reciprocal interconnections, suggesting a close functional relation (Schwartz and Goldman-Rakic 1984). This may explain the observation that individuals with deficit forms of schizophrenia have greater impairment in cognitive performance (Buchanan et al. 1994, 1997). Another study in patients with predominantly negative symptoms implicated the medial prefrontal, dorsolateral, and prefrontal cortices (Potkin et al. 2002). Lower activity also was noted in the thalamus (Tamminga et al. 1992), particularly the mediodorsal nucleus of the thalamus (Hazlett et al. 2004). The amygdala, a key component in the circuit of emotion, is implicated in emotional processing in schizophrenia (R.E. Gur et al. 2002). The neural system we propose for the negative symptom cluster includes the dorsolateral prefrontal cortex, parietal cortex, amygdala, anterior hippocampus, thalamus, ventral pallidum, striatum, and substantia nigra/ventral tegmental area.

Cognitive Deficit Neural Circuit

Abnormalities seen in the frontal lobes of schizophrenic patients may be the result of a problem of integration across regions and not a single regional abnormality (Jennings et al. 1998; Spence et al. 2000). rCBF increases in prefrontal regions with greater working memory demands, but if working memory capacity is exceeded, the activation decreases (Callicott et al. 1999). In separate studies, disorganization was associated with flow in anterior cingulate and mediodorsal thalamus (Liddle et al. 1992), whereas apomorphine, a dopamine agonist that has antipsychotic properties, normalizes anterior cingulate blood flow of schizophrenic persons during verbal fluency task performance (Dolan et al. 1995). We propose that a neural system for cognitive deficits

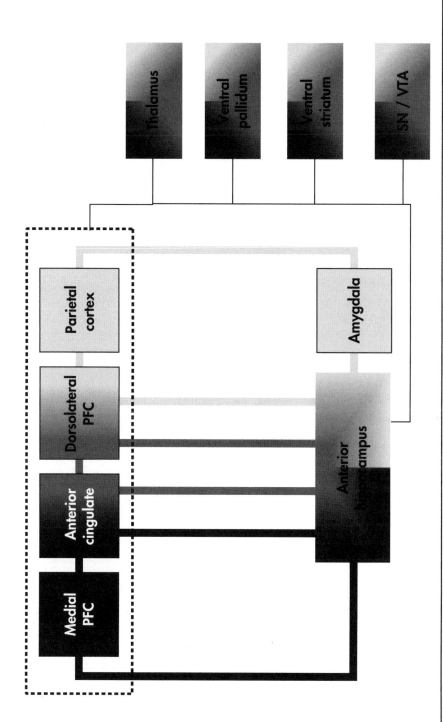

FIGURE 14–3. Hypothetical neural circuits underlying the three symptom domains of schizophrenia.

See Appendix for color version. In this model, a specific neural circuit underlies each of the symptom domains—the psychosis circuit (*dark shading*), cognitive deficit circuit (*medium shading*), and negative symptom circuit (*light shading*). The *dotted line* represents neocortex. Core deficits in the anterior hippocampus can influence functional integrity of each of these circuits. PFC = prefrontal cortex; SN/VTA = substantia nigra/ventral tegmental area.

involves the dorsolateral prefrontal cortex, anterior hippocampus, anterior cingulate, thalamus, ventral pallidum, striatum, and substantia nigra/ventral tegmental area.

SYNTHESIS

CLINICAL OBSERVATIONS ABOUT SCHIZOPHRENIA IMPORTANT FOR FORMULATING PATHOPHYSIOLOGY

Several characteristics of schizophrenic illness are strikingly consistent across clinics, laboratories, and cultures, such that any theory of the illness must take them into account. These include but are not limited to the following: schizophrenic symptoms are clear and their clustering is common but not exclusive; symptoms fluctuate during the course of illness and may disappear entirely between episodes but then reappear; and the illness is most often lifelong, with the most flagrant symptoms and psychosocial deterioration appearing early in the illness, showing a plateau during middle years, and frequently ending with some degree of symptom resolution in later years. The illness has a genetic component but is by no means fully genetically determined. Each candidate risk gene confers a small degree of risk, and it is likely that gene-environment interactions play a crucial etiological role in the disease. Although no traditional anatomical or biochemical change has come to be pathognomonic of the illness, it is in the limbic system (especially the hippocampus and entorhinal and cingulate cortices) and prefrontal cortices that anatomical and functional changes, albeit of a varied pathological nature, are highly concentrated.

Schizophrenic subjects, even when they are performing equivalently to healthy control subjects on a task, use similar brain areas but activate them prematurely and not in relation to difficulty. Evidence of consistent, highly replicable biochemical change in the brain in schizophrenia has yet evaded the study of this illness. This does not mean that these parameters should not be studied, but it might suggest that only a composite biochemical change will give a clue (see, e.g., Issa et al. 1994a, 1994b)

or that an entirely new (perhaps functional) approach is needed.

PITFALLS AND CONFOUNDS IN SCHIZOPHRENIA STUDIES

Schizophrenia is a difficult disease to study biologically for methodological and theoretical reasons. The brain is a highly protected organ whose tissue or integrated function cannot easily be sampled in vivo, even in illness. Schizophrenic individuals themselves often have compromised cognitive ability, and they may not be able to collaborate fully with a demanding research study. The long-term use of neuroleptic drugs is almost ubiquitous in schizophrenia and regularly confounds biological study. This long-term treatment alters much of the brain neurochemistry, as well as aspects of its structure, portions of its function, and probably more. Neuroleptic withdrawal for biological study is difficult because it frequently results in symptom reemergence. Symptom diversity is a hallmark of the illness, as is symptom fluctuation over time and within single individuals. Moreover, this diversity and fluctuation are most often masked by neuroleptic treatment in what we would have to assume is a complex manner. Although they are difficult to manage for experimental designs, these issues can be worked with through careful clinical, pharmacological, genetic, and imaging assessment. Certainly these areas are always important parameters to assess in evaluating study results.

TOWARD A PATHOPHYSIOLOGY OF SCHIZOPHRENIA

Our understanding of the pathophysiology of schizophrenia is still obscure, and it is becoming evident that schizophrenia is not one disease but rather a syndrome. The identification of candidate risk genes, specific developmental environmental factors, and the effects of gene-environment interactions speaks to the heterogeneity we can expect to find in schizophrenia. A shift in conceptual framework from searching for a specific protein defect in schizophrenia to a search for defects in neural networks may represent a plausible biological approach to investigating the pathophysiology of schizophrenia. Identification of relevant neural systems and an understanding of the dynamics of the systems would provide a model to test function. As an initial formulation, we have proposed neural networks for each of the symptom domains. This formulation proposes that core pathology in the hippocampus influences the function of networks involving distinct cortical regions and subcortical structures.

Studies of schizophrenia are proceeding on many fronts. Investigators use information from patients, family members, birth records, and life histories, along with in vivo imaging, postmortem tissue, and phenomenological presentation, to formulate hypotheses. Translational research techniques with high sensitivity and resolution are now becoming available. Moreover, the techniques are broad and use molecular and functional probes as well as traditional measures. Productive leads are being used to target novel drug discovery, and new information in this area may inform our ideas of pathophysiology and etiology. Although the exact nature of schizophrenia is now unknown, it is not likely to remain unknown for long.

RECOMMENDED READINGS

Harrison PJ, Weinberger DR: Schizophrenia genes, gene expression, and neuropathology: on the matter of their convergence. Mol Psychiatry 10:40–68, 2005

Maki P, Veijola J, Jones PB, et al: Predictors of schizophrenia: a review. Br Med Bull 73–74:1–15, 2005

REFERENCES

Abi-Dargham A, Gil R, Krystal J, et al: Increased striatal dopamine transmission in schizophrenia: confirmation in a second cohort. Am J Psychiatry 155:761–767, 1998

Abi-Dargham A, Rodenhiser J, Printz D, et al: Increased baseline occupancy of D_2 receptors by dopamine in schizophrenia. Proc Natl Acad Sci USA 97:8104–8109, 2000

Adams ME, Kramarcy N, Krall SP, et al: Absence of alpha-syntrophin leads to structurally aberrant neuromuscular synapses deficient in utrophin. J Cell Biol 150:1385–1398, 2000

Addington AM, Gornick M, Sporn AL, et al: Polymorphisms in the 13q33.2 gene G72/G30 are associated with childhood-onset schizophrenia and psychosis not otherwise specified. Biol Psychiatry 55:976–980, 2004

Akbarian S, Kim JJ, Potkin SG, et al: Gene expression for glutamic acid decarboxylase is reduced without loss of neurons in prefrontal cortex of schizophrenics. Arch Gen Psychiatry 52:258–266, 1995

Alexander GE, Crutcher MD: Functional architecture of basal ganglia circuits: neural substrates of parallel processing. Trends Neurosci 13:266–271, 1990

Alexander GE, DeLong MR, Strick PL: Parallel organization of functionally segregated circuits linking basal ganglia and cortex. Annu Rev Neurosci 9:357–381, 1986

American Psychiatric Association: Diagnostic and Statistical Manual of Mental Disorders, 4th Edition, Text Revision. Washington, DC, American Psychiatric Association, 2000

Andreasen NC, Rezai K, Alliger R, et al: Hypofrontality in neuroleptic-naive patients and in patients with chronic schizophrenia. Arch Gen Psychiatry 49:943–958, 1992

Andreasen NC, Arndt S, Swayze V II, et al: Thalamic abnormalities in schizophrenia visualized through magnetic resonance image averaging. Science 266:294–298, 1994

Andreasen NC, Arndt S, Alliger R, et al: Symptoms of schizophrenia: methods, meanings, and mechanisms. Arch Gen Psychiatry 52:341–351, 1995

Andreasson S, Allebeck P, Engstrom A, et al: Cannabis and schizophrenia: a longitudinal study of Swedish conscripts. Lancet 2:1483–1486, 1987

Arndt S, Alliger RJ, Andreasen NC: The distinction of positive and negative symptoms: the failure of a two-dimensional model. Br J Psychiatry 158:317–322, 1991

Arnsten AFT: Adrenergic targets for the treatment of cognitive deficits in schizophrenia. Psychopharmacology (Berl) 174:25–31, 2004

Arseneault L, Cannon M, Poulton R, et al: Cannabis use in adolescence and risk for adult psychosis: longitudinal prospective study. BMJ 325:1212–1213, 2002

Artiges E, Salame P, Recasens C, et al: Working memory control in patients with schizophrenia: a PET study during a random number generation task. Am J Psychiatry 157:1517–1519, 2000

Avila MT, Hong E, Thaker GK: Current progress in schizophrenia research: eye movement abnormalities in schizophrenia: what is the nature of the deficit? J Nerv Ment Dis 190:479–480, 2002

Barnes TR, Liddle PF: Evidence for the validity of negative symptoms. Mod Probl Pharmacopsychiatry 24:43–72, 1990

Barr CE, Mednick SA, Munk-Jorgensen P: Exposure to influenza epidemics during gestation and adult schizophrenia: a 40-year study. Arch Gen Psychiatry 47:869–874, 1990

Barta PE, Pearlson GD, Powers RE, et al: Auditory hallucinations and smaller superior temporal gyral volume in schizophrenia. Am J Psychiatry 146:1457–1462, 1990

Bebbington P, Wilkins S, Jones P, et al: Life events and psychosis: initial results from the Camberwell Collaborative Psychosis Study. Br J Psychiatry 162:72–79, 1993

Benes FM, Berretta S: GABAergic interneurons: implications for understanding schizophrenia and bipolar disorder. Neuropsychopharmacology 25:1–27, 2001

Benwell MEM, Balfour DJK, Anderson JM: Evidence that tobacco smoking increases the density of [3H]nicotine binding sites in human brain. J Neurochem 50:1243–1247, 1988

Bertolino A, Caforio G, Blasi G, et al: Interaction of *COMT* (Val(108/158)Met) genotype and olanzapine treatment on prefrontal cortical function in patients with schizophrenia. Am J Psychiatry 161:1798–1805, 2004

Blackwood DH, St Clair DM, Muir WJ, et al: Auditory P300 and eye tracking dysfunction in schizophrenic pedigrees. Arch Gen Psychiatry 48:899–909, 1991

Bleuler M: The Schizophrenic Disorders: Long-Term Patient and Family Studies. Translated by Clemens SM. New Haven, CT, Yale University Press, 1978

Bogerts B: Recent advances in the neuropathology of schizophrenia. Schizophr Bull 19:431–445, 1993

Bogerts B, Ashtari M, Degreef G, et al: Reduced temporal limbic structure volumes on magnetic resonance images in first episode schizophrenia. Psychiatry Res 35:1–13, 1990

Braff DL, Geyer MA: Sensorimotor gating and schizophrenia: human and animal model studies. Arch Gen Psychiatry 47:181–188, 1990

Braff DL, Heaton R, Kuck J, et al: The generalized pattern of neuropsychological deficits in outpatients with chronic schizophrenia with heterogeneous Wisconsin Card Sorting Test results. Arch Gen Psychiatry 48:891–898, 1991

Breier A, Buchanan RW, Elkashef A, et al: Brain morphology and schizophrenia: a magnetic resonance imaging study of limbic, prefrontal cortex, and caudate structures. Arch Gen Psychiatry 49:921–926, 1992

Buchanan RW, Strauss ME, Kirkpatrick B, et al: Neuropsychological impairments in deficit vs nondeficit forms of schizophrenia. Arch Gen Psychiatry 51:804–811, 1994

Buchanan RW, Strauss ME, Breier A, et al: Attentional impairments in deficit and nondeficit forms of schizophrenia. Am J Psychiatry 154:363–370, 1997

Buchanan RW, Breier A, Kirkpatrick B, et al: Positive and negative symptom response to clozapine in schizophrenic patients with and without the deficit syndrome. Am J Psychiatry 155:751–760, 1998

Callicott JH, Mattay VS, Bertolino A, et al: Physiological characteristics of capacity constraints in working memory as revealed by functional MRI. Cereb Cortex 9:20–26, 1999

Callicott JH, Straub RE, Pezawas L, et al: Variation in *DISC1* affects hippocampal structure and function and increases risk for schizophrenia. Proc Natl Acad Sci USA 102:8627–8632, 2005

Cannon M, Jones PB, Murray RM: Obstetric complications and schizophrenia: historical and meta-analytic review. Am J Psychiatry 159:1080–1092, 2002

Cardno AG, Gottesman II: Twin studies of schizophrenia: from bow-and-arrow concordances to star wars Mx and functional genomics. Am J Med Genet 97:12–17, 2000

Cantor-Graae E, Selten JP: Schizophrenia and migration: a meta-analysis and review. Am J Psychiatry 162:12–24, 2005

Carlsson A, Lindquist M: Effect of chlorpromazine and haloperidol on formation of 3-methoxytyramine and normetanephrine in mouse brain. Acta Pharmacol Toxicol 20:140–144, 1963

Carlsson A, Waters N, Holm-Waters S, et al: Interactions between monoamines, glutamate, and GABA in schizophrenia: new evidence. Annu Rev Pharmacol Toxicol 41:237–260, 2001

Carpenter WT Jr, Buchanan RW: Domains of psychopathology relevant to the study of etiology and treatment in schizophrenia, in Schizophrenia: Scientific Progress. Edited by Schulz SC, Tamminga CA. New York, Oxford University Press, 1989, pp 13–22

Carpenter WT Jr, Buchanan RW: Schizophrenia. N Engl J Med 330:681–690, 1994

Carpenter WT Jr, Buchanan RW, Kirkpatrick B, et al: Strong inference, theory testing and the neuroanatomy of schizophrenia. Arch Gen Psychiatry 50:825–831, 1993

Caspi A, Moffitt TE, Cannon M, et al: Moderation of the effect of adolescent-onset cannabis use on adult psychosis by a functional polymorphism in the catechol-O-methyltransferase gene: longitudinal evidence of a gene × environment interaction. Biol Psychiatry 57:1117–1127, 2005

Chen X, Wang X, O'Neill AF, et al: Variants in the catechol-O-methyltransferase (COMT) gene are associated with schizophrenia in Irish high-density families. Mol Psychiatry 9:962–967, 2004

Chowdari KV, Mirnics K, Semwal P, et al: Association and linkage analyses of RGS4 polymorphisms in schizophrenia. Hum Mol Genet 11:1373–1380, 2002

Chumakov I, Blumenfeld M, Guerassimenko O, et al: Genetic and physiological data implicating the new human gene G72 and the gene for D-amino acid oxidase in schizophrenia. Proc Natl Acad Sci USA 99:13675–13680, 2002

Ciompi L, Müller C: Lebensweg und Alter der Schizophrenen: Eine katamnestische Langzeitstudie bis ins Senium. Berlin, Springer-Verlag, 1976

Colter N, Battal S, Crow TJ: White matter reduction in the parahippocampal gyrus of patients with schizophrenia. Arch Gen Psychiatry 44:1023–1026, 1987

Copolov DL, Seal ML, Maruff P, et al: Cortical activation associated with the experience of auditory hallucinations and perception of human speech in schizophrenia: a PET correlation study. Psychiatry Res 122:139–152, 2003

Corvin AP, Morris DW, McGhee K, et al: Confirmation and refinement of an "at-risk" haplotype for schizophrenia suggests the EST cluster, Hs.97362, as a potential susceptibility gene at the Neuregulin-1 locus. Mol Psychiatry 9:208–213, 2004

Coyle JT: The nagging question of the function of N-acetylaspartylglutamate. Neurobiol Dis 4:231–238, 1997

Coyle JT, Tsai G: The NMDA receptor glycine modulatory site: a therapeutic target for improving cognition and reducing negative symptoms in schizophrenia. Psychopharmacology (Berl) 174:32–38, 2004

Csernansky JG, Joshi S, Wang L, et al: Hippocampal morphometry in schizophrenia by high dimensional brain mapping. Proc Natl Acad Sci USA 95:11406–11411, 1998

Csernansky JG, Schindler MK, Splinter NR, et al: Abnormalities of thalamic volume and shape in schizophrenia. Am J Psychiatry 161:896–902, 2004

Davis KL, Kahn RS, Ko G, et al: Dopamine in schizophrenia: a review and reconceptualization. Am J Psychiatry 148:1474–1486, 1991

de Frias CM, Annerbrink K, Westberg L, et al: COMT gene polymorphism is associated with declarative memory in adulthood and old age. Behav Genet 34:533–539, 2004

Delay J, Deniker P: Le traitement des psychoses par une méthode neurolytique dérivée de l'hibernothérapie, in Congress des Médecins Aliénistes et Neurologistes de France. Luxembourg, 1952, pp 497–502

DeLong MR: Primate models of movement disorders of basal ganglia origin. Trends Neurosci 13:281–285, 1990

de Paulis T: M-100907 (Aventis). Curr Opin Investig Drugs 2:123–132, 2001

Dolan RJ, Fletcher P, Frith CD, et al: Dopaminergic modulation of impaired cognitive activation in the anterior cingulate cortex in schizophrenia. Nature 378:180–182, 1995

Dracheva S, McGurk SR, Haroutunian V: mRNA expression of AMPA receptors and AMPA receptor binding proteins in the cerebral cortex of elderly schizophrenics. J Neurosci Res 79:868–878, 2005

Egan MF, Goldberg TE, Kolachana BS, et al: Effect of COMT Val108/158 Met genotype on frontal lobe function and risk for schizophrenia. Proc Natl Acad Sci USA 98:6917–6922, 2001

Egan MF, Straub RE, Goldberg TE, et al: Variation in GRM3 affects cognition, prefrontal glutamate, and risk for schizophrenia. Proc Natl Acad Sci USA 101:12604–12609, 2004

Ekelund J, Hovatta I, Parker A, et al: Chromosome 1 loci in Finnish schizophrenia families. Hum Mol Genet 10:1611–1617, 2001

Ekelund J, Hennah W, Hiekkalinna T, et al: Replication of 1q42 linkage in Finnish schizophrenia pedigrees. Mol Psychiatry 9:1037–1041, 2004

Elkashef AM, Issa F, Wyatt RJ: The biochemical basis of schizophrenia, in Contemporary Issues in the Treatment of Schizophrenia. Edited by Shriqui CL, Nasrallah HA. Washington, DC, American Psychiatric Press, 1995, pp 3–41, 863

Falkai P, Bogerts B: Cell loss in the hippocampus of schizophrenics. Eur Arch Psychiatry Neurol Sci 236:154–161, 1986

Farde L, Wiesel FA, Stone-Elander S, et al: D_2 dopamine receptors in neuroleptic-naive schizophrenic patients: a positron emission tomography study with 11C raclopride. Arch Gen Psychiatry 47:213–219, 1990

Fergusson DM, Horwood LJ, Swain-Campbell NR: Cannabis dependence and psychotic symptoms in young people. Psychol Med 33:15–21, 2003

Freedman DX: LSD, psychotogenic procedures, and brain neurohumors. Psychopharmacol Bull 11:42–43, 1975

Freedman R: Electrophysiological phenotypes. Methods Mol Med 77:215–225, 2003

Friedman JI: Cholinergic targets for cognitive enhancement in schizophrenia: focus on cholinesterase inhibitors and muscarinic agonists. Psychopharmacology (Berl) 174:45–53, 2004

Friston KJ: The dorsolateral prefrontal cortex, schizophrenia and PET. J Neural Transm Suppl 37:79–93, 1992

Frith CD, Friston KJ, Herold S, et al: Regional brain activity in chronic schizophrenic patients during the performance of a verbal fluency task. Br J Psychiatry 167:343–349, 1995

Fujii Y, Shibata H, Kikuta R, et al: Positive associations of polymorphisms in the metabotropic glutamate receptor type 3 gene (*GRM3*) with schizophrenia. Psychiatr Genet 13:71–76, 2003

Funke B, Finn CT, Plocik AM, et al: Association of the *DTNBP1* locus with schizophrenia in a U.S. population. Am J Hum Genet 75:891–898, 2004

Gao X-M, Sakai K, Roberts RC, et al: Ionotropic glutamate receptors and expression of *N*-methyl-D-aspartate receptor subunits in subregions of human hippocampus: effects of schizophrenia. Am J Psychiatry 157:1141–1149, 2000

Geyer MA, Tamminga CA: Measurement and treatment research to improve cognition in schizophrenia: neuropharmacological aspects. Psychopharmacology (Berl) 174:1–2, 2004

Ghose S, Weickert CS, Colvin SM, et al: Glutamate carboxypeptidase II gene expression in the human frontal and temporal lobe in schizophrenia. Neuropsychopharmacology 29:117–125, 2004

Giuliani NR, Calhoun VD, Pearlson GD, et al: Voxel-based morphometry versus region of interest: a comparison of two methods for analyzing gray matter differences in schizophrenia. Schizophr Res 74:135–147, 2005

Glatt SJ, Faraone SV, Tsuang MT: Association between a functional catechol O-methyltransferase gene polymorphism and schizophrenia: meta-analysis of case-control and family based studies. Am J Psychiatry 160:469–476, 2003

Gold J, Goldberg T, Weinberger D: Prefrontal function and schizophrenic symptoms. Neuropsychiatry Neuropsychol Behav Neurol 5:253–261, 1992

Gold JM, Hermann BP, Randolph C, et al: Schizophrenia and temporal lobe epilepsy: a neuropsychological analysis. Arch Gen Psychiatry 51:265–272, 1994

Goldberg TE, Weinberger DR, Berman KF, et al: Further evidence for dementia of the prefrontal type in schizophrenia? A controlled study of teaching the Wisconsin Card Sorting Test. Arch Gen Psychiatry 44:1008–1014, 1987

Goldberg TE, Ragland D, Torrey EF, et al: Neuropsychological assessment of monozygotic twins discordant for schizophrenia. Arch Gen Psychiatry 47:1066–1072, 1990

Goldberg TE, Egan MF, Gscheidle T, et al: Executive subprocesses in working memory: relationship to catechol-O-methyltransferase Val158Met genotype and schizophrenia. Arch Gen Psychiatry 60:889–896, 2003

Goldman-Rakic PS: Working memory dysfunction in schizophrenia. J Neuropsychiatry Clin Neurosci 6:348–357, 1994

Goldman-Rakic PS: Psychopathology and neuropathology of prefrontal cortex in schizophrenia, in Schizophrenia: An Integrated View. Alfred Benzon Symposium 38. Edited by Fog R, Gerlach J, Hemmingsen R. Copenhagen, Denmark, Munksgaard, 1995, pp 126–138

Goldman-Rakic PS, Castner SA, Svensson TH, et al: Targeting the dopamine D1 receptor in schizophrenia: insights for cognitive dysfunction. Psychopharmacology 174:3–16, 2004

Gottesman II, Gould T: The endophenotype concept in psychiatry: etymology and strategic intentions. Am J Psychiatry 160:636–645, 2003

Gottesman II, Shields J: A polygenic theory of schizophrenia. Proc Natl Acad Sci U S A 58:199–205, 1967

Gottesman II, Shields J: Schizophrenia: The Epigenetic Puzzle. New York, Cambridge University Press, 1982

Grady RM, Grange RW, Lau KS, et al: Role for alpha-dystrobrevin in the pathogenesis of dystrophin-dependent muscular dystrophies. Nat Cell Biol 1:215–220, 1999

Grady RM, Zhou H, Cunningham JM, et al: Maturation and maintenance of the neuromuscular synapse: genetic evidence for roles of the dystrophin–glycoprotein complex. Neuron 25:279–293, 2000

Green MF, Marder SR, Glynn SM, et al: The neurocognitive effects of low-dose haloperidol: a two-year comparison with risperidone. Biol Psychiatry 51:972–978, 2002

Gruzelier J, Seymour K, Wilson L: Impairments on neuropsychotic tests of temporohippocampal and frontohippocampal functions and word fluency in remitting schizophrenia and affective disorders. Arch Gen Psychiatry 45:623–629, 1988

Gur RC, Saykin AJ, Gur RE: Neuropsychological study of schizophrenia. Schizophr Res 1:153–162, 1991

Gur RE, McGrath C, Chan RM, et al: An fMRI study of facial emotion processing in patients with schizophrenia. Am J Psychiatry 159:1992–1999, 2002

Hall W, Degenhardt L: Cannabis use and psychosis: a review of clinical and epidemiological evidence. Aust N Z J Psychiatry 34:26–34, 2000

Harrison PJ: The neuropathology of schizophrenia: a critical review of the data and their interpretation. Brain 122:593–624, 1999

Harrison PJ, Law AJ: Neuregulin 1 and schizophrenia: genetics, gene expression, and neurobiology. Biol Psychiatry 60:132–140, 2006

Harrison PJ, Weinberger DR: Schizophrenia genes, gene expression, and neuropathology: on the matter of their convergence. Mol Psychiatry 10:40–68, 2005

Hazlett EA, Buchsbaum MS, Kemether E, et al: Abnormal glucose metabolism in the mediodorsal nucleus of the thalamus in schizophrenia. Am J Psychiatry 161:305–314, 2004

Heckers S, Heinsen H, Heinsen YC, et al: Cortex, white matter, and basal ganglia in schizophrenia: a volumetric postmortem study. Biol Psychiatry 29:556–566, 1991

Heckers S, Rauch SL, Goff D, et al: Impaired recruitment of the hippocampus during conscious recollection in schizophrenia. Nat Neurosci 1:318–323, 1998

Hennah W, Varilo T, Kestila M, et al: Haplotype transmission analysis provides evidence of association for *DISC1* to schizophrenia and suggests sex-dependent effects. Hum Mol Genet 12:3151–3159, 2003

Hietala J, Syvälahti E, Vuorio K: Striatal dopamine D_2 receptor density in neuroleptic-naive schizophrenics studied with positron emission tomography, in Biological Psychiatry, Vol 2. Edited by Racagni G, Brunello N, Fukuda T. Amsterdam, The Netherlands, Excerpta Medica, 1991, pp 386–387

Hill K, Mann L, Laws KR, et al: Hypofrontality in schizophrenia: a meta-analysis of functional imaging studies. Acta Psychiatr Scand 110:243–256, 2004

Hirsch S, Bowen J, Emami J, et al: A one year prospective study of the effect of life events and medication in the aetiology of schizophrenic relapse. Br J Psychiatry 168:49–56, 1996

Hodgkinson CA, Goldman D, Jaeger J, et al: Disrupted in schizophrenia 1 (*DISC1*): association with schizophrenia, schizoaffective disorder, and bipolar disorder. Am J Hum Genet 75:862–872, 2004

Holcomb HH, Links J, Smith C, et al: Positron emission tomography: measuring the metabolic and neurochemical characteristics of the living human nervous system, in Brain Imaging Applications in Psychiatry. Edited by Andreasen NC. Washington, DC, American Psychiatric Press, 1989, pp 235–370

Holzman PS, Solomon CM, Levin S, et al: Pursuit eye movement dysfunctions in schizophrenia: family evidence for specificity. Arch Gen Psychiatry 41:136–139, 1984

Hughes JR, Hatsukami DK, Mitchell JE, et al: Prevalence of smoking among psychiatric outpatients. Am J Psychiatry 143:993–997, 1986

Hutchinson G, Takei N, Fahy TA, et al: Morbid risk of schizophrenia in first-degree relatives of white and African-Caribbean patients with psychosis. Br J Psychiatry 169:776–780, 1996

Huttunen MO, Niskanen P: Prenatal loss of father and psychiatric disorders. Arch Gen Psychiatry 35:429–431, 1978

Hyde TM, Crook JM: Cholinergic systems and schizophrenia: primary pathology or epiphenomena? J Chem Neuroanat 22(1–2):53–63, 2001

Ibrahim HM, Hogg AJ Jr, Healy DJ, et al: Ionotropic glutamate receptor binding and subunit mRNA expression in thalamic nuclei in schizophrenia. Am J Psychiatry 157:1811–1823, 2000

Issa F, Gerhardt GA, Bartko JJ, et al: A multidimensional approach to analysis of cerebrospinal fluid biogenic amines in schizophrenia, I: comparisons with healthy control subjects and neuroleptic-treated/unmedicated pairs analyses. Psychiatry Res 52:237–249, 1994a

Issa F, Kirch DG, Gerhardt GA, et al: A multidimensional approach to analysis of cerebrospinal fluid biogenic amines in schizophrenia, II: correlations with psychopathology. Psychiatry Res 52:251–258, 1994b

Iwata N, Suzuki T, Ikeda M, et al: No association with the neuregulin 1 haplotype to Japanese schizophrenia. Mol Psychiatry 9:126–127, 2004

Jennings JM, McIntosh AR, Kapur S, et al: Functional network differences in schizophrenia: a rCBF study of semantic processing. Neuroreport 9:1697–1700, 1998

Jeste DV, Lohr JB: Hippocampal pathologic findings in schizophrenia. Arch Gen Psychiatry 46:1019–1026, 1989

Johnstone EC, Crow TJ, Frith DC, et al: Cerebral ventricular size and cognitive impairment in schizophrenia. Lancet 2:924–926, 1976

Joober R, Gauthier J, Lal S, et al: Catechol-O-methyltransferase Val-108/158-Met gene variants associated with performance on the Wisconsin Card Sorting Test. Arch Gen Psychiatry 59:662–663, 2002

Kamiya A, Kubo K, Tomoda T, et al: A schizophrenia-associated mutation of *DISC1* perturbs cerebral cortex development. Nat Cell Biol 7:1067–1078, 2005

Karlsson P, Farde L, Halldin C, et al: PET study of D(1) dopamine receptor binding in neuroleptic-naive patients with schizophrenia. Am J Psychiatry 159:761–767, 2002

Kay SR, Sevy S: Pyramidical model of schizophrenia. Schizophr Bull 16:537–545, 1990

Kegeles LS, Abi-Dargham A, Zea-Ponce Y, et al: Modulation of amphetamine-induced striatal dopamine release by ketamine in humans: implications for schizophrenia. Biol Psychiatry 48:627–640, 2000

Kendell RE, Kemp IW: Maternal influenza in the etiology of schizophrenia. Arch Gen Psychiatry 46:878–882, 1989

Kety SS: The significance of genetic factors in the etiology of schizophrenia: results from the national study of adoptees in Denmark. J Psychiatr Res 21:423–429, 1987

Kirov G, Ivanov D, Williams NM, et al: Strong evidence for association between the dystrobrevin binding protein 1 gene (*DTNBP1*) and schizophrenia in 488 parent-offspring trios from Bulgaria. Biol Psychiatry 55:971–975, 2004

Krystal JH, Abi-Saab W, Perry E, et al: Preliminary evidence of attenuation of the disruptive effects of the NMDA glutamate receptor antagonist, ketamine, on working memory by pretreatment with the group II metabotropic glutamate receptor agonist, LY354740, in healthy human subjects. Psychopharmacology (Berl) 179:303–309, 2005

Kuperberg GR, Broome MR, McGuire PK, et al: Regionally localized thinning of the cerebral cortex in schizophrenia. Arch Gen Psychiatry 60:878–888, 2003

Lahti AC, Holcomb HH, Medoff DR, et al: Ketamine activates psychosis and alters limbic blood flow in schizophrenia. Neuroreport 6:869–872, 1995a

Lahti AC, Koffel B, LaPorte D, et al: Subanesthetic doses of ketamine stimulate psychosis in schizophrenia. Neuropsychopharmacology 13:9–19, 1995b

Laruelle M, Abi-Dargham A, van Dyck CH, et al: Single photon emission computerized tomography imaging of amphetamine-induced dopamine release in drug-free schizophrenic subjects. Proc Natl Acad Sci USA 93:9235–9240, 1996

Laruelle M, Abi-Dargham A, Gil R, et al: Increased dopamine transmission in schizophrenia: relationship to illness phases. Biol Psychiatry 46:56–72, 1999

Lawrie SM, Whalley HC, Abukmeil SS, et al: Temporal lobe volume changes in people at high risk of schizophrenia with psychotic symptoms. Br J Psychiatry 181:138–143, 2002

Lenzenweger MF, Dworkin RH, Wethington E: Examining the underlying structure of schizophrenic phenomenology: evidence for a three-process model. Schizophr Bull 17:515–524, 1991

Lesch A, Bogerts B: The diencephalon in schizophrenia: evidence for reduced thickness of the periventricular grey matter. Eur Arch Psychiatry Neurol Sci 234:212–219, 1984

Lewis DA, Lund JS: Heterogeneity of chandelier neurons in monkey neocortex: corticotropin-releasing factor- and parvalbumin-immunoreactive populations. J Comp Neurol 293:599–615, 1990

Lewis DA, Volk DW, Hashimoto T: Selective alterations in prefrontal cortical GABA neurotransmission in schizophrenia: a novel target for the treatment of working memory dysfunction. Psychopharmacology (Berl) 174:143–150, 2004

Lewis DA, Hashimoto T, Volk DW: Cortical inhibitory neurons and schizophrenia. Nat Rev Neurosci 6:312–324, 2005

Liddle PF: The symptoms of chronic schizophrenia: a re-examination of the positive-negative dichotomy. Br J Psychiatry 151:145–151, 1987

Liddle PF, Morris DL: Schizophrenic syndromes and frontal lobe performance. Br J Psychiatry 158:340–345, 1991

Liddle PF, Friston KJ, Frith CD, et al: Patterns of cerebral blood flow in schizophrenia. Br J Psychiatry 160:179–186, 1992

Lisberger SG, Morris EJ, Tychsen L: Visual motion processing and sensory-motor integration for smooth pursuit eye movements. Annu Rev Neurosci 10:97–129, 1987

Luby ED, Cohen BD, Rosenbaum G, et al: Study of a new schizophrenomimetic drug; sernyl. Arch Neurol Psychiatr 81:363–369, 1959

Ma J, Qin W, Wang XY, et al: Further evidence for the association between G72/G30 genes and schizophrenia in two ethnically distinct populations. Mol Psychiatry 11:479–487, 2006

Malhotra AK, Kestler LJ, Mazzanti C, et al: A functional polymorphism in the COMT gene and performance on a test of prefrontal cognition. Am J Psychiatry 159:652–654, 2002

Marti SB, Cichon S, Propping P, et al: Metabotropic glutamate receptor 3 (GRM3) gene variation is not associated with schizophrenia or bipolar affective disorder in the German population. Am J Med Genet 114:46–50, 2002

Martin LF, Kem WR, Freedman R: Alpha-7 nicotinic receptor agonists: potential new candidates for the treatment of schizophrenia. Psychopharmacology (Berl) 174:55–64, 2004

Martinot JL, Peron-Magnan P, Huret JD, et al: Striatal D_2 dopaminergic receptors assessed with positron emission tomography and [^{76}Br]bromospiperone in untreated schizophrenic patients. Am J Psychiatry 147:44–50, 1990

Martinot JL, Paillère-Martinot ML, Loch C, et al: The estimated density of D_2 striatal receptors in schizophrenia: a study with positron emission tomography and 76Br-bromolisuride. Br J Psychiatry 158:346–350, 1991

McCarley RW, Shenton ME, O'Donnell BF, et al: Auditory P300 abnormalities and left posterior superior temporal gyrus volume reduction in schizophrenia. Arch Gen Psychiatry 50:190–197, 1993

McGue M, Gottesman II: A single dominant gene still cannot account for the transmission of schizophrenia. Arch Gen Psychiatry 46:478–480, 1989

Meador-Woodruff JH, Healy DJ: Glutamate receptor expression in schizophrenic brain. Brain Res Brain Res Rev 31:288–294, 2000

Mednick SA, Machon RA, Huttunen MO, et al: Adult schizophrenia following prenatal exposure to an influenza epidemic. Arch Gen Psychiatry 45:189–192, 1988

Meltzer HY, McGurk SR: The effects of clozapine, risperidone, and olanzapine on cognitive function in schizophrenia. Schizophr Bull 25:233–255, 1999

Meltzer HY, Sumiyoshi T: Atypical antipsychotic drugs improve cognition in schizophrenia. Biol Psychiatry 53:265–267, 2003

Menon RR, Barta PE, Aylward EH, et al: Posterior superior temporal gyrus in schizophrenia: grey matter changes and clinical correlates. Schizophr Res 16:127–135, 1995

Mirnics K, Middleton FA, Stanwood GD, et al: Disease-specific changes in regulator of G-protein signaling 4 (RGS4) expression in schizophrenia. Mol Psychiatry 6:293–301, 2001

Moghaddam B: Targeting metabotropic glutamate receptors for treatment of the cognitive symptoms of schizophrenia. Psychopharmacology (Berl) 174:39–44, 2004

Moghaddam B, Adams BW: Reversal of phencyclidine effects by a group II metabotropic glutamate receptor agonist in rats. Science 281:1349–1352, 1998

Morris DW, McGhee KA, Schwaiger S, et al: No evidence for association of the dysbindin gene [DTNBP1] with schizophrenia in an Irish population-based study. Schizophr Res 60:167–172, 2003

Neale JH, Bzdega T, Wroblewska B: N-Acetylaspartylglutamate: the most abundant peptide neurotransmitter in the mammalian central nervous system. J Neurochem 75:443–452, 2000

Nemeroff CB, Youngblood W, Manberg PJ, et al: Regional brain concentrations of neuropeptides in Huntington's chorea and schizophrenia. Science 221:972–975, 1983

Niznikiewicz M, Donnino R, McCarley RW, et al: Abnormal angular gyrus asymmetry in schizophrenia. Am J Psychiatry 157:428–437, 2000

Nuechterlein KH, Dawson ME, Gitlin M, et al: Developmental processes in schizophrenic disorders: longitudinal studies of vulnerability and stress. Schizophr Bull 18:387–425, 1992

Numakawa T, Yagasaki Y, Ishimoto T, et al: Evidence of novel neuronal functions of dysbindin, a susceptibility gene for schizophrenia. Hum Mol Genet 13:2699–2708, 2004

O'Callaghan E, Larkin C, Kinsella A, et al: Familial, obstetric, and other clinical correlates of minor physical anomalies in schizophrenia. Am J Psychiatry 148:479–483, 1991

Owen MJ, Craddock N, O'Donovan MC: Schizophrenia: genes at last? Trends Genet 21:518–525, 2005

Pakkenberg B: Postmortem study of chronic schizophrenic brains. Br J Psychiatry 151:744–752, 1987

Pakkenberg B: Pronounced reduction of total neuron number in mediodorsal thalamic nucleus and nucleus accumbens in schizophrenics. Arch Gen Psychiatry 47:1023–1028, 1990

Park S, Holzman PS: Schizophrenics show spatial working memory deficits. Arch Gen Psychiatry 49:975–982, 1992

Pearlson GD, Marsh L: Magnetic resonance imaging in psychiatry, in American Psychiatric Press Review of Psychiatry, Vol 12. Edited by Oldham JM, Riba MB, Tasman A. Washington, DC, American Psychiatric Association, 1993, pp 347–381

Pfefferbaum A, Wenegrat BG, Ford JM, et al: Clinical application of the P3 component of event-related potentials, II: dementia, depression and schizophrenia. Electroencephalogr Clin Neurophysiol 59:104–124, 1984

Potkin SG, Alva G, Fleming K, et al: A PET study of the pathophysiology of negative symptoms in schizophrenia. Am J Psychiatry 159:227–237, 2002

Read J, Van Os J, Morrison AP, et al: Childhood trauma, psychosis and schizophrenia: a literature review with theoretical and clinical implications. Acta Psychiatr Scand 112:330–350, 2005

Reynolds GP: Increased concentrations and lateral asymmetry of amygdala dopamine in schizophrenia. Nature 305:527–529, 1983

Reynolds GP, Mason SL: Absence of detectable striatal dopamine D4 receptors in drug-treated schizophrenia. Eur J Pharmacol 281:R5–R6, 1995

Rosenthal R, Bigelow LB: Quantitative brain measurements in chronic schizophrenia. Br J Psychiatry 121:259–264, 1972

Ross RG, Olincy A, Mikulich SK, et al: Admixture analysis of smooth pursuit eye movements in probands with schizophrenia and their relatives suggests gain and leading saccades are potential endophenotypes. Psychophysiology 39:809–819, 2002

Roth BL, Hanizavareh SM, Blum AE: Serotonin receptors represent highly favorable molecular targets for cognitive enhancement in schizophrenia and other disorders. Psychopharmacology (Berl) 174:17–24, 2004

Sanders AR, Rusu I, Duan J, et al: Haplotypic association spanning the 22q11.21 genes COMT and ARVCF with schizophrenia. Mol Psychiatry 10:353–365, 2005

Sartorius N: The International Pilot Study of Schizophrenia. Schizophr Bull (Winter):21–34, 1974

Saykin AJ, Gur RC, Gur RE, et al: Neuropsychological function in schizophrenia: selective impairment in memory and learning. Arch Gen Psychiatry 48:618–624, 1991

Scarr E, Beneyto M, Meador-Woodruff JH, et al: Cortical glutamatergic markers in schizophrenia. Neuropsychopharmacology 30:1521–1531, 2005

Scheibel AB, Kovelman JA: Disorientation of the hippocampal pyramidal cell and its processes in schizophrenia patients. Biol Psychiatry 16:101–102, 1981

Schroeder J, Buchsbaum MS, Siegel BV, et al: Patterns of cortical activity in schizophrenia. Psychol Med 24:947–955, 1994

Schumacher J, Jamra RA, Freudenberg J, et al: Examination of G72 and D-amino-acid oxidase as genetic risk factors for schizophrenia and bipolar affective disorder. Mol Psychiatry 9:203–207, 2004

Schwab SG, Knapp M, Mondabon S, et al: Support for association of schizophrenia with genetic variation in the 6p22.3 gene, dysbindin, in sib-pair families with linkage and in an additional sample of triad families. Am J Hum Genet 72:185–190, 2003

Schwartz ML, Goldman-Rakic PS: Callosal and intrahemispheric connectivity of the prefrontal association cortex in rhesus monkey: relation between intraparietal and principal sulcal cortex. J Comp Neurol 226:403–420, 1984

Shelton RC, Weinberger DR: Brain morphology in schizophrenia, in Psychopharmacology: The Third Generation of Progress. Edited by Meltzer HY. New York, Raven, 1987, pp 773–781

Shenton ME, Kikinis R, Jolesz FA, et al: Abnormalities of the left temporal lobe and thought disorder in schizophrenia: a quantitative magnetic resonance imaging study. N Engl J Med 327:604–612, 1992

Shifman S, Bronstein M, Sternfeld M, et al: A highly significant association between a COMT haplotype and schizophrenia. Am J Hum Genet 71:1296–1302, 2002

Silbersweig DA, Stern E, Frith C, et al: A functional neuroanatomy of hallucinations in schizophrenia. Nature 378:176–179, 1995

Smith GS, Schloesser R, Brodie JD, et al: Glutamate modulation of dopamine measured in vivo with positron emission tomography (PET) and 11C-raclopride in normal human subjects. Neuropsychopharmacology 18:18–25, 1998

Spence SA, Brooks DJ, Hirsch SR, et al: A PET study of voluntary movement in schizophrenic patients experiencing passivity phenomena (delusions of alien control). Brain 120:1997–2011, 1997

Spence SA, Liddle PF, Stefan MD, et al: Functional anatomy of verbal fluency in people with schizophrenia and those at genetic risk: focal dysfunction and distributed disconnectivity reappraised. Br J Psychiatry 176:52–60, 2000

St Clair D, Blackwood D, Muir W, et al: Association within a family of a balanced autosomal translocation with major mental illness. Lancet 336:13–16, 1990

Stefansson H, Sigurdsson E, Steinthorsdottir V, et al: Neuregulin 1 and susceptibility to schizophrenia. Am J Hum Genet 71:877–892, 2002

Stefansson H, Sarginson J, Kong A, et al: Association of neuregulin 1 with schizophrenia confirmed in a Scottish population. Am J Hum Genet 72:83–87, 2003

Straub RE, Jiang Y, MacLean CJ, et al: Genetic variation in the 6p22.3 gene DTNBP1, the human ortholog of the mouse dysbindin gene, is associated with schizophrenia. Am J Hum Genet 71:337–348, 2002

Suddath RL, Casanova MF, Goldberg TE: Temporal lobe pathology in schizophrenia: a quantitative magnetic resonance imaging study. Am J Psychiatry 146:464–472, 1989

Suddath RL, Christison GW, Torrey EF, et al: Anatomical abnormalities in the brains of monozygotic twins discordant for schizophrenia. N Engl J Med 322:789–794, 1990

Sugarman PA, Craufurd D: Schizophrenia in the Afro-Caribbean community. Br J Psychiatry 164:474–480, 1994

Sullivan EV, Shear PK, Zipursky RB, et al: A deficit profile of executive, memory, and motor functions in schizophrenia. Biol Psychiatry 36:641–653, 1994

Susser E, Neugebauer R, Hoek HW, et al: Schizophrenia after prenatal famine: further evidence. Arch Gen Psychiatry 53:25–31, 1996

Sweeney JA, Luna B, Srinivasagam NM, et al: Eye tracking abnormalities in schizophrenia: evidence for dysfunction in the frontal eye fields. Biol Psychiatry 44:698–708, 1998

Swerdlow NR, Geyer MA: Using an animal model of deficient sensorimotor gating to study the pathophysiology and new treatments of schizophrenia. Schizophr Bull 24:285–301, 1998

Swerdlow NR, Braff DL, Taaid N, et al: Assessing the validity of an animal model of deficient sensorimotor gating in schizophrenic patients. Arch Gen Psychiatry 51:139–154, 1994

Swerdlow NR, Braff DL, Geyer MA: Cross-species studies of sensorimotor gating of the startle reflex. Ann N Y Acad Sci 877:202–216, 1999

Talbot K, Eidem WL, Tinsley CL, et al: Dysbindin-1 is reduced in intrinsic, glutamatergic terminals of the hippocampal formation in schizophrenia. J Clin Invest 113:1353–1363, 2004

Tamminga CA: Schizophrenia and glutamatergic transmission. Crit Rev Neurobiol 12:21–36, 1998

Tamminga CA, Thaker GK, Buchanan R, et al: Limbic system abnormalities identified in schizophrenia using positron emission tomography with fluorodeoxyglucose and neocortical alterations with deficit syndrome. Arch Gen Psychiatry 49:522–530, 1992

Tang JX, Chen WY, He G, et al: Polymorphisms within 5' end of the neuregulin 1 gene are genetically associated with schizophrenia in the Chinese population. Mol Psychiatry 9:11–12, 2004

Taylor SF, Tandon R, Koeppe RA: Global cerebral blood flow increase reveals focal hypoperfusion in schizophrenia. Neuropsychopharmacology 21:368–371, 1999

Thaker GK, Nguyen JA, Tamminga CA: Increased saccadic distractibility in tardive dyskinesia: functional evidence for subcortical GABA dysfunction. Biol Psychiatry 25:49–59, 1989

Thaker GK, Ross DE, Cassady SL, et al: Saccadic eye movement abnormalities in relatives of patients with schizophrenia. Schizophr Res 45:235–244, 2000

Thiselton DL, Webb BT, Neale BM, et al: No evidence for linkage or association of neuregulin-1 (*NRG1*) with disease in the Irish study of high-density schizophrenia families (ISHDSF). Mol Psychiatry 9:777–783, 2004

Tienari PJ, Wynne LC: Adoption studies of schizophrenia. Ann Med 26:233–237, 1994

Treff WM, Hempel KJ: Die Zelidichte bei Schizophrenen und klinisch Gesunden. J Hirnforsch 4:314–369, 1958

Tregellas JR, Tanabe JL, Miller DE, et al: Neurobiology of smooth pursuit eye movement deficits in schizophrenia: an fMRI study. Am J Psychiatry 161:315–321, 2004

Tsai G, Passani LA, Slusher BS, et al: Abnormal excitatory neurotransmitter metabolism in schizophrenic brains. Arch Gen Psychiatry 52:829–836, 1995

Tsuang MT, Stone WS, Faraone SV: Toward reformulating the diagnosis of schizophrenia. Am J Psychiatry 157:1041–1050, 2000

Van Den Bogaert A, Schumacher J, Schulze TG, et al: The DTNBP1 (dysbindin) gene contributes to schizophrenia, depending on family history of the disease. Am J Hum Genet 73:1438–1443, 2003

Van Os J, Selten JP: Prenatal exposure to maternal stress and subsequent schizophrenia: the May 1940 invasion of the Netherlands. Br J Psychiatry 172:324–326, 1998

Van Os J, Bak M, Hanssen M, et al: Cannabis use and psychosis: a longitudinal population-based study. Am J Epidemiol 156:319–327, 2002

van Praag HM: CSF 5-HIAA and suicide in nondepressed schizophrenics. Lancet 2:977–978, 1983

Volk DW, Austin MC, Pierri JN, et al: Decreased glutamic acid decarboxylase67 messenger RNA expression in a subset of prefrontal cortical gamma-aminobutyric acid neurons in subjects with schizophrenia. Arch Gen Psychiatry 57:237–245, 2000

Volkow ND, Wolf AP, Van Gelder P, et al: Phenomenological correlates of metabolic activity in 18 patients with chronic schizophrenia. Am J Psychiatry 144:151–158, 1987

Wahlberg KE, Wynne LC, Oja H, et al: Gene-environment interaction in vulnerability to schizophrenia: findings from the Finnish Adoptive Family Study of Schizophrenia. Am J Psychiatry 154:355–362, 1997

Wang X, He G, Gu N, et al: Association of G72/G30 with schizophrenia in the Chinese population. Biochem Biophys Res Commun 319:1281–1286, 2004

Weickert CS, Straub RE, McClintock BW, et al: Human dysbindin (*DTNBP1*) gene expression in normal brain and in schizophrenic prefrontal cortex and midbrain. Arch Gen Psychiatry 61:544–555, 2004

Weickert TW, Goldberg TE, Mishara A, et al: Catechol-O-methyltransferase val108/158met genotype predicts working memory response to antipsychotic medications. Biol Psychiatry 56:677–682, 2004

Weinberger DR, Berman KF, Suddath R, et al: Evidence of dysfunction of a prefrontal-limbic network in schizophrenia: a magnetic resonance imaging and regional cerebral blood flow study of discordant monozygotic twins. Am J Psychiatry 149:890–897, 1992

Weiser M, Knobler HY, Noy S, et al: Clinical characteristics of adolescents later hospitalized for schizophrenia. Am J Med Genet 114:949–955, 2002

Whitfield CL, Dube SR, Felitti VJ, et al: Adverse childhood experiences and hallucinations. Child Abuse Negl 29:797–810, 2005

Wicks S, Hjern A, Gunnell D, et al: Social adversity in childhood and the risk of developing psychosis: a national cohort study. Am J Psychiatry 162:1652–1657, 2005

Widerlöv E, Lindstrom LH, Bissette G, et al: Subnormal CSF levels of neurotensin in a subgroup of schizophrenic patients: normalization after neuroleptic treatment. Am J Psychiatry 139:1122–1126, 1982

Williams NM, Preece A, Spurlock G, et al: Support for genetic variation in neuregulin 1 and susceptibility to schizophrenia. Mol Psychiatry 8:485–487, 2003

Williams NM, Preece A, Morris DW, et al: Identification in 2 independent samples of a novel schizophrenia risk haplotype of the dystrobrevin binding protein gene (*DTNBP1*). Arch Gen Psychiatry 61:336–344, 2004

Wolkin A, Sanfilipo M, Wolf AP, et al: Negative symptoms and hypofrontality in chronic schizophrenia. Arch Gen Psychiatry 49:959–965, 1992

Wong DF, Wagner HN Jr, Tune LE, et al: Positron emission tomography reveals elevated D_2 dopamine receptors in drug-naïve schizophrenics [published erratum appears in Science 235:623, 1987]. Science 234:1558–1563, 1986

Wonnacott S: The paradox of nicotinic acetylcholine receptor up-regulation by nicotine. Trends Pharmacol Sci 11:216–219, 1990

World Health Organization: International Statistical Classification of Diseases and Related Health Problems, 10th Revision. Geneva, Switzerland, World Health Organization, 1992

Yang JZ, Si TM, Ruan Y, et al: Association study of neuregulin 1 gene with schizophrenia. Mol Psychiatry 8:706–709, 2003

Zammit S, Allebeck P, Andreasson S, et al: Self reported cannabis use as a risk factor for schizophrenia in Swedish conscripts of 1969: historical cohort study. BMJ 325:1199, 2002

Zhang F, Sarginson J, Crombie C, et al: Genetic association between schizophrenia and the *DISC1* gene in the Scottish population. Am J Med Genet B Neuropsychiatr Genet 141:155–159, 2006

Zhao X, Shi Y, Tang J, et al: A case control and family based association study of the neuregulin 1 gene and schizophrenia. J Med Genet 41:31–34, 2004

Zou F, Li C, Duan S, et al: A family-based study of the association between the *G72/G30* genes and schizophrenia in the Chinese population. Schizophr Res 73:257–261, 2005

15

NEUROPSYCHIATRIC ASPECTS OF MOOD DISORDERS

Paul E. Holtzheimer III, M.D.

Helen S. Mayberg, M.D.

Mood disorders are characterized by abnormalities of mood regulation, cognition, motor activity, sleep, appetite, and other drive states (e.g., libido). Neuropsychiatric disorders are commonly associated with disturbances of mood and affect, especially depressive syndromes. A growing database supports a similar neurobiological basis for mood disorders, regardless of etiology. However, rather than defining a single causative "lesion" or neurochemical abnormality, current models propose dysfunction within an integrated set of neural systems. In this chapter, we review the neuropsychiatric aspects of mood disorders within this neural systems framework.

CLINICAL FEATURES

TYPES OF MOOD DISORDERS

Mood disorders are characterized by *mood episodes* that can occur over the course of the illness, and each mood disorder and episode can be associated with several qualifiers (American Psychiatric Association 2000). This classification of mood disorders is useful for both clinical and research purposes. However, the simplicity of this schema belies the phenomenological complexity of mood disorders. For example, two patients with major depressive disorder (MDD) may present with very different symptoms of a major depressive episode. One may have decreased sleep with early-morning awakening, severe psychomotor retardation, profound anhedonia, absence of mood reactivity, and a distinct quality of "depressed" mood that actually "feels" different from normal sadness (i.e., *melancholic features*). The other may present with sad mood and *atypical features* consisting of increased sleep, appetite, and mood reactivity. When mood disorders present in the context of neuropsychiatric conditions (such as Parkinson's disease), there can be even greater phenomenological variability. Because of this heterogeneity, this section is organized by specific symptom clusters rather than specific mood disorder diagnoses.

MOOD AND AFFECT

Every mood disorder requires a specific and primary alteration of mood or affect to justify the diagnosis (with the exception of MDD, which allows for no alteration of mood as long as anhedonia is present). The term *mood* is used to refer to the subjective emotional state experienced by an individual (e.g., the subject *feels* happy, sad, anxious, numb). *Affect* is more objective and refers to the individual's emotional state as it appears to an outside observer (e.g., the subject *looks* happy, sad, anxious, numb). Importantly, affect also can be defined by the range of emotional states shown by a subject (e.g., during an interview), its stability and consistency over time, and how appropriate affect is, given the conversation, stated mood, and so forth. Typically, mood and affect will correspond (i.e., a sad patient reports depressed mood and looks sad, a manic patient reports euphoria and looks elated). However, patients with neuropsychiatric disease may present with mood dissociated from affect. For example, a patient with Parkinson's disease may deny depressed mood or other symptoms of depression but present with severely restricted affect that looks depressed. Other neurological patients may deny feelings of depression or euphoria but present with prominent affective instability (e.g., inappropriate crying spells, laughing) called *pseudobulbar affect*. These observed dissociations between mood and affect suggest these symptoms are controlled by related but distinct neural systems.

INTEREST AND MOTIVATION

Mood episodes are commonly associated with disturbances of interest and motivation. Depressive states are typically characterized by both anhedonia and apathy (*anhedonia* is a decreased ability to experience pleasure, whereas *apathy* represents decreased drive to engage in self-directed activity). Manic patients typically have an exaggerated interest level; clinically, this may present as increased goal-directed activity (e.g., vigorous writing or cleaning) or engagement in pleasurable activity regardless of risks (e.g., promiscuity or substance abuse).

In the absence of a mood disorder, interest and motivation also may be disturbed. Apathy without associated depression is common in neuropsychiatric patients, especially those with Parkinson's disease, dementia, or traumatic brain injury. Furthermore, some neurological patients (often patients with traumatic brain injury, stroke, or dementia) show increased pleasure-seeking or disinhibition without other symptoms associated with mania.

SLEEP

Depressed patients often complain of decreased sleep characterized by difficulty falling asleep (early insomnia), frequent awakenings during the sleep cycle (middle insomnia), or early-morning awakening (late insomnia). Other patients describe hypersomnia. Manic/hypomanic patients typically report decreased *need* for sleep—that is, they feel capable of functioning "normally" on little or no sleep at all—in addition to a decreased amount of sleep. As with disturbances of affect, interest, and motivation, sleep abnormalities in the absence of a mood disorder are common in neuropsychiatric patients.

APPETITE

In patients with depression, appetite may be decreased, increased, or unchanged. The most common abnormality is a decrease in appetite with weight loss; however, some patients report increased appetite and weight gain. In mania, appetite change is not a specific criterion for the disorder, although a decreased appetite (or decreased intake) is commonly observed. As with sleep abnormalities, appetite abnormalities are common in neuropsychiatric disease in the absence of other mood disorder symptoms.

PSYCHOMOTOR ACTIVITY

Motor and psychomotor deficits in depression involve a range of behaviors, including changes in motility, mental activity, and speech. Depressed patients typically report fatigue and slowing of thought processes, often observed as psychomotor retardation. At the extreme, a depressed patient may present with catatonia. Conversely, mania almost always involves an increase in psychomotor speed (reported as "racing" thoughts and observed as pressured speech and agitation).

Many neuropsychiatric illnesses are associated with a slowing of thought and motor activity without other symptoms of depression (e.g., Parkinson's disease). Agitation is also a common but nonspecific symptom in neuropsychiatric patients. Although agitation may be indicative of a manic episode, it may arise as a response to pain or a medication side effect (e.g., akathisia from antipsychotic medications).

EMOTIONAL BIAS

Patients with mood disorders commonly show mood-congruent emotional bias in cognitive processing (Murphy et al. 1999). For example, depressed subjects show better recall for negative words (Teasdale and Russell 1983) and are faster than nondepressed individuals at identifying negative adjectives as self-descriptive (Alloy et al. 1999). Depressed patients show worsened performance in the context of negative feedback (Elliott et al. 1997b), and negative bias in emotional processing may predict treatment resistance (Levitan et al. 1998). In mania, subjects may have a strong positive emotional bias that presents as grandiosity and overfriendliness.

Neuroticism (as defined in the five-factor model of personality [McCrae and Costa 1987]) involves temperamental hypersensitivity to negative stimuli and the tendency to experience exaggerated negative mood in situations of emotional instability (Santor et al. 1997). High levels of neuroticism may indicate a predisposition to developing depression (Fanous et al. 2002). Cloninger et al. (2006) used a different model of personality and suggested that personality traits involving negative bias (such as high "harm avoidance" and low "self-directedness") predict development of depression (Cloninger et al. 2006). In the extreme, negative emotional bias in depression may present as excessive guilt and suicidal ideation.

COGNITION

Cognitive abnormalities typically seen in depressed patients include slowed thought processes and impaired attention/concentration. Depressed patients often have impaired executive functioning (planning, organization, short-term memory). Manic patients also show impaired concentration, attention, and executive functioning (including disinhibition and impulsivity). Cognitive deficits in mood disorders are typically mild to moderate but can become severe in intractable depression. Some patients, especially those with late-life depression, may develop "pseudodementia" (Raskind 1998). In contrast to deficits associated with many neurological disorders, language, perception, and spatial abilities are not usually impaired in patients with idiopathic mood disorders. In the absence of mood disorders, neurological patients commonly show cognitive impairment such that these symptoms may be nonspecific; this impairment may be exacerbated in patients with a comorbid mood disorder.

MOOD DISORDERS ASSOCIATED WITH NEUROPSYCHIATRIC CONDITIONS

DIFFICULTIES IN DIAGNOSIS

Correctly diagnosing a mood disorder in the neuropsychiatric patient can be difficult because symptoms of the neurological illness may mimic or mask the symptoms of mood disturbance. As discussed earlier, patients with neuropsychiatric disease may present with one or more symptoms without meeting other criteria for a mood episode. Thus, when evaluating patients with neuropsychiatric disease, it is important to be vigilant for any and all symptoms of depression and to pay particular attention to symptoms that are less likely to be independently associated with the underlying neurological illness.

DEPRESSION

Depression is the most common mood disorder associated with neuropsychiatric illness. In patients with neurological illness, depression may result from the pathophysiology or treatment of the underlying neurological disease, reaction to the psychosocial stress of having the underlying illness, recurrence of a premorbid depressive disorder, or some combination of these. Table 15–1 lists common associations of depression with various neuropsychiatric illnesses and treatments.

MANIA

Mania is seen less commonly than depression in neuropsychiatric patients. As with depression, mania can have a multifactorial etiology (Table 15–2).

NEUROBIOLOGY OF MOOD DISORDERS

The neurobiology of mood disorders can be approached in two general ways: 1) defining the neurobiology of a mood episode or disorder as a distinct entity—a syndrome-specific approach, or 2) defining the neurobiology of specific phenomenological aspects of mood disorders (e.g., assessment of neuroanatomical correlates of sad mood)—a symptom-specific approach.

SYNDROME-SPECIFIC FINDINGS

Several studies have investigated the neurophysiological and neuroanatomical correlates of specific mood disorders and mood episodes. These data suggest that mood disorders, regardless of etiology, share a similar neurobiology. However, these findings also highlight that no single neurochemical or neuroanatom-

TABLE 15–1. Common associations with depression in neuropsychiatric patients

Psychiatric (idiopathic)
  Major depressive disorder
  Bipolar disorder
  Dysthymia
  Cyclothymia
Neurological
  Basal ganglia disease, especially:
    Parkinson's disease
    Huntington's disease
    Wilson's disease
  Cerebrovascular disease, especially:
    Frontal cortical/subcortical stroke
    Basal ganglia stroke
  Multiple sclerosis
  Infectious encephalitis
  Neoplasm
  Paraneoplastic syndrome
  Traumatic brain injury
  Dementia
  Epilepsy
Pharmacological/iatrogenic
  Corticosteroids
  Thyroid ablation
  Interferon-α
  Deep brain stimulation (especially of subthalamic nucleus)
  Substance intoxication or withdrawal
Other
  Hypothyroidism
  Cushing's syndrome
  Vitamin deficiency (e.g., B_{12})
  Autoimmune disease

ical abnormality fully explains the pathophysiology of mood disorders.

Neurochemical Findings

In depression, the main focus of neurochemical research has been driven by the "mono-

TABLE 15–2.   Common associations with mania in neuropsychiatric patients

Psychiatric (idiopathic)

Bipolar disorder

Cyclothymia

Neurological

Basal ganglia disease

Huntington's disease

Wilson's disease

Cerebrovascular disease

Frontal cortical/subcortical stroke

Basal ganglia stroke

Multiple sclerosis

Infectious encephalitis

Neoplasm

Paraneoplastic syndrome

HIV encephalopathy

Epilepsy

Pharmacological/iatrogenic

Dopaminergic agents

Corticosteroids

Substance intoxication or withdrawal

Surgical treatments, especially:

Pallidotomy

Deep brain stimulation

Antidepressant medications

Other

Cushing's syndrome

Vitamin deficiencies (e.g., B_{12} or niacin)

Hyperthyroidism

Systemic infections

Uremia

Electrolyte abnormality (e.g., hypocalcemia)

amine hypothesis" of depression (Schildkraut 1965). Of the major monoamine neurotransmitter systems (serotonin, norepinephrine, and dopamine), the strongest evidence indicates serotonergic dysfunction plays a major role in the pathophysiology of depression. Although data are not unequivocal, patients with depression (compared with nondepressed subjects) show lower cerebrospinal fluid (CSF) levels of serotonin metabolites (Asberg et al. 1976; Mann et al. 1996), decreased serotonin transporter binding (Malison et al. 1998), and serotonin receptor abnormalities (D'Haenen et al. 1992; Sargent et al. 2000). Medications that specifically target serotonin neurotransmission are effective in treating depression in up to 60% of patients (Nelson 1999). Tryptophan depletion, which results in an acute but transient decrease in available serotonin, can result in depressive relapse (Neumeister et al. 2004). Gene-environment interaction studies suggest that subjects exposed to environmental stress are more likely to develop depression if they have at least one allele for a "low-efficiency" version of the serotonin transporter (Caspi et al. 2003; Kendler et al. 2005).

Data supporting norepinephrine and dopamine dysfunction in the pathophysiology of depression are more limited but still compelling. Medications that increase noradrenergic neurotransmission are effective in treating depression (Arroll et al. 2005). In depressed patients taking noradrenergic antidepressants and some euthymic patients with a history of depression, catecholamine depletion can result in depressive relapse (Berman et al. 1999). CSF and urine concentrations of dopamine metabolites are decreased in depressed patients (Roy et al. 1992). Dopamine transporter activity may be reduced in patients with depression (Meyer et al. 2001). Medications targeting the dopamine system, such as psychostimulants and pramipexole, have shown antidepressant efficacy (Goldberg et al. 2004; Nierenberg et al. 1998).

Neuroendocrine systems have also been implicated in the pathophysiology of mood disorders. The hypothalamic-pituitary-adrenal (HPA) axis is dysfunctional in at least some patients with depression (Posener et al. 2000). HPA axis dysregulation may be an important marker of vulnerability to various types of mood disorders, and HPA axis abnormalities may be causal for certain types of depression rather than the reverse (Heim et al. 2000). Corticotropin-releasing factor (CRF) has been shown to be an important modulator of monoaminergic activity and vice versa (Ruggiero et al. 1999). The hypothalamic-pituitary-thyroid axis has also been linked with depression (Banki et al. 1988; Nemeroff et al. 1985) and thyroid hormone augmentation may be effective in treating antidepressant-resistant depression (Joffe and Sokolov 2000).

A role for other neuromodulatory systems in the pathophysiology of depression is likely. For example, glutamate and γ-aminobutyric acid dysfunction have been found in depressed patients and animal models of depression (Choudary et al. 2005). The neurokinin system (known to be involved in nociception) also may play a role in depression (Bondy et al. 2003).

A growing database supports a role for inflammatory processes in mood disorders, especially depression (Raison et al. 2006). Immune mediators, such as corticosteroids and interferon-α, have been clearly associated with mood disorder symptoms (Brown and Suppes 1998; Loftis and Hauser 2004). Also, depressed patients have higher levels of circulating inflammatory markers compared with nondepressed subjects (O'Brien et al. 2004). Inflammatory pathways may interact with stress-response systems (i.e., HPA axis) to mediate effects on mood and behavior (Raison et al. 2006).

An increasing number of studies have focused on dysregulation of second messenger systems, gene transcription, various neurotrophic factors, and cell turnover in mood disorders (Manji et al. 2001). Such pathways have been more extensively studied in bipolar disorder, where medications (such as lithium) may directly affect these systems (Einat and Manji 2006).

Genetics

The heritability of depression is 33%–50% (Levinson 2006), and the heritability of bipolar disorder may be as high as 80%–90% (Kieseppa et al. 2004). These illnesses likely involve multiple genes and important genetic-environmental interactions.

Several genes involved in monoamine function have been implicated in the vulnerability to depression and bipolar disorders (Levinson 2006). One of the most consistent findings in genetic studies of mood disorders has been increased rates of depression in subjects with an "inefficient" form of the serotonin transporter (resulting from a functional single-nucleotide polymorphism in the promoter region for the transporter gene) who are also exposed to stressful life events (Caspi et al. 2003; Kendler et al. 2005); however, a meta-analysis of similar studies suggested that this relationship may be more complex (Risch et al. 2009). Serotonin transporter gene polymorphisms also have been implicated in bipolar disorder, although the data are contradictory (Levinson 2005). Some data suggest that such polymorphisms may be associated with specific personality traits and symptoms of mood disorders, including neuroticism (Schinka et al. 2004) and suicidality (Levinson 2005).

Because monoamine dysfunction cannot fully explain the neurobiology of mood disorders, genes for other neuromodulators are another focus of investigation (Levinson 2006). For example, a functional polymorphism of the promoter region for the brain-derived neurotrophic factor gene may cause susceptibility to mood disorders, especially bipolar disorder (Strauss et al. 2004).

Neuroanatomical Findings

Advances in structural and functional neuroimaging have allowed increasingly detailed investigation of brain anatomy and have greatly advanced our understanding of how parts of the brain are involved in the pathophysiology of depression. The most common structural abnormalities associated with depression include decreased volumes of the prefrontal cortex, hippocampus, amygdala, and basal ganglia, although the data are inconsistent (Sheline 2003). Some studies have also shown decreased volume of the subgenual medial frontal cortex in patients with depression (Botteron et al. 2002; Drevets et al. 1997). Data suggest structural differences in depressed patients may be partially determined by gender (Botteron et al. 2002), age (Ballmaier et al. 2004), and genetic factors (Pezawas et al. 2005).

The most common functional abnormality associated with depression is decreased activity (blood flow or metabolism) in multiple regions of the prefrontal cortex (Baxter et al. 1989; Bench et al. 1992; Videbech 2000), and prefrontal cortex activity has been inversely correlated with overall depression severity (Baxter et al. 1989; Drevets et al. 1992). Increased activity has been frequently described in various limbic-paralimbic subcortical regions (amygdala, anterior temporal region, insula, basal ganglia, thalamus), but the data are less consistent than with the prefrontal findings (Drevets et al. 1992; Mayberg et al. 1997). Hypoactivity in dorsal portions of the anterior cingulate cortex and hyperactivity in ventral regions have been frequently identified (Bench et al. 1992; Kennedy et al. 2001; Mayberg et al. 1997; Videbech et al. 2002), although not all studies have agreed (Drevets et al. 2002; Pizzagalli et al. 2004). Also, hyperactivity of the prefrontal cortex has been reported (Drevets et al. 1992; Goldapple et al. 2004).

The neuroanatomy of bipolar disorder has been less well studied (for a review, see Strakowski et al. 2005). Generally, brain regions implicated in bipolar depression significantly overlap with those identified in unipolar depression (Sheline 2003). Neuroanatomical findings in mania are even more limited. Interestingly, during mania, activity of prefrontal cortical regions may decrease (as often seen in depression), perhaps suggesting a valence-independent change in cortical activity during mood episodes (Strakowski et al. 2005).

It should be recognized that although there is a good deal of consistency across neuroanatomical studies of mood disorders, there is also notable variability. Although some of this variability might be explained by differences in imaging technique and analysis (Videbech 2000; Videbech et al. 2002), this discordance likely results from underlying biological heterogeneity among patients.

Taken together, these data suggest that mood disorders are best characterized not by any single functional abnormality but rather by a pattern of abnormalities involving a largely consistent network of brain regions presumably involved in normal and abnormal mood regulation (Mayberg 2003).

Neurobiology of Mood Disorders in Neuropsychiatric Patients

Depression in patients with neurological disease is associated with similar neurochemical findings as in patients with idiopathic major depression. All three monoamines are disrupted in Parkinson's disease, which is highly associated with depression (Mayberg and Solomon 1995). Serotonergic dysfunction also has been linked to poststroke depression (Mayberg et al. 1988). Huntington's disease has been less clearly associated with monoaminergic abnormalities, but abnormalities of CRF and glutamate function have been suggested (Slaughter et al. 2001).

The structural and functional neuroanatomy of depression associated with neurological disease also shares similarities with findings in idiopathic depression. Computed tomography and magnetic resonance imaging (MRI) studies in stroke patients with and without mood disorders have documented a high association of mood changes with infarctions of the frontal lobe and basal ganglia, particularly those occurring in close proximity to the frontal pole or involving the caudate nucleus (R.G. Robinson et al. 1984; Starkstein et al. 1987). Reports of patients with traumatic frontal lobe injury indicate a high correlation between affective disturbances and right hemisphere pathology (Grafman et al. 1986). Late-onset depression has been linked with MRI-defined white matter abnormalities likely to be related to otherwise subclinical ischemic changes (Alexopoulos et al. 1997). Secondary mania, although rare, is most consistently seen with right-sided basal frontal-temporal or subcortical damage (Starkstein et al. 1990). Studies of patients with head trauma, brain tumors, or ablative neurosurgery (Grafman et al. 1986; Stuss and Benson 1986) further suggest that dorsolateral lesions are associated with depression and depressive-like symptoms such as apathy and psychomotor slowing.

Several functional imaging studies of depressed patients with neurological disease have been conducted in which functional abnormalities would not be confounded by gross cortical lesions. These studies typically have included Parkinson's disease, Huntington's disease, and lacunar strokes of the basal ganglia—disorders with known or identifiable neurochemical, neurodegenerative, or focal changes in which the primary pathology spares frontal cortex (the region repeatedly implicated in idiopathic depression studies). These data have shown that depressed patients with Parkinson's disease have selective hypometabolism involving the caudate nucleus and prefrontal and orbitofrontal cortices (Jagust et al. 1992; Mayberg et al. 1990). Depressed patients with Huntington's disease show decreases in paralimbic orbitofrontal and inferior prefrontal cortices (as well as caudate abnormalities inherent to the disease) (Mayberg et al. 1992). Patients with depression following unilateral lacunar subcortical stroke also show cortical hypometabolism (Mayberg 1994), suggesting that subcortical lesions can affect function throughout a network of brain regions involved in mood regulation. These data suggest that the depressive syndrome, regardless of etiology, is associated with similar regional brain changes (Figure 15–1).

SYMPTOM-SPECIFIC FINDINGS

Another approach to the study of mood disorders has been to focus on the neurobiology of specific symptom clusters. In this section, we review the neurobiological bases for different symptoms and symptom clusters associated with mood disorders.

Mood and Affect

Broadly speaking, it has been shown that emotional processing occurs within neural networks that include predominantly ventral frontal brain structures (Phillips et al. 2003a, 2003b). In particular, sad mood has been correlated with increased activity in the ventral medial frontal cortex, with several studies implicating Brodmann area 25 of the subgenual cingulate cortex as a critical node in this network (Damasio et al. 2000; Levesque et al. 2003b; Liotti et al. 2000; Talbot and Cooper 2006), and changes in this region have been associated with antidepressant treatments (Mayberg 2003; Mayberg et al. 2005).

Suppression of sadness in healthy subjects has been associated with activity of the dorsolateral prefrontal cortex (Levesque et al. 2003a), possibly suggesting a normal compensatory response in healthy subjects that may be abnormal in depressed patients. Positive mood is associated with similar frontal, especially prefrontal, brain structures (Damasio et al. 2000; Habel et al. 2005). Temporal lobe structures, especially the amygdala, also have been implicated in emotional processing (Phelps and LeDoux 2005). Furthermore, cortical-amygdalar interactions may be involved in emotional reactivity, with variability between persons explained in part by genetic differences (Pezawas et al. 2005). Some investigators have suggested that the brain has lateralized networks for emotional regulation, such that processing of positive emotions is more strongly associated with left-sided brain function and processing of negative emotions is more strongly associated with right-sided neural systems (Davidson 1995).

Disturbance of affect (as distinct from mood) has been associated with dysfunction within the basal ganglia and related structures. Patients with Parkinson's disease, for example, may have "depressive" affect in the absence of other depressive symptoms; furthermore, patients with Parkinson's disease may have greater difficulty demonstrating and recognizing facial expressions of emotion (Jacobs et al. 1995). Electrical stimulation of the subthalamic nucleus has been associated with pseudobulbar crying (Okun et al. 2004). Pseudobulbar affect in general (e.g., pathological crying or laughing) is associated with neurological diseases involving diverse brain structures (Schiffer and Pope 2005). However, lesions almost always occur in motor neural systems (Schiffer and Pope 2005).

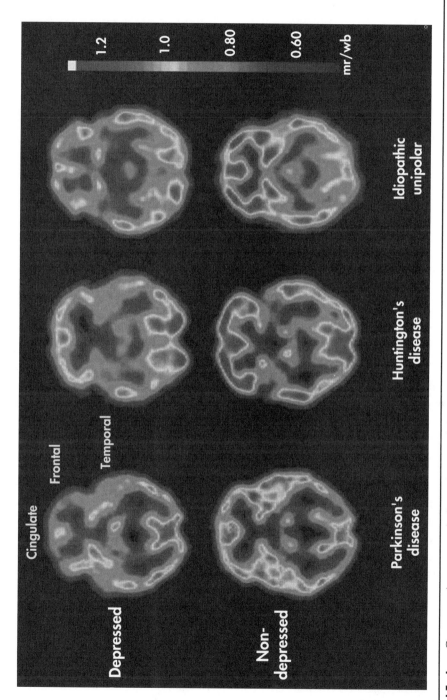

FIGURE 15–1. Common glucose metabolic positron emission tomography findings in neurological and idiopathic depression.

See Appendix for color version. Decreased prefrontal, dorsal cingulate, and temporal cortical metabolism is a common finding across different depressive syndromes, including patients with Parkinson's disease, Huntington's disease, and idiopathic unipolar depression.

The neurochemical bases of mood and affect are not clear, although the involvement of monoaminergic systems has been suggested. Acute depletion of tryptophan (resulting in decreased available serotonin) can lead to a recurrence of depressive symptoms in vulnerable patients (Booij et al. 2002). Successful SSRI treatment is associated with decreased activation of specific brain regions in response to sad stimuli in depressed patients (Fu et al. 2004). Dopamine function has been associated with positive mood states (Burgdorf and Panksepp 2006).

Interest and Motivation

Studies of interest and motivation implicate function within ventral striatal and cortical systems, with the dopamine system likely involved. Ventral striatal dopaminergic pathways appear to play a critical role in motivation (Tremblay et al. 2005; Wise 2005). Interestingly, dopamine may be more important for motivation (seeking) behavior than for hedonic response or reward (S. Robinson et al. 2005). Orbitofrontal, anterior cingulate, and prefrontal cortices, as well as ventral basal ganglia (nucleus accumbens, ventral caudate, and ventral putamen), appear to be involved in the neurobiology of interest and hedonic response (Roesch and Olson 2004; Tremblay et al. 2005).

In depressed patients, anhedonia has been associated with decreased activity in ventral basal ganglia and ventral prefrontal cortical regions (Dunn et al. 2002; Keedwell et al. 2005), and altered reward processing has been identified with a dopaminergic probe (Tremblay et al. 2005). A study of hedonic response in schizophrenia patients (compared with healthy control subjects) found that patients failed to activate ventral cortical-subcortical regions (including insular cortex, nucleus accumbens, and parahippocampal gyrus) during an unpleasant experience but instead showed increased metabolism in frontal cortical regions (Crespo-Facorro et al. 2001). Studies of apathy (separate from depression and anhedonia) have implicated similar, but more dorsal, prefrontal and subcortical brain regions (van Reekum et al. 2005).

In summary, anhedonia and apathy appear to be mediated by overlapping brain regions that primarily include ventral cortical and subcortical areas. These regions largely overlap those involved in mood regulation.

Sleep

Sleep physiology has been extensively studied in depressed patients. Sleep electroencephalogram abnormalities reported in depression include prolonged sleep latency, decreased slow-wave sleep, and reduced rapid eye movement (REM) latency with disturbances in the relative time spent in both REM and non-REM sleep (Benca et al. 1992). Reduced REM latency is the best-studied and most reproducible sleep-related electroencephalography finding in depressed patients, and this abnormality is reversed by most antidepressants (Sharpley and Cowen 1995). Sleep deprivation, particularly if instituted in the second half of the night, has an effect similar to that of medication, although the rapid, dramatic improvement in depressive symptoms is short-lived (Wu and Bunney 1990). Imaging data have suggested that increased pretreatment activity in the ventral anterior cingulate cortex and ventromedial prefrontal cortex may predict antidepressant response to sleep deprivation (Wu et al. 1999). Changes in nocturnal body temperature and attenuation of the normal fluctuations in core body temperature during sleep further suggest a more generalized dysregulation of normal circadian rhythms in patients with depression (Benca 1994). To date, however, none of these markers has proven to be specific to depression, suggesting a neural system underlying sleep and circadian rhythms that is involved but not specific to mood disorder syndromes.

The physiology of sleep disturbances in patients with mania and bipolar depression is less well characterized. Clinically, it has long been observed that sleep deprivation is a common precipitant of manic episodes, again suggesting an important biological link between sleep and affective symptoms. Patients with bipolar depression presenting with hypersomnia do not show a consistent reduction in REM latency (Nofzinger et al. 1991). Marked changes in sleep continuity and other REM measures comparable to those seen in patients with MDD also have been described, however (Benca 1994).

Appetite

The neurobiology of appetite disturbance in mood disorder and/or neuropsychiatric disease is not well understood. As described earlier, appetite and weight changes are common in these conditions. Also, medications used for treatment (e.g., anticonvulsants, lithium, neuroleptics) have effects on appetite, body weight, and metabolism. Brain regions involved in regulation of appetite and feeding include the hypothalamus and amygdala, and neuromodulatory systems involved include leptin (a peripheral hormone with central nervous system activity), melanocortin, neuropeptide Y, the HPA axis, and the monoamines (especially dopamine) (Kishi and Elmquist 2005).

Psychomotor Activity

Psychomotor abnormalities have largely been linked to monoaminergic neurotransmission (especially dopamine) and dorsal cortical and subcortical brain activity. For example, patients with Parkinson's disease have decreased psychomotor activity that clearly improves with dopaminergic therapies. Mice bred to underexpress the gene for the dopamine transporter (leading to a hyperdopaminergic state) show hyperactivity in novel environments (but not in a home cage situation) (Zhuang et al. 2001). Decreased dopamine in the basal ganglia has been associated with psychomotor retardation in depressed patients (Martinot et al. 2001). Dorsolateral prefrontal cortex activity correlates with psychomotor activity in depressed patients (Videbech et al. 2002).

Emotional Bias

Processing of positive and negative information (such as rewards and punishments) has been linked to the ventral prefrontal cortex, ventral striatum, midbrain, and hippocampus (Elliott et al. 2000) and to dopamine function (Wise 2002). Depressed patients have shown abnormal activity in ventral cortical and subcortical brain regions associated with processing of feedback (Elliott et al. 1998) and negative emotional stimuli (Elliott et al. 2002). Depressed patients also may have heightened sensitivity to the rewarding effects of dextroamphetamine compared with healthy controls (suggesting a hypodopaminergic state); this sensitivity is associated with altered brain activity in ventral cortical and subcortical regions (Tremblay et al. 2005).

Emotional bias is treated here as a separate symptom, but it may also be described as a cognitive process applied to emotional stimuli. As such, it is not unreasonable to expect that emotional bias may reflect an interaction of neural systems involved in mood and cognition. For example, older patients with depression have shown slower performance on the emotional Stroop Test (compared with matched control subjects) as well as slower response for negative than for neutral or positive words (a pattern not seen in matched control subjects) (Dudley et al. 2002). Depressed patients show a different pattern of frontal-limbic brain activity during the standard and emotional Stroop Test compared with healthy control subjects (George et al. 1997), and interference on the emotional Stroop Test has been correlated with increased ventral anterior cingulate activity (Whalen et al. 1998) as opposed to increased dorsal anterior cingulate activity with interference on a nonemotional Stroop Test (Bush et al. 1998).

Suicidal ideation might be viewed as an extreme of negative emotional bias. Postmortem brain studies of depressed people who committed suicide reported changes in several serotonin markers (Arango et al. 2003).

Cognition

Cognitive processes disturbed in patients with mood disorders involve primarily dorsal frontal and subcortical brain regions. Working memory, planning, and organization are executive functions linked with dorsolateral prefrontal cortical function and known to be abnormal in depression (Rogers et al. 2004). Depressed patients have shown blunting of an expected left anterior cingulate increase during performance of a cognitive interference task (the Stroop Test) (George et al. 1997). These patients also have shown a corresponding increase in function within the dorsolateral prefrontal cortex (a region not normally recruited during this task) (George et al. 1997), suggesting altered compensatory activity. During a planning task, depressed patients show poor activation of the dorsal prefrontal cortex, anterior cingulate cortex, and dorsal caudate (Elliott et al. 1997a). Poor performance on the standard Stroop task in patients with late-life depression has been specifically associated with abnormalities in dorsal subcortical white matter (Alexopoulos et al. 2002).

Disinhibition (commonly seen in mania) has been associated with ventral cortical structures (Cummings 1995). Disinhibition in dementia, for example, is associated with tissue loss in the subgenual cingulate cortex (Rosen et al. 2005). Manic patients show poor activation in the orbitofrontal cortex during a response inhibition task that reliably increases orbitofrontal activity in nonmanic control subjects (Altshuler et al. 2005).

CONCLUSION

Several distinct but interconnected neural systems regulate mood, affect, cognition, sleep, appetite, psychomotor activity, emotional regulation, and homeostatic/drive states. When these systems are disrupted, the resulting symptomatic presentation is broadly defined as a "mood disorder." Mood disorders may be associated with distinct neurological illnesses or other medical abnormalities (e.g., hypothyroidism), or they may be idiopathic. The etiologies of mood disorders may be diverse, but the neural dysfunction underlying the clinical manifestations is presumed to be the same. On this basis, models of brain systems involved in mood disorders can be developed and tested.

RECOMMENDED READINGS

Drevets WC: Prefrontal cortical-amygdalar metabolism in major depression. Ann N Y Acad Sci 877:614–637, 1999

Mayberg HS: Modulating dysfunctional limbic-cortical circuits in depression: towards development of brain-based algorithms for diagnosis and optimised treatment. Br Med Bull 65:193–207, 2003

McDonald WM, Richard IH, DeLong MR: Prevalence, etiology, and treatment of depression in Parkinson's disease. Biol Psychiatry 54:363–375, 2003

REFERENCES

Alexopoulos GS, Meyers BS, Young RC, et al: "Vascular depression" hypothesis. Arch Gen Psychiatry 54:915–922, 1997

Alexopoulos GS, Kiosses DN, Choi SJ, et al: Frontal white matter microstructure and treatment response of late-life depression: a preliminary study. Am J Psychiatry 159:1929–1932, 2002

Alloy LB, Abramson LY, Whitehouse WG, et al: Depressogenic cognitive styles: predictive validity, information processing and personality characteristics, and developmental origins. Behav Res Ther 37:503–531, 1999

Altshuler LL, Bookheimer SY, Townsend J, et al: Blunted activation in orbitofrontal cortex during mania: a functional magnetic resonance imaging study. Biol Psychiatry 58:763–769, 2005

American Psychiatric Association: Diagnostic and Statistical Manual of Mental Disorders, 4th Edition, Text Revision. Washington, DC, American Psychiatric Association, 2000

Arango V, Huang YY, Underwood MD, et al: Genetics of the serotonergic system in suicidal behavior. J Psychiatr Res 37:375–386, 2003

Arroll B, Macgillivray S, Ogston S, et al: Efficacy and tolerability of tricyclic antidepressants and SSRIs compared with placebo for treatment of depression in primary care: a meta-analysis. Ann Fam Med 3:449–456, 2005

Asberg M, Thoren P, Traskman L, et al: "Serotonin depression"—a biochemical subgroup within the affective disorders? Science 191:478–480, 1976

Ballmaier M, Toga AW, Blanton RE, et al: Anterior cingulate, gyrus rectus, and orbitofrontal abnormalities in elderly depressed patients: an MRI-based parcellation of the prefrontal cortex. Am J Psychiatry 161:99–108, 2004

Banki CM, Bissette G, Arato M, et al: Elevation of immunoreactive CSF TRH in depressed patients. Am J Psychiatry 145:1526–1531, 1988

Baxter LR Jr, Schwartz JM, Phelps ME, et al: Reduction of prefrontal cortex glucose metabolism common to three types of depression. Arch Gen Psychiatry 46:243–250, 1989

Benca RM: Mood disorders, in Principles and Practice of Sleep Medicine. Edited by Kryger MH, Roth T, Dement WC. Philadelphia, PA, WB Saunders, 1994, pp 899–913

Benca RM, Obermeyer WH, Thisted RA, et al: Sleep and psychiatric disorders: a meta-analysis. Arch Gen Psychiatry 49:651–668; discussion 669–670, 1992

Bench CJ, Friston KJ, Brown RG, et al: The anatomy of melancholia: focal abnormalities of cerebral blood flow in major depression. Psychol Med 22:607–615, 1992

Berman RM, Narasimhan M, Miller HL, et al: Transient depressive relapse induced by catecholamine depletion: potential phenotypic vulnerability marker? Arch Gen Psychiatry 56:395–403, 1999

Bondy B, Baghai TC, Minov C, et al: Substance P serum levels are increased in major depression: preliminary results. Biol Psychiatry 53:538–542, 2003

Booij L, Van der Does W, Benkelfat C, et al: Predictors of mood response to acute tryptophan depletion: a reanalysis. Neuropsychopharmacology 27:852–861, 2002

Botteron KN, Raichle ME, Drevets WC, et al: Volumetric reduction in left subgenual prefrontal cortex in early onset depression. Biol Psychiatry 51:342–344, 2002

Brown ES, Suppes T: Mood symptoms during corticosteroid therapy: a review. Harv Rev Psychiatry 5:239–246, 1998

Burgdorf J, Panksepp J: The neurobiology of positive emotions. Neurosci Biobehav Rev 30:173–187, 2006

Bush G, Whalen PJ, Rosen BR, et al: The counting Stroop: an interference task specialized for functional neuroimaging—validation study with functional MRI. Hum Brain Mapp 6:270–282, 1998

Caspi A, Sugden K, Moffitt TE, et al: Influence of life stress on depression: moderation by a polymorphism in the 5-HTT gene. Science 301(5631):386–389, 2003

Choudary PV, Molnar M, Evans SJ, et al: Altered cortical glutamatergic and GABAergic signal transmission with glial involvement in depression. Proc Natl Acad Sci U S A 102:15653–15658, 2005

Cloninger CR, Svrakic DM, Przybeck TR: Can personality assessment predict future depression? A twelve-month follow-up of 631 subjects. J Affect Disord 92:35–44, 2006

Crespo-Facorro B, Paradiso S, Andreasen NC, et al: Neural mechanisms of anhedonia in schizophrenia: a PET study of response to unpleasant and pleasant odors. JAMA 286:427–435, 2001

Cummings JL: Anatomic and behavioral aspects of frontal-subcortical circuits. Ann N Y Acad Sci 769:1–13, 1995

Damasio AR, Grabowski TJ, Bechara A, et al: Subcortical and cortical brain activity during the feeling of self-generated emotions. Nat Neurosci 3:1049–1056, 2000

Davidson R: Cerebral asymmetry, emotion, and affective style, in Brain Asymmetry. Edited by Davidson RJ, Hugdahl K. Cambridge, MA, MIT Press, 1995, pp 361–387

D'Haenen H, Bossuyt A, Mertens J, et al: SPECT imaging of serotonin2 receptors in depression. Psychiatry Res 45:227–237, 1992

Drevets WC, Videen TO, Price JL, et al: A functional anatomical study of unipolar depression. J Neurosci 12:3628–3641, 1992

Drevets WC, Price JL, Simpson JR Jr, et al: Subgenual prefrontal cortex abnormalities in mood disorders. Nature 386(6627):824–827, 1997

Drevets WC, Bogers W, Raichle ME: Functional anatomical correlates of antidepressant drug treatment assessed using PET measures of regional glucose metabolism. Eur Neuropsychopharmacol 12:527–544, 2002

Dudley R, O'Brien J, Barnett N, et al: Distinguishing depression from dementia in later life: a pilot study employing the emotional Stroop task. Int J Geriatr Psychiatry 17:48–53, 2002

Dunn RT, Kimbrell TA, Ketter TA, et al: Principal components of the Beck Depression Inventory and regional cerebral metabolism in unipolar and bipolar depression. Biol Psychiatry 51:387–399, 2002

Einat H, Manji HK: Cellular plasticity cascades: genes-to-behavior pathways in animal models of bipolar disorder. Biol Psychiatry 59:1160–1171, 2006

Elliott R, Baker SC, Rogers RD, et al: Prefrontal dysfunction in depressed patients performing a complex planning task: a study using positron emission tomography. Psychol Med 27:931–942, 1997a

Elliott R, Sahakian BJ, Herrod JJ, et al: Abnormal response to negative feedback in unipolar depression: evidence for a diagnosis specific impairment. J Neurol Neurosurg Psychiatry 63:74–82, 1997b

Elliott R, Sahakian BJ, Michael A, et al: Abnormal neural response to feedback on planning and guessing tasks in patients with unipolar depression. Psychol Med 28:559–571, 1998

Elliott R, Friston KJ, Dolan RJ: Dissociable neural responses in human reward systems. J Neurosci 20:6159–6165, 2000

Elliott R, Rubinsztein JS, Sahakian BJ, et al: The neural basis of mood-congruent processing biases in depression. Arch Gen Psychiatry 59:597–604, 2002

Fanous A, Gardner CO, Prescott CA, et al: Neuroticism, major depression and gender: a population-based twin study. Psychol Med 32:719–728, 2002

Fu CH, Williams SC, Cleare AJ, et al: Attenuation of the neural response to sad faces in major depression by antidepressant treatment: a prospective, event-related functional magnetic resonance imaging study. Arch Gen Psychiatry 61:877–889, 2004

George MS, Ketter TA, Parekh PI, et al: Blunted left cingulate activation in mood disorder subjects during a response interference task (the Stroop). J Neuropsychiatry Clin Neurosci 9:55–63, 1997

Goldapple K, Segal Z, Garson C, et al: Modulation of cortical-limbic pathways in major depression: treatment-specific effects of cognitive behavior therapy. Arch Gen Psychiatry 61:34–41, 2004

Goldberg JF, Burdick KE, Endick CJ: Preliminary randomized, double-blind, placebo-controlled trial of pramipexole added to mood stabilizers for treatment-resistant bipolar depression. Am J Psychiatry 161:564–566, 2004

Grafman J, Vance SC, Weingartner H, et al: The effects of lateralized frontal lesions on mood regulation. Brain 109 (pt 6):1127–1148, 1986

Habel U, Klein M, Kellermann T, et al: Same or different? Neural correlates of happy and sad mood in healthy males. Neuroimage 26:206–214, 2005

Heim C, Newport DJ, Heit S, et al: Pituitary-adrenal and autonomic responses to stress in women after sexual and physical abuse in childhood. JAMA 284:592–597, 2000

Jacobs DH, Shuren J, Bowers D, et al: Emotional facial imagery, perception, and expression in Parkinson's disease. Neurology 45:1696–1702, 1995

Jagust WJ, Reed BR, Martin EM, et al: Cognitive function and regional cerebral blood flow in Parkinson's disease. Brain 115 (pt 2):521–537, 1992

Joffe RT, Sokolov ST: Thyroid hormone treatment of primary unipolar depression: a review. Int J Neuropsychopharmacol 3:143–147, 2000

Keedwell PA, Andrew C, Williams SC, et al: The neural correlates of anhedonia in major depressive disorder. Biol Psychiatry 58:843–853, 2005

Kendler KS, Kuhn JW, Vittum J, et al: The interaction of stressful life events and a serotonin transporter polymorphism in the prediction of episodes of major depression: a replication. Arch Gen Psychiatry 62:529–535, 2005

Kennedy SH, Evans KR, Kruger S, et al: Changes in regional brain glucose metabolism measured with positron emission tomography after paroxetine treatment of major depression. Am J Psychiatry 158:899–905, 2001

Kieseppa T, Partonen T, Haukka J, et al: High concordance of bipolar I disorder in a nationwide sample of twins. Am J Psychiatry 161:1814–1821, 2004

Kishi T, Elmquist JK: Body weight is regulated by the brain: a link between feeding and emotion. Mol Psychiatry 10:132–146, 2005

Levesque J, Eugene F, Joanette Y, et al: Neural circuitry underlying voluntary suppression of sadness. Biol Psychiatry 53:502–510, 2003a

Levesque J, Joanette Y, Mensour B, et al: Neural correlates of sad feelings in healthy girls. Neuroscience 121:545–551, 2003b

Levinson DF: Meta-analysis in psychiatric genetics. Curr Psychiatry Rep 7:143–151, 2005

Levinson DF: The genetics of depression: a review. Biol Psychiatry 60:84–92, 2006

Levitan RD, Rector NA, Bagby RM: Negative attributional style in seasonal and nonseasonal depression. Am J Psychiatry 155:428–430, 1998

Liotti M, Mayberg HS, Brannan SK, et al: Differential limbic-cortical correlates of sadness and anxiety in healthy subjects: implications for affective disorders. Biol Psychiatry 48:30–42, 2000

Loftis JM, Hauser P: The phenomenology and treatment of interferon-induced depression. J Affect Disord 82:175–190, 2004

Malison RT, Price LH, Berman R, et al: Reduced brain serotonin transporter availability in major depression as measured by [^{123}I]-2 beta-carbomethoxy-3 beta-(4-iodophenyl)tropane and single photon emission computed tomography. Biol Psychiatry 44:1090–1098, 1998

Manji HK, Drevets WC, Charney DS: The cellular neurobiology of depression. Nat Med 7:541–547, 2001

Mann JJ, Malone KM, Psych MR [sic], et al: Attempted suicide characteristics and cerebrospinal fluid amine metabolites in depressed inpatients. Neuropsychopharmacology 15:576–586, 1996

Martinot M, Bragulat V, Artiges E, et al: Decreased presynaptic dopamine function in the left caudate of depressed patients with affective flattening and psychomotor retardation. Am J Psychiatry 158:314–316, 2001

Mayberg HS: Frontal lobe dysfunction in secondary depression. J Neuropsychiatry Clin Neurosci 6:428–442, 1994

Mayberg HS: Modulating dysfunctional limbic-cortical circuits in depression: towards development of brain-based algorithms for diagnosis and optimised treatment. Br Med Bull 65:193–207, 2003

Mayberg HS, Solomon DH: Depression in Parkinson's disease: a biochemical and organic viewpoint. Adv Neurol 65:49–60, 1995

Mayberg HS, Robinson RG, Wong DF, et al: PET imaging of cortical S2 serotonin receptors after stroke: lateralized changes and relationship to depression. Am J Psychiatry 145:937–943, 1988

Mayberg HS, Starkstein SE, Sadzot B, et al: Selective hypometabolism in the inferior frontal lobe in depressed patients with Parkinson's disease. Ann Neurol 28:57–64, 1990

Mayberg HS, Starkstein SE, Peyser CE, et al: Paralimbic frontal lobe hypometabolism in depression associated with Huntington's disease. Neurology 42:1791–1797, 1992

Mayberg HS, Brannan SK, Mahurin RK, et al: Cingulate function in depression: a potential predictor of treatment response. Neuroreport 8:1057–1061, 1997

Mayberg HS, Lozano AM, Voon V, et al: Deep brain stimulation for treatment-resistant depression. Neuron 45:651–660, 2005

McCrae RR, Costa PT Jr: Validation of the five-factor model of personality across instruments and observers. J Pers Soc Psychol 52:81–90, 1987

Meyer JH, Kruger S, Wilson AA, et al: Lower dopamine transporter binding potential in striatum during depression. Neuroreport 12:4121–4125, 2001

Murphy FC, Sahakian BJ, Rubinsztein JS, et al: Emotional bias and inhibitory control processes in mania and depression. Psychol Med 29:1307–1321, 1999

Nelson JC: A review of the efficacy of serotonergic and noradrenergic reuptake inhibitors for treatment of major depression. Biol Psychiatry 46:1301–1308, 1999

Nemeroff CB, Simon JS, Haggerty JJ Jr, et al: Antithyroid antibodies in depressed patients. Am J Psychiatry 142:840–843, 1985

Neumeister A, Nugent AC, Waldeck T, et al: Neural and behavioral responses to tryptophan depletion in unmedicated patients with remitted major depressive disorder and controls. Arch Gen Psychiatry 61:765–773, 2004

Nierenberg AA, Dougherty D, Rosenbaum JF: Dopaminergic agents and stimulants as antidepressant augmentation strategies. J Clin Psychiatry 59 (suppl 5):60–63; discussion 64, 1998

Nofzinger EA, Thase ME, Reynolds CF 3rd, et al: Hypersomnia in bipolar depression: a comparison with narcolepsy using the multiple sleep latency test. Am J Psychiatry 148:1177–1181, 1991

O'Brien SM, Scott LV, Dinan TG: Cytokines: abnormalities in major depression and implications for pharmacological treatment. Hum Psychopharmacol 19:397–403, 2004

Okun MS, Raju DV, Walter BL, et al: Pseudobulbar crying induced by stimulation in the region of the subthalamic nucleus. J Neurol Neurosurg Psychiatry 75:921–923, 2004

Pezawas L, Meyer-Lindenberg A, Drabant EM, et al: 5-HTTLPR polymorphism impacts human cingulate-amygdala interactions: a genetic susceptibility mechanism for depression. Nat Neurosci 8:828–834, 2005

Phelps EA, LeDoux JE: Contributions of the amygdala to emotion processing: from animal models to human behavior. Neuron 48:175–187, 2005

Phillips ML, Drevets WC, Rauch SL, et al: Neurobiology of emotion perception, I: the neural basis of normal emotion perception. Biol Psychiatry 54:504–514, 2003a

Phillips ML, Drevets WC, Rauch SL, et al: Neurobiology of emotion perception, II: implications for major psychiatric disorders. Biol Psychiatry 54:515–528, 2003b

Pizzagalli DA, Oakes TR, Fox AS, et al: Functional but not structural subgenual prefrontal cortex abnormalities in melancholia. Mol Psychiatry 9:393–405, 2004

Posener JA, DeBattista C, Williams GH, et al: 24-Hour monitoring of cortisol and corticotropin secretion in psychotic and nonpsychotic major depression. Arch Gen Psychiatry 57:755–760, 2000

Raison CL, Capuron L, Miller AH: Cytokines sing the blues: inflammation and the pathogenesis of depression. Trends Immunol 27:24–31, 2006

Raskind MA: The clinical interface of depression and dementia. J Clin Psychiatry 59 (suppl 10):9–12, 1998

Risch N, Herrell R, Lehner T, et al: Interaction between the serotonin transporter gene (5-HTTLPR), stressful life events, and risk of depression: a meta-analysis. JAMA 301:2462–2471, 2009

Robinson RG, Kubos KL, Starr LB, et al: Mood disorders in stroke patients: importance of location of lesion. Brain 107 (pt 1):81–93, 1984

Robinson S, Sandstrom SM, Denenberg VH, et al: Distinguishing whether dopamine regulates liking, wanting, and/or learning about rewards. Behav Neurosci 119:5–15, 2005

Roesch MR, Olson CR: Neuronal activity related to reward value and motivation in primate frontal cortex. Science 304(5668):307–310, 2004

Rogers MA, Kasai K, Koji M, et al: Executive and prefrontal dysfunction in unipolar depression: a review of neuropsychological and imaging evidence. Neurosci Res 50:1–11, 2004

Rosen HJ, Allison SC, Schauer GF, et al: Neuroanatomical correlates of behavioural disorders in dementia. Brain 128 (pt 11):2612–2625, 2005

Roy A, Karoum F, Pollack S: Marked reduction in indexes of dopamine metabolism among patients with depression who attempt suicide. Arch Gen Psychiatry 49:447–450, 1992

Ruggiero DA, Underwood MD, Rice PM, et al: Corticotropic-releasing hormone and serotonin interact in the human brainstem: behavioral implications. Neuroscience 91:1343–1354, 1999

Santor DA, Bagby RM, Joffe RT: Evaluating stability and change in personality and depression. J Pers Soc Psychol 73:1354–1362, 1997

Sargent PA, Kjaer KH, Bench CJ, et al: Brain serotonin1A receptor binding measured by positron emission tomography with [11C] WAY-100635: effects of depression and antidepressant treatment. Arch Gen Psychiatry 57:174–180, 2000

Schiffer R, Pope LE: Review of pseudobulbar affect including a novel and potential therapy. J Neuropsychiatry Clin Neurosci 17:447–454, 2005

Schildkraut JJ: The catecholamine hypothesis of affective disorders: a review of supporting evidence. Am J Psychiatry 122:509–522, 1965

Schinka JA, Busch RM, Robichaux-Keene N: A meta-analysis of the association between the serotonin transporter gene polymorphism (5-HTTLPR) and trait anxiety. Mol Psychiatry 9:197–202, 2004

Sharpley AL, Cowen PJ: Effect of pharmacologic treatments on the sleep of depressed patients. Biol Psychiatry 37:85–98, 1995

Sheline YI: Neuroimaging studies of mood disorder effects on the brain. Biol Psychiatry 54:338–352, 2003

Slaughter JR, Martens MP, Slaughter KA: Depression and Huntington's disease: prevalence, clinical manifestations, etiology, and treatment. CNS Spectr 6:306–326, 2001

Starkstein SE, Robinson RG, Price TR: Comparison of cortical and subcortical lesions in the production of poststroke mood disorders. Brain 110 (pt 4):1045–1059, 1987

Starkstein SE, Mayberg HS, Berthier ML, et al: Mania after brain injury: neuroradiological and metabolic findings. Ann Neurol 27:652–659, 1990

Strakowski SM, Delbello MP, Adler CM: The functional neuroanatomy of bipolar disorder: a review of neuroimaging findings. Mol Psychiatry 10:105–116, 2005

Strauss J, Barr CL, George CJ, et al: BDNF and COMT polymorphisms: relation to memory phenotypes in young adults with childhood-onset mood disorder. Neuromolecular Med 5:181–192, 2004

Stuss DT, Benson DF: The Frontal Lobes. New York, Raven, 1986

Talbot PS, Cooper SJ: Anterior cingulate and subgenual prefrontal blood flow changes following tryptophan depletion in healthy males. Neuropsychopharmacology 31:1757–1767, 2006

Teasdale JD, Russell ML: Differential effects of induced mood on the recall of positive, negative and neutral words. Br J Clin Psychol 22 (pt 3): 163–171, 1983

Tremblay LK, Naranjo CA, Graham SJ, et al: Functional neuroanatomical substrates of altered reward processing in major depressive disorder revealed by a dopaminergic probe. Arch Gen Psychiatry 62:1228–1236, 2005

van Reekum R, Stuss DT, Ostrander L: Apathy: why care? J Neuropsychiatry Clin Neurosci 17:7–19, 2005

Videbech P: PET measurements of brain glucose metabolism and blood flow in major depressive disorder: a critical review. Acta Psychiatr Scand 101:11–20, 2000

Videbech P, Ravnkilde B, Pedersen TH, et al: The Danish PET/depression project: clinical symptoms and cerebral blood flow: a regions-of-interest analysis. Acta Psychiatr Scand 106:35–44, 2002

Whalen PJ, Bush G, McNally RJ, et al: The emotional counting Stroop paradigm: a functional magnetic resonance imaging probe of the anterior cingulate affective division. Biol Psychiatry 44:1219–1228, 1998

Wise RA: Brain reward circuitry: insights from unsensed incentives. Neuron 36:229–240, 2002

Wise RA: Forebrain substrates of reward and motivation. J Comp Neurol 493:115–121, 2005

Wu JC, Bunney WE: The biological basis of an antidepressant response to sleep deprivation and relapse: review and hypothesis. Am J Psychiatry 147:14–21, 1990

Wu J, Buchsbaum MS, Gillin JC, et al: Prediction of antidepressant effects of sleep deprivation by metabolic rates in the ventral anterior cingulate and medial prefrontal cortex. Am J Psychiatry 156:1149–1158, 1999

Zhuang X, Oosting RS, Jones SR, et al: Hyperactivity and impaired response habituation in hyperdopaminergic mice. Proc Natl Acad Sci U S A 98:1982–1987, 2001

16

NEUROPSYCHIATRIC ASPECTS OF ANXIETY DISORDERS

Dan J. Stein, M.D., Ph.D.

Scott L. Rauch, M.D.

Although it has long been recognized that specific neurological lesions may lead to anxiety symptoms, only in the past several years have advances in research allowed particular neuroanatomical hypotheses to be put forward about each of the different anxiety disorders. In this chapter, we review these developments in our understanding of the anxiety disorders. We begin by reviewing neurological disorders that may present with anxiety symptoms and then outline neuroanatomical models of each of the principal anxiety disorders (panic disorder, social phobia [social anxiety disorder], posttraumatic stress disorder [PTSD], generalized anxiety disorder [GAD], and obsessive-compulsive disorder [OCD]).

NEUROLOGICAL DISORDERS WITH ANXIETY SYMPTOMS

Neurological conditions that affect a range of different neuroanatomical structures may be associated with anxiety symptoms or disorders. Given that temporolimbic regions, striatum, and prefrontal cortex all likely play an important role in the pathogenesis of certain anxiety disorders, we begin by reviewing the association between lesions in these areas and subsequent anxiety symptoms before moving on to disorders with more widespread pathology.

Various lesions of temporolimbic regions have been associated with the subsequent development of panic disorder. Temporal lobe

Dr. Stein is supported by the Medical Research Council of South Africa.

seizures, tumors, arteriovenous malformation, lobectomy, and parahippocampal infarction all have been reported to present with panic attacks. The association seems particularly strong with right-sided lesions. (Conversely, removal of the amygdala results in both placidity toward previously feared objects [Klüver and Bucy 1939] and deficits in fear conditioning [Bechara et al. 1995].)

This literature, taken together with clinical observations that panic disorder may be accompanied by dissociation and depersonalization and possibly by electroencephalographic abnormalities and temporal abnormalities, as well as preliminary data that panic disorder can respond to anticonvulsants, raises the question of whether partially overlapping mechanisms may be at work in both temporal lobe seizure disorder and panic disorder. Certainly, it has been suggested that electroencephalography (EEG) and anticonvulsant trials may be appropriate in patients with panic disorder refractory to conventional treatment (Kinrys and Wygant 2005).

Lesions of the basal ganglia have been associated with obsessions and compulsions, a finding that has been crucial to the development of a "cortico-striatal-thalamic-cortical" (CSTC) hypothesis of OCD. An early "striatal topography" hypothesis was that caudate lesions in particular are associated with OCD, whereas putamen lesions result in tics (Rauch and Baxter 1998). On the other hand, there is also evidence that OCD is mediated by a range of CSTC circuits, and particular projection fields or cell types may be associated with specific kinds of symptoms.

The 1915–1926 pandemic of viral encephalitis lethargica provided early evidence of a specific neurological basis for OCD. The outbreak was followed by the presentation of numerous patients with a somnolent-like state and parkinsonian features. Various focal brain lesions, including involvement of the basal ganglia, were documented in these cases, and patients also were observed to have obsessive-compulsive symptoms and tics (Cheyette and Cummings 1995).

OCD symptoms also have been reported in a range of other basal ganglia lesions of various etiologies. Thus, OCD symptoms may be seen in Huntington's disease, Parkinson's disease, spasmodic torticollis, and basal ganglia lesions of a range of etiologies, including calcification, infarction, intoxication, and trauma. In this context, it is noteworthy that the basal ganglia may be particularly sensitive to prenatal and perinatal hypoxic-ischemic injury (in twins with Tourette syndrome, for example, an association exists between lower birth weight and increased severity of Tourette syndrome).

Furthermore, early studies suggested a link between Sydenham's chorea and OCD symptoms, and a study by Swedo et al. (1989) reported that rheumatic fever patients with Sydenham's chorea had significantly more OCD symptoms than did those without chorea. This work has formed the basis for an autoimmune theory of at least some cases of OCD. Swedo and colleagues have coined the term *PANDAS*, or pediatric autoimmune neuropsychiatric disorders associated with streptococcal infections, to describe patients who present with acute obsessive-compulsive or tic symptoms, hypothetically after developing antistriatal antibodies in response to infection.

Some of the most promising research on the association between OCD and a movement disorder has focused on the relation of OCD to Tourette syndrome. Gilles de la Tourette's 1885 initial description of the syndrome included a patient with tics, vocalizations, and perhaps obsessions. Increasing evidence suggests that a subgroup of patients with Tourette syndrome also has OCD. Conversely, a subgroup of OCD patients has tics. Furthermore, family studies have found a high rate of OCD and/or tics in relatives of patients with Tourette syndrome and a high rate of Tourette syndrome and/or tics in relatives of OCD patients.

Anxiety symptoms other than OCD may, however, also be seen in striatal disorders. In Huntington's disease, for example, anxiety has been reported as a common prodromal symptom, with later development of several different anxiety disorders including OCD. Anxiety symptoms and disorders are also common in Parkinson's disease and may correlate inversely with left striatal dopamine transporter availability.

Lesions of the frontal cortex may be associated with a range of perseverative symptoms. In the classic case of Phineas Gage, in addition to impairment in executive functions, the patient had perseverative symptoms and hoarding behaviors. Ames et al. (1994) reviewed the literature on frontal lobe degeneration and subsequent obsessive-compulsive symptoms and noted descriptions of a range of repetitive behaviors from motor stereotypies to OCD.

Anxiety symptoms and disorders can, of course, be seen in a range of neurological disorders that affect multiple brain regions, including frontal cortex. In multiple sclerosis, for example, anxiety symptoms may be found in up to 37% of subjects, and anxiety disorders are not uncommon. Similarly, anxiety symptoms have been noted to be common in Alzheimer's disease and in other dementias, including vascular and frontotemporal dementias.

Although the prevalence of depression after stroke has been well studied, less research has focused on anxiety after stroke. In one study, however, of 309 admissions to a stroke unit, DSM-III-R (American Psychiatric Association 1987) GAD was present in 26.9% of the patients (Castillo et al. 1993). The authors reported that anxiety plus depression was associated with left cortical lesions, whereas anxiety alone was associated with right hemisphere lesions. Also, worry was associated with anterior and GAD with right posterior lesions. Longitudinal studies have found that GAD can persist for several years after the stroke. Agoraphobia is also common after stroke.

Anxiety disorders also have been reported in the aftermath of traumatic brain injury. In one study, prevalence rates were 19% for PTSD, 15% for OCD, 14% for panic disorder, 10% for phobias, and 9% for GAD (Hibbard et al. 1998). Some evidence indicates relations between areas affected and risk for anxiety (Vasa et al. 2004). PTSD can develop even when the patient has neurogenic amnesia for the trau-

matic event; this finding may suggest that implicit memories of trauma are sufficient for later PTSD to emerge, although subsequent appraisal processes also may be relevant. In either event, PTSD in such patients may be unusual because reexperiencing symptoms are absent.

NEUROANATOMY OF ANXIETY DISORDERS

In the following sections, we consider the neuropsychiatry of each of the major anxiety disorders. Each section begins by sketching a simplistic neuroanatomical model of the relevant anxiety disorder. This sketch is then used as a framework for attempting a more complex integration of animal data, clinical biological research (e.g., pharmacological probe studies), and brain imaging studies.

GENERALIZED ANXIETY DISORDER

Neuroanatomical models of GAD have not been well delineated to date. However, it may be speculated that GAD involves 1) a general "limbic circuit," including paralimbic cortex (e.g., anterior temporal cortex, posterior medial orbitofrontal cortex) and related subcortical structures (e.g., amygdala), which may be activated across a range of different anxiety disorders, and 2) perhaps some degree of prefrontal hyperactivity, which may represent an attempt across the anxiety disorders to suppress subcortically mediated anxiety or which may arguably reflect more specific GAD symptoms of excessive worrying and planning (Figure 16–1). In reviewing research relevant to this speculative model, we consider first neurochemical studies and then neuroanatomical findings.

Neurochemical Studies

Serotonergic mediation of GAD is supported by several findings. Reduced cerebrospinal fluid levels of serotonin and reduced platelet paroxetine binding have been observed. Administration of the pharmacological probe *m*-chlorophenylpiperazine (m-CPP), a sero-

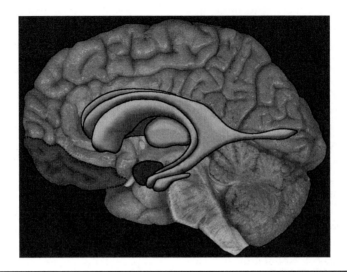

FIGURE 16–1.   Neuroanatomical model of generalized anxiety disorder.

See Appendix for color version. Note the increased activity in temporolimbic areas (Tiihonen et al. 1997b; Wu et al. 1991) as well as in prefrontal areas (Rauch et al. 1997; Wu et al. 1991).

Source.   Reprinted from Stein DJ: *False Alarm! How to Conquer the Anxiety Disorders.* Cape Town, South Africa, University of Stellenbosch, 2000. Used with permission.

tonergic agonist, results in increased anxiety. Serotonergic compounds appear effective in the pharmacotherapy for GAD; buspirone, a serotonin type 1A (5-HT$_{1A}$) receptor partial agonist, is effective in some studies, and the selective serotonin reuptake inhibitors (SSRIs) are well studied in GAD.

Animal work has long established involvement of the locus coeruleus–norepinephrine–sympathetic nervous system in fear and arousal. In GAD, increased plasma norepinephrine and 3-methoxy-4-hydroxyphenylglycol (MHPG) and reduced platelet α_2-adrenergic peripheral receptor binding sites have been reported. Administration of more dynamic adrenergic probes has, however, indicated reduced adrenergic receptor sensitivity, perhaps an adaptation to high circulating catecholamines. Dual serotonin and noradrenergic reuptake inhibitors have been shown effective in GAD. The locus coeruleus system projects to the amygdala and to other structures involved in anxiety responses, so that noradrenergic involvement is not inconsistent with the neuroanatomical model outlined earlier.

Involvement of the γ-aminobutyric acid (GABA)–benzodiazepine receptor complex in GAD is supported by several studies, including studies showing responsiveness of this disorder to benzodiazepine treatment. Anxious subjects and GAD patients have reduced benzodiazepine binding capacity, with normalization of findings after benzodiazepine treatment. GABA is the brain's predominant inhibitory neurotransmitter, and GABAergic pathways are widely distributed; nevertheless, the distribution of GABA and benzodiazepine receptors is particularly dense in limbic and paralimbic areas.

Neuroanatomical Studies

Neuroimaging research on GAD remains at a relatively preliminary stage. Nevertheless, findings are consistent with involvement of limbic, paralimbic, and prefrontal regions. Work with positron emission tomography found that GAD patients had increased relative metabolic rates in right posterior temporal lobe, right precentral frontal gyrus, and left inferior area 17 in the occipital lobe but

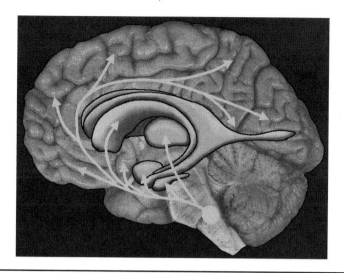

FIGURE 16–2. Serotonergic circuits project to key regions (prefrontal cortex, orbitofrontal cortex, anterior cingulate, amygdala, hippocampus, basal ganglia, thalamus) involved in the mediation of anxiety disorders.

See Appendix for color version.

Source. Reprinted from Stein DJ: *False Alarm! How to Conquer the Anxiety Disorders.* Cape Town, South Africa, University of Stellenbosch, 2000. Used with permission.

reduced absolute basal ganglia metabolic rates (Wu et al. 1991). Benzodiazepine treatment resulted in decreases in absolute metabolic rates for limbic system and cortical surface. Studies with magnetic resonance imaging and spectroscopy have provided additional data on the role of these circuits in GAD.

Preliminary imaging data on receptor binding in GAD are also available. In a study of female GAD patients, for example, left temporal pole benzodiazepine receptor binding was significantly reduced. Imaging studies do not suggest dysregulation of the serotonin transporter in GAD. Nevertheless, serotonergic neurons branch widely throughout the brain, affecting each of the main regions postulated to mediate anxiety symptoms (Figure 16–2); and SSRI treatment may result in a normalization of neuronal activity in pooled anxiety disorder subjects and in GAD patients.

OBSESSIVE-COMPULSIVE DISORDER

Current neuroanatomical models of OCD emphasize the role of CSTC circuits (Figure 16–3). There is a growing realization of the importance of various CSTC loops in a range of behavior disorders; ventral cognitive circuits, involving anterior and lateral orbitofrontal cortex, ventromedial caudate, and dorsomedial nuclei of the thalamus, appear to play a role in response inhibition, particularly in relation to certain kinds of cognitive-affective cues, and appear most relevant to OCD. This kind of model of OCD was first suggested by early findings of an association between neurological lesions of the striatum and OCD and has been supported by a range of subsequent additional studies.

Similar CSTC circuits also have been hypothesized to be involved in various putative obsessive-compulsive spectrum disorders (such as Tourette syndrome). An early "striatal topography" model of obsessive-compulsive spectrum disorders suggested that whereas the ventral cognitive system mediated symptoms of OCD, the sensorimotor cortex and putamen would instead be involved in Tourette syndrome and perhaps trichotillomania (Rauch

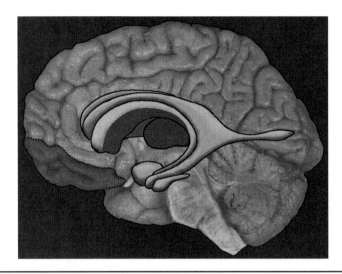

FIGURE 16–3.   Neuroanatomical model of obsessive-compulsive disorder.

See Appendix for color version. Note the increased activity in the ventromedial cortico-striatal-thalamic-cortical circuit (Rauch and Baxter 1998).

Source.   Reprinted from Stein DJ: *False Alarm! How to Conquer the Anxiety Disorders.* Cape Town, South Africa, University of Stellenbosch, 2000. Used with permission.

and Baxter 1998). It is possible, however, that particular striatal projection fields or cell types are involved in specific kinds of symptoms.

Neurochemical Studies

Interest in the neurochemical substrate of OCD received significant impetus from the early finding that the disorder responded to clomipramine, a serotonin reuptake inhibitor. Subsequent studies confirmed that clomipramine is more effective than desipramine, a noradrenergic reuptake inhibitor, in OCD. Each of the SSRIs studied to date has been effective for the treatment of OCD. After effective treatment with a serotonin reuptake inhibitor, cerebrospinal fluid 5-hydroxyindoleacetic acid decreases, and exacerbation of OCD symptoms by m-CPP is no longer seen.

The serotonergic system innervates not only the basal ganglia but also the orbitofrontal cortex. Animal work shows that downregulation of serotonin terminal autoreceptors in orbitofrontal cortex occurs only after a relatively long time and with relatively high doses of medication. This parallels clinical findings that

OCD pharmacotherapy differs from that used for depression.

Many OCD patients do not respond to serotonin reuptake inhibitors, suggesting that other neurochemical systems are also important. Administration of dopamine agonists results in stereotypic behavior in animals and in tics in humans, and conversely, dopamine blockers are effective for the treatment of tics. OCD patients with comorbid tics are less likely to respond to serotonin reuptake inhibitors but more likely to respond to augmentation of serotonin reuptake inhibitors with typical neuroleptics.

Given the dopaminergic innervation of the striatum and the interaction between the serotonin and the dopaminergic systems, these findings are consistent with the CSTC model. Indeed, infusion of dopamine into the caudate results in stereotyped orofacial behaviors in animals. Infusion of dopamine blockers into the same areas reduces amphetamine-induced stereotypy. Dopaminergic striatal circuits may be particularly important in OCD patients with tics and in patients with obsessive-compulsive spectrum disorders, such as Tourette syndrome, that are characterized by involuntary movements.

Other neurochemical systems, including glutamate and GABA, also play an important role in CSTC circuits. In the future, manipulation of such systems may turn out to be useful for the pharmacotherapy of OCD.

Neuroanatomical Studies

A range of evidence indicates that corticostriatal circuits are important in mediating stereotypic behavior. Isolation of primates during development, for example, results in basal ganglia cytoarchitectural abnormalities and stereotypic behavior. MacLean (1973) noted that lesions of the striatum resulted in stereotypic behavior and suggested that the striatum was a repository for fixed action patterns or inherited motor sequences (e.g., grooming, nestbuilding). Indeed, the animal literature on stereotypies and disorders of grooming parallels not only the phenomenology of OCD but also its psychopharmacology.

There is, however, a growing appreciation of the role of the striatum in cognition and learning. In particular, striatal function has increasingly been associated with the development, maintenance, and selection of motoric and cognitive procedural strategies. Different terms given to allude to this group of functions include *habit system*, *response set*, and *procedural mobilization*. Basal ganglia may play a particularly important role in the implicit learning of procedural strategies and their subsequent automatic execution. Neurological soft sign abnormalities and neuropsychological dysfunction in patients with OCD are consistent with dysfunction in CSTC circuits.

Structural imaging studies are also consonant with a role for CSTC circuits in OCD. An early study found reduced caudate volume in OCD patients, but not all subsequent research has replicated this finding. The finding that patients with PANDAS have increased basal ganglia volume may partly explain this inconsistency; in some OCD patients, basal ganglia volume initially may be increased, with subse-

quent reduction over time. Structural studies also have shown neuronal abnormalities or volume loss in orbitofrontal cortex, cingulate, amygdala, and thalamus in OCD. Also, putamen volume may be reduced in certain putative obsessive-compulsive spectrum disorders such as Tourette syndrome and trichotillomania.

Functional imaging studies, however, provide some of the most persuasive evidence of the role of CSTC circuits in OCD. OCD patients at rest, and especially when exposed to feared stimuli, show increased activity in the orbitofrontal cortex, anterior cingulate, and basal ganglia. A range of functional abnormalities also have been found in Tourette syndrome; one study, for example, found increased metabolism in the orbitofrontal cortex and putamen that correlated with complex behavioral and cognitive features.

Functional imaging findings may have particular explanatory power when they also integrate cognitive neuroscience constructs and findings. Rauch and colleagues (1997), for example, have shown that during brain imaging of an implicit sequence learning task, control subjects without OCD showed striatal activation, but patients with OCD instead appeared to recruit medial temporal regions. These latter regions are typically involved in conscious cognitive-affective processing. Control subjects can process procedural strategies outside of awareness, but in OCD, these strategies intrude into consciousness.

A further important set of findings that relate to the CSTC hypothesis of OCD emerges from work on neurosurgical treatments for OCD. Several different procedures have been used, but the general effect of these interventions is to interrupt CSTC circuits.

The "standard" neuroanatomical model of OCD may, however, be insufficiently complex to account for all cases. There is, for example, a literature on temporal lobe involvement in OCD. In some cases of OCD, temporal EEG abnormalities are seen, and anticonvulsants may on occasion be useful. Although OCD is in many ways a homogeneous entity, further research is necessary to delineate different neurobiological mechanisms, including divergent mediating neuronal circuitry, in symptom dimensions and subtypes of the disorder (Saxena and Rauch 2000).

Several studies have successfully integrated neurochemical and neuroimaging data. In OCD, preliminary evidence now indicates alterations in components of the glutamatergic and serotonergic systems in frontostriatal circuitry and disturbances in striatal dopamine transporter function. In Tourette syndrome, evidence also indicates alterations in striatal dopamine functioning (e.g., higher striatal binding to the dopamine transporter on imaging and in postmortem studies) and perhaps also disruptions in serotonin transporter function. Finally, a seminal publication reported that patients with OCD treated with either serotonin reuptake inhibitors or behavior therapy had normalization of activity in CSTC circuits (Baxter et al. 1992); effective interventions appear to work via a final common pathway of specific brain structures.

Nevertheless, several important questions remain unresolved about the CSTC model of OCD. It is unclear, for example, how presumptive lesions to the CSTC occur. Despite the documentation of cases of PANDAS, the extent to which autoimmune processes contribute to OCD in general is not known. Also, there may be differential pathogenic mechanisms across different obsessive-compulsive spectrum disorders. Genetic variability may play some role; for example, some studies have found differences in polymorphisms in dopamine pathway candidate genes in OCD patients with and without tics.

Additionally, questions remain about the precise nature of CSTC dysfunction in OCD and its normalization by effective treatment. It is interesting, for example, that decreased orbitofrontal activity in OCD predicts positive response to pharmacotherapy, whereas higher orbitofrontal activity predicts positive response to behavior therapy (Brody et al. 1998). Further work to consolidate fully a neuroanatomical model of both pharmacological and behavioral interventions in OCD is necessary.

PANIC DISORDER

Over the past decade or two, models of panic disorder have become increasingly sophisticated. Current neuroanatomical models of panic disorder (Figure 16–4) emphasize 1) afferents from viscerosensory pathways to thalamus to the lateral nucleus of the amygdala, as well as from thalamus to cortical association areas to the lateral nucleus of the amygdala; 2) the extended amygdala, which is thought to play a central role in conditioned fear (Le Doux 1998) and anxiety (Davis and Whalen 2001); 3) the hippocampus, which is thought crucial for conditioning to the context of the fear (and so perhaps for phobic avoidance); and 4) efferent tracts from the amygdala to the hypothalamus and brain stem structures, which mediate many of the symptoms of panic. Thus, efferents of the central nucleus of the amygdala include the lateral nucleus (autonomic arousal and sympathetic discharge) and paraventricular nucleus (increased adrenocorticoid release) of the hypothalamus and the locus coeruleus (increased norepinephrine release), parabrachial nucleus (increased respiratory rate), and periaqueductal gray (defensive behaviors and postural freezing) in the brain stem.

Neurochemical Studies

Early animal studies found that the locus coeruleus plays a key role in fear and anxiety (Redmond 1986), with both electrical and pharmacological stimulation resulting in fear responses. The locus coeruleus contains the highest concentration of noradrenergic-producing neurons in the brain. Viscerosensory input reaches the locus coeruleus via the nucleus tractus solitarius and the medullary nucleus paragigantocellularis, and the locus coeruleus sends efferents to a range of important structures, including the amygdala, hypothalamus, and brain stem periaqueductal gray.

Several clinical studies of panic disorder provide support for the role of the locus coeruleus; administration of yohimbine, for example, resulted in greater increases in MHPG in panic disorder patients than in control subjects without panic disorder. However, not all stud-

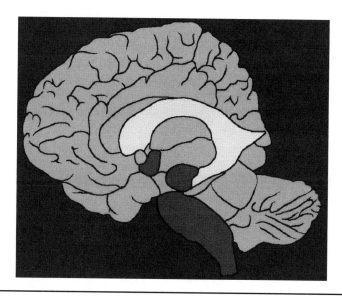

FIGURE 16–4. Neuroanatomical model of panic disorder.

See Appendix for color version. Note the activation of the amygdala, which has efferents to hypothalamus and brain stem sites (Gorman et al. 2000).

Source. Reprinted from Stein DJ: *False Alarm! How to Conquer the Anxiety Disorders.* Cape Town, South Africa, University of Stellenbosch, 2000. Used with permission.

ies have replicated such findings, and studies of noradrenergic function in lactate-induced panic also have been inconsistent, suggesting that additional neurochemical factors are important in the mediation of panic attacks.

Increasing evidence indicates that the serotonergic system plays a crucial role in panic disorder. A range of studies provide evidence for this; for example, several studies have found that m-CPP administration leads to an acute exacerbation of panic symptoms in panic disorder patients. Also, a good deal of evidence supports the efficacy of the SSRIs in panic disorder.

The serotonergic system interacts at several points with neuroanatomical structures thought important in panic disorder. First, serotonergic projections from the dorsal raphe nucleus generally inhibit the locus coeruleus, whereas projections from the locus coeruleus stimulate dorsal raphe nucleus serotonergic neurons and inhibit median raphe nucleus neurons. Furthermore, the dorsal raphe nucleus sends projections to prefrontal cortex, amygdala, hypothalamus, and periaqueductal gray, among other structures. Thus, modulation of the serotonin system has the potential to influence the major regions of the panic disorder circuit, resulting in decreased noradrenergic activity, diminished release of corticotropin-releasing factor, and modification of defense and escape behaviors.

Peripheral benzodiazepine receptor binding is decreased in panic disorder, and benzodiazepines are effective in treating this condition. In animal models, direct administration of a benzodiazepine agonist into the amygdala produces anxiolytic effects, which are weakened by pretreatment with a benzodiazepine receptor antagonist. GABA and benzodiazepine receptors are widely distributed in the brain, but the basolateral and lateral amygdala nucleus and the hippocampus, as well as frontal and occipital cortex, have high densities.

A consideration of the various afferents to the locus coeruleus and amygdala is relevant to the extensive literature on panicogenic stimuli. It has been argued that respiratory panicogens (e.g., carbon dioxide), baroceptor stimulation (β agonists), and circulating peptides (cholecystokinin) promote panic via a limbic viscero-receptor pathway. In contrast, panic attacks that are conditioned by visuospatial, auditory, or cognitive cues may be mediated by pathways from cortical association areas to the amygdala. Ultimately, it may be possible to determine particular genetic loci that are involved in contextual fear conditioning, allowing for an integration of the neurochemical, genetic, and environmental data on panic disorder.

Neuroanatomical Studies

Preliminary studies in nonanxious control subjects reported activation of the amygdala and periamygdaloid cortical areas during conditioned fear acquisition and extinction. Furthermore, in patients with panic disorder, increasing evidence suggests temporal or amygdalar-hippocampal abnormalities, as well as frontal abnormalities. Although hypocapnia-induced vasoconstriction has made the results of certain imaging studies in panic disorder difficult to interpret, it is noteworthy that imaging data may predict response to panicogens.

Advances in brain imaging methods have begun to allow the integration of neuroanatomical and neurochemical data. Thus, evidence indicates altered midbrain $5\text{-}HT_{1A}$ receptor binding and serotonin transporter levels in panic disorder. Several studies also have shown decreased benzodiazepine binding in temporal and frontal regions. Preliminary data suggest that both pharmacotherapy and cognitive-behavioral therapy act to normalize the neurocircuitry thought to mediate panic disorder.

POSTTRAUMATIC STRESS DISORDER

Features of current neuroanatomical models of PTSD (Figure 16–5) include the following: 1) amygdalothalamic pathways are involved in the rapid, automatic (implicit) processing of incoming information; 2) hyperactivation of the amygdala, which sends afferents to other regions involved in the anxiety response (hypothalamus, brain stem nuclei), occurs; 3) the hippocampus is involved in (explicitly) remembering the context of traumatic memo-

ries; and 4) activity is decreased in certain frontal cortical areas, consistent with decreased verbalization during processing of trauma (e.g., deactivation of Broca's area), failure of fear extinction (e.g., failure to recruit medial and ventral prefrontal areas), and an inability to override automatic amygdala processing.

Neurochemical Studies

A range of neurochemical findings in PTSD are consistent with sensitization of various neurotransmitter systems. In particular, there is evidence of hyperactive noradrenergic function and dopaminergic sensitization. Such sensitization is also consistent with the role of environmental traumas in PTSD; dopamine agonists and environmental traumas act as cross-sensitizers of each other. Evidence indicates that the amygdala and related limbic regions may play a particularly important role in the final common pathway of such hyperactivation.

Also, growing evidence suggests the importance of the serotonin system in mediating PTSD symptoms. Clinical studies of abnormal paroxetine binding and exacerbations of symptoms in response to administration of m-CPP are certainly consistent with a role for serotonin in PTSD. Furthermore, there is evidence for the efficacy of serotonin reuptake inhibitors in PTSD. These agents may act on amygdala circuits, helping to inhibit efferents to structures such as hypothalamus and brain stem nuclei, which mediate fear.

A third set of neurochemical findings in PTSD is focused on the hypothalamic-pituitary-adrenal (HPA) system. PTSD is characterized by decreased plasma levels of cortisol, as well as increased glucocorticoid receptor responsiveness, suggesting that negative feedback inhibition may play an important role in the pathogenesis of the disorder. Such findings differ from those found in other anxiety disorders and in depression. Notably, cortisol-releasing factor receptors are also prominent in the amygdala, particularly in the central nucleus.

One important implication of the HPA findings is the possibility that dysfunction in this system results in neuronal damage, partic-

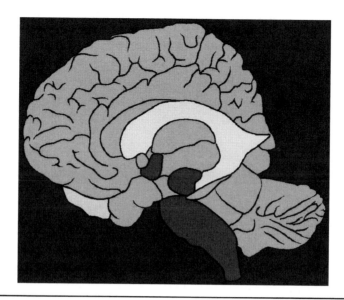

FIGURE 16–5. Neuroanatomical model of posttraumatic stress disorder.

See Appendix for color version. Note the increased activity in the amygdala and decreased activity in prefrontal areas (not anatomically to scale).

Source. Reprinted from Stein DJ: *False Alarm! How to Conquer the Anxiety Disorders.* Cape Town, South Africa, University of Stellenbosch, 2000. Used with permission.

ularly to the hippocampus. Animal studies have documented hippocampal damage after exposure to either glucocorticoids or naturalistic psychosocial stressors. Parallel neurotoxicity in human PTSD could account for some of the cognitive impairments that are characteristic of this disorder.

Neuroanatomical Studies

A range of structural imaging studies are in fact consistent with the possibility of hippocampal dysfunction occurring in PTSD. A meta-analysis of magnetic resonance imaging studies emphasized the consistent finding of decreased hippocampal volume in PTSD (Kitayama et al. 2005). Nevertheless, evidence also shows that decreased hippocampal volume may precede the onset of PTSD and thus constitutes a risk factor for the development of this condition. In addition, there are now increasing data suggesting decreased volume in medial and ventral prefrontal cortex (Rauch et al. 2006).

Functional imaging studies have provided additional information in support of a neuroan-atomical model of PTSD. Several studies in control subjects without PTSD have provided evidence for subcortical processing of masked emotional stimuli by the amygdala. PTSD patients exposed to audiotaped traumatic and neutral scripts had increases in neuronal activity in limbic and paralimbic areas. Also, areas of decreased activity may mediate symptoms; for example, decreased activity in Broca's area during exposure to trauma in PTSD is consistent with patients' inability to verbally process traumatic memories. Subsequent studies have extended the work to address abnormalities during cognitive-affective processing of tasks in PTSD. The data support a view that there is deficient recruitment of medial and ventral prefrontal cortex in PTSD, consistent with dysfunction in fear extinction (Rauch et al. 2006).

Once again, modern techniques have allowed for the integration of neurochemical and neuroanatomical data, with increasing numbers of receptor binding studies in PTSD. During treatment of PTSD with SSRIs, normalization of structure and activity in the limbic neurocir-

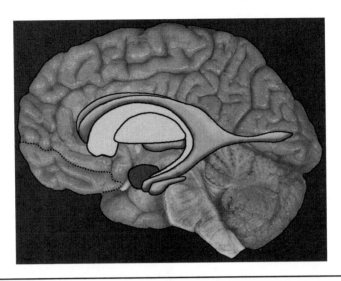

FIGURE 16–6.   Neuroanatomical model of social phobia.

See Appendix for color version. Note the increased temporolimbic activity (van der Linden et al. 2000), decreased basal ganglia dopaminergic activity (Tiihonen et al. 1997a), and perhaps some increased prefrontal activity (Rauch et al. 1997; van der Linden et al. 2000).

Source.   Reprinted from Stein DJ: *False Alarm! How to Conquer the Anxiety Disorders.* Cape Town, South Africa, University of Stellenbosch, 2000. Used with permission.

cuitry occurs and is likely to mediate symptoms (Seedat et al. 2004; Vermetten et al. 2003).

SOCIAL PHOBIA (SOCIAL ANXIETY DISORDER)

Detailed neuroanatomical models of social phobia remain to be fully delineated. Nevertheless, it may be hypothesized again that temporolimbic circuitry is important in mediating the fear responses that characterize this disorder. Furthermore, serotonin and dopamine neurocircuitry, presumably involving prefrontal and basal ganglia regions, may also play a crucial role (Figure 16–6).

Neurochemical Studies

A range of evidence supports the role of serotonergic and dopaminergic circuits in social phobia. For example, patients with social phobia had an augmented cortisol response to fenfluramine administration, and social phobia may develop in the context of Parkinson's disease or after the administration of neuroleptics.

Evidence that the HPA axis may be dysfunctional in social phobia is inconsistent to date. However, socially subordinate baboons have been reported to have elevated basal cortisol and to be less responsive to dexamethasone inhibition. Also, children with a high frequency of wary behavior during peer play and behavioral inhibition had relatively high morning salivary cortisol levels.

Neuroanatomical Studies

Increasing evidence suggests that patients with social phobia have selective activation of the amygdala when exposed to potentially fear-relevant stimuli. Subjects with behavioral inhibition, when studied as adults, also had heightened amygdala responses to novel fear-relevant stimuli. Nonphobic control subjects with a particular variant in the serotonin transporter gene that is associated with anxiety traits, as well as subjects with social phobia, also have decreased volume or increased activity in amygdala or related circuitry. Treatment with an SSRI or with cognitive-behavioral therapy is able to normalize neuronal activity in such neurocircuitry.

Several molecular imaging studies provide additional data that are relevant to an integrated model of social phobia. Thus, evidence indicates that striatal dopamine reuptake site densities are markedly lower in patients with social phobia than in nonphobic control subjects. Other findings confirm abnormalities in components of the striatal dopaminergic system, supporting the hypothesis that social phobia may be associated with a dysfunction of the striatal dopaminergic system.

CONCLUSION

Several lessons emerge from a review of the neuropsychiatry of anxiety disorders. First, the anxiety disorders are common and disabling disorders not only in general clinical settings but also in patients with neurological illnesses such as Alzheimer's disease, stroke, and traumatic brain injury. Although the link between depression and neuropsychiatric disorders is increasingly recognized, the importance of anxiety disorders in this context has perhaps been relatively overlooked, paralleling their underdiagnosis and undertreatment in primary care settings. The anxiety disorders deserve to be carefully diagnosed, thoroughly assessed, and rigorously treated.

Second, both animal and clinical studies increasingly indicate that the amygdala and paralimbic structures play important roles in conditioned fear and in anxiety disorders. Amygdala lesions are classically associated with decreased fear responses, and conversely, limbic hyperactivation is characteristic of several different anxiety disorders. Paralimbic regions such as the anterior cingulate appear to play a key role at the interface of cognition and emotion. The apparent centrality of such systems to different anxiety disorders may account in part for their high comorbidity. Other limbic involvement may be specific to particular disorders (e.g., decreased hippocampal volume in PTSD or parahippocampal asymmetry in panic disorder).

Models of anxiety disorders increasingly integrate data from genetics, brain imaging, and treatment studies. Thus, particular genetic variants appear to be associated with increased activation of specific neuronal circuits during functional imaging, and effective pharmacotherapy and psychotherapy may act to normalize such circuitry. Serotonin reuptake inhibitors and cognitive-behavioral therapy are increasingly viewed as first-line treatments for anxiety disorders. Innervation of amygdala and paralimbic structures by serotonergic neurons may be crucial in explaining their efficacy. Further advances in our understanding of the neurobiological bases of fear conditioning and extinction may lead to new therapeutic interventions (Ressler et al. 2004).

Finally, CSTC pathways are crucial in OCD, and data increasingly support a role for putative obsessive-compulsive spectrum disorders such as Tourette syndrome. It is particularly remarkable that CSTC pathways can be normalized by pharmacotherapy, by psychotherapy, and by neurosurgery. It can be argued that although OCD was once viewed as the key to a psychodynamic understanding of the mind, OCD and some obsessive-compulsive spectrum disorders such as Tourette syndrome are now the neuropsychiatric disorders par excellence. Certainly, such disorders provide a key paradigm and challenge for those who are interested in integrating "brain" and "mind" approaches to psychiatric disorders.

RECOMMENDED READINGS

Gorman JM, Kent JM, Sullivan GM, et al: Neuroanatomical hypothesis of panic disorder, revised. Am J Psychiatry 157:493–505, 2000

Rauch SL, Shin LM, Phelps EA: Neurocircuitry models of posttraumatic stress disorder and extinction: human neuroimaging research: past, present, and future. Biol Psychiatry 60:376–382, 2006

Saxena S, Rauch SL: Functional neuroimaging and the neuroanatomy of obsessive-compulsive disorder. Psychiatr Clin North Am 23:563–586, 2000

Shin LM, Liberzon I: The neurocircuitry of fear, stress, and anxiety disorders. Neuropsychopharmacology 35:169–191, 2010

REFERENCES

American Psychiatric Association: Diagnostic and Statistical Manual of Mental Disorders, 3rd Edition, Revised. Washington, DC, American Psychiatric Association, 1987

Ames D, Cummings JL, Wirshing WC, et al: Repetitive and compulsive behavior in frontal lobe degenerations. J Neuropsychiatry Clin Neurosci 6:100–113, 1994

Baxter LR, Schwartz JM, Bergman KS, et al: Caudate glucose metabolic rate changes with both drug and behavior therapy for OCD. Arch Gen Psychiatry 49:681–689, 1992

Bechara A, Tranel D, Damasio H, et al: Double dissociation of conditioning and declarative knowledge relative to the amygdala and hippocampus in humans. Science 269:1115–1118, 1995

Brody AL, Saxena S, Schwartz JM, et al: FDG-PET predictors of response to behavioral therapy and pharmacotherapy in obsessive compulsive disorder. Psychiatry Res 84:1–6, 1998

Castillo CS, Starkstein SE, Fedoroff JP, et al: Generalized anxiety disorder after stroke. J Nerv Ment Dis 181:100–106, 1993

Cheyette SR, Cummings JL: Encephalitis lethargica: lessons for contemporary neuropsychiatry. J Neuropsychiatry Clin Neurosci 7:125–135, 1995

Davis M, Whalen PJ: The amygdala: vigilance and emotion. Mol Psychiatry 6:13–34, 2001

Gorman JM, Kent JM, Sullivan GM, et al: Neuroanatomical hypothesis of panic disorder, revised. Am J Psychiatry 157:493–505, 2000

Hibbard MR, Uysal S, Kepler K, et al: Axis I psychopathology in individuals with traumatic brain injury. J Head Trauma Rehabil 13:24–39, 1998

Kinrys G, Wygant LE: Anticonvulsants in anxiety disorders. Curr Psychiatry Rep 7:258–267, 2005

Kitayama N, Vaccarino V, Kutner M, et al: Magnetic resonance imaging (MRI) measurement of hippocampal volume in posttraumatic stress disorder: a meta-analysis. J Affect Disord 88:79–86, 2005

Klüver H, Bucy PC: Preliminary analysis of functions of the temporal lobes in monkeys. AMA Arch Neurol Psychiatry 42:979–1000, 1939

Le Doux J: Fear and the brain: where have we been, and where are we going? Biol Psychiatry 44:1229–1238, 1998

MacLean PD: A Triune Concept of the Brain and Behavior. Toronto, ON, University of Toronto Press, 1973

Rauch SL, Baxter LR: Neuroimaging in obsessive-compulsive and related disorders, in Obsessive-Compulsive Disorders: Practical Management, 3rd Edition. Edited by Jenike MA, Baer L, Minichiello WE. St. Louis, MO, Mosby, 1998, pp 289–316

Rauch SL, Savage CR, Alpert NM, et al: Probing striatal function in obsessive compulsive disorder: a PET study of implicit sequence learning. J Neuropsychiatry Clin Neurosci 9:568–573, 1997

Rauch SL, Shin LM, Phelps EA: Neurocircuitry models of posttraumatic stress disorder and extinction: human neuroimaging research—past, present, and future. Biol Psychiatry 60:376–382, 2006

Redmond DE Jr: The possible role of locus coeruleus noradrenergic activity in anxiety-panic. Clin Neuropharmacol 9 (suppl 4):40–42, 1986

Ressler KJ, Rothbaum BO, Tannenbaum L, et al: Cognitive enhancers as adjuncts to psychotherapy: use of D-cycloserine in phobic individuals to facilitate extinction of fear. Arch Gen Psychiatry 61:1136–1144, 2004

Saxena S, Rauch SL: Functional neuroimaging and the neuroanatomy of obsessive-compulsive disorder. Psychiatr Clin North Am 23:563–586, 2000

Seedat S, Warwick J, van Heerden B, et al: Single photon emission computed tomography in posttraumatic stress disorder before and after treatment with a selective serotonin reuptake inhibitor. J Affect Disord 80:45–53, 2004

Swedo SE, Rapoport JL, Cheslow DL, et al: High prevalence of obsessive-compulsive symptoms in patients with Sydenham's chorea. Am J Psychiatry 146:246–249, 1989

Tiihonen J, Kuikka J, Bergstrom K, et al: Dopamine reuptake site densities in patients with social phobia. Am J Psychiatry 154:239–242, 1997a

Tiihonen JF, Kuikka J, Rasanen P, et al: Cerebral benzodiazepine receptor binding and distribution in generalized anxiety disorder: a fractal analysis. Mol Psychiatry 2:463–471, 1997b van der Linden G, van Heerden B, Warwick J, et al: Functional brain imaging and pharmacotherapy in social phobia: single photon emission computed tomography before and after treatment with the selective serotonin reuptake inhibitor citalopram. Prog Neuropsychopharmacol Biol Psychiatry 24:419–438, 2000

Vasa RA, Grados M, Slomine B, et al: Neuroimaging correlates of anxiety after pediatric traumatic brain injury. Biol Psychiatry 55:208–216, 2004

Vermetten E, Vythilingam M, Southwick SM, et al: Long-term treatment with paroxetine increases verbal declarative memory and hippocampal volume in posttraumatic stress disorder. Biol Psychiatry 54:693–702, 2003

Wu JC, Buchsbaum MS, Hershey TG, et al: PET in generalized anxiety disorder. Biol Psychiatry 29:1181–1199, 1991

17

PSYCHOPHARMACOLOGICAL TREATMENTS FOR PATIENTS WITH NEUROPSYCHIATRIC DISORDERS

Paul E. Holtzheimer III, M.D.

Mark Snowden, M.D., M.P.H.

Peter P. Roy-Byrne, M.D.

Modern neuropsychiatry is concerned with the understanding and treatment of cognitive, emotional, and behavioral syndromes in patients with known neurological illness or central nervous system (CNS) dysfunction. Although some psychiatric syndromes in patients with neurological disease are clinically similar to those seen in patients experiencing the syndrome de novo, treatment response may be quite different.

Despite dissimilarities in the pathophysiology, clinical presentation, and treatment response of neuropsychiatric and "idiopathic" psychiatric syndromes, the treatment of neuropsychiatric illness has largely been modeled on known treatments of idiopathic psychiatric disorders. In addition to identifying efficacious treatments, attention to altered side-effect sensitivity and pertinent interactions with commonly used neurological drugs is an especially important aspect of the treatment of neuropsychiatric patients.

APPROACH TO THE NEUROPSYCHIATRIC PATIENT

The psychiatrist who is asked to assess a neuropsychiatric patient for pharmacological treatment must first have a familiarity with the pathophysiology and treatment of the underlying neurological illness. Other medical conditions and treatments, recent surgeries, and health habits should also be considered. Importantly, history of alcohol and drug use must be explored because substance abuse, intoxication, and withdrawal can lead to a vast array of psychiatric symptoms (Rosse et al. 1997).

Establishing good rapport will increase the integrity of data obtained via the patient and history, as well as adherence to recommendations. Presenting the pharmacological intervention as a way to optimize treatment of the primary neurological disease can be helpful. However, realistic expectations, including the possibility of incomplete remission of symptoms, should be conveyed from the outset.

The neuropsychiatrist must also be aware of his or her own desire to help—even in the absence of data to guide treatment. The frequent urge to "do something…anything" must be resisted. Some symptoms may be long-standing and unlikely to resolve quickly, whereas others may result from an adjustment disorder that may dissipate without pharmacological treatment; and the treatments themselves may not be benign.

When assessing the patient, the clinician must look beyond DSM-IV-TR (American Psychiatric Association 2000) criteria when appropriate. A careful, detailed focus on identifying problematic symptoms may establish clear symptom clusters (e.g., anhedonia, apathy, poor energy) that may respond to pharmacological intervention, even when specific diagnostic criteria for a particular disorder (e.g., major depression) are not fully met.

Optimal treatment must also take into account whether the psychiatric symptoms appeared before the neurological disorder or arose as a neurologically or psychologically mediated result of the neurological disease. Because CNS insults, particularly in the frontal lobe, can amplify underlying character traits (Prigatano 1992), it may not be possible to eradicate completely behaviors that at first appear to be a direct result of the neurological insult. In addition, certain premorbid traits, such

as IQ, may have important implications for course of illness (Palsson et al. 1999).

During the patient interview, the clinician must remember that the neurological disorder may dampen (or heighten) the patient's emotional expressivity. Importantly, patients and their caregivers may disagree about which symptoms are most troubling; for example, a patient often reports cognitive difficulties as more disabling, whereas family members may view the patient's emotional or behavior changes as more problematic (Hendryx 1989). Careful prospective documentation of symptoms will help in tracking what are often slow improvements that seem subjectively inconsequential to the patient and caregiver but lead to noticeable improvements in overall functioning. Although it may be impractical to document all symptoms completely, specific target symptoms and functional goals should be measured in as much detail as possible.

A basic tenet of treating psychiatric symptoms in patients with neurological disorders is to limit polypharmacy. Patients with CNS pathology are more susceptible to CNS side effects. Treatment of symptoms secondary to the primary neurological disorder, such as pain and sleep disturbance, may decrease psychiatric symptoms sufficiently to allow avoidance of further psychopharmacotherapy. For example, analgesia has been shown to alleviate agitation, irritability, and anger in both patients and caregivers (Perry et al. 1991). Similarly, appropriate treatment of psychiatric symptoms early in presentation may prevent exacerbation of the underlying neurological disorder. For example, emotional distress has been shown to precipitate and/or worsen multiple sclerosis exacerbations (Grant et al. 1989).

Detailed knowledge of the patient's stage in rehabilitation as well as the patient's current social, occupational, and interpersonal status is required to tailor the pharmacological regimen to specific practical needs and limitations. For example, starting a potentially sedating medication when rigorous physical therapy is being initiated or during reentry into the workplace would be ill-advised. Social and interpersonal status can affect access to treatment (Ferrando et al. 1999), ability of caregivers to participate in treatment (Donaldson et al. 1998), vulnerability of patients to domestic violence (Diaz-Olavarrieta et al. 1999), and psychiatric outcome (Max et al. 1998).

Because of susceptibility to medication side effects, the clinician should typically start at a lower dose of medication and titrate more slowly, though the patient may ultimately require the same dosage as the non-neurological patient (i.e., "Start low and go slow…but go!"). Side effects should be well documented, and standardized measures should be used whenever possible. Because neurological patients may have cognitive deficits, the anticipated benefit of the medication, the dosing regimen, and any potential side effects must be thoroughly explained to the patient and caregiver as well as all other physicians caring for the patient.

Once medication has been initiated, all available tools to subjectively monitor pharmacokinetics and pharmacological efficacy must be considered. Objective rating scales for symptoms and side effects should be considered. Additionally, monitoring medication blood levels and physiological response (such as vital signs), as well as other laboratory monitoring when appropriate, can be helpful. Medication blood levels do not always correlate with medication efficacy but can still give information about compliance, drug metabolism, and potential toxicity. It should be remembered that some neuropsychiatric patients with impaired cognition or communication ability may not be able to convey information adequately about efficacy and side effects, requiring more objective monitoring.

DEPRESSION, APATHY, AND "DEFICIT" STATES

Major depression and dysthymia are among the most common psychiatric disorders, including in neurological patients. The common etiologies and pathophysiology of depressive states

are discussed in Chapter 15. Untreated depression can have a significant negative impact on quality of life and management of the underlying neurological disease; therefore, timely identification and treatment are essential. As the symptoms of depression overlap significantly with symptoms of many neurological conditions, confirming the presence or absence of depression in the neuropsychiatric patient can be quite difficult.

TREATMENT

Several open and small placebo-controlled studies suggest efficacy for a range of typical antidepressant medications (especially tricyclic antidepressants [TCAs], selective serotonin reuptake inhibitors [SSRIs], and some monoamine oxidase inhibitors [MAOIs]) in a range of neuropsychiatric patients.

Parkinson's disease studies generally report response rates somewhat lower than in non–medically ill depressed patients. However, many studies have purposely used lower doses, which may have affected efficacy; unfortunately, higher doses can be associated with more side effects in these populations, underscoring the need to titrate medications slowly.

SSRIs may have a more favorable side-effect profile compared with TCAs in neuropsychiatric patients. Sedation, postural hypotension, modest hypertension, and seizure threshold–lowering effects are common with TCAs and may be more pronounced in medically ill, especially neuropsychiatric, patients. SSRIs also have been shown to improve "emotional incontinence" in neuropsychiatric patients (Iannaccone and Ferini-Strambi 1996; Muller et al. 1999; Nahas et al. 1998; Tan and Dorevitch 1996).

Given their side-effect burden, potential for adverse events, and potential for serious interaction with multiple other medications, there would seem to be little reason to use nonselective MAOIs in treating depressed neuropsychiatric patients. Selegiline, a selective monoamine oxidase–B (MAO-B) inhibitor, would seem to be a good choice for Parkinson's disease patients because it has primary effects on the underlying illness. However, the lower doses used to treat Parkinson's disease symptoms generally have not been effective in studies of primary major depression, which usually requires higher doses that also inhibit monoamine oxidase–A (MAO-A). Finally, bupropion was found to be effective in fewer than half of Parkinson's disease patients in one study (Goetz et al. 1984); also, bupropion can lower the seizure threshold, which may limit its usefulness in many neuropsychiatric patients.

Dopaminergic agents have been recommended for treating apathy—for example, in Parkinson's disease patients without accompanying depression (Chatterjee and Fahn 2002). Parkinson's disease patients do not experience euphoria with methylphenidate, possibly reflecting decreased dopamine availability secondary to dopaminergic neuron loss (Cantello et al. 1989). However, more direct-acting agonists such as bromocriptine and amantadine have been found effective in these patients (Jouvent et al. 1983) as well as patients with traumatic brain injury (TBI)–associated apathy (Van Reekum et al. 1995). Pramipexole, a dopamine agonist, may be effective in treating depression in Parkinson's disease patients (Moller et al. 2005; Rektorova et al. 2003). Stimulants such as methylphenidate have shown efficacy in treating apathy related to dementia and stroke, can work quickly, and may enhance functional recovery due to greater participation in rehabilitation programs. Patients with HIV-related apathetic depression have done particularly well with methylphenidate in case reports (White et al. 1992). However, other reports have claimed that even though dopaminergic agents improve affect and cognitive function, they may be less effective on core symptoms of apathy such as lack of initiative (Salloway 1994), and they could provoke psychosis in Parkinson's disease and other vulnerable patients.

A growing database suggests that various brain stimulation techniques may have efficacy in treating depression, although they have not been extensively studied in neuropsychiatric patients. Electroconvulsive therapy (ECT) is an effective treatment for depression in Parkinson's disease patients that can also transiently improve core motor symptoms (Fall et al. 1995; Moellentine et al. 1998). Five of six patients with Huntington's disease also improved with ECT, although two patients developed notable side effects (Ranen et al. 1994). Reports of a high rate of ECT-induced delirium in Parkinson's disease patients have been interpreted as being due to denervation supersensitivity of dopamine receptors, and reduction of dopaminergic drugs before ECT has been advised (Rudorfer et al. 1992).

Repetitive transcranial magnetic stimulation (rTMS) has shown antidepressant efficacy (Burt et al. 2002; Holtzheimer et al. 2001; O'Reardon et al. 2007), and some data suggest efficacy in depressed patients with Parkinson's disease (Fregni et al. 2004) and poststroke depression (Jorge et al. 2004). Vagus nerve stimulation (VNS) has led to mood improvements in patients with epilepsy (Elger et al. 2000) and was recently approved by the U.S. Food and Drug Administration (FDA) for treatment-resistant depression (George et al. 2005; Rush et al. 2005). Deep brain stimulation (DBS) of the subthalamic nucleus or internal globus pallidus has shown efficacy in treating motor symptoms associated with Parkinson's disease (Deep Brain Stimulation for Parkinson's Disease Study Group 2001), essential tremor (Schuurman et al. 2000), and dystonia (Lozano and Abosch 2004) but has also been associated with negative mood changes (Bejjani et al. 1999; Berney et al. 2002). Studies of DBS of the white matter adjacent to the subgenual cingulate region or the ventral striatum/anterior internal capsule have shown antidepressant efficacy in patients without neurological disease (Lozano et al. 2008; Malone et al. 2009; Mayberg et al. 2005).

In summary, SSRIs are generally considered the treatment of choice in neuropsychiatric patients with depression. SSRIs with relatively shorter half-lives (paroxetine, fluvoxamine) or absence of inhibition of select microsomal enzyme systems (citalopram, sertraline, paroxetine, fluvoxamine) may be advantageous in some cases. Because of the potentially activating properties of the SSRIs, they should be started at about half the usual starting dose and titrated up to standard antidepressant doses in the first 1–3 weeks. Venlafaxine at lower doses is less likely to cause hypertension but also acts more like a pure SSRI, with noradrenergic properties requiring higher (225 mg or greater) doses. Mirtazapine's effect of increased appetite could be advantageous in patients with wasting, although sedative side effects may limit its use. Apathetic states could be treated with dopaminergic strategies, including bupropion, bromocriptine, amantadine, and stimulants. TCAs, if used, should probably be limited to desipramine (lowest anticholinergic effects) and nortriptyline (lowest hypotensive effects, low anticholinergic effects). Nonselective MAOIs should probably be avoided in neuropsychiatric patients. Table 17–1 lists characteristic antidepressants recommended in this section, dose ranges, side effects, and relevant drug interactions.

In severely ill patients who do not respond or cannot tolerate pharmacological treatments, ECT is a reasonable treatment option. Other brain stimulation techniques (rTMS, VNS, DBS) have shown promising results in treating depression but require further study before their utility in neuropsychiatric patients can be determined.

PSYCHOSIS

Psychotic states (hallucinations, delusions, and formal thought disorder) occur principally in schizophrenia and less commonly in mania and depression. Psychosis occurs less frequently overall in neurological patients than does depression, agitation, or cognitive impairment and often may be associated with and result from cognitive impairment. Psychosis can have a serious effect on patient care, such that rapid, definitive, and independent treatment is warranted. The common etiologies and pathophysiology of psychotic states are discussed in Chapter 14.

TREATMENT

Neuroleptic (antipsychotic) medications remain the mainstay in the pharmacological treatment of psychosis. Although typical neuroleptics (e.g., haloperidol, perphenazine, chlorpromazine) have proven efficacy in the treatment of psychosis, side effects including the risk of severe adverse reactions (such as tardive dyskinesia and neuroleptic malignant syndrome) can limit their usefulness. Alternatively, the atypical neuroleptics (clozapine, risperidone, olanzapine, quetiapine, ziprasidone, and aripiprazole) have been shown to be as effective as typical neuroleptics in the treatment of psychosis and are generally associated with different, somewhat more tolerable side effects. These advantages are even more relevant in neuropsychiatric patients, who are more prone to neurological side effects. However, the association of atypical neuroleptics with metabolic alterations (hyperglycemia, hyperlipidemia) may present difficulties for long-term use. These medications have also been associated with tardive dyskinesia and neuroleptic malignant syndrome, though at much lower rates than typical neuroleptics.

Typical neuroleptics have been most often studied in the mixed psychosis and agitation of dementia patients. One placebo-controlled study showed superiority of both haloperidol (mean dose = 4.6 mg) and loxapine (mean dose = 22 mg) in these patients, but reported that only one-third showed significant improvement (Petrie et al. 1982). A later study (Devanand et al. 1998) showed a response rate of 55%–60% with 2–3 mg of haloperidol, superior to a 30% response rate with 0.5 mg. Despite a long history of typical neuroleptic use in epilepsy-related psychosis, there are few data to support this indication. Chronic interictal psychosis should be treated with neuroleptics, with careful attention to effects on seizure frequency. In one report (Onuma et al. 1991), only 11 of 21 patients (52%) showed aggravation of symptoms with decrease or discontinuation of neuroleptics. This suggests that patients should be carefully monitored to determine whether ongoing neuroleptics are required.

TABLE 17–1. Antidepressants

Drug	Starting daily dose (mg)	Target daily dose (mg)	Neuropsychiatric side effects	Neuropsychiatric drug interactions	Comments
Tricyclic antidepressants (TCAs)					
Nortriptyline	10	30–100	Dizziness, fatigue, drowsiness, tremor, nervousness, confusion, insomnia, headache, seizures, anticholinergic effects	Increased blood levels with SSRIs, neuroleptics, methylphenidate, VPA, opioids	Low, but present, anticholinergic and hypotensive potential
Desipramine	25	75–200			Blood level monitoring available
Amitriptyline	10	50–150		Decreased blood levels with CBZ, phenytoin, barbiturates	Antiarrhythmic properties
Imipramine	10	50–200	Other: orthostatic hypotension, ECG alterations, cardiac conduction delay, tachycardia, sexual dysfunction, weight gain	Increased blood levels of neuroleptics, CBZ, opioids	Analgesic effects, even at low doses, for neuropathic pain
Clomipramine	25	75–200		Decreased blood levels of levodopa	
Doxepin	10	50–200		Additive anticholinergic effects with neuroleptics, antiparkinsonian agents, antihistamines	
Protriptyline	2.5	10–30			

TABLE 17–1.   Antidepressants (continued)

Drug	Starting daily dose (mg)	Target daily dose (mg)	Neuropsychiatric side effects	Neuropsychiatric drug interactions	Comments
SSRIs and SNRIs					
Fluoxetine	5	10–80	Drowsiness (especially with paroxetine, fluvoxamine), nervousness or agitation (especially with fluoxetine), fatigue (especially with paroxetine), insomnia, tremor, dizziness, headache, confusion, paresthesia Other: nausea, diarrhea, sexual dysfunction, weight loss, hyponatremia, blood pressure changes (especially with venlafaxine)	Increased sedation with hypnotics, chloral hydrate, antihistamines Lethargy, impaired consciousness with metoprolol, propranolol Excitation and hallucinations with narcotics EPS with neuroleptics Neurotoxicity with lithium Serotonergic effects with lithium, buspirone, sumatriptan Serotonin syndrome with other serotonergic drugs (e.g., TCAs, MAOIs, atypical neuroleptics, opioids) Contraindicated with MAOIs (hypertensive crisis) Increased blood levels with valproate Decreased blood levels with CBZ Increased blood levels of TCAs, neuroleptics, BZDs, CBZ, valproate, phenytoin, propranolol (especially with fluoxetine, paroxetine)	Fluoxetine: may require up to 8 weeks to reach steady state; most inhibition of hepatic cytochrome P450 2D6 enzymes; also inhibits 2C and 3A4; potential use in cataplexy; antimyoclonic adjunct with oxitriptan Sertraline: increased blood level with food; most likely to cause diarrhea; least inhibition of cytochrome P450 2D6 but does inhibit 2C and 3A4 Paroxetine: more sedating, less stimulating, and shorter half-life than fluoxetine, sertraline; withdrawal syndrome more likely/severe; inhibition of cytochrome P450 2D6 but not 2C and 3A4; can inhibit trazodone metabolism Fluvoxamine: use twice-daily administration; most sedating and shortest half-life of SSRIs; withdrawal syndrome most likely; least bound to plasma proteins and no inhibition of hepatic cytochrome P450 2D6 enzymes; does inhibit 1A2, 2C, and 3A4 enzymes; less ejaculatory delay compared with fluoxetine, sertraline, paroxetine Citalopram: Minimal to no cytochrome inhibition; most purely serotonergic in vitro Venlafaxine: hypertensive exacerbation likely dose related; extended-release formulation much better tolerated than immediate release Duloxetine: cytochrome P450 inhibition similar to fluoxetine; less hypertensive exacerbation than venlafaxine
Sertraline	25	50–200			
Paroxetine	10	20–50			
Fluvoxamine	25	50–300			
Citalopram	10	20–60			
Escitalopram	5–10	10–20			
Venlafaxine	37.5	150–300			
Duloxetine	20–30	60			

TABLE 17–1. Antidepressants *(continued)*

Drug	Starting daily dose (mg)	Target daily dose (mg)	Neuropsychiatric side effects	Neuropsychiatric drug interactions	Comments
Other antidepressants					
Bupropion	75–150	200–450	Nervousness, tremor, dizziness, insomnia, headache, confusion, paresthesia, drowsiness, seizures	Contraindicated with MAOIs Decreased blood level with CBZ	Risk of seizures, especially with dosages >450 mg/day, >150 mg/dose Contraindicated in seizure disorders, bulimia, anorexia nervosa Fewer drug interactions than SSRIs
Mirtazapine	15	30–60	Sedation (less with higher doses); weight gain, agranulocytosis (very rare)	Contraindicated with MAOIs	No in vitro cytochrome enzyme inhibition May be more effective at higher doses (>60 mg/day) but few controlled data
Psychostimulants					
Methylphenidate	5–30	10–90	Nervousness, insomnia, dizziness, headache, dyskinesia, drowsiness, confusion, delusions, rebound depression, hallucinations, Tourette's, tics Other: anorexia, palpitations, blood pressure and pulse changes, cardiac arrhythmia, weight loss	Hypertension with MAOIs Increased blood levels of TCAs, phenytoin, phenobarbital, primidone Antagonistic effect by neuroleptics, phenobarbital	Contraindicated in marked anxiety, tension, agitation Fast onset of action Give early in day, divided doses (methylphenidate three times daily, dextroamphetamine twice daily) Dependence rare in medically ill May precipitate or worsen Tourette's or dyskinesia
Dextroamphetamine	2.5–20	5–60			

Note. BZDs = benzodiazepines; CBZ = carbamazepine; ECG = electrocardiogram; EPS = extrapyramidal side effects; MAOIs = monoamine oxidase inhibitors; SNRIs = serotonin-norepinephrine reuptake inhibitors; SSRIs = selective serotonin reuptake inhibitors; TCAs = tricyclic antidepressants; VPA = valproic acid.

Much of the literature on atypical antipsychotics in neuropsychiatric patients has focused on Parkinson's disease patients with psychotic side effects from antiparkinsonian medications. Double-blind, placebo-controlled trials of clozapine at a dosage less than 50 mg/day confirmed antipsychotic benefit without worsening of Parkinson's symptoms (Pollak et al. 2004; Parkinson Study Group 1999). However, clozapine is also associated with significant weight gain, abnormalities in glucose and cholesterol metabolism, and autonomic reactions (increased salivation, increased heart rate, constipation, hypotension). There is an approximately 1% risk of agranulocytosis with clozapine, and close monitoring of white blood cell counts is required. Clozapine significantly lowers the seizure threshold (Malow et al. 1994; Welch et al. 1994). In schizophrenic patients, seizures are dose dependent (Haller and Binder 1990), and both slow titration and lower ceiling doses (below 600 mg) may reduce the risk. In neuropsychiatric patients, lower doses may provoke seizures. Both seizures and myoclonus due to clozapine may respond to valproate (Meltzer and Ranjan 1994). Reports in neuropsychiatric groups suggest that preexisting electroencephalographic abnormalities predict likelihood of developing delirium with clozapine (Duffy and Kant 1996).

Placebo-controlled data for olanzapine suggest no benefit for psychosis (and worsening of motor symptoms in Parkinson's disease) (Breier et al. 2002). Several chart reviews and open or active medication comparison studies suggest that quetiapine may be useful in treating psychosis in Parkinson's disease patients (Fernandez et al. 1999; Reddy et al. 2002). Open-label data suggest risperidone may have antipsychotic efficacy in Parkinson's disease patients (Mohr et al. 2000), although risperidone may worsen parkinsonian symptoms more than clozapine (Ellis et al. 2000). One open-label study did not support benefit for aripiprazole in Parkinson's disease psychosis (Fernandez et al. 2004). A case report (Connemann and Schonfeldt-Lecuona 2004) and two small open studies (Gomez-Esteban et al.

2005; Oechsner and Korchounov 2005) suggest a potential benefit for ziprasidone.

Thus, the data to date suggest clozapine as the most efficacious atypical antipsychotic for psychosis in Parkinson's disease, though side effects and risks limit its use.

Beyond clozapine, quetiapine and risperidone have the next strongest database in Parkinson's disease psychosis, though no placebo-controlled data exist. Quetiapine and risperidone have both been associated with weight gain and metabolic abnormalities but to a lesser degree than clozapine; also, the risk of agranulocytosis appears to be much lower with these medications. Risperidone may worsen parkinsonism to a greater degree than clozapine does (and possibly quetiapine), but this risk is lower than with typical neuroleptics.

There is growing evidence for the efficacy of atypical antipsychotics in dementia-related psychoses, with risperidone and olanzapine supported by the strongest database (Sink et al. 2005). Reports in severe Lewy body dementia suggest the potential for marked confusion with clozapine (Burke et al. 1998) and intolerance in three of eight patients taking olanzapine (Walker et al. 1999); however, other reports with risperidone and clozapine suggest good tolerability (Allen et al. 1995; Chacko et al. 1993). Atypical antipsychotics may increase the risk of stroke in patients with dementia (Sink et al. 2005).

Results are mixed in other neuropsychiatric patient groups. Singh et al. (1997) reported substantial efficacy without extrapyramidal side effects (EPS) for risperidone in 20 of 21 psychotic HIV patients, and Lera and Zirulnik (1999) reported good efficacy for clozapine in psychotic HIV patients who experienced EPS with typical neuroleptics. Other reports have shown EPS with risperidone and akathisia with olanzapine (Meyer et al. 1998). For Huntington's disease, atypical antipsychotics can benefit the movement disorder as well as the psychiatric complications, although the database is limited (Bonelli et al. 2004). Some data suggest that atypical antipsychotics may be beneficial in Huntington's disease only when doses equivalent to 6 mg of risperidone are used (Dallocchio et al. 1999; Parsa et al. 1997), and Huntington's disease patients may have difficulty tolerating these doses. With clozapine, marked disability was seen in most patients at doses of 150 mg—lower than needed for maximal benefit (van Vugt et al. 1997). Atypical antipsychotics are considered first-line agents for the treatment of psychosis in patients with TBI (McAllister and Ferrell 2002). Risperidone has been effective in 5 of 6 patients with TBI without EPS (Duffy and Kant 1996). In other reports, risperidone was superior to conventional neuroleptics in improving TBI psychosis, sleep and daytime alertness (Schreiber et al. 1998), and psychosis following ischemic brain damage (Zimnitzky et al. 1996). Finally, risperidone has been effective for psychosis associated with neurosarcoidosis (Popli 1997).

Few novel treatments for psychosis are available. One report noted good antipsychotic efficacy without worsening of motor symptoms in 15 of 16 Parkinson's disease patients given the 5-HT$_3$ antagonist antiemetic ondansetron at dosages of 12–24 mg/day (Zoldan et al. 1995). However, this drug has not been found to be effective in schizophrenia (Newcomer et al. 1992). Glutamatergic medications offer a potential avenue for antipsychotic effects in Parkinson's disease patients (Goff et al. 1999; Lange and Riederer 1994). ECT may improve treatment-resistant psychosis, especially if the psychosis presents acutely and/or within the context of a mood disorder.

In summary, neuroleptic medications should be considered first-line agents for the treatment of psychosis across the full range of neuropsychiatric conditions. Many neuropsychiatric patients will show exaggerated sensitivity to motor side effects, making atypical antipsychotics the treatment of choice. Clozapine is least likely to have motor side effects, although seizure threshold–lowering and other side effects may be problematic. It may be preferred in unusually EPS-sensitive patients with Parkinson's disease, Huntington's disease, or other conditions with basal ganglia involvement. Table 17–2 lists characteristic antipsychotics

recommended in this section, dose ranges, side effects, and relevant drug interactions.

AGITATED STATES, INCLUDING ANXIETY AND MANIA

Agitation and anxiety occur in a wide spectrum of psychiatric illness, including mood disorders, anxiety disorders, psychosis, dementia, and impulse-control disorders. The differential diagnosis of prominent agitation remains broad and may include agitated depression, mixed bipolar states, severe anxiety, delirium, medication side effects (e.g., akathisia), and pain.

TREATMENT

An important step in treating agitated states in neuropsychiatric patients is identifying and addressing both medical factors (e.g., infection, electrolyte imbalance, or metabolic abnormalities) and pharmacological factors (e.g., corticosteroids, thyroid hormone replacements, antiemetics, or anticholinergics) that may be causing or contributing to symptoms. Although specific pharmacological management of the agitated state still may be required, it is equally if not more important to treat associated medical conditions and stop offending medications if possible.

Numerous medications have been used in the treatment of agitated states in neuropsychiatric patients, although few double-blind, placebo-controlled studies are available. Across multiple neuropsychiatric syndromes associated with agitation, anticonvulsants (particularly carbamazepine and valproate) have shown consistent efficacy and reasonable tolerability. Anticonvulsants have been recommended for secondary mania–associated "neurological" factors, including substance abuse (Pope et al. 1988). Scattered reports have suggested efficacy for carbamazepine in mentally retarded manic patients (Glue 1989), in patients with HIV-related mania resistant to lithium (Halman et al. 1993), in TBI patients with agitation (Azouvi et al. 1999), and in patients with Alzheimer's-related agitation resistant to neuroleptics (Olin et al. 2001). A placebo-controlled trial in 51 agitated patients with dementia showed a 77% response rate for carbamazepine compared with a 21% response for placebo (Tariot et al. 1998a).

Valproate has shown efficacy in mentally retarded manic patients (Sovner 1989) and in agitated patients with brain injury (Horne and Lindley 1995). Valproate has shown potential efficacy in agitated patients with dementia (Kunik et al. 1998); however, a large randomized, placebo-controlled trial showed no efficacy (Tariot et al. 2005). Blood levels have varied widely (14–107 µg/mL), though some studies showed response at levels lower than 50 µg/mL. One placebo-controlled trial with open follow-up showed good efficacy and reasonable tolerability for valproate in agitated demented patients (Porsteinsson et al. 2001, 2003). It is of interest that one survey noted that valproate is preferred by clinicians to carbamazepine (Expert Consensus Panel for Agitation in Dementia 1998); this is perhaps related to more clinical experience with valproate (given its widespread use in bipolar disorder).

Because of the potential for bone marrow suppression with carbamazepine and for hepatotoxicity and thrombocytopenia with valproate, complete blood cell count and liver function tests should be monitored. Carbamazepine and valproate blood levels do not necessarily correlate with clinical response but should be used to monitor compliance and drug metabolism.

A very preliminary database suggests a possible role for gabapentin in the treatment of agitation in neuropsychiatric patients. Given its relatively mild side-effect profile and few drug-drug interactions, gabapentin would be an attractive treatment option if efficacy could be documented. Several case reports and case series have shown that gabapentin has potential efficacy for agitation in patients with dementia (Miller 2001; Roane et al. 2000), stroke (Low and Brandes 1999), or mental retardation (Bozikas et al. 2001). However,

other reports have shown gabapentin to be minimally effective in agitated dementia patients (Herrmann et al. 2000) or associated with increases in anxiety and restlessness in TBI patients (Childers and Holland 1997). No placebo-controlled data are available. Several other anticonvulsants are available (including oxcarbazepine, topiramate, tiagabine, zonisamide, levetiracetam) but have not been well studied in neuropsychiatric patients. Lamotrigine has a growing database showing efficacy in treating patients with bipolar disorder (Bowden et al. 2003; Calabrese et al. 1999) but limited data supporting its use in other neuropsychiatric patients.

Lithium, a first-line agent in the management of mania and bipolar disorder in younger patients, has been used successfully in manic patients with neurological illness but may have significantly more side effects in this population (Himmelhoch et al. 1980; Kemperman et al. 1989). These side effects can include tremor, gastrointestinal complaints, increased thirst, cardiac abnormalities, muscle weakness, and fatigue. Neurological side effects of lithium may be greater in patients with underlying neurological disease. Finally, the narrow therapeutic window may make it difficult to use lithium appropriately in patients who have poor medication compliance (because of memory problems and confusion), who have decreased renal clearance, or who are taking concomitant medications that may result in clinically significant interactions (such as thiazide diuretics). Two reports have shown that lithium, even at low levels, was less effective and produced severe side effects in bipolar patients after head trauma (Hornstein and Seliger 1989). Lithium also has been shown to be inadequate without clozapine augmentation in Parkinson's disease (Kim et al. 1994) and to be less effective in patients with mental retardation (Glue 1989). Except for a possibly unique effect on steroid-induced mania and agitation (Falk et al. 1979), lithium would appear not to be considered a first-line choice for many neuropsychiatric patients. Its proconvulsant effect (Sacristan et al. 1991) and ability to cause or

TABLE 17–2. Antipsychotics/neuroleptics

Drug	Starting daily dose (mg)	Target daily dose (mg)	Neuropsychiatric side effects	Neuropsychiatric drug interactions	Comments
Typical neuroleptics					
Haloperidol	1–5	2–20	Parkinsonism, dystonia, akathisia, perioral (rabbit) tremor, anticholinergic effects, sedation, confusion, impaired psychomotor performance, TD, NMS, orthostatic hypotension, ejaculatory inhibition, priapism, dysphagia, urinary incontinence, temperature dysregulation, sudden death (possibly due to cardiac arrhythmia) Other: slowed cardiac repolarization, photosensitivity, hyperthermia, hyperprolactinemia, weight gain	Additive CNS depressant effects with other CNS depressants Additive anticholinergic effects with other anticholinergic drugs Increased EPS with SSRIs, lithium, buspirone Neurotoxicity with lithium Increased blood level of TCAs, valproate, phenytoin, β-adrenergic blockers Decreased blood level with lithium, CBZ, phenytoin, phenobarbital, antiparkinsonian agents Increased blood level with TCAs, SSRIs, MAOIs, alprazolam, buspirone, β-adrenergic blockers	Haloperidol: most EPS potential, especially with low calcium, akathisia with low iron; intravenous route provides rapid onset of action with potentially lower risk of EPS; available in decanoate form; useful in Huntington's, Tourette's Perphenazine: available in decanoate form
Perphenazine	4–16	8–40			
Atypical antipsychotics					
Risperidone	0.25–1	2–6	Sedation, insomnia, agitation, EPS, headache, anxiety, dizziness, aggressive reaction, NMS Other: anticholinergic side effects, weight gain, possible glucose control and cholesterol abnormalities	May antagonize effects of levodopa and dopamine agonists Increased blood level with clozapine, inhibitor of cytochrome P450 2D6 Decreased blood level with CBZ	Maximum efficacy for most patients at 4–6 mg/day Less EPS potential than haloperidol but more than other atypical agents Typically use two divided daily doses

TABLE 17-2.   Antipsychotics/neuroleptics (continued)

Drug	Starting daily dose (mg)	Target daily dose (mg)	Neuropsychiatric side effects	Neuropsychiatric drug interactions	Comments
Clozapine	15–50	200–600	Drowsiness, dizziness, headache, tremor, syncope, insomnia, restlessness, hypokinesia/akinesia, agitation, seizures, rigidity, akathisia, confusion, fatigue, hyperkinesia, weakness, lethargy, ataxia, slurred speech, depression, abnormal movements, anxiety, EPS, NMS, obsessive-compulsive symptoms Other: salivation, weight gain, glucose intolerance, hypercholesterolemia, agranulocytosis	Additive CNS depressant effects with other CNS depressants Occasional collapse (hypotension, respiratory depression, loss of consciousness) with BZDs Increased risk of bone marrow suppression with CBZ, possibly lithium Increased risk of NMS with other antipsychotics, lithium, CBZ Decreased blood level with CBZ, phenytoin Serotonin syndrome with other serotonergic drugs	Initially monitor WBC count weekly; may increase interval if stable for several months; lower risk of EPS, TD, NMS, and higher risk of lowering seizure threshold than typical neuroleptics have May improve motor function in Tourette's, Huntington's, drug-induced persistent dyskinesia, spasmodic torticollis, essential tremor
Olanzapine	5	10–20	Somnolence, headache, dizziness, NMS Other: dry mouth, weight gain, glucose control abnormalities, hypercholesterolemia, nausea, constipation, elevated transaminase	Additive CNS depressant effects with other CNS depressants Increased blood level with fluoxetine, duloxetine Decreased blood level with smoking and CBZ	Once-daily dosing
Quetiapine	12.5–25	300–450	Sedation, EPS, dizziness, agitation Other: moderate weight gain, postural hypotension, dry mouth, elevated transaminase, glucose control abnormalities, lipid abnormalities	Additive CNS depressant effects with other CNS depressants	Very sedating; often used in low doses for treating insomnia

TABLE 17-2. Antipsychotics/neuroleptics (*continued*)

Drug	Starting daily dose (mg)	Target daily dose (mg)	Neuropsychiatric side effects	Neuropsychiatric drug interactions	Comments
Ziprasidone	20–40	120–160	Agitation, akathisia, insomnia, NMS Other: QT prolongation possible, may affect lipid and glucose metabolism	Serotonin syndrome with other serotonergic drugs Increased cardiac rhythm effects with other medications that affect conduction	Use divided daily doses Appears to cause little weight gain and few effects on glucose and lipid metabolism
Aripiprazole	5–15	20–30	Agitation, akathisia, insomnia, NMS	Decreased blood level with barbiturates, CBZ	Appears to cause little weight gain and few effects on glucose and lipid metabolism Long half-life

Note. BZDs = benzodiazepines; CBZ = carbamazepine; CNS = central nervous system; EPS = extrapyramidal side effects; MAOIs = monoamine oxidase inhibitors; NMS = neuroleptic malignant syndrome; SSRIs = selective serotonin reuptake inhibitors; TCAs = tricyclic antidepressants; TD = tardive dyskinesia; WBC = white blood cell.

aggravate EPS (Lecamwasam et al. 1994) are other shortcomings. In dementia, most reports show that it has minimal effect (Holton and George 1985), although it may be useful in certain HIV-related manic syndromes (Halman et al. 1993).

Benzodiazepines are acutely effective for mania and anxiety. However, in agitated states secondary to neurological illness, these agents can cause confusion, cognitive impairment, psychomotor slowing, and disinhibition; also, short- and long-term efficacy have not been established. Benzodiazepines are generally inferior to typical neuroleptics in the treatment of behavioral disturbances (Coccaro et al. 1990; Herz et al. 1992). A double-blind study in hospitalized patients with acquired immunodeficiency syndrome (AIDS) and delirium showed that lorazepam was markedly inferior to both haloperidol and chlorpromazine and was associated with such severe, treatment-limiting adverse effects that this arm of the study was prematurely terminated (Breitbart et al. 1996). A drug discontinuation study showed that dementia patients tapered from long-term use of benzodiazepines had improved memory without worsening of anxiety (Salzman 2000). Despite these findings, the judicious use of benzodiazepines could be considered in extremely difficult cases that do not respond to other interventions. Low doses and careful titration are necessary to minimize side effects, and agents with short half-lives and without active metabolites are preferred.

Typical neuroleptics have been used frequently to treat nonspecific agitation with reasonably good effect in some studies (Breitbart et al. 1996). However, the side effects discussed above limit their use, and several placebo-controlled studies have shown these drugs to be only marginally effective in the absence of more classic psychotic symptoms (Lonergan et al. 2002). In general, typical neuroleptics have largely been replaced by the atypical antipsychotics in clinical practice (Alexopoulos et al. 2004). Risperidone was effective at a low dose in two placebo-controlled studies (Brodaty et al. 2003; Katz et al. 1999),

though the data are inconsistent (De Deyn et al. 1999). Other studies have shown efficacy for olanzapine (Meehan et al. 2001; Street et al. 2000), although, again, the data are not consistent (De Deyn et al. 2004). Atypical antipsychotics may be associated with increased mortality when used in agitated patients with dementia (Schneider et al. 2005). However, it should be recognized that untreated agitation is also associated with significant risks, including danger to the patient and caregivers and loss of living situation. Thus, risks must be carefully weighed against the potential benefits of use.

Typical antidepressant medications have shown mixed efficacy in treating agitation in neuropsychiatric patients. Citalopram was effective for anxiety, fear, and panic in 65 Alzheimer's dementia (AD) patients but not in 24 patients with vascular dementia (Nyth and Gottfries 1990). Fluoxetine was no more effective than placebo or haloperidol in reducing agitation in Alzheimer's patients in another small study (Auchus and Bissey-Black 1997). Although SSRIs are known to cause agitation as a side effect in primary depression, they work equally well in patients with agitated and retarded primary depression (Tollefson et al. 1994). Other reports have noted utility for TCAs in TBI-related agitation (Mysiw et al. 1988), pathological emotional lability in stroke (Robinson et al. 1993), and agitation in multiple sclerosis (Schiffer et al. 1985). Fluoxetine also has reportedly been effective for emotional lability in stroke, multiple sclerosis, brain injury, amyotrophic lateral sclerosis, and encephalitis (Iannaccone and Ferini-Strambi 1996; Sloan et al. 1992; W.C. Tsai et al. 1998). Sertraline also may be effective (Burns et al. 1999; Peterson et al. 1996), though data are mixed (Lanctot et al. 2002). Although some studies have suggested trazodone may be helpful in treating agitation in patients with dementia (Lawlor et al. 1994; Sultzer et al. 1997), an analysis of double-blind, placebo-controlled data found the data were insufficient to support this indication (Martinon-Torres et al. 2004).

A number of other agents may be effective for treating agitation, though confirmatory data are lacking. β-Adrenergic blockers have shown efficacy in patients with TBI (Fleminger et al. 2003). Cholinergic medications may also have antiagitation effects (Mega et al. 1999). Buspirone has shown efficacy in agitated states associated with dementia (Colenda 1988; Cooper 2003) and TBI (Levine 1988), especially when no severe motor or cognitive deficits were present (Gualtieri 1991). In Huntington's disease, one study reported improvement in both agitation and choreoathetoid movements with buspirone 120 mg/day (Hamner et al. 1996). In developmentally delayed patients, 16 of 22 had a good response to buspirone 15–45 mg/day (Buitelaar et al. 1998). One study showed that low-dose buspirone was modestly superior to haloperidol in agitated dementia (Cantillon et al. 1996).

In summary, several pharmacological agents have some data supporting efficacy in the treatment of agitation and anxiety in neuropsychiatric patients, though well-designed clinical trials are needed to better guide treatment. The anticonvulsants carbamazepine and valproate have a reasonably strong database supporting their use in treating agitation and anxiety across a range of neuropsychiatric conditions and generally would be considered first-line agents; however, the side effects and risks associated with these medications are not inconsequential. In the presence of prominent anxiety or an underlying depressive syndrome, antidepressant medications should be considered. Benzodiazepines should be reserved for severe or treatment-resistant cases; when used, agents with shorter half-lives and no active metabolites should be chosen, and doses should be started very low and titrated carefully. In the absence of clear mania, lithium is not supported as a first- or second-line agent. Neuroleptics, a mainstay in the treatment of agitated neuropsychiatric patients, are coming under closer scrutiny given recent concerns about increased mortality risk when they are used in agitated patients with dementia. However, these agents, especially the atypical antipsychotics, have shown efficacy in treating agitation across a range of conditions. Before using these agents, a careful risk-benefit analysis should be performed, and informed consent should be carefully documented. Tables 17–3 and 17–4 list characteristic mood stabilizers and anxiolytics recommended in this section, with dose ranges, side effects, and relevant drug interactions.

AGGRESSION, IMPULSIVITY, AND BEHAVIORAL DYSCONTROL

Behavioral dyscontrol is a common complication in neuropsychiatric patients and includes aggressive acts, paraphilias, compulsions, rituals, self-mutilation, and other socially inappropriate behaviors. Such symptoms can be associated with psychosis, agitation, mania, depression, or cognitive impairment. They may also be part of acute delirium or chronic severe brain dysfunction. Less often, behavioral dyscontrol (e.g., aggression, hypersexuality) may result from specific neurological lesions.

TREATMENT

Treatment for behavioral dyscontrol should primarily target the clinical syndrome associated with the maladaptive behavior. Thus, the irritable, depressed patient should first be given an antidepressant; the agitated, paranoid patient should receive a trial of a neuroleptic; and the agitated, angry patient may benefit from an anticonvulsant. However, common side effects of medications used to treat anger and aggression can themselves exacerbate the symptoms (e.g., benzodiazepine-induced disinhibition), and anticholinergic agents can aggravate cognitive deficits, lower seizure threshold, and promote delirium, particularly when combined with other delirium-promoting agents.

β-Adrenergic blockers have been studied in a wide range of neuropsychiatric disorders and shown to be efficacious (Alpert et al. 1990; Connor et al. 1997; Greendyke and Kanter 1986; Ratey et al. 1992b); however, not all data are consistent (Silver et al. 1999). β-Blockers are effective in reducing anger and aggression in patients with acute TBI (Fleminger et al. 2003) and patients with developmental disability (Connor et al. 1997). Secondary depression resulting from β-blockers appears to be a rare occurrence, but these medications are contraindicated in patients with certain medical conditions (e.g., chronic obstructive pulmonary disease, type 1 diabetes). Yudofsky et al. (1987) proposed titrating the dose of propranolol as high as 12 mg/kg or up to 800 mg and maintaining maximum tolerable dosages for up to 8 weeks to achieve the desired clinical response, although dosages between 160 and 320 mg/day have also been effective.

Parenteral benzodiazepines are often used to manage both acute aggression and behavioral dyscontrol and can be as effective as neuroleptics (Dorevitch et al. 1999). However, they can also produce disinhibition, which worsens agitation and arousal (Yudofsky et al. 1987). Benzodiazepines with rapid onset of action and relatively short half-lives that can be given intramuscularly or intravenously, such as lorazepam, are most useful in the acute situation. Diazepam and chlordiazepoxide are less reliably and rapidly absorbed intramuscularly (Garza-Trevino et al. 1989). Although longer-acting benzodiazepines, such as clonazepam (Freinhar and Alvarez 1986), can be useful in patients with more chronic agitation and aggression, particularly when symptoms of anxiety coexist, their use in treating or preventing more chronic aggression is not supported (Salzman 1988). Impairment of cognitive function by benzodiazepines could potentially aggravate aggression by increasing confusion.

Buspirone can reduce anxiety-associated agitation and has a benign side-effect profile. It has been reported to be effective in treating aggression in patients with head injury (Gualtieri 1991), developmental disability (Verhoeven and Tuinier 1996), dementia (Colenda 1988; Tiller et al. 1988), and Huntington's disease (Byrne et al. 1994). Although the effect of buspirone on anxiety can reduce agitation, its effect on aggression is probably independent of anxiolysis. The usual dose is between 30 and 60 mg (Verhoeven and Tuinier 1996), but

lower doses (5–15 mg) have been useful in some reports (Ratey et al. 1992a).

Serotonergic antidepressants also have been effective in the treatment of aggression and behavioral dyscontrol. Open trials support efficacy for SSRIs (typically at standard dosages) in patients with TBI (Sobin et al. 1989), Huntington's disease (Ranen et al. 1996), dementia (Pollock et al. 1997; Swartz et al. 1997), and mental retardation/developmental disability (Cook et al. 1992; Davanzo et al. 1998; Hellings et al. 1996; McDougle et al. 1996). Trazodone may be effective in reducing aggression secondary to organic mental disorders and dementia (Greenwald et al. 1986; Pinner and Rich 1988).

Although anticonvulsants are particularly effective in treating mood lability, impulsivity, and aggression in patients with seizure disorders, lack of electroencephalographic abnormalities does not preclude potential benefit (Mattes 1990). Carbamazepine has been effective in managing aggression and irritability in a variety of neuropsychiatric patients (Chatham-Showalter 1996; Mattes 1990; McAllister 1985), though a placebo-controlled trial in children with conduct disorder showed no benefit (Cueva et al. 1996). Valproate has been found to be effective for aggression in patients with mental retardation (Ruedrich et al. 1999), TBI (Wroblewski et al. 1997), and dementia (Haas et al. 1997); however, placebo-controlled data are generally lacking (Lindenmayer and Kotsaftis 2000). Blood levels below 50 μg/mL have been effective in some reports (Mazure et al. 1992) but not others (Sival et al. 2002). A review of 17 reports showed a 77% response rate with normal blood level range (Lindenmayer and Kotsaftis 2000). Phenytoin has been effective for impulsive aggression in inmates (Barratt 1993; Stanford et al. 2005). Limited data are available for other anticonvulsants.

Lithium was effective in treating aggressive behavior and affective instability in brain-injured patients (Glenn et al. 1989) and in a double-blind, placebo-controlled trial with 42 adult mentally retarded patients (M. Craft et al. 1987). Open trials in aggressive children

TABLE 17–3. Mood stabilizers

Drug	Starting daily dose (mg)	Target daily dose (mg)	Neuropsychiatric side effects	Neuropsychiatric drug interactions	Comments
Lithium	300–900	600–2,400	Lethargy, fatigue, muscle weakness, tremor, headache, confusion, dulled senses, ataxia, dysarthria, aphasia, muscle hyperirritability, hyperactive deep tendon reflexes, hypertonia, choreoathetoid movements, cogwheel rigidity, dizziness, drowsiness, disturbed accommodation, dystonia, seizures, EPS Other: nausea, diarrhea, polyuria, nephrogenic diabetes insipidus, hypothyroidism, hyperparathyroidism, T-wave depression, acne, leukocytosis	EPS and NMS with neuroleptics Neurotoxicity with SSRIs, neuroleptics, CBZ, valproate, phenytoin, calcium channel blockers Increased blood level with SSRIs, NSAIDs, dehydration Increased or decreased blood levels with diuretics Increased or decreased blood level of neuroleptics	Lowers seizure threshold Predominantly renally excreted Once-daily dosing more tolerable with less renal toxicity Blood levels correlate with therapeutic response and toxicity Used in Huntington's, cluster headaches, torticollis, Tourette's, SIADH, leukopenia
Carbamazepine	200–600	400–2,000	Dizziness, drowsiness, incoordination, confusion, headache, fatigue, blurred vision, hallucinations, diplopia, oculomotor disturbance, nystagmus, speech disturbance, abnormal involuntary movement, peripheral neuritis, paresthesia, depression, agitation, talkativeness, tinnitus, hyperacusis Other: nausea, bone marrow suppression, hepatotoxicity, SIADH	Additive CNS depressant effects with other CNS depressants Contraindicated with MAOIs Neurotoxicity with lithium, neuroleptics Bone marrow suppression with clozapine Increased blood level with SSRIs, verapamil Decreased blood level with TCAs, haloperidol, valproate, phenytoin, phenobarbital Decreased blood levels of TCAs, BZDs, neuroleptics, valproate, phenytoin, phenobarbital, methadone, propranolol	Induces own hepatic metabolism (2–5 weeks) Monitor CBC, LFTs, electrolytes Blood level of approximately 4–12 µg/mL Useful in trigeminal neuralgia, neuropathic pain, sedative–hypnotic withdrawal

TABLE 17–3.   Mood stabilizers (continued)

Drug	Starting daily dose (mg)	Target daily dose (mg)	Neuropsychiatric side effects	Neuropsychiatric drug interactions	Comments
Valproate	250–750	500–3,000	Sedation, tremor, paresthesia, headache, lethargy, dizziness, diplopia, confusion, incoordination, ataxia, dysarthria, psychosis, nystagmus, asterixis, "spots before eyes" Other: nausea, hair loss, thrombocytopenia, impaired platelet aggregation, elevated liver transaminases, hepatotoxicity, pancreatitis	Additive CNS depressant effects with other CNS depressants Increased blood level with chlorpromazine Decreased blood level with SSRIs, CBZ, phenytoin, phenobarbital Increased blood level of TCAs, chlorpromazine, CBZ, phenytoin, phenobarbital, primidone, BZDs	Monitor CBC with platelets, LFTs Blood level of approximately 50–150 µg/mL Useful in neuropathic pain

Note.   BZDs = benzodiazepines; CBC = complete blood count; CBZ = carbamazepine; CNS = central nervous system; EPS = extrapyramidal side effects; LFTs = liver function tests; MAOIs = monoamine oxidase inhibitors; NMS = neuroleptic malignant syndrome; NSAIDs = nonsteroidal anti-inflammatory drugs; SIADH = syndrome of inappropriate antidiuretic hormone; SSRIs = selective serotonin reuptake inhibitors; TCAs = tricyclic antidepressants.

TABLE 17–4. Anxiolytics and sedative-hypnotics

Drug	Starting daily dose (mg)	Target daily dose (mg)	Neuropsychiatric side effects	Neuropsychiatric drug interactions	Comments
Benzodiazepines					
Alprazolam	0.25–0.50	0.75–6.00	Drowsiness, incoordination, confusion, dysarthria, fatigue, agitation, dizziness, akathisia, anterograde amnesia (especially alprazolam, lorazepam) Other: sexual dysfunction	Augments respiratory depression with opioids	May develop tolerance to psychotropic and anticonvulsant effects
Lorazepam	0.5–1.0	1.5–12.0		Neurotoxicity and sexual dysfunction with lithium	Do not induce own metabolism
Clonazepam	0.25–0.50	1–5		Additive CNS depressant effects with other CNS depressants	Addictive potential
				Increased blood level with SSRIs, phenytoin	May cause withdrawal syndrome
				Decreased blood level with CBZ	May cause EEG changes
				Decreased blood level of levodopa, phenytoin	May worsen delirium and dementia
					May be useful in treating akathisia
					Clonazepam may accumulate in bloodstream
					May have utility in pain syndromes, movement disorders
Others					
Buspirone	10–15	15–60	Nervousness, headache, confusion, weakness, numbness, drowsiness, tremor, paresthesia, incoordination	EPS with neuroleptics	Has antidepressant effects as adjunct to SSRI but may produce dysphoria at higher doses
				Hypertension with MAOIs	Slow onset of action
				Increased ALT with trazodone	Nonaddictive
				Increased blood level of BZDs, haloperidol	Usually does not impair psychomotor performance

TABLE 17–4.   Anxiolytics and sedative-hypnotics (continued)

Drug	Starting daily dose (mg)	Target daily dose (mg)	Neuropsychiatric side effects	Neuropsychiatric drug interactions	Comments
Diphenhy-dramine	25–50	25–200	Drowsiness, fatigue, dizziness, confusion, anticholinergic effects, incoordination, tremor, nervousness, insomnia, euphoria, paresthesia	Additive CNS depressant effects with other CNS depressants Increased anticholinergic effects with MAOIs, TCAs	Minimal effects on EEG Anticholinergic effects may decrease EPS but may exacerbate delirium May help with insomnia; tolerance may develop Unpredictable anxiolytic properties
Clonidine	0.05–0.20	0.15–0.80	Nervousness, agitation, depression, headache, insomnia, vivid dreams or nightmares, behavior changes, restlessness, anxiety, hallucinations, delirium, sedation, weakness, fatigue	Additive CNS depressant effects with other CNS depressants Impaired blood pressure control with neuroleptics Decreased blood level with TCAs	Useful in opiate withdrawal, Tourette's, and possibly mania, anxiety, akathisia, ADHD, aggression Available in transdermal form

Note. ADHD = attention-deficit/hyperactivity disorder; ALT = alanine aminotransferase; BZDs = benzodiazepines; CBZ = carbamazepine; CNS = central nervous system; EEG = electroencephalogram; EPS = extrapyramidal side effects; MAOIs = monoamine oxidase inhibitors; SSRIs = selective serotonin reuptake inhibitors; TCAs = tricyclic antidepressants.

with mental retardation and patients chronically hospitalized for severe aggression also support its use (Bellus et al. 1996; Campbell et al. 1995). Although higher plasma levels are more likely to result in clinical improvement, the potential for lower serum levels of lithium to cause neurotoxicity in neuropsychiatric patients may limit its use.

Neuroleptics are effective in treating aggression in neuropsychiatric patients (Rao et al. 1985). They should generally be reserved, however, for patients who have psychotic symptoms or who require rapid behavioral control. Although typical neuroleptics may decrease arousal and agitation in the acute setting, the extrapyramidal and anticholinergic properties of these medications can further increase agitation, particularly when the agents are combined with other drugs with anticholinergic properties (Tune et al. 1992). Akathisia can be confused with worsening aggression, thus prompting a detrimental increase in neuroleptic dose. Neuroleptics can also, in some cases, impair executive cognitive functioning (Medalia et al. 1988). In the chronically aggressive psychotic patient, clozapine at doses of 300–500 mg may be the most effective antipsychotic (Cohen and Underwood 1994). Open studies showed good effects for risperidone in autistic (Horrigan and Barnhill 1997) and mentally retarded (Cohen et al. 1998) patients. Overall, risperidone, olanzapine, and quetiapine have data to support their use in patients with dementia, although side effects can still limit their use (Kindermann et al. 2002; Lawlor 2004; Tariot et al. 2004b); also, the potentially increased mortality of patients with dementia taking atypical antipsychotics raises serious questions about the use of these agents. Various atypical antipsychotics have also shown efficacy in treating aggression in patients with developmental disability and mental retardation (Barnard et al. 2002; McCracken et al. 2002; Posey and McDougle 2000); again, side effects and potential long-term risks should be considered.

Other medications, such as amantadine, a dopamine agonist, and clonidine, an α-adrener-

gic agonist, have been used to treat aggression. Gualtieri et al. (1989) used amantadine successfully in dosages of 50–400 mg/day in agitated patients recovering from coma. Clonidine at 0.6 mg/day reduced violent outbursts in an autistic adult (Koshes and Rock 1994), but its depressogenic and hypotensive risks may be problematic in the neurological patient.

COGNITIVE DISTURBANCE

Cognitive disturbance is almost always the result of etiologically identifiable brain dysfunction. However, difficulties with concentration, memory, and more complicated executive cognitive functions occur not just as primary components of neurological disease but also as epiphenomena in the course of major mood disturbance (i.e., pseudodementia) and as a core feature of schizophrenia and chronic bipolar disorder; cognitive disturbance can also be secondary to medications used to treat neurological and other medical illnesses. Treating cognitive disturbance can lead to improvements in quality of life, and even minor improvements in cognition can produce substantial health care cost savings (Ernst and Hay 1997).

TREATMENT

Most treatment studies have focused on Alzheimer's dementia (AD), the most prevalent cause of cognitive impairment in the U.S. population. A substantial database has documented the palliative efficacy of reversible cholinesterase inhibitors in these patients. Available FDA-approved agents include donepezil, rivastigmine, and galantamine, and all have better tolerability than tacrine hydrochloride. The available cholinesterase inhibitors have shown similar efficacy and tolerability (Farlow et al. 2000; Greenberg et al. 2000; Wilkinson and Murray 2001). Evidence also suggests beneficial psychotropic effects in patients with problematic depression, psychosis, agitation, and disinhibition, although other patients without obvious behavior problems may experience behavioral worsening (Mega et al. 1999). These medications may also have efficacy in vascular dementia (Erkinjuntti et al. 2002; Mendez et al. 1999; Wilkinson et al. 2003) and for psychotropic-induced memory loss in patients without dementia (Jacobsen and Comas-Diaz 1999).

The N-methyl-D-aspartate (NMDA) receptor antagonist memantine reduces glutamatergic CNS toxicity and has been approved for use in moderate to severe AD. Compared with placebo, memantine improves activities of daily living scores and global function (Reisberg et al. 2003). This improvement was modest and of the magnitude seen in cholinesterase inhibitor trials. When memantine was added to donepezil, limited data suggest significantly better outcomes in activities of daily living function compared to donepezil plus placebo (Tariot et al. 2004a).

Selegiline, an MAO-B inhibitor commonly used in Parkinson's disease, was initially shown at an open daily dose of 20 mg to improve cognitive performance of 14 AD patients (Schneider et al. 1991). Subsequently, double-blind studies of selegiline at low 10-mg doses likely to act principally by increasing CNS dopamine showed superiority to placebo (Finali et al. 1991), to phosphatidylserine (Monteverde et al. 1990), and to oxiracetam (Falsaperla et al. 1990) on a variety of cognitive tests. However, as summarized in a negative crossover study (Tariot et al. 1998b), positive effects of this drug on agitation and depression in some patients make it difficult to separate mood state–dependent effects on cognition from a primary cognitive effect. One other study showed no effect (Freedman et al. 1998), and still another showed a modest effect on delaying functional impairment (Sano et al. 1997).

Several naturalistic case–control studies have shown that anti-inflammatory drugs may help AD patients. In one study, patients taking daily NSAIDs or aspirin had shorter duration of illness and better cognitive performance (Rich et al. 1995). In another study, the onset of AD in monozygotic twin pairs was inversely proportional to prior use of steroids or corticotropin (Breitner et al. 1994). Finally, a third naturalistic study (Prince et al. 1998) showed that

NSAID use was associated with less cognitive decline, particularly in younger subjects. One placebo-controlled study of 44 patients supported an effect for indomethacin (Rogers et al. 1993), and NSAIDs are associated with histopathological evidence of slowed progression of AD (Alafuzoff et al. 2000). However, another study failed to show an effect for diclofenac/misoprostol (Scharf et al. 1999), and a study of prednisone also had negative findings (Aisen et al. 2000), although the dose was quite low, and adverse effects on hippocampal cells could have counteracted anti-inflammatory effects. A meta-analysis of six prospective studies found NSAID use was associated with a decreased risk of AD (Szekely et al. 2008). However, a randomized, placebo-controlled trial found no benefit for naproxen and celecoxib in the treatment of AD (B.K. Martin et al. 2008). Although no reports have examined effects of therapy aimed at the cytokine-related inflammatory pathways in HIV disease patients, this strategy also holds some promise.

Two studies support very modest effects of antioxidants. Le Bars et al. (1997) showed that ginkgo biloba was superior to placebo in a mixed Alzheimer's and vascular dementia group, but with a small clinical effect. These results are inferior to those seen with tacrine or donepezil, and the predominance of mild cases makes the generalizability of results unclear. A meta-analysis of studies with this agent (Oken et al. 1998) showed that few reports were well designed with clearly described patient groups, although these few also showed similar modest effects. An increase in bleeding risk, especially for patients taking anticoagulants, warrants caution, however. A second study (Sano et al. 1997) showed that 2,000 IU of α-tocopherol slowed functional decline in Alzheimer's disease patients, with a delay of about a half-year over a 2-year period. However, no cognitive improvements were noted, despite these functional benefits.

Initial studies showing that fewer Alzheimer's and vascular dementia patients take replacement estrogen than do matched control subjects (Mortel and Meyer 1995) and that

TABLE 17–5.   Cognitive agents

Drug	Starting daily dose (mg)	Target daily dose (mg)	Neuropsychiatric side effects	Neuropsychiatric drug interactions	Comments
Acetylcholinesterase inhibitors					
Donepezil	5	10	Headache, fatigue, dizziness, insomnia	Effects antagonized by anticholinergic drugs	Donepezil has once-daily dosing
Rivastigmine	3	12	Other: nausea, diarrhea, weight loss, muscle cramps, joint pain		Rivastigmine and galantamine have twice-daily dosing; once-daily formulation for galantamine also available
Galantamine	8	24			
NMDA antagonist					
Memantine	5	20	Fatigue, headache, dizziness, psychosis, confusion Other: nausea, diarrhea, pain, increased blood pressure	Carbonic anhydrase inhibitors (such as acetazolamide) may increase blood levels Possible interactions with other NMDA antagonists (such as amantadine) are unknown	Twice-daily dosing

Note.   NMDA = *N*-methyl-D-aspartate.

those who do have better cognitive function than those who do not (Henderson et al. 1994) have been replicated in several other uncontrolled naturalistic designs showing that estrogen use is associated with reduced incidence of Alzheimer's disease (Slooter et al. 1999). These associations were convergent with preclinical studies showing genomic and receptor-mediated effects of estrogen on learning, memory, and neuronal growth and connections (Shaywitz and Shaywitz 2000). Unfortunately, well-designed treatment studies (Henderson et al. 2000; Mulnard et al. 2000) failed to show a beneficial effect of estrogen supplements for mildly to moderately impaired elderly women with Alzheimer's disease, although beneficial effects in postmenopausal women without dementia (Kampen and Sherwin 1994) suggest that preventive effects might be possible.

Based on the possibility that calcium blockade will slow mechanisms of neuronal death that depend on increased free intracellular calcium in Alzheimer's disease, studies of 90 mg/day of nimodipine in patients have shown some promise. Ban et al. (1990) showed 12 weeks of nimodipine to be more effective than placebo for improvement on the Mini-Mental State Examination and the Wechsler Memory Scale; improvement continued between 60 and 90 days. Tollefson (1990) showed that the same dose improved recall on the Buschke test, although 180 mg proved worse than placebo. However, one naturalistic study showed that elderly patients taking calcium channel blockers are more likely to develop dementia (Maxwell et al. 1999). Unique calcium channel effects of nimodipine could explain some of these differences.

A variety of other agents have been studied. Stimulants improved cognitive performance of HIV disease patients in an open trial (Angrist et al. 1992) and a placebo-controlled crossover trial (van Dyck et al. 1997). Stimulants can be useful in patients with distractibility, impaired attention, impulsivity, and irritability (Mooney and Haas 1993). These medications are generally well tolerated in the neurological patient (Kaufmann et al. 1984), do not appear to lower

the seizure threshold at therapeutic doses (Wroblewski et al. 1992), and may even enhance cortical recovery (Feeney et al. 1982). However, they should be used with caution because of their potential to aggravate irritability and delusional thought content. Opiate antagonists helped improve TBI-associated memory impairment in one case series (Tennant and Wild 1987). The serotonergic antidepressant fluvoxamine has improved memory impairment in Korsakoff's dementia in two studies (P.R. Martin et al. 1989, 1995). Clonidine variably improved memory in Korsakoff's dementia, and this was correlated with increased cingulate gyrus and thalamic blood flow (Moffoot et al. 1994). Both clonidine and another α_2 agonist, guanfacine, improve various aspects of cognition in healthy humans (Jakala et al. 1999a, 1999b, 1999c).

Phosphatidylserine, a lipid membrane processor, improved several cognitive measures in AD patients (Crook et al. 1992). Citicoline, a metabolic intermediate that enhances the formation of neural membranes and promotes acetylcholine biosynthesis, improved verbal memory in older individuals with "inefficient" memories who did not have dementia (Spiers et al. 1996). Milacemide, a prodrug for glycine (Dysken et al. 1992), did not work in AD patients despite the plausibility of NMDA-glutamate theories of cognition (Ingram et al. 1994), though it had increased word retrieval in young and old subjects without dementia (Schwartz et al. 1991). However, cycloserine improved cognition, relative to placebo, in 17 Alzheimer's disease patients, suggesting that NMDA strategies need to be pursued further (G.E. Tsai et al. 1999). Finally, preliminary studies show a beneficial effect for both insulin and somatostatin acutely administered to Alzheimer's disease patients (S. Craft et al. 1999), whereas peptide T may be associated with improved performance in more cognitively impaired HIV disease patients with relatively preserved immunological status (Heseltine et al. 1998).

In conclusion, only a few approved treatments for cognitive impairment, principally in

AD, are available. Donepezil, rivastigmine, and galantamine are generally well tolerated, with modest efficacy at slowing cognitive decline. Memantine may have benefit in patients with moderate to severe dementia and as a combination therapy. It is actively being studied as a potential neuroprotective agent. Other agents have been investigated, but data are too limited to provide strong recommendations. Table 17–5 (p. 518) lists characteristic cognitive agents recommended in this section and the dose ranges, side effects, and relevant drug interactions for each.

RECOMMENDED READINGS

Charney D, Nestler E (eds): Neurobiology of Mental Illness, 2nd Edition. New York, Oxford University Press, 2005

Davis KL, Charney D, Coyle JT, et al (eds): Neuropsychopharmacology: The Fifth Generation of Progress. American College of Neuropsychopharmacology. Philadelphia, PA, Lippincott Williams & Wilkins, 2002

Nestler EJ, Hyman SE, Malenka RC (eds): Molecular Basis of Neuropharmacology: A Foundation for Clinical Neuroscience. New York, McGraw-Hill, 2001

REFERENCES

Aisen PS, Davis KL, Berg JD, et al: A randomized controlled trial of prednisone in Alzheimer's disease. Alzheimer's Disease Cooperative Study. Neurology 54:588–593, 2000

Alafuzoff I, Overmyer M, Helisalmi S, et al: Lower counts of astroglia and activated microglia in patients with Alzheimer's disease with regular use of non-steroidal anti-inflammatory drugs. J Alzheimers Dis 2:37–46, 2000

Alexopoulos GS, Streim J, Carpenter D, et al: Using antipsychotic agents in older patients. J Clin Psychiatry 65 (suppl 2):5–99, 2004

Allen RL, Walker Z, D'Ath PJ, et al: Risperidone for psychotic and behavioural symptoms in Lewy body dementia. Lancet 346:185, 1995

Alpert M, Allan ER, Citrome L, et al: A double-blind, placebo-controlled study of adjunctive nadolol in the management of violent psychiatric patients. Psychopharmacol Bull 26:367–371, 1990

Angrist B, d'Hollosy M, Sanfilipo M, et al: Central nervous system stimulants as symptomatic treatments for AIDS-related neuropsychiatric impairment. J Clin Psychopharmacol 12:268–272, 1992

Auchus AP, Bissey-Black C: Pilot study of haloperidol, fluoxetine, and placebo for agitation in Alzheimer's disease. J Neuropsychiatry Clin Neurosci 9:591–593, 1997

Azouvi P, Jokic C, Attal N, et al: Carbamazepine in agitation and aggressive behaviour following severe closed-head injury: results of an open trial. Brain Inj 13:797–804, 1999

Ban TA, Morey L, Aguglia E, et al: Nimodipine in the treatment of old age dementias. Prog Neuropsychopharmacol Biol Psychiatry 14:525–551, 1990

Barnard L, Young AH, Pearson J, et al: A systematic review of the use of atypical antipsychotics in autism. J Psychopharmacol 16:93–101, 2002

Barratt ES: The use of anticonvulsants in aggression and violence. Psychopharmacol Bull 29:75–81, 1993

Bejjani BP, Damier P, Arnulf I, et al: Transient acute depression induced by high-frequency deep-brain stimulation. N Engl J Med 340:1476–1480, 1999

Bellus SB, Stewart D, Vergo JG, et al: The use of lithium in the treatment of aggressive behaviours with two brain-injured individuals in a state psychiatric hospital. Brain Inj 10:849–860, 1996

Berney A, Vingerhoets F, Perrin A, et al: Effect on mood of subthalamic DBS for Parkinson's disease: a consecutive series of 24 patients. Neurology 59:1427–1429, 2002

Bonelli RM, Wenning GK, Kapfhammer HP: Huntington's disease: present treatments and future therapeutic modalities. Int Clin Psychopharmacol 19:51–62, 2004

Bowden CL, Calabrese JR, Sachs G, et al: A placebo-controlled 18-month trial of lamotrigine and lithium maintenance treatment in recently manic or hypomanic patients with bipolar I disorder. Arch Gen Psychiatry 60:392–400, 2003

Bozikas V, Bascialla F, Yulis P, et al: Gabapentin for behavioral dyscontrol with mental retardation. Am J Psychiatry 158:965–966, 2001

Breier A, Sutton VK, Feldman PD, et al: Olanzapine in the treatment of dopamimetic-induced psychosis in patients with Parkinson's disease. Biol Psychiatry 52:438–445, 2002

Breitbart W, Marotta R, Platt MM, et al: A double-blind trial of haloperidol, chlorpromazine, and lorazepam in the treatment of delirium in hospitalized AIDS patients. Am J Psychiatry 153:231–237, 1996

Breitner JC, Gau BA, Welsh KA, et al: Inverse association of anti-inflammatory treatments and Alzheimer's disease: initial results of a co-twin control study. Neurology 44:227–232, 1994

Brodaty H, Ames D, Snowdon J, et al: A randomized placebo-controlled trial of risperidone for the treatment of aggression, agitation, and psychosis of dementia. J Clin Psychiatry 64:134–143, 2003

Buitelaar JK, van der Gaag RJ, van der Hoeven J: Buspirone in the management of anxiety and irritability in children with pervasive developmental disorders: results of an open-label study. J Clin Psychiatry 59:56–59, 1998

Burke WJ, Pfeiffer RF, McComb RD: Neuroleptic sensitivity to clozapine in dementia with Lewy bodies. J Neuropsychiatry Clin Neurosci 10:227–229, 1998

Burns A, Russell E, Stratton-Powell H, et al: Sertraline in stroke-associated lability of mood. Int J Geriatr Psychiatry 14:681–685, 1999

Burt T, Lisanby SH, Sackeim HA: Neuropsychiatric applications of transcranial magnetic stimulation: a meta-analysis. Int J Neuropsychopharmacol 5:73–103, 2002

Byrne A, Martin W, Hnatko G: Beneficial effects of buspirone therapy in Huntington's disease (letter). Am J Psychiatry 151:1097, 1994

Calabrese JR, Bowden CL, Sachs GS, et al: A double-blind placebo-controlled study of lamotrigine monotherapy in outpatients with bipolar I depression. Lamictal 602 Study Group. J Clin Psychiatry 60:79–88, 1999

Campbell M, Kafantaris V, Cueva JE: An update on the use of lithium carbonate in aggressive children and adolescents with conduct disorder. Psychopharmacol Bull 31:93–102, 1995

Cantello R, Aguggia M, Gilli M, et al: Major depression in Parkinson's disease and the mood response to intravenous methylphenidate: possible role of the "hedonic" dopamine synapse. J Neurol Neurosurg Psychiatry 52:724–731, 1989

Cantillon M, Brunswick R, Molina D, et al: A double-blind trial for agitation in a nursing home population with Alzheimer's disease. Am J Geriatr Psychiatry 4:263–267, 1996

Chacko RC, Hurley RA, Jankovic J: Clozapine use in diffuse Lewy body disease. J Neuropsychiatry Clin Neurosci 5:206–208, 1993

Chatham-Showalter PE: Carbamazepine for combativeness in acute traumatic brain injury. J Neuropsychiatry Clin Neurosci 8:96–99, 1996

Chatterjee A, Fahn S: Methylphenidate treats apathy in Parkinson's disease. J Neuropsychiatry Clin Neurosci 14:461–462, 2002

Childers MK, Holland D: Psychomotor agitation following gabapentin use in brain injury. Brain Inj 11:537–540, 1997

Coccaro EF, Kramer E, Zemishlany Z, et al: Pharmacologic treatment of noncognitive behavioral disturbances in elderly demented patients. Am J Psychiatry 147:1640–1645, 1990

Cohen SA, Underwood MT: The use of clozapine in a mentally retarded and aggressive population. J Clin Psychiatry 55:440–444, 1994

Cohen SA, Ihrig K, Lott RS, et al: Risperidone for aggression and self-injurious behavior in adults with mental retardation. J Autism Dev Disord 28:229–233, 1998

Colenda CC 3rd: Buspirone in treatment of agitated demented patient (letter). Lancet 1:1169, 1988

Connemann BJ, Schonfeldt-Lecuona C: Ziprasidone in Parkinson's disease psychosis (letter). Can J Psychiatry 49:73, 2004

Connor DF, Ozbayrak KR, Benjamin S, et al: A pilot study of nadolol for overt aggression in developmentally delayed individuals. J Am Acad Child Adolesc Psychiatry 36:826–834, 1997

Cook EH Jr, Rowlett R, Jaselskis C, et al: Fluoxetine treatment of children and adults with autistic disorder and mental retardation. J Am Acad Child Adolesc Psychiatry 31:739–745, 1992

Cooper JP: Buspirone for anxiety and agitation in dementia (letter). J Psychiatry Neurosci 28:469, 2003

Craft M, Ismail IA, Krishnamurti D, et al: Lithium in the treatment of aggression in mentally handicapped patients: a double-blind trial. Br J Psychiatry 150:685–689, 1987

Craft S, Asthana S, Newcomer JW, et al: Enhancement of memory in Alzheimer disease with insulin and somatostatin, but not glucose. Arch Gen Psychiatry 56:1135–1140, 1999

Crook T, Petrie W, Wells C, et al: Effects of phosphatidylserine in Alzheimer's disease. Psychopharmacol Bull 28:61–66, 1992

Cueva JE, Overall JE, Small AM, et al: Carbamazepine in aggressive children with conduct disorder: a double-blind and placebo-controlled study. J Am Acad Child Adolesc Psychiatry 35:480–490, 1996

Dallocchio C, Buffa C, Tinelli C, et al: Effectiveness of risperidone in Huntington chorea patients. J Clin Psychopharmacol 19:101–103, 1999

Davanzo PA, Belin TR, Widawski MH, et al: Paroxetine treatment of aggression and self-injury in persons with mental retardation. Am J Ment Retard 102:427–437, 1998

De Deyn PP, Rabheru K, Rasmussen A, et al: A randomized trial of risperidone, placebo, and haloperidol for behavioral symptoms of dementia. Neurology 53:946–955, 1999

De Deyn PP, Carrasco MM, Deberdt W, et al: Olanzapine versus placebo in the treatment of psychosis with or without associated behavioral disturbances in patients with Alzheimer's disease. Int J Geriatr Psychiatry 19:115–126, 2004

Deep Brain Stimulation for Parkinson's Disease Study Group: Deep-brain stimulation of the subthalamic nucleus or the pars interna of the globus pallidus in Parkinson's disease. N Engl J Med 345:956–963, 2001

Devanand DP, Marder K, Michaels KS, et al: A randomized, placebo-controlled dose-comparison trial of haloperidol for psychosis and disruptive behaviors in Alzheimer's disease. Am J Psychiatry 155:1512–1520, 1998

Diaz-Olavarrieta C, Campbell J, Garcia de la Cadena C, et al: Domestic violence against patients with chronic neurologic disorders. Arch Neurol 56:681–685, 1999

Donaldson C, Tarrier N, Burns A: Determinants of carer stress in Alzheimer's disease. Int J Geriatr Psychiatry 13:248–256, 1998

Dorevitch A, Katz N, Zemishlany Z, et al: Intramuscular flunitrazepam versus intramuscular haloperidol in the emergency treatment of aggressive psychotic behavior. Am J Psychiatry 156:142–144, 1999

Duffy JD, Kant R: Clinical utility of clozapine in 16 patients with neurological disease. J Neuropsychiatry Clin Neurosci 8:92–96, 1996

Dysken MW, Mendels J, LeWitt P, et al: Milacemide: a placebo-controlled study in senile dementia of the Alzheimer type. J Am Geriatr Soc 40:503–506, 1992

Elger G, Hoppe C, Falkai P, et al: Vagus nerve stimulation is associated with mood improvements in epilepsy patients. Epilepsy Res 42:203–210, 2000

Ellis T, Cudkowicz ME, Sexton PM, et al: Clozapine and risperidone treatment of psychosis in Parkinson's disease. J Neuropsychiatry Clin Neurosci 12:364–369, 2000

Erkinjuntti T, Kurz A, Gauthier S, et al: Efficacy of galantamine in probable vascular dementia and Alzheimer's disease combined with cerebrovascular disease: a randomised trial. Lancet 359:1283–1290, 2002

Ernst RL, Hay JW: Economic research on Alzheimer disease: a review of the literature. Alzheimer Dis Assoc Disord 11 (suppl 6):135–145, 1997

Expert Consensus Panel for Agitation in Dementia: Treatment of agitation in older persons with dementia. Postgrad Med Spec No:1–88, 1998

Falk WE, Mahnke MW, Poskanzer DC: Lithium prophylaxis of corticotropin-induced psychosis. JAMA 241:1011–1012, 1979

Fall PA, Ekman R, Granerus AK, et al: ECT in Parkinson's disease: changes in motor symptoms, monoamine metabolites and neuropeptides. J Neural Transm Park Dis Dement Sect 10(2–3):129–140, 1995

Falsaperla A, Monici Preti PA, Oliani C: Selegiline versus oxiracetam in patients with Alzheimer-type dementia. Clin Ther 12:376–384, 1990

Farlow M, Anand R, Messina J Jr, et al: A 52-week study of the efficacy of rivastigmine in patients with mild to moderately severe Alzheimer's disease. Eur Neurol 44:236–241, 2000

Feeney DM, Gonzalez A, Law WA: Amphetamine, haloperidol, and experience interact to affect rate of recovery after motor cortex injury. Science 217:855–857, 1982

Fernandez HH, Friedman JH, Jacques C, et al: Quetiapine for the treatment of drug-induced psychosis in Parkinson's disease. Mov Disord 14:484–487, 1999

Fernandez HH, Trieschmann ME, Friedman JH: Aripiprazole for drug-induced psychosis in Parkinson disease: preliminary experience. Clin Neuropharmacol 27:4–5, 2004

Ferrando SJ, Rabkin JG, de Moore GM, et al: Antidepressant treatment of depression in HIV-seropositive women. J Clin Psychiatry 60:741–746, 1999

Finali G, Piccirilli M, Oliani C, et al: L-deprenyl therapy improves verbal memory in amnesic Alzheimer patients. Clin Neuropharmacol 14:523–536, 1991

Fleminger S, Greenwood RJ, Oliver DL: Pharmacological management for agitation and aggression in people with acquired brain injury. Cochrane Database Syst Rev (1): CD003299, 2003

Freedman M, Rewilak D, Xerri T, et al: L-deprenyl in Alzheimer's disease: cognitive and behavioral effects. Neurology 50:660–668, 1998

Fregni F, Santos CM, Myczkowski ML, et al: Repetitive transcranial magnetic stimulation is as effective as fluoxetine in the treatment of depression in patients with Parkinson's disease. J Neurol Neurosurg Psychiatry 75:1171–1174, 2004

Freinhar JP, Alvarez WA: Clonazepam treatment of organic brain syndromes in three elderly patients. J Clin Psychiatry 47:525–526, 1986

Garza-Trevino ES, Hollister LE, Overall JE, et al: Efficacy of combinations of intramuscular antipsychotics and sedative-hypnotics for control of psychotic agitation. Am J Psychiatry 146:1598–1601, 1989

George MS, Rush AJ, Marangell LB, et al: A one-year comparison of vagus nerve stimulation with treatment as usual for treatment-resistant depression. Biol Psychiatry 58:364–373, 2005

Glenn MB, Wroblewski B, Parziale J, et al: Lithium carbonate for aggressive behavior or affective instability in ten brain-injured patients. Am J Phys Med Rehabil 68:221–226, 1989

Glue P: Rapid cycling affective disorders in the mentally retarded. Biol Psychiatry 26:250–256, 1989

Goetz CG, Tanner CM, Klawans HL: Bupropion in Parkinson's disease. Neurology 34:1092–1094, 1984

Goff DC, Tsai G, Levitt J, et al: A placebo-controlled trial of D-cycloserine added to conventional neuroleptics in patients with schizophrenia. Arch Gen Psychiatry 56:21–27, 1999

Gomez-Esteban JC, Zarranz JJ, Velasco F, et al: Use of ziprasidone in parkinsonian patients with psychosis. Clin Neuropharmacol 28:111–114, 2005

Grant I, Brown GW, Harris T, et al: Severely threatening events and marked life difficulties preceding onset or exacerbation of multiple sclerosis. J Neurol Neurosurg Psychiatry 52:8–13, 1989

Greenberg SM, Tennis MK, Brown LB, et al: Donepezil therapy in clinical practice: a randomized crossover study. Arch Neurol 57:94–99, 2000

Greendyke RM, Kanter DR: Therapeutic effects of pindolol on behavioral disturbances associated with organic brain disease: a double-blind study. J Clin Psychiatry 47:423–426, 1986

Greenwald BS, Marin DB, Silverman SM: Serotoninergic treatment of screaming and banging in dementia. Lancet 2:1464–1465, 1986

Gualtieri CT: Buspirone for the behavior problems of patients with organic brain disorders. J Clin Psychopharmacol 11:280–281, 1991

Gualtieri T, Chandler M, Coons TB, et al: Amantadine: a new clinical profile for traumatic brain injury. Clin Neuropharmacol 12:258–270, 1989

Haas S, Vincent K, Holt J, et al: Divalproex: a possible treatment alternative for demented, elderly aggressive patients. Ann Clin Psychiatry 9:145–147, 1997

Haller E, Binder RL: Clozapine and seizures. Am J Psychiatry 147:1069–1071, 1990

Halman MH, Worth JL, Sanders KM, et al: Anticonvulsant use in the treatment of manic syndromes in patients with HIV-1 infection. J Neuropsychiatry Clin Neurosci 5:430–434, 1993

Hamner M, Huber M, Gardner VT 3rd: Patient with progressive dementia and choreoathetoid movements treated with buspirone. J Clin Psychopharmacol 16:261–262, 1996

Hellings JA, Kelley LA, Gabrielli WF, et al: Sertraline response in adults with mental retardation and autistic disorder. J Clin Psychiatry 57:333–336, 1996

Henderson VW, Paganini-Hill A, Emanuel CK, et al: Estrogen replacement therapy in older women: comparisons between Alzheimer's disease cases and nondemented control subjects. Arch Neurol 51:896–900, 1994

Henderson VW, Paganini-Hill A, Miller BL, et al: Estrogen for Alzheimer's disease in women: randomized, double-blind, placebo-controlled trial. Neurology 54:295–301, 2000

Hendryx PM: Psychosocial changes perceived by closed-head-injured adults and their families. Arch Phys Med Rehabil 70:526–530, 1989

Herrmann N, Lanctot K, Myszak M: Effectiveness of gabapentin for the treatment of behavioral disorders in dementia. J Clin Psychopharmacol 20:90–93, 2000

Herz LR, Volicer L, Ross V, et al: Pharmacotherapy of agitation in dementia. Am J Psychiatry 149:1757–1758, 1992

Heseltine PN, Goodkin K, Atkinson JH, et al: Randomized double-blind placebo-controlled trial of peptide T for HIV-associated cognitive impairment. Arch Neurol 55:41–51, 1998

Himmelhoch JM, Neil JF, May SJ, et al: Age, dementia, dyskinesias, and lithium response. Am J Psychiatry 137:941–945, 1980

Holton A, George K: The use of lithium in severely demented patients with behavioural disturbance. Br J Psychiatry 146:99–100, 1985

Holtzheimer PE 3rd, Russo J, Avery DH: A meta-analysis of repetitive transcranial magnetic stimulation in the treatment of depression [published erratum appears in Psychopharmacol Bull 37:5, 2003]. Psychopharmacol Bull 35:149–169, 2001

Horne M, Lindley SE: Divalproex sodium in the treatment of aggressive behavior and dysphoria in patients with organic brain syndromes. J Clin Psychiatry 56:430–431, 1995

Hornstein A, Seliger G: Cognitive side effects of lithium in closed head injury. J Neuropsychiatry Clin Neurosci 1:446–447, 1989

Horrigan JP, Barnhill LJ: Risperidone and explosive aggressive autism. J Autism Dev Disord 27:313–323, 1997

Iannaccone S, Ferini-Strambi L: Pharmacologic treatment of emotional lability. Clin Neuropharmacol 19:532–535, 1996

Ingram DK, Spangler EL, Iijima S, et al: New pharmacological strategies for cognitive enhancement using a rat model of age-related memory impairment. Ann N Y Acad Sci 717:16–32, 1994

Jacobsen FM, Comas-Diaz L: Donepezil for psychotropic-induced memory loss. J Clin Psychiatry 60:698–704, 1999

Jakala P, Riekkinen M, Sirvio J, et al: Clonidine, but not guanfacine, impairs choice reaction time performance in young healthy volunteers. Neuropsychopharmacology 21:495–502, 1999a

Jakala P, Riekkinen M, Sirvio J, et al: Guanfacine, but not clonidine, improves planning and working memory performance in humans. Neuropsychopharmacology 20:460–470, 1999b

Jakala P, Sirvio J, Riekkinen M, et al: Guanfacine and clonidine, alpha 2-agonists, improve paired associates learning, but not delayed matching to sample, in humans. Neuropsychopharmacology 20:119–130, 1999c

Jorge RE, Robinson RG, Tateno A, et al: Repetitive transcranial magnetic stimulation as treatment of poststroke depression: a preliminary study. Biol Psychiatry 55:398–405, 2004

Jouvent R, Abensour P, Bonnet AM, et al: Antiparkinsonian and antidepressant effects of high doses of bromocriptine: an independent comparison. J Affect Disord 5:141–145, 1983

Kampen DL, Sherwin BB: Estrogen use and verbal memory in healthy postmenopausal women. Obstet Gynecol 83:979–983, 1994

Katz IR, Jeste DV, Mintzer JE, et al: Comparison of risperidone and placebo for psychosis and behavioral disturbances associated with dementia: a randomized, double-blind trial. Risperidone Study Group. J Clin Psychiatry 60:107–115, 1999

Kaufmann MW, Cassem NH, Murray GB, et al: Use of psychostimulants in medically ill patients with neurological disease and major depression. Can J Psychiatry 29:46–49, 1984

Kemperman CJ, Gerdes JH, De Rooij J, et al: Reversible lithium neurotoxicity at normal serum level may refer to intracranial pathology. J Neurol Neurosurg Psychiatry 52:679–680, 1989

Kim E, Zwil AS, McAllister TW, et al: Treatment of organic bipolar mood disorders in Parkinson's disease. J Neuropsychiatry Clin Neurosci 6:181–184, 1994

Kindermann SS, Dolder CR, Bailey A, et al: Pharmacological treatment of psychosis and agitation in elderly patients with dementia: four decades of experience. Drugs Aging 19:257–276, 2002

Koshes RJ, Rock NL: Use of clonidine for behavioral control in an adult patient with autism. Am J Psychiatry 151:1714, 1994

Kunik ME, Puryear L, Orengo CA, et al: The efficacy and tolerability of divalproex sodium in elderly demented patients with behavioral disturbances. Int J Geriatr Psychiatry 13:29–34, 1998

Lanctot KL, Herrmann N, van Reekum R, et al: Gender, aggression and serotonergic function are associated with response to sertraline for behavioral disturbances in Alzheimer's disease. Int J Geriatr Psychiatry 17:531–541, 2002

Lange KW, Riederer P: Glutamatergic drugs in Parkinson's disease. Life Sci 55:2067–2075, 1994

Lawlor BA: Behavioral and psychological symptoms in dementia: the role of atypical antipsychotics. J Clin Psychiatry 65 (suppl 11):5–10, 2004

Lawlor BA, Radcliffe J, Molchan SE, et al: A pilot placebo-controlled study of trazodone and buspirone in Alzheimer's disease. Int J Geriatr Psychiatry 9:55–59, 1994

Le Bars PL, Katz MM, Berman N, et al: A placebo-controlled, double-blind, randomized trial of an extract of Ginkgo biloba for dementia. North American EGb Study Group. JAMA 278:1327–1332, 1997

Lecamwasam D, Synek B, Moyles K, et al: Chronic lithium neurotoxicity presenting as Parkinson's disease. Int Clin Psychopharmacol 9:127–129, 1994

Lera G, Zirulnik J: Pilot study with clozapine in patients with HIV-associated psychosis and drug-induced parkinsonism. Mov Disord 14:128–131, 1999

Levine AM: Buspirone and agitation in head injury. Brain Inj 2:165–167, 1988

Lindenmayer JP, Kotsaftis A: Use of sodium valproate in violent and aggressive behaviors: a critical review. J Clin Psychiatry 61:123–128, 2000

Lonergan E, Luxenberg J, Colford J: Haloperidol for agitation in dementia. Cochrane Database Syst Rev (2):CD002852, 2002

Low RA Jr, Brandes M: Gabapentin for the management of agitation. J Clin Psychopharmacol 19:482–483, 1999

Lozano AM, Abosch A: Pallidal stimulation for dystonia. Adv Neurol 94:301–308, 2004

Lozano AM, Mayberg HS, Giacobbe P, et al: Subcallosal cingulate gyrus deep brain stimulation for treatment-resistant depression. Biol Psychiatry 64:461–467, 2008

Malone DA Jr, Dougherty DD, Rezai AR, et al: Deep brain stimulation of the ventral capsule/ventral striatum for treatment-resistant depression. Biol Psychiatry 65:267–275, 2009

Malow BA, Reese KB, Sato S, et al: Spectrum of EEG abnormalities during clozapine treatment. Electroencephalogr Clin Neurophysiol 91:205–211, 1994

Martin BK, Szekely C, Brandt J, et al: Cognitive function over time in the Alzheimer's Disease Anti-inflammatory Prevention Trial (ADAPT): results of a randomized, controlled trial of naproxen and celecoxib. Arch Neurol 65:896–905, 2008

Martin PR, Adinoff B, Eckardt MJ, et al: Effective pharmacotherapy of alcoholic amnestic disorder with fluvoxamine: preliminary findings. Arch Gen Psychiatry 46:617–621, 1989

Martin PR, Adinoff B, Lane E, et al: Fluvoxamine treatment of alcoholic amnestic disorder. Eur Neuropsychopharmacol 5:27–33, 1995

Martinon-Torres G, Fioravanti M, Grimley EJ: Trazodone for agitation in dementia. Cochrane Database Syst Rev (4):CD004990, 2004

Mattes JA: Comparative effectiveness of carbamazepine and propranolol for rage outbursts. J Neuropsychiatry Clin Neurosci 2:159–164, 1990

Max JE, Robin DA, Lindgren SD, et al: Traumatic brain injury in children and adolescents: psychiatric disorders at one year. J Neuropsychiatry Clin Neurosci 10:290–297, 1998

Maxwell CJ, Hogan DB, Ebly EM: Calcium-channel blockers and cognitive function in elderly people: results from the Canadian Study of Health and Aging. CMAJ 161:501–506, 1999

Mayberg HS, Lozano AM, Voon V, et al: Deep brain stimulation for treatment-resistant depression. Neuron 45:651–660, 2005

Mazure CM, Druss BG, Cellar JS: Valproate treatment of older psychotic patients with organic mental syndromes and behavioral dyscontrol. J Am Geriatr Soc 40:914–916, 1992

McAllister TW: Carbamazepine in mixed frontal lobe and psychiatric disorders. J Clin Psychiatry 46:393–394, 1985

McAllister TW, Ferrell RB: Evaluation and treatment of psychosis after traumatic brain injury. NeuroRehabilitation 17:357–368, 2002

McCracken JT, McGough J, Shah B, et al: Risperidone in children with autism and serious behavioral problems. N Engl J Med 347:314–321, 2002

McDougle CJ, Naylor ST, Cohen DJ, et al: A double-blind, placebo-controlled study of fluvoxamine in adults with autistic disorder. Arch Gen Psychiatry 53:1001–1008, 1996

Medalia A, Gold J, Merriam A: The effects of neuroleptics on neuropsychological test results of schizophrenics. Arch Clin Neuropsychol 3:249–271, 1988

Meehan K, Zhang F, David S, et al: A double-blind, randomized comparison of the efficacy and safety of intramuscular injections of olanzapine, lorazepam, or placebo in treating acutely agitated patients diagnosed with bipolar mania. J Clin Psychopharmacol 21:389–397, 2001

Mega MS, Masterman DM, O'Connor SM, et al: The spectrum of behavioral responses to cholinesterase inhibitor therapy in Alzheimer disease. Arch Neurol 56:1388–1393, 1999

Meltzer HY, Ranjan R: Valproic acid treatment of clozapine-induced myoclonus. Am J Psychiatry 151:1246–1247, 1994

Mendez MF, Younesi FL, Perryman KM: Use of donepezil for vascular dementia: preliminary clinical experience. J Neuropsychiatry Clin Neurosci 11:268–270, 1999

Meyer JM, Marsh J, Simpson G: Differential sensitivities to risperidone and olanzapine in a human immunodeficiency virus patient. Biol Psychiatry 44:791–794, 1998

Miller LJ: Gabapentin for treatment of behavioral and psychological symptoms of dementia. Ann Pharmacother 35:427–431, 2001

Moellentine C, Rummans T, Ahlskog JE, et al: Effectiveness of ECT in patients with parkinsonism. J Neuropsychiatry Clin Neurosci 10:187–193, 1998

Moffoot A, O'Carroll RE, Murray C, et al: Clonidine infusion increases uptake of 99mTc-exametazime in anterior cingulate cortex in Korsakoff's psychosis. Psychol Med 24:53–61, 1994

Mohr E, Mendis T, Hildebrand K, et al: Risperidone in the treatment of dopamine-induced psychosis in Parkinson's disease: an open pilot trial. Mov Disord 15:1230–1237, 2000

Moller JC, Oertel WH, Koster J, et al: Long-term efficacy and safety of pramipexole in advanced Parkinson's disease: results from a European multicenter trial. Mov Disord 20:602–610, 2005

Monteverde A, Gnemmi P, Rossi F, et al: Selegiline in the treatment of mild to moderate Alzheimer-type dementia. Clin Ther 12:315–322, 1990

Mooney GF, Haas LJ: Effect of methylphenidate on brain injury-related anger. Arch Phys Med Rehabil 74:153–160, 1993

Mortel KF, Meyer JS: Lack of postmenopausal estrogen replacement therapy and the risk of dementia. J Neuropsychiatry Clin Neurosci 7:334–337, 1995

Muller U, Murai T, Bauer-Wittmund T, et al: Paroxetine versus citalopram treatment of pathological crying after brain injury. Brain Inj 13:805–811, 1999

Mulnard RA, Cotman CW, Kawas C, et al: Estrogen replacement therapy for treatment of mild to moderate Alzheimer disease: a randomized controlled trial. Alzheimer's Disease Cooperative Study. JAMA 283:1007–1015, 2000

Mysiw WJ, Jackson RD, Corrigan JD: Amitriptyline for post-traumatic agitation. Am J Phys Med Rehabil 67:29–33, 1988

Nahas Z, Arlinghaus KA, Kotrla KJ, et al: Rapid response of emotional incontinence to selective serotonin reuptake inhibitors. J Neuropsychiatry Clin Neurosci 10:453–455, 1998

Newcomer JW, Faustman WO, Zipursky RB, et al: Zacopride in schizophrenia: a single-blind serotonin type 3 antagonist trial. Arch Gen Psychiatry 49:751–752, 1992

Nyth AL, Gottfries CG: The clinical efficacy of citalopram in treatment of emotional disturbances in dementia disorders: a Nordic multicentre study. Br J Psychiatry 157:894–901, 1990

Oechsner M, Korchounov A: Parenteral ziprasidone: a new atypical neuroleptic for emergency treatment of psychosis in Parkinson's disease? Hum Psychopharmacol 20:203–205, 2005

Oken BS, Storzbach DM, Kaye JA: The efficacy of Ginkgo biloba on cognitive function in Alzheimer disease. Arch Neurol 55:1409–1415, 1998

Olin JT, Fox LS, Pawluczyk S, et al: A pilot randomized trial of carbamazepine for behavioral symptoms in treatment-resistant outpatients with Alzheimer disease. Am J Geriatr Psychiatry 9:400–405, 2001

Onuma T, Adachi N, Hisano T, et al: 10-Year follow-up study of epilepsy with psychosis. Jpn J Psychiatry Neurol 45:360–361, 1991

O'Reardon JP, Solvason HB, Janicak PG, et al: Efficacy and safety of transcranial magnetic stimulation in the acute treatment of major depression: a multisite randomized controlled trial. Biol Psychiatry 62:1208–1216, 2007

Palsson S, Aevarsson O, Skoog I: Depression, cerebral atrophy, cognitive performance and incidence of dementia: population study of 85-year-olds. Br J Psychiatry 174:249–253, 1999

Parkinson Study Group: Low-dose clozapine for the treatment of drug-induced psychosis in Parkinson's disease. N Engl J Med 340:757–763, 1999

Parsa MA, Szigethy E, Voci JM, et al: Risperidone in treatment of choreoathetosis of Huntington's disease. J Clin Psychopharmacol 17:134–135, 1997

Perry EK, McKeith I, Thompson P, et al: Topography, extent, and clinical relevance of neurochemical deficits in dementia of Lewy body type, Parkinson's disease, and Alzheimer's disease. Ann N Y Acad Sci 640:197–202, 1991

Peterson KA, Armstrong S, Moseley J: Pathologic crying responsive to treatment with sertraline (letter). J Clin Psychopharmacol 16:333, 1996

Petrie WM, Ban TA, Berney S, et al: Loxapine in psychogeriatrics: a placebo- and standard-controlled clinical investigation. J Clin Psychopharmacol 2:122–126, 1982

Pinner E, Rich CL: Effects of trazodone on aggressive behavior in seven patients with organic mental disorders. Am J Psychiatry 145:1295–1296, 1988

Pollak P, Tison F, Rascol O, et al: Clozapine in drug induced psychosis in Parkinson's disease: a randomised, placebo controlled study with open follow up. J Neurol Neurosurg Psychiatry 75:689–695, 2004

Pollock BG, Mulsant BH, Sweet R, et al: An open pilot study of citalopram for behavioral disturbances of dementia: plasma levels and real-time observations. Am J Geriatr Psychiatry 5:70–78, 1997

Pope HG Jr, McElroy SL, Satlin A, et al: Head injury, bipolar disorder, and response to valproate. Compr Psychiatry 29:34–38, 1988

Popli AP: Risperidone for the treatment of psychosis associated with neurosarcoidosis. J Clin Psychopharmacol 17:132–133, 1997

Porsteinsson AP, Tariot PN, Erb R, et al: Placebo-controlled study of divalproex sodium for agitation in dementia. Am J Geriatr Psychiatry 9:58–66, 2001

Porsteinsson AP, Tariot PN, Jakimovich LJ, et al: Valproate therapy for agitation in dementia: open-label extension of a double-blind trial. Am J Geriatr Psychiatry 11:434–440, 2003

Posey DJ, McDougle CJ: The pharmacotherapy of target symptoms associated with autistic disorder and other pervasive developmental disorders. Harv Rev Psychiatry 8:45–63, 2000

Prigatano GP: Personality disturbances associated with traumatic brain injury. J Consult Clin Psychol 60:360–368, 1992

Prince M, Rabe-Hesketh S, Brennan P: Do antiarthritic drugs decrease the risk for cognitive decline? An analysis based on data from the MRC treatment trial of hypertension in older adults. Neurology 50:374–379, 1998

Ranen NG, Peyser CE, Folstein SE: ECT as a treatment for depression in Huntington's disease. J Neuropsychiatry Clin Neurosci 6:154–159, 1994

Ranen NG, Lipsey JR, Treisman G, et al: Sertraline in the treatment of severe aggressiveness in Huntington's disease. J Neuropsychiatry Clin Neurosci 8:338–340, 1996

Rao N, Jellinek HM, Woolston DC: Agitation in closed head injury: haloperidol effects on rehabilitation outcome. Arch Phys Med Rehabil 66:30–34, 1985

Ratey JJ, Leveroni CL, Miller AC, et al: Low-dose buspirone to treat agitation and maladaptive behavior in brain-injured patients: two case reports. J Clin Psychopharmacol 12:362–364, 1992a

Ratey JJ, Sorgi P, O'Driscoll GA, et al: Nadolol to treat aggression and psychiatric symptomatology in chronic psychiatric inpatients: a double-blind, placebo-controlled study. J Clin Psychiatry 53:41–46, 1992b

Reddy S, Factor SA, Molho ES, et al: The effect of quetiapine on psychosis and motor function in parkinsonian patients with and without dementia. Mov Disord 17:676–681, 2002

Reisberg B, Doody R, Stoffler A, et al: Memantine in moderate-to-severe Alzheimer's disease. N Engl J Med 348:1333–1341, 2003

Rektorova I, Rektor I, Bares M, et al: Pramipexole and pergolide in the treatment of depression in Parkinson's disease: a national multicentre prospective randomized study. Eur J Neurol 10:399–406, 2003

Rich JB, Rasmusson DX, Folstein MF, et al: Nonsteroidal anti-inflammatory drugs in Alzheimer's disease. Neurology 45:51–55, 1995

Roane DM, Feinberg TE, Meckler L, et al: Treatment of dementia-associated agitation with gabapentin. J Neuropsychiatry Clin Neurosci 12:40–43, 2000

Robinson RG, Parikh RM, Lipsey JR, et al: Pathological laughing and crying following stroke: validation of a measurement scale and a double-blind treatment study. Am J Psychiatry 150:286–293, 1993

Rogers J, Kirby LC, Hempelman SR, et al: Clinical trial of indomethacin in Alzheimer's disease. Neurology 43:1609–1611, 1993

Rosse RB, Riggs RL, Dietrich AM, et al: Frontal cortical atrophy and negative symptoms in patients with chronic alcohol dependence. J Neuropsychiatry Clin Neurosci 9:280–282, 1997

Rudorfer MV, Manji HK, Potter WZ: ECT and delirium in Parkinson's disease. Am J Psychiatry 149:1758–1759; author reply 1759–1760, 1992

Ruedrich S, Swales TP, Fossaceca C, et al: Effect of divalproex sodium on aggression and self-injurious behaviour in adults with intellectual disability: a retrospective review. J Intellect Disabil Res 43 (pt 2):105–111, 1999

Rush AJ, Marangell LB, Sackeim HA, et al: Vagus nerve stimulation for treatment-resistant depression: a randomized, controlled acute phase trial. Biol Psychiatry 58:347–354, 2005

Sacristan JA, Iglesias C, Arellano F, et al: Absence seizures induced by lithium: possible interaction with fluoxetine. Am J Psychiatry 148:146–147, 1991

Salloway SP: Diagnosis and treatment of patients with "frontal lobe" syndromes. J Neuropsychiatry Clin Neurosci 6:388–398, 1994

Salzman C: Treatment of agitation, anxiety, and depression in dementia. Psychopharmacol Bull 24:39–42, 1988

Salzman C: Cognitive improvement after benzodiazepine discontinuation (letter). J Clin Psychopharmacol 20:99, 2000

Sano M, Ernesto C, Thomas RG, et al: A controlled trial of selegiline, alpha-tocopherol, or both as treatment for Alzheimer's disease. The Alzheimer's Disease Cooperative Study. N Engl J Med 336:1216–1222, 1997

Scharf S, Mander A, Ugoni A, et al: A double-blind, placebo-controlled trial of diclofenac/misoprostol in Alzheimer's disease. Neurology 53:197–201, 1999

Schiffer RB, Herndon RM, Rudick RA: Treatment of pathologic laughing and weeping with amitriptyline. N Engl J Med 312:1480–1482, 1985

Schneider LS, Pollock VE, Zemansky MF, et al: A pilot study of low-dose L-deprenyl in Alzheimer's disease. J Geriatr Psychiatry Neurol 4:143–148, 1991

Schneider LS, Dagerman KS, Insel P: Risk of death with atypical antipsychotic drug treatment for dementia: meta-analysis of randomized placebo-controlled trials. JAMA 294:1934–1943, 2005

Schreiber S, Klag E, Gross Y, et al: Beneficial effect of risperidone on sleep disturbance and psychosis following traumatic brain injury. Int Clin Psychopharmacol 13:273–275, 1998

Schuurman PR, Bosch DA, Bossuyt PM, et al: A comparison of continuous thalamic stimulation and thalamotomy for suppression of severe tremor. N Engl J Med 342:461–468, 2000

Schwartz BL, Hashtroudi S, Herting RL, et al: Glycine prodrug facilitates memory retrieval in humans. Neurology 41:1341–1343, 1991

Shaywitz BA, Shaywitz SE: Estrogen and Alzheimer disease: plausible theory, negative clinical trial. JAMA 283:1055–1056, 2000

Silver JM, Yudofsky SC, Slater JA, et al: Propranolol treatment of chronically hospitalized aggressive patients. J Neuropsychiatry Clin Neurosci 11:328–335, 1999

Singh AN, Golledge H, Catalan J: Treatment of HIV-related psychotic disorders with risperidone: a series of 21 cases. J Psychosom Res 42:489–493, 1997

Sink KM, Holden KF, Yaffe K: Pharmacological treatment of neuropsychiatric symptoms of dementia: a review of the evidence. JAMA 293:596–608, 2005

Sival RC, Haffmans PM, Jansen PA, et al: Sodium valproate in the treatment of aggressive behavior in patients with dementia—a randomized placebo controlled clinical trial. Int J Geriatr Psychiatry 17:579–585, 2002

Sloan RL, Brown KW, Pentland B: Fluoxetine as a treatment for emotional lability after brain injury. Brain Inj 6:315–319, 1992

Slooter AJ, Bronzova J, Witteman JC, et al: Estrogen use and early onset Alzheimer's disease: a population-based study. J Neurol Neurosurg Psychiatry 67:779–781, 1999

Sobin P, Schneider L, McDermott H: Fluoxetine in the treatment of agitated dementia (letter). Am J Psychiatry 146:1636, 1989

Sovner R: The use of valproate in the treatment of mentally retarded persons with typical and atypical bipolar disorders. J Clin Psychiatry 50(suppl):40–43, 1989

Spiers PA, Myers D, Hochanadel GS, et al: Citicoline improves verbal memory in aging. Arch Neurol 53:441–448, 1996

Stanford MS, Helfritz LE, Conklin SM, et al: A comparison of anticonvulsants in the treatment of impulsive aggression. Exp Clin Psychopharmacol 13:72–77, 2005

Street JS, Clark WS, Gannon KS, et al: Olanzapine treatment of psychotic and behavioral symptoms in patients with Alzheimer disease in nursing care facilities: a double-blind, randomized, placebo-controlled trial. The HGEU Study Group. Arch Gen Psychiatry 57:968–976, 2000

Sultzer DL, Gray KF, Gunay I, et al: A double-blind comparison of trazodone and haloperidol for treatment of agitation in patients with dementia. Am J Geriatr Psychiatry 5:60–69, 1997

Swartz JR, Miller BL, Lesser IM, et al: Frontotemporal dementia: treatment response to serotonin selective reuptake inhibitors. J Clin Psychiatry 58:212–216, 1997

Szekely CA, Green RC, Breitner JC, et al: No advantage of A beta 42–lowering NSAIDs for prevention of Alzheimer dementia in six pooled cohort studies. Neurology 70:2291–2298, 2008

Tan I, Dorevitch M: Emotional incontinence: a dramatic response to paroxetine (letter). Aust N Z J Med 26:844, 1996

Tariot PN, Erb R, Podgorski CA, et al: Efficacy and tolerability of carbamazepine for agitation and aggression in dementia. Am J Psychiatry 155:54–61, 1998a

Tariot PN, Goldstein B, Podgorski CA, et al: Short-term administration of selegiline for mild-to-moderate dementia of the Alzheimer's type. Am J Geriatr Psychiatry 6:145–154, 1998b

Tariot PN, Farlow MR, Grossberg GT, et al: Memantine treatment in patients with moderate to severe Alzheimer disease already receiving donepezil: a randomized controlled trial. JAMA 291:317–324, 2004a

Tariot PN, Profenno LA, Ismail MS: Efficacy of atypical antipsychotics in elderly patients with dementia. J Clin Psychiatry 65 (suppl 11):11–15, 2004b

Tariot PN, Raman R, Jakimovich L, et al: Divalproex sodium in nursing home residents with possible or probable Alzheimer disease complicated by agitation: a randomized, controlled trial. Am J Geriatr Psychiatry 13:942–949, 2005

Tennant FS Jr, Wild J: Naltrexone treatment for postconcussional syndrome. Am J Psychiatry 144:813–814, 1987

Tiller JW, Dakis JA, Shaw JM: Short-term buspirone treatment in disinhibition with dementia (letter). Lancet 2:510, 1988

Tollefson GD: Short-term effects of the calcium channel blocker nimodipine (Bay-e-9736) in the management of primary degenerative dementia. Biol Psychiatry 27:1133–1142, 1990

Tollefson GD, Greist JH, Jefferson JW, et al: Is baseline agitation a relative contraindication for a selective serotonin reuptake inhibitor: a comparative trial of fluoxetine versus imipramine. J Clin Psychopharmacol 14:385–391, 1994

Tsai GE, Yang P, Chung LC, et al: D-serine added to clozapine for the treatment of schizophrenia. Am J Psychiatry 156:1822–1825, 1999

Tsai WC, Lai JS, Wang TG: Treatment of emotionalism with fluoxetine during rehabilitation. Scand J Rehabil Med 30:145–149, 1998

Tune L, Carr S, Hoag E, et al: Anticholinergic effects of drugs commonly prescribed for the elderly: potential means for assessing risk of delirium. Am J Psychiatry 149:1393–1394, 1992

van Dyck CH, McMahon TJ, Rosen MI, et al: Sustained-release methylphenidate for cognitive impairment in HIV-1-infected drug abusers: a pilot study. J Neuropsychiatry Clin Neurosci 9:29–36, 1997

Van Reekum R, Bayley M, Garner S, et al: N of 1 study: amantadine for the amotivational syndrome in a patient with traumatic brain injury. Brain Inj 9:49–53, 1995

van Vugt JP, Siesling S, Vergeer M, et al: Clozapine versus placebo in Huntington's disease: a double blind randomised comparative study. J Neurol Neurosurg Psychiatry 63:35–39, 1997

Verhoeven WM, Tuinier S: The effect of buspirone on challenging behaviour in mentally retarded patients: an open prospective multiple-case study. J Intellect Disabil Res 40 (pt 6):502–508, 1996

Walker Z, Grace J, Overshot R, et al: Olanzapine in dementia with Lewy bodies: a clinical study. Int J Geriatr Psychiatry 14:459–466, 1999

Welch J, Manschreck T, Redmond D: Clozapine-induced seizures and EEG changes. J Neuropsychiatry Clin Neurosci 6:250–256, 1994

White JC, Christensen JF, Singer CM: Methylphenidate as a treatment for depression in acquired immunodeficiency syndrome: an N-of-1 trial. J Clin Psychiatry 53:153–156, 1992

Wilkinson D, Murray J: Galantamine: a randomized, double-blind, dose comparison in patients with Alzheimer's disease. Int J Geriatr Psychiatry 16:852–857, 2001

Wilkinson D, Doody R, Helme R, et al: Donepezil in vascular dementia: a randomized, placebo-controlled study. Neurology 61:479–486, 2003

Wroblewski BA, Leary JM, Phelan AM, et al: Methylphenidate and seizure frequency in brain injured patients with seizure disorders. J Clin Psychiatry 53:86–89, 1992

Wroblewski BA, Joseph AB, Kupfer J, et al: Effectiveness of valproic acid on destructive and aggressive behaviours in patients with acquired brain injury. Brain Inj 11:37–47, 1997

Yudofsky SC, Silver JM, Schneider SE: Pharmacologic treatment of aggression. Psychiatr Ann 17:397–407, 1987

Zimnitzky BM, DeMaso DR, Steingard RJ: Use of risperidone in psychotic disorder following ischemic brain damage. J Child Adolesc Psychopharmacol 6:75–78, 1996

Zoldan J, Friedberg G, Livneh M, et al: Psychosis in advanced Parkinson's disease: treatment with ondansetron, a 5-HT$_3$ receptor antagonist. Neurology 45:1305–1308, 1995

18

COGNITIVE REHABILITATION AND BEHAVIOR THERAPY FOR PATIENTS WITH NEUROPSYCHIATRIC DISORDERS

Michael D. Franzen, Ph.D.

Mark R. Lovell, Ph.D.

Increasing evidence indicates that the treatment of central nervous system (CNS) disorders is a viable and productive endeavor even for traumatic brain injury (Cicerone et al. 2000; NIH Consensus Statement 1998). Psychiatry plays a central role in the assessment and treatment of individuals with neurological impairment. There is an increasing need for a broad-based understanding of methods of promoting recovery from brain injury and disease. The role of the psychiatrist in diagnosis and treatment has become a crucial one with the continued development of sophisticated neuropharmacological treatments for both the cognitive and the psychosocial components of brain impairment (Gualtieri 1988).

The recent application of selective serotonin reuptake inhibitors with brain-injured patients appears to hold some promise. An understanding of nonpharmacological, behavioral methods of assessment, together with a pharmacological approach, can greatly enhance the patient's recovery. In this chapter, we review the role of psychological treatments for the neuropsychological (cognitive) and behavioral consequences of CNS dysfunction.

In response to the increase in the number of patients requiring treatment for CNS dysfunction, there has been a proliferation of treatment agencies, as well as an increase in research efforts designed to assess the efficacy of these treatment programs. With evidence of the beneficial effects of rehabilitation have come modest increases in reimbursement, which in turn have fueled the increase in availability of services. Additionally, there has been an increasing awareness of the potential neuropsychological effects of disorders of other somatic systems that have some effect on CNS operations, such as cancer (Anderson-Hanley et al. 2003) and hypertension (Muldoon et al. 2002), as well as potential neuropsychological side effects of the treatment for those disorders.

NEUROANATOMICAL AND NEUROPHYSIOLOGICAL DETERMINANTS OF RECOVERY

Recovery from brain injury or disease involves a number of separate but interacting processes. A complete discussion of existing research concerning neuroanatomical and neurophysiological aspects of the recovery process is beyond the scope of this chapter; we provide here a brief review.

After an acute brain injury, some degree of improvement is likely because of a lessening of the temporary or treatable consequences of the injury. Factors such as degree of cerebral edema and extent of increased intracranial pressure are well known to temporarily affect brain function after a closed head injury or stroke (Lezak 1995). Extracellular changes after injury to the cell also have been shown to affect neural functioning. In addition, the regrowth of neural tissue to compensate for an injured area has been shown to occur to some minimal extent in animal studies on both anatomical (Kolata 1983) and physiological (Wall and Egger 1971) levels and may have some limited relevance for humans. With many acute brain injuries, functioning improves as these temporary effects subside. However, with degenerative illnesses, the condition actually worsens over time.

The differences in prognosis among various neurological disorders obviously affect the structure of the rehabilitation program. For example, a rehabilitation program for patients with head injury will be different from a program for patients with Alzheimer's disease. Similarly, the goals will vary as a function of the severity of memory impairment in patients with closed head injury. A program designed for patients with head injury and consequent moderate memory impairment is likely to focus on teaching alternative strategies for remembering new information. In contrast, a program designed for a patient with Alzheimer's disease would probably focus on improving the patient's functioning with regard to activities of daily living. Some intriguing data suggest that at least for stroke, brain reorganization for motor skills may be possible even a decade past the time of the stroke (Liepert et al. 2000).

COGNITIVE REHABILITATION OF PATIENTS WITH NEUROPSYCHIATRIC DISORDERS

The terms *cognitive rehabilitation* and *cognitive retraining* have been variously used to describe treatments designed to maximize recovery of the individual's abilities. The techniques used to improve cognitive functioning after a neurological event are a heterogeneous group of procedures that vary widely in their focus according to the nature of the patient's cognitive difficulties, the specific skills and training of the staff members, and the medium through which information is presented (e.g., computer vs. individual therapy vs. group therapy). Ideally, treatment should be tailored to each patient's particular needs based on a thorough neuropsychological assessment of cognitive and behavioral deficits, as well as an estimation of how these deficits affect daily life.

Because patients with different neurological or neuropsychiatric syndromes often have different cognitive deficits, the focus of the treatment is likely to vary greatly. For disorders with changing parameters such as the progressive neurological disorders, the stage of the illness and degree of impairment may also play a role in the development of a rehabilitation treatment plan. Sinforiani et al. (2004) reported that a cognitive rehabilitation program was effective in reversing the cognitive deficits associated with the early stages of Parkinson's disease, but it may be unlikely that such a program would be effective in later stages.

Attention to psychiatric problems in patients with neurological impairment is an important component of rehabilitation efforts (e.g., Robinson 1997). The use of pharmacological agents in the treatment of affective and behavior changes following traumatic brain injury has been reported in case studies (Khouzam and Donnelly 1998; Mendez et al. 1999). Carbamazepine has been used in the treatment of behavioral agitation following severe traumatic brain injury (Azouvi et al. 1999).

The systematic research concerning the effectiveness of cognitive and behavioral treatment strategies in this group is increasing. Medd and Tate (2000) reported the effects of anger management training in individuals with traumatic brain injury. In addition to psychologically based methods, pharmacological methods have been used to treat the physical and emotional symptoms (Holzer 1998; McIntosh 1997; Wroblewski et al. 1997). Although amantadine was at first promising, it has not provided robust effects in improving cognitive and behavioral functioning in brain-injured subjects (Schneider et al. 1999). The treatment of frontal lobe injury with dopaminergic agents may beneficially affect other rehabilitation efforts (Kraus and Maki 1997). Furthermore, the use of psychostimulants in facilitating treatment effects has been reported for pediatric subjects with traumatic brain injury (Williams et al. 1998) as well as for adults (Glen 1998). Most of our information comes from experience with patients in rehabilitation settings.

The results of psychological treatment methods for the cognitive deficits associated with traumatic brain injury generally show larger effects for skills as measured by standardized tests than as measured by ecologically relevant behaviors (Ho and Bennett 1997). Future research is needed to investigate the variables that govern generalizability and ecological validity.

There has been some interest in the cognitive rehabilitation of individuals with schizophrenia. Flesher (1990) presented an intriguing discussion of an approach to using this type of intervention with schizophrenic patients; however, there have been limited reports of applications, an exception being that by Benedict et al. (1994), who used computer vigilance training to treat the attentional deficits shown by a group of schizophrenic patients. Although it may be too early to critically evaluate the efficacy of this approach (Bellak and Mueser 1993), it certainly bears watching. In contrast, the use of behavioral methods for training in social skills in schizophrenic patients is well documented.

ATTENTIONAL PROCESSES

Recognition and treatment of attentional disorders are extremely important because an inability to focus and sustain attention may directly limit the patient's ability to actively participate in the rehabilitation program. A number of components of attention have been identified, including alertness and the ability to selectively attend to incoming information, as well as the capacity to focus and maintain attention or vigilance (Posner and Rafal 1987).

Rehabilitation programs designed to improve attention usually attempt to address all of these processes. For example, the Orientation Remedial program (Ben-Yishay and Diller 1981) consists of five separate tasks that are presented by microcomputer and vary in degree of difficulty; they involve training in the following areas:

1. Attending and reacting to environmental signals
2. Timing responses in relation to changing environmental cues
3. Being actively vigilant
4. Estimating time
5. Synchronizing of response with complex rhythms

Progress on these tasks is a prerequisite for further training on higher-level tasks. Modafinil has been found to improve performance on measures of attention, reaction time, and executive function in healthy subjects who have been sleep deprived (Walsh et al. 2004), but the generalizability of these findings to individuals with CNS injury has yet to be demonstrated.

MEMORY

Within the field of cognitive rehabilitation, much emphasis has been placed on the development of treatment approaches to improve memory. Franzen and Haut (1991) divided the strategies into three basic categories: 1) the use of spared skills in the form of mnemonic devices or alternative functional systems, 2) the use of direct retraining with repetitive practice and drills, and 3) the use of behavioral prosthetics or external devices or strategies to improve memory.

Use of Spared Skills

Mnemonic strategies are approaches to memory rehabilitation that are specifically designed to promote the encoding and remembering of a specific type of information, depending on the patient's particular memory impairment, by capitalizing on the spared skills. Visual imagery (Glisky and Schacter 1986) involves the use of visual images to assist in the learning and retention of verbal information. Probably the oldest and best-known visual imagery strategy is the method of loci, which involves the association of verbal information to be remembered with locations that are familiar to the patient (e.g., the room in a house or the location on a street). When recall of the information is required, the patient visualizes each room and the items that are to be remembered in each location (Moffat 1984). Initial research suggested that this method may be particularly useful for elderly patients (Robertson-Tchabo et al. 1976).

Peg mnemonics requires the patient to learn a list of peg words and to associate these words with a given visual image, such as "one bun," "two shoe," and so on. After the learned asso-

ciation of the numbers with the visual image, sequential information can be remembered in order by association with the visual image (Gouvier et al. 1986). This strategy has been widely used by professional mnemonists and showed some early promise in patients with brain injuries (Patten 1972). More recent research, however, suggested that this approach may not be highly effective because patients with brain injuries are unable to generate visual images (Crovitz et al. 1979) and have difficulty maintaining this information over time.

Face-name association has been used by patients with brain injuries to promote the remembering of people's names based on visual cues. For example, the name "Angela Harper" might be encoded by the patient by visualizing an angel playing a harp. Obviously, the ease with which this method can be used by patients with brain injuries depends on their ability to form internal visual images, as well as the ease with which the name can be transferred into a distinct visual image.

A series of single-subject experiments reported by Wilson (1987) indicated that the strategy of visual imagery to learn people's names may be differentially effective for different individuals, even when the etiology of memory impairment is similar.

In addition to the extensive use of visual imagery strategies for improving memory in patients with brain injuries, the use of verbally based mnemonic strategies also has become quite popular, particularly with patients who have difficulty using visual imagery. One such procedure, semantic elaboration, involves constructing a story out of new information to be remembered. This type of procedure may be particularly useful in patients who are unable to use imagery strategies because of a reduced ability to generate internal visual images.

Rhyming strategies involve remembering verbal information by incorporating the information into a rhyme. This procedure was originally demonstrated by Gardner (1977) with a globally amnesic patient who was able to recall pertinent personal information by the learning and subsequent singing of the following rhyme:

Henry's my name/Memory's my game/
   I'm in the V.A. in Jamaica Plain.
My bed's on 7D/The year is '73/
   Every day I make a little gain.

For patients who have difficulty learning and remembering written information, Glasgow et al. (1977) used a structured procedure called *PQRST*. This strategy involves application of the following five steps:

1. **P**review the information.
2. Form **Q**uestions about the information.
3. **R**ead the information.
4. **S**tate the questions.
5. **T**est for retention by answering the questions after the material has been read.

REPETITIVE PRACTICE

Cognitive rehabilitation strategies that emphasize repetitive practice of information are extremely popular in rehabilitation settings despite little experimental evidence of lasting improvement in memory. Repetitive practice strategies rely heavily on the use of drills and appear to be based on a mental muscle conceptualization of memory (Harris and Sunderland 1981) in which it is assumed that memory can be improved merely by repeated exposure to the information to be learned. Patients with brain injuries can learn specific pieces of information through repeated exposure, but studies designed to show generalization of this training to new settings or tasks have not been encouraging. (For a review, see Schacter and Glisky 1986.)

Glisky and Schacter (1986) suggested that attempts to remedy memory disorders should be focused on the acquisition of domain-specific knowledge that is likely to be relevant to everyday functioning. This approach differs from the use of traditional cognitive remediation strategies in that 1) the goal of this treatment is not to improve memory functioning in general but rather to deal with specific problems associated with memory impairment, 2) the information acquired through this treatment has practical value to the individual, and 3) the information learned through training exercises is chosen on the basis of having some practical value in the patient's natural environment. Initial research has established that even patients with severe brain injuries are indeed capable of acquiring discrete pieces of information that are important to their ability to function on a daily basis (Glasgow et al. 1977; Wilson 1982). Chiaravalloti et al. (2003) found that repetition was not helpful in remediating the memory deficits of individuals with multiple sclerosis (MS), who instead may benefit from other rehabilitation strategies in addition to the repetition.

EXTERNAL MEMORY AIDS

External aids to memory can take various forms, but generally they fall into the two categories of memory storage devices and memory-cuing strategies (Harris 1984). Schmitter-Edgecombe et al. (1995) supported the efficacy of memory notebook training to improve memory for everyday activities, although there was no difference in laboratory-based memory tasks, and the gains were not maintained as well at a 6-month follow-up evaluation.

Handheld electronic storage devices allow for the storage of large amounts of information, but their often complicated operation requirements may obviate their use in all but the mildest cases of brain injury or disease. Another problem is that the devices must be consulted at the appropriate time in order to be useful. This may be a difficult task for the patient with brain injury and often requires the use of cuing strategies that remind the patient to engage in a behavior at a given time.

The application of cuing involves the use of prompts designed to remind the patient to engage in a specific behavioral sequence at a given time. To be maximally effective, the cue should be given as close as possible to the time that the behavior is required, must be active rather than passive, and should provide a reminder of the specific behavior that is desired (Harris 1984). One particularly useful cuing device currently in use is the alarm wristwatch.

VISUAL-PERCEPTUAL DISORDERS

Deficits in visual perception are most common in patients who have undergone right hemisphere cerebrovascular accidents (Gouvier et al. 1986). Given the importance of visual-perceptual processing to many occupational tasks and to the safe operation of an automobile (Sivak et al. 1985), the rehabilitation of deficits in this area could have important implications for the recovery of neuropsychiatric patients.

Hemispatial neglect syndrome, common in stroke patients, is an inability to recognize stimuli in the contralateral visual field and has been treated with visual scanning training (Diller and Weinberg 1977; Gianutsos et al. 1983). A light board with 20 colored lights and a target that can be moved around the board at different speeds is used to train the patient to attend to the neglected visual field. This procedure, with the addition of other tasks (e.g., a size estimation and body awareness task), was found to be effective (Gordon et al. 1985). Other researchers have produced similar therapeutic gains in scanning and other aspects of visual-perceptual functioning through rehabilitation strategies. (For a more complete review of this area, see Gianutsos and Matheson 1987 and Gordon et al. 1985.)

PROBLEM SOLVING AND EXECUTIVE FUNCTIONS

Patients often experience a breakdown in their ability to reason, to form concepts, to solve problems, to execute and terminate behavioral sequences, and to engage in other complex cognitive activities (F.C. Goldstein and Levin 1987). Executive dysfunction correlates with white matter changes seen in diffusion tensor magnetic resonance imaging of patients with vascular dementia (O'Sullivan et al. 2004). These deficits are debilitating because they often underlie changes in the basic abilities to function interpersonally, socially, and vocationally. Executive function appears to have a relationship to other, simpler tasks—for example, lower-extremity coordination and walking speed in older healthy individuals (Ble et al. 2005). Because of increasing evidence that executive function affects lower-order tasks, more effort has been dedicated to the systematic development of rehabilitation programs to ameliorate these disorders. These treatment programs can be difficult to plan and implement, partly due to the complex and multifaceted nature of intellectual and executive functions.

Intellectual and executive functioning involve numerous processes that include motivation, abstract thinking, and concept formation, as well as the ability to plan, reason, and execute and terminate behaviors. Breakdowns in intellectual and executive functioning can occur for various reasons depending on the underlying core deficit(s) and the area of the brain that is injured. For example, injury to the parieto-occipital area is likely to result in a problem-solving deficit secondary to difficulty with comprehension of logical-grammatical structure, whereas a frontal lobe injury may impede problem solving by disrupting the individual's ability to plan and to carry out the series of steps necessary to process the grammatical material (Luria and Tsvetkova 1990). Executive dysfunction may also affect capacity to consent to medical treatment in patients with Alzheimer's disease (Marson and Harrell 1999).

An apparent breakdown in the patient's ability to function intellectually also can occur secondary to deficits in other related areas, such as attention, memory, and language. The type of rehabilitation strategy best suited for such a patient depends on the underlying core deficit that needs to be addressed. The goal of rehabilitation for a patient with a left parieto-occipital lesion might be to help the patient develop the skill to correctly analyze the grammatical structure of the problem. Rehabilitation efforts for a patient with frontal lobe injury might emphasize impulse control and execution of the appropriate behavioral sequence to solve the problem.

Rehabilitation programs frequently involve attempts to address these deficits in a hierarchical manner, as originally proposed by Luria (1963). Ben-Yishay and Diller (1983) developed a two-tiered approach that defines five basic deficit areas—arousal and attention, memory, impairment in underlying skill structure, language and thought, and feeling tone—and two domains of higher-level problem solving. Deficits in the higher-level skills are often produced by core deficits, and the patient's behavior is likely to depend on an interaction between the two domains (F.C. Goldstein and Levin 1987). Stablum et al. (2000) reported the effects of a treatment of executive dysfunction by training and practice in a dual-task procedure. They found improvements in executive function for both patients with closed head injury and patients with anterior communicating artery (ACoA) aneurysms, with maintenance of the gains at 3 months for patients with closed head injury and at 12 months for ACoA aneurysm patients.

SPEECH AND LANGUAGE

Disorders of speech and language are common when the dominant (usually left) hemisphere is injured. In most rehabilitation settings, speech and language therapies have traditionally been the province of speech pathologists. Therapy has often involved a wide variety of treatments depending on the training, interest, and theoretic orientation of the therapist. The goal of therapy has variously been the improvement of comprehension (receptive language) and expression (expressive language), and it has been shown that patients who receive speech therapy after a stroke improve more than patients who do not (Basso et al. 1979).

In treating speech and language impairment, it is important to consider the reason for the observed speech deficit in designing the treatment; that is, it is not sufficient simply to identify the behavioral deficit and attempt to increase the rate of production (Franzen 1991). For example, Giles et al. (1988) increased appropriate verbalizations in a patient with head injury by providing cuing to keep verbalization short and to pause in planning his speech. Here the remediation attempted to affect the mediating behavior rather than to decrease unwanted behavior through extinction.

MOLAR BEHAVIORS

The final test of rehabilitation efforts is frequently the change in ecologically relevant molar behaviors—that is, in behaviors that would be used in the open environment. Standardized testing may account for most of the variance reported for molar behaviors such as driving skill (Galski et al. 1997). However, the improvement in these molar behaviors also may depend on treatment aimed directly at the production of the behaviors, even when the component cognitive skills have been optimized. Giles et al. (1997) used behavioral techniques to improve washing and dressing skills in a series of individuals with severe brain injury.

USE OF COMPUTERS IN COGNITIVE REHABILITATION

The microcomputer has great potential for use in rehabilitation settings (Gourlay et al. 2000; Grimm and Bleiberg 1986). Microcomputers may have the advantage of being potentially self-instructional and self-paced, of requiring less direct staff time, and of accurately providing direct feedback to the patient about performance. Microcomputers also facilitate research by accurately and consistently recording the large amounts of potentially useful data that are generated during the rehabilitation process.

It must be emphasized that the microcomputer is merely a tool (albeit a highly sophisticated one), and its usefulness is limited by the availability of software that meets the needs of the individual patient and the skill of the therapist in implementing the program(s). As noted by Harris (1984), the danger is that cognitive rehabilitation will become centered around the software that is available. Also, microcomputers are not capable of simulating human social interaction and should not be used in lieu of human therapeutic contact.

Despite these challenges, there is a significant potential advantage in the capacity to present precise stimuli and conditions and to readily measure and record the effects of the treatments (Rizzo and Buckwalter 1997), and the use of computer programs in cognitive rehabilitation is increasing in quantity and quality (Gontkovsky et al. 2002). There are reports of the effectiveness of computerized rehabilitation programs for patients with Parkinson's disease (Sinforiani et al. 2004), closed head injury (Grealy et al. 1999), and schizophrenia (Bellucci et al. 2003; da Costa and de Carvalho 2004).

DISORDERS AND ASSOCIATED TREATMENTS

Birnboim and Miller (2004) reported that patients with MS have specific deficits in working strategies and that interventions aimed at improving the capacity to develop and use these strategies may necessarily precede other cognitive rehabilitation interventions. Amato and Zipoli (2003) review limited evidence in support of existing programs that attempt to moderate the cognitive impairment associated with MS, and also provide suggestions for future attempts and report optimism on the part of investigators involved in current research. Cuesta (2003) reviewed published studies involving the treatment of memory impairment following stroke and reported generally positive but moderate results. Particular interest has been focused on treatment of the dementias, especially Alzheimer's dementia (Clare et al. 2003). Some of these advances have involved novel pharmacological approaches, such as nicotinic substances, that can be combined with behavioral approaches (Newhouse et al. 1997). Another study involved the combination of cognitive rehabilitation methods with the use of cholinesterase inhibitors (Loewenstein et al. 2004). In this study, gains were reported at the end of 12 weeks of treatment and were maintained at a 3-month follow-up. Certain disorders may have their own specific considerations. For ex-

ample, greater awareness of deficit is associated with greater improvement from cognitive rehabilitation in patients with Alzheimer's disease (Clare et al. 2002, 2004).

Patients with schizophrenia demonstrate significant cognitive impairment, and cognitive dysfunction is a prominent symptom of the disorder. This cognitive impairment can interfere with other treatment efforts, and cognitive rehabilitation has been reported to improve general aspects of other symptoms and problems exhibited by patients with schizophrenia (L. Lewis et al. 2003). A review of attempts to rehabilitate the attention deficits associated with schizophrenia indicates generally positive results (Suslow et al. 2001). The evidence is mixed regarding the extent to which brain perfusion changes as a result of cognitive rehabilitation in schizophrenia (Penades et al. 2000). However, a quantitative review of studies indicates that cognitive rehabilitation not only improves cognitive operations on the experimental tasks but also generalizes to improvement on tasks outside the experimental setting (Krabbendam and Aleman 2003).

BEHAVIORAL DYSFUNCTION AFTER BRAIN INJURY

Relatively few follow-up studies to date have systematically investigated the efficacy of neuropsychiatric treatment programs. In addition, as with the literature on cognitive rehabilitation, much of what is known comes from studies conducted in rehabilitation settings rather than in hospitals specifically designed to treat patients with neuropsychiatric disorders. Studies have focused primarily on patients with traumatic brain injuries but also on other neurological disorders such as cerebrovascular accidents and progressive dementing disorders. Despite the relatively sparse amount of literature on treatment outcome in this area, the studies that have been reported have been useful in guiding the development of practical strategies for dealing with the behavioral-psychiatric consequences of brain injury. In particular, behaviorally based treatments have been heavily used. Research studies (Levin et al. 1982; Lishman 1978; Weddell et al. 1980) have shown that behavioral dysfunction is often associated with reduced abilities to comply with rehabilitation programs, to return to work, to engage in recreational and leisure activities, and to sustain positive interpersonal relationships.

Levin and Grossman (1978) reported behavior problems that were present 1 month after traumatic brain injury and that occurred in areas such as emotional withdrawal, conceptual disorganization, motor slowing, unusual thought content, blunt affect, excitement, and disorientation. At 6 months after injury, those patients who had poor social and occupational recovery continued to manifest significant cognitive and behavioral disruption. Complaints of tangential thinking, fragmented speech, slowness of thought and action, depressed mood, increased anxiety, and marital and/or family conflict also were frequently noted (Levin et al. 1979). Other behavioral changes reported to have the potential to cause psychosocial disruption include increased irritability (Rosenthal 1983), social inappropriateness (F.D. Lewis et al. 1988), aggression (Mungas 1988), and expansiveness, helplessness, suspiciousness, and anxiety (Grant and Alves 1987). Rapoport et al. (2005) describe the deleterious effect of depressive reactions on cognitive functions in individuals who have experienced mild to moderate closed head injury.

Patients with lesions in specific brain regions secondary to other pathological conditions also can have characteristic patterns of dysfunctional behavior. For example, frontal lobe dysfunction secondary to stroke, tumor, or other disease processes is often associated with a cluster of symptoms, including social disinhibition, reduced attention, distractibility, impaired judgment, affective lability, and more pervasive mood disorder (Bond 1984; Stuss and Benson 1984). In contrast, Prigatano (1987) noted that individuals with temporal lobe dysfunction can show heightened interpersonal sensitivity, which can evolve into frank paranoid ideation.

In addition to differences between patients with different types of brain injury or disease, the variability in the severity and extent of behavioral disruption after injury within each patient group is remarkable (Eames and Wood 1985). Perhaps not too surprisingly, individuals with mild head injuries are less prone to debilitating behavioral changes but still can experience physical, cognitive, and affective changes of sufficient magnitude to affect their ability to return to preaccident activities (Dikmen et al. 1986; Levin et al. 1987).

It seems clear that adjustment after brain injury appears to be related to a multitude of neurological and nonneurological factors, each of which requires consideration in the choice of an appropriate intervention. In addition to the extent and severity of the neurological injury itself, some of the other factors that can contribute to the presence and type of behavioral dysfunction include the amount of time elapsed since the injury, premorbid psychiatric and psychosocial adjustment, financial resources, social supports, and personal awareness of (and reaction to) acquired deficits (Eames 1988; G. Goldstein and Ruthven 1983; Gross and Schutz 1986; Meier et al. 1987).

Given the large number of factors that influence recovery from brain injury, a multidimensional approach to the behavioral treatment of patients with brain injury is likely to result in an optimal recovery. Individuals with more severe cognitive impairments are more likely to profit from highly structured behavioral programs. Those whose neuropsychological functioning is more intact, in contrast, may profit from interventions with a more active cognitive component that requires them to use abstract thought as well as self-evaluative and self-corrective processes. Not surprisingly, therapeutic approaches that fall under the general heading of behavior therapy represent an approach that is gaining increasing interest as a component of the overall treatment plan for patients with neuropsychiatric impairment. Ackerman (2004) presents a case study of treatment for a patient with mild traumatic brain injury and posttraumatic stress disorder in which the treatment required coordinated application of cognitive rehabilitation techniques, biofeedback, and psychotherapy.

BEHAVIOR THERAPY FOR PATIENTS WITH BRAIN IMPAIRMENT

Behavioral assessment and treatment have been adapted for use with numerous special populations, most recently including persons with brain injuries (Bellack and Hersen 1985a; Haynes 1984; Hersen and Bellack 1985, 1988; Kazdin 1979).

Despite a broadening scope that has included the treatment of patients with neurological impairment, behavioral approaches remain committed to the original principles derived from experimental and social psychology. They also emphasize the empirical and objective implementation and evaluation of treatment (Bellack and Hersen 1985b).

The general assumptions about the nature of behavior disorders that form the basis of behavioral approaches include the following (Haynes 1984):

- Disordered behavior can be expressed through overt actions, thoughts, verbalizations, and physiological reactions.
- These reactions do not necessarily vary in the same way for different individuals or for different behavior disorders.
- Changing one specific behavior may result in changes in other related behaviors.
- Environmental conditions play an important role in the initiation, maintenance, and alteration of behavior.

These assumptions have led to approaches emphasizing the objective evaluation of observable aspects of the individual and his or her interaction with the environment. The range of observable events is limited only by the clinician's ability to establish a reliable, valid quantification of the target behavior or environmental condition. As previously noted, this could range from a specific physiological reaction,

such as heart rate, to a self-report of the number of obsessive thoughts occurring during a 24-hour period.

Intervention focuses on the active interaction between the individual and the environment. The goal of treatment is to alter those aspects of the environment that have become associated with the initiation or maintenance of maladaptive behaviors or to alter the patient's response to those aspects of the environment in some way.

The application of a behavioral intervention with a neuropsychiatric patient requires careful consideration of both the neuropsychological and the environmental aspects of the presenting problem. Few clinicians have the training, time, or energy to become and remain equally competent in both neuropsychology and behavioral psychology.

At present, the accumulated body of evidence remains limited regarding the specific types of behavioral interventions that are most effective in treating the various dysfunctional behaviors observed in individuals with different kinds of brain injuries. Despite this limitation, there is optimism, based on the current literature, that behavior therapy can be effective for patients with brain injuries (Horton and Miller 1985). Indeed, an increasing number of books, primarily on the rehabilitation of patients with brain injuries, describe the potential applications of behavioral approaches for persons with neurological impairment (Edelstein and Couture 1984; G. Goldstein and Ruthven 1983; Seron 1987; Wood 1984). Such sources provide an excellent introduction to the basic models, methods, and limitations of behavioral treatments of patients with brain injuries.

Behavioral approaches can be broadly classified into at least three general models (Calhoun and Turner 1981): 1) a traditional behavioral approach, 2) a social learning approach, and 3) a cognitive-behavioral approach. The degree to which the client or patient is required to participate actively in the identification and alteration of the environmental conditions assumed to be supporting the maladaptive behavior varies across these models.

TRADITIONAL BEHAVIORAL APPROACH

The traditional behavioral approach emphasizes the effects of environmental events that occur after (consequences), as well as before (antecedents), a particular behavior of interest. We address these two aspects of environmental influence separately.

Interventions Aimed at the Consequences of Behavior

A consequence that increases the probability of a specific behavior occurring again under similar circumstances is termed a *reinforcer*. Consequences can either increase or decrease the likelihood of a particular behavior occurring again.

A behavior followed by an environmental consequence that increases the likelihood that the behavior will occur again is called a *positive reinforcer*. A behavior followed by the removal of a negative or aversive environmental condition is called a *negative reinforcer*. A behavior followed by an aversive environmental event is termed a *punishment*. The effect of punishment is to reduce the probability that the behavior will occur under similar conditions. There has often been confusion concerning the difference between negative reinforcers and punishments. It is useful to remember that reinforcers (positive or negative) always increase the likelihood of the behavior occurring again, whereas punishments decrease the likelihood of a behavior occurring again. When the reliable relation between a specific behavior and an environmental consequence is removed, the behavioral effect is to reduce the target behavior to a near-zero level of occurrence. This process is called *extinction*. Self-management skills (relaxation training, biofeedback) have been used in the treatment of ataxia (Guercio et al. 1997).

Interventions Aimed at the Antecedents of Behavior

Behavior is controlled or affected not only by the consequences that follow it but also by events that precede it. These events are called *antecedents*. For example, an aggressive patient may have outbursts only in the presence of the nursing staff and never in the presence of the physician. In this case, a failure to search for potential antecedents (e.g., female sex or physical size) that may be eliciting the behavior may leave half of the behavioral assessment undone and may result in difficulty decreasing the aggressive behavior. This type of approach may be particularly useful in patients for whom the behavior is disruptive enough that approaches aimed at manipulation of consequences hold some danger for staff and family (e.g., in the case of a patient with explosive or violent outbursts). In this situation, treatment is structured to decrease the likelihood of an outburst by restructuring the events that lead to the violent behavior. Some patients are able to learn to anticipate these antecedents themselves, whereas for others, it becomes the task of the treatment staff to identify and modify the antecedents that lead to unwanted behavior. For example, if the stress of verbal communication leads to aggressive behavior in an aphasic patient, the patient may be initially trained to use an alternative form of communication, such as writing or sign language (Franzen and Lovell 1987).

Other Behavioral Approaches

Yet another class of approaches involves the use of differential reinforcement of other behaviors. In this approach, the problem behavior is not consequated. Instead, another behavior that is inconsistent with the problem target behavior is reinforced. As the other behavior increases in frequency, the problem behavior decreases. Hegel and Ferguson (2000) reported the successful use of this approach in reducing aggressive behavior in a subject with brain injury. Differential reinforcement of low rates of responding also may be used to reduce undesired behaviors (Alderman and Knight 1997). Finally, noncontingent reinforcement in the form of increased attention to a subject resulted in a decrease in aggression toward others and a decrease in self-injurious behaviors (Persel et al. 1997).

SOCIAL LEARNING APPROACH

With the social learning approach, cognitive processes that mediate between environmental conditions and behavioral responses are included in explanations of the learning process. Social learning approaches take advantage of learning through modeling—by systematically arranging opportunities for patients to observe socially adaptive examples of social interaction. Emphasis is also placed on practicing the components of social skills in role-playing situations, where the patient can receive corrective feedback. Intervention that focuses on social skills training is one example of a treatment that is often useful for patients with brain injuries who have lost the ability to effectively monitor their behavior and to respond appropriately in a given situation.

Socially skilled behavior is generally divided into three components: 1) social perception, 2) social problem solving, and 3) social expression. Training can occur at any one of these levels. For the patient who has lost the ability to interact appropriately with conversational skills, this behavior may be modeled by staff members. (For a comprehensive review, see Bandura 1977.)

COGNITIVE-BEHAVIORAL APPROACH

The term *cognitive-behavioral approach* refers to a heterogeneous group of procedures that emphasizes the individual's cognitive mediation (self-messages) in explaining behavioral responses within environmental contexts. Treatment focuses on changing maladaptive beliefs and increasing an individual's self-control within the current social environment by changing maladaptive thoughts or beliefs. This approach is particularly useful with patients who have relatively intact language and self-evaluative abilities.

Cognitive-behavioral treatments originally were designed to treat affective disorders and symptoms. However, the use of the approach has widened to include anxiety, personality disorders, and skills deficits. For example, Suzman et al. (1997) used cognitive-behavioral methods to improve the problem-solving skills of children with cognitive deficits following traumatic brain injury.

ASSESSMENT OF TREATMENT EFFECTS

In addition to providing a set of methodologies to affect the disordered behavior produced by cognitive deficits, the literature on behavior therapy has provided a conceptual scheme for evaluating the effects of intervention. One of the most influential products of the tradition of behavior therapy has been the development of single-subject designs to evaluate the effect of interventions. Although originally conceived as a method of evaluating the effect of environmental interventions, the single-subject design has been successfully applied in the evaluation of pharmacological interventions as well. Because each patient is an individual and treatment of cognitive dysfunction is still a relatively nascent endeavor, interventions often need to be specifically tailored to the individual patient. Interventions often must be applied before the period of spontaneous recovery has ended, and a method to distinguish the effects of intervention from the effects of recovery from acute physiological disturbance is needed. The multiple-baseline design is a single-subject design that addresses these issues (Franzen and Iverson 1990).

The design of multiple baselines across behaviors involves the evaluation of more than one behavior taking place at the same time. However, only one of the behaviors is targeted for intervention at a time. In this way, the non-targeted behaviors are used as control comparisons for the targeted behaviors. For example, behavior A is targeted for intervention first, and monitors on behaviors B and C are used as control comparisons. After completion of the treatment phase for behavior A, an intervention is implemented for behavior B, and monitors on behaviors A and C are used as control comparisons.

The graph shown in Figure 18–1 presents an example of a multiple baseline design for the treatment of an individual with brain injury and

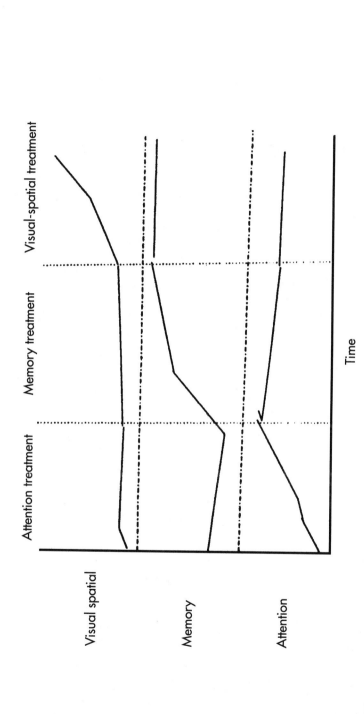

FIGURE 18–1. Multiple-baseline design for the treatment of a patient with brain injury and deficits in attention, memory, and visual-spatial processing.

Attention, memory, and visual-spatial skills are each treated in sequence; improvement is seen in one area before beginning the next phase of treatment, and performance in untreated skill areas is used as a comparison for the treated areas. The vertical axis represents level of performance in each skill area (visual spatial, memory, and attention). The passage of time is represented on the horizontal axis. The dotted vertical lines are those times at which treatment was switched from the previous focus to the current focus, such as from attention training to memory training.

deficits in memory, attention, and visual-spatial processing. The attention skills receive treatment in the first phase, with a concomitant improvement in skill level. At the second phase, memory skills are treated, with a concomitant improvement. Finally, visual-spatial skills are treated at the third phase, and improvement is seen there. At each phase, performance in the other untreated skill areas is used as a control comparison for the treated skill areas.

In an application of the multiple-baseline design to the treatment of a patient with brain injury, Franzen and Harris (1993) reported a case in which a patient had deficits in attention-based memory and in abstraction and planning as the result of a closed head injury. This patient was first seen 23 days after the closed head injury occurred. He was seen for a series of weekly appointments. At these appointments, the emotional adjustment was discussed and support was provided. Additionally, the patient received psychotherapy in the form of anger control training and social reinforcement for increasing his daily level of activity and self-initiated social interactions, two areas identified as problems during the evaluation. Finally, cognitive retraining exercises were implemented and taught to the patient and his family so that home practice could take place on a daily basis. The family was instructed in the methods used to record the scores from the exercises, which were then entered into a daily log.

CONCLUSION

Neuropsychological and behavioral dysfunction associated with brain injury can be varied and complex. Effective intervention requires an integrated interdisciplinary approach that focuses on the individual patient and his or her specific needs. There may be an interactive effect in that improvement in cognitive operations may result in improvement in emotional and behavioral adaptation. Behaviorally based formulations can provide a valuable framework from which to understand the interaction between an individual with compromised physical, neuropsychological, and emotional

functioning, as well as the psychosocial environment in which he or she is trying to adjust.

Much work remains to define the most effective cognitive and behaviorally based treatments for various neuropsychiatric disorders. There is increasing evidence that computerized approaches may be helpful. A combined behavioral and pharmacological approach may be more effective than either strategy alone. The evidence to date suggests that cognitive rehabilitation is indeed an area worthy of continued pursuit.

RECOMMENDED READINGS

Halligan PW, Wade DT (eds): The Effectiveness of Rehabilitation for Cognitive Deficits. New York, Oxford University Press, 2005

High WM Jr, Sander AM, Struchen MA, et al (eds): Rehabilitation for Traumatic Brain Injury. New York, Oxford University Press, 2005

Klein R, McNamara P, Albert ML): Neuropharmacologic approaches to cognitive rehabilitation. Behav Neurol 17:1–3, 2006

León-Carrión J, von Wild KRH, Zitnay GA (eds): Brain Injury Treatment: Theories and Practices. New York, Taylor & Francis, 2006

Loewenstein D, Acevedo A: Training of cognitive and functionally relevant skills in Mild Alzheimer's disease: an integrated approach, in Geriatric Neuropsychology: Assessment and Intervention. Edited by Attix DK, Welsh-Bohmer KA. New York, Guilford, 2006, pp 261–274

Murrey GJ: Alternate Therapies in the Treatment of Brain Injury and Neurobehavioral Disorders: A Practical Guide. New York, Haworth Press, 2006

REFERENCES

Ackerman RJ: Applied psychophysiology, clinical biofeedback, and rehabilitation neuropsychology: a case study—mild traumatic brain injury and post-traumatic stress disorder. Phys Med Rehabil Clin N Am 15:919–931, 2004

Alderman N, Knight C: The effectiveness of DRL in the management of severe behaviour disorders following brain injury. Brain Inj 11:79–101, 1997

Amato MP, Zipoli V: Clinical management of cognitive impairment in multiple sclerosis: a review of current evidence. Int MS J 1072–1083, 2003

Anderson-Hanley C, Sherman ML, Riggs R, et al: Neuropsycholgoical effects of treatments for adults with cancer: a meta-analysis and review of the literature. J Int Neuropsychol Soc 9:967–982, 2003

Azouvi P, Jokic C, Attal N, et al: Carbamazepine in agitation and aggressive behaviour following severe closed-head injury. Brain Inj 13:797–804, 1999

Bandura A: Social Learning Theory. Englewood Cliffs, NJ, Prentice-Hall, 1977

Basso A, Capotani E, Vignolo L: Influence of rehabilitation on language skills in aphasic patients. Arch Neurol 36:190–196, 1979

Bellack AS, Hersen M: Dictionary of Behavior Therapy Techniques. New York, Pergamon, 1985a

Bellack AS, Hersen M: General considerations, in Handbook of Clinical Behavior Therapy With Adults. Edited by Hersen M, Bellack AS. New York, Plenum, 1985b, pp 3–19

Bellack AS, Mueser KT: Psychosocial treatment for schizophrenia. Schizophr Bull 19:317–336, 1993

Bellucci DM, Glaberman K, Haslam N: Computer assisted cognitive rehabilitation reduces negative symptoms in the severely mentally ill. Schizophr Res 59:225–232, 2003

Ben-Yishay Y, Diller L: Cognitive deficits, in Rehabilitation of the Head-Injured Adult. Edited by Griffith EA, Bond M, Miller J. Philadelphia, PA, FA Davis, 1983, pp 167–183

Ben-Yishay Y, Diller L: Rehabilitation of cognitive and perceptual deficits in people with traumatic brain damage. Int J Rehabil Res 4:208–210, 1981

Benedict RH, Harris AE, Markow T, et al: Effects of attention training on information processing in schizophrenia. Schizophr Bull 20:537–546, 1994

Birnboim S, Miller A: Cognitive strategies application of multiple sclerosis patients. Mult Scler 10:67–73, 2004

Ble A, Volpato S, Zuliani G, et al: Executive function correlates with walking speed in older person: the InCHIANTI study. J Am Geriatr Soc 3:410–415, 2005

Bond M: The psychiatry of closed head injury, in Closed Head Injury: Psychosocial, Social and Family Consequences. Edited by Brooks PN. Oxford, England, Oxford University Press, 1984, pp 148–178

Calhoun KS, Turner SM: Historical perspectives and current issues in behavior therapy, in Handbook of Clinical Behavior Therapy. Edited by Turner SM, Calhoun KS, Adams HE. New York, Wiley, 1981, pp 1–11

Chiaravalloti ND, Demaree H, Gaudino EA, et al: Can the repetition effect maximize learning multiple sclerosis? Clin Rehabil 17:58–68, 2003

Cicerone KD, Dahlberg C, Kalmar K, et al: Evidence-based cognitive rehabilitation: recommendations for clinical practice. Arch Phys Med Rehabil 81:1596–1615, 2000

Clare L, Wilson BA, Carter G, et al: Relearning face-name associations in early Alzheimer's disease. Neuropsychology 16:538–547, 2002

Clare L, Carter G, Hodges JR: Cognitive rehabilitation as a component of early intervention in Alzheimer's disease: a single case study. Aging Ment Health 7:15–21, 2003

Clare L, Wilson BA, Carter G, et al: Awareness in early stage Alzheimer's disease: relation to outcome of cognitive rehabilitation. J Clin Exp Neuropsychol 26:215–226, 2004

Crovitz H, Harvey M, Horn R: Problems in the acquisition of imagery mnemonics: three brain damaged cases. Cortex 15:225–234, 1979

Cuesta GM: Cognitive rehabilitation of memory following stroke. Adv Neurol 92:415–421, 2003

da Costa RM, de Carvalho LA: The acceptance of virtual realist devices for cognitive rehabilitation: a report of positive results with schizophrenia. Comput Methods Programs Biomed 73:173–182, 2004

Dikmen S, McLean A, Temkin N: Neuropsychological and psychosocial consequences of minor head injury. J Neurol Neurosurg Psychiatry 49:1227–1232, 1986

Diller L, Weinberg J: Hemi-inattention in rehabilitation: the evolution of a rational remediation program. Adv Neurol 18:63–82, 1977

Eames P: Behavior disorders after severe head injury: their nature, causes and strategies for management. J Head Trauma Rehabil 3:1–6, 1988

Eames P, Wood R: Rehabilitation after severe brain injury: a follow-up study of a behavior modification approach. J Neurol Neurosurg Psychiatry 48:613–619, 1985

Edelstein BA, Couture ET: Behavioral Assessment and Rehabilitation of the Traumatically Brain-Damaged. New York, Plenum, 1984

Flesher S: Cognitive habilitation in schizophrenia: a theoretical review and model of treatment. Neuropsychol Rev 1:223–246, 1990

Franzen MD: Behavioral assessment and treatment of brain-impaired individuals, in Progress in Behavior Modification. Edited by Hersen M, Eisler RM. Newbury Park, CA, Sage, 1991, pp 56–85

Franzen MD, Harris CV: Neuropsychological rehabilitation: application of a modified multiple baseline design. Brain Inj 7:525–534, 1993

Franzen MD, Haut MW: The psychological treatment of memory impairment: a review of empirical studies. Neuropsychol Rev 2:29–63, 1991

Franzen MD, Iverson GL: Applications of single subject design to cognitive rehabilitation, in Neuropsychology Across the Lifespan. Edited by Horton AM. New York, Springer, 1990, pp 155–174

Franzen MD, Lovell MR: Behavioral treatments of aggressive sequelae of brain injury. Psychiatr Ann 17:389–396, 1987

Galski T, Ehle HT, Williams JB: Off-road driving evaluations for persons with cerebral injury: a factor analytic study of predriver and simulator testing. Am J Occup Ther 51:352–359, 1997

Gardner H: The Shattered Mind: The Person After Brain Damage. London, Routledge & Kegan Paul, 1977

Gianutsos R, Matheson P: The rehabilitation of visual perceptual disorders attributable to brain injury, in Neuropsychological Rehabilitation. Edited by Meier MJ, Benton AL, Diller L. New York, Guilford, 1987, pp 202–241

Gianutsos R, Glosser D, Elbaum J, et al: Visual imperception in brain injured adults: multifaceted measures. Arch Phys Med Rehabil 64:456–461, 1983

Giles GM, Pussey I, Burgess P: The behavioral treatment of verbal interaction skills following severe head injury: a single case study. Brain Inj 2:75–79, 1988

Giles GM, Ridley JE, Dill A, et al: A consecutive series of adults with brain injury treated with a washing and dressing retraining program. Am J Occup Ther 51:256–266, 1997

Glasgow RE, Zeiss RA, Barrera M, et al: Case studies on remediating memory deficits in brain damaged individuals. J Clin Psychol 33:1049–1054, 1977

Glen MB: Methylphenidate for cognitive and behavioral dysfunction after traumatic brain injury. J Head Trauma Rehabil 13:87–90, 1998

Glisky EL, Schacter DL: Remediation of organic memory disorders: current status and future prospects. J Head Trauma Rehabil 4:54–63, 1986

Goldstein FC, Levin HS: Disorders of reasoning and problem solving ability, in Neuropsychological Rehabilitation. Edited by Meier MJ, Benton AL, Diller L. New York, Guilford, 1987, pp 327–354

Goldstein G, Ruthven L: Rehabilitation of the Brain-Damaged Adult. New York, Plenum, 1983

Gontkovsky ST, McDonald NB, Clark PG, et al: Current directions in computer-assisted cognitive rehabilitation. NeuroRehabilitation 17:195–199, 2002

Gordon W, Hibbard M, Egelko S, et al: Perceptual remediation in patients with right brain damage: a comprehensive program. Arch Phys Med Rehabil 66:353–359, 1985

Gourlay D, Lun KC, Liya G: Telemedicinal virtual reality for cognitive rehabilitation. Stud Health Technol Inform 77:1181–1186, 2000

Gouvier WD, Webster JS, Blanton PD: Cognitive retraining with brain damaged patients, in The Neuropsychology Handbook: Behavioral and Clinical Perspectives. Edited by Wedding D, Horton AM, Webster J. New York, Springer, 1986, pp 278–324

Grant I, Alves W: Psychiatric and psychosocial disturbances in head injury, in Neurobehavioral Recovery From Head Injury. Edited by Levin HS, Grafman J, Eisenberg HM. New York, Oxford University Press, 1987, pp 222–246

Grealy MA, Johnson DA, Rushton SK: Improving cognitive function after brain injury: the use of exercise and virtual reality. Arch Phys Med Rehabil 80:661–667, 1999

Grimm BH, Bleiberg J: Psychological rehabilitation in traumatic brain injury, in Handbook of Clinical Neuropsychology, Vol 2. Edited by Filskov SB, Boll TJ. New York, Wiley, 1986, pp 495–560

Gross Y, Schutz LF: Intervention models in neuropsychology, in Clinical Neuropsychology of Intervention. Edited by Uzzell BP, Gross Y. Boston, MA, Martinus Highoff, 1986, pp 179–204

Gualtieri CT: Pharmacotherapy and the neurobehavioral sequelae of traumatic brain injury. Brain Inj 2:101–109, 1988

Guercio J, Chittum R, McMorrow M: Self-management in the treatment of ataxia: a case study in reducing ataxic tremor through relaxation and biofeedback. Brain Inj 11:353–362, 1997

Harris JE: Methods of improving memory, in Clinical Management of Memory Problems. Edited by Wilson BA, Moffat N. Rockville, MD, Aspen, 1984, pp 46–62

Harris JE, Sunderland A: A brief survey of the management of memory disorders in rehabilitation units in Britain. Int Rehabil Med 3:206–209, 1981

Haynes SN: Behavioral assessment of adults, in Handbook of Psychological Assessment. Edited by Goldstein G, Hersen M. New York, Pergamon, 1984, pp 369–401

Hegel MT, Ferguson RJ: Differential reinforcement of other behavior (DRO) to reduce aggressive behavior following traumatic brain injury. Behav Modif 24:94–101, 2000

Hersen M, Bellack AS: Handbook of Clinical Behavior Therapy With Adults. New York, Plenum, 1985

Hersen M, Bellack AS: Dictionary of Behavioral Assessment Techniques. New York, Pergamon, 1988

Ho MR, Bennett TL: Efficacy of neuropsychological rehabilitation of mild-moderate traumatic brain injury. Arch Clin Neuropsychol 12:1–11, 1997

Holzer JC: Buspirone and brain injury (letter). J Neuropsychiatry Clin Neurosci 10:113, 1998

Horton AM, Miller WA: Neuropsychology and behavior therapy, in Progress in Behavior Modifications. Edited by Hersen M, Eisler R, Miller PM. New York, Academic Press, 1985, pp 1–55

Kazdin AE: Fictions, factions, and functions of behavior therapy. Behav Ther 10:629–654, 1979

Khouzam HR, Donnelly NJ: Remission of traumatic brain injury-induced compulsions during venlafaxine treatment. Gen Hosp Psychiatry 20:62–63, 1998

Kolata G: Brain-grafting work shows promise (letter). Science 221:1277, 1983

Krabbendam L, Aleman A: Cognitive remediation in schizophrenia: a quantitative review of controlled studies. Psychopharmacology 169:376–382, 2003

Kraus MF, Maki M: Effect of amantadine hydrochloride on symptoms of frontal lobe dysfunction in brain injury: case studies and review. J Neuropsychiatry Clin Neurosci 9:222–230, 1997

Levin HS, Grossman RG: Behavioral sequelae of closed head injury: a quantitative study. Arch Neurol 35:720–727, 1978

Levin HS, Grossman RG, Ross JE, et al: Long-term neuropsychological outcome of closed head injury. J Neurosurg 50:412–422, 1979

Levin HS, Benton AL, Grossman RG: Neurobehavioral Consequences of Closed Head Injury. New York, Oxford University Press, 1982

Levin HS, Mattis S, Ruff R, et al: Neurobehavioral outcome following minor head injury: a three center study. J Neurosurg 66:234–243, 1987

Lewis FD, Nelson J, Nelson C, et al: Effects of three feedback contingencies on the socially inappropriate talk of a brain-injured adult. Behav Ther 19:203–211, 1988

Lewis L, Unkefer EP, O'Neal SK, et al: Cognitive rehabilitation with patients having severe psychiatric disabilities. Psychiatr Rehabil J 26:325–331, 2003

Lezak MD: Neuropsychological Assessment, 3rd Edition. New York, Oxford University Press, 1995

Liepert J, Bauder H, Miltner WHR, et al: Treatment-induced cortical reorganization after stroke in humans. Stroke 31:1210–1216, 2000

Lishman WA: Organic Psychiatry. St. Louis, MO, Blackwell Scientific, 1978

Loewenstein DA, Acevedo AS, Czaja SJ, et al: Cognitive rehabilitation of mildly impaired Alzheimer's disease patients on cholinesterase inhibitors. Am J Geriatr Psychiatry 12:395–402, 2004

Luria AR: Restoration of Function After Brain Injury. New York, Macmillan, 1963

Luria AR, Tsvetkova LS: The Neuropsychological Analysis of Problem Solving. Orlando, FL, Paul Deutsch, 1990

Marson D, Harrell L: Executive dysfunction and loss of capacity to consent to medical treatment in patients with Alzheimer's disease. Semin Clin Neuropsychiatry 4:41–49, 1999

McIntosh GC: Medical management of noncognitive sequelae of minor traumatic brain injury. Appl Neuropsychol 4:62–68, 1997

Medd J, Tate RL: Evaluation of anger management therapy programme following acquired brain injury: a preliminary study. Neuropsychol Rehabil 10:185–201, 2000

Meier MJ, Strauman S, Thompson WG: Individual differences in neuropsychological recovery: an overview, in Neuropsychological Rehabilitation. Edited by Meier MJ, Benton AL, Diller L. New York, Guilford, 1987, pp 71–110

Mendez MF, Nakawatase TV, Brown CV: Involuntary laughter and inappropriate hilarity. J Neuropsychiatry Clin Neurosci 11:253–258, 1999

Moffat N: Strategies of memory therapy, in Clinical Management of Memory Problems. Edited by Wilson BA, Moffat N. Rockville, MD, Aspen, 1984, pp 63–88

Muldoon MF, Waldstein SR, Ryan CM, et al: Effects of six anti-hypertensive medications on cognitive performance. J Hypertens 20:1643–1652, 2002

Mungas D: Psychometric correlates of episodic violent behavior: a multidimensional neuropsychological approach. Br J Psychiatry 152:180–187, 1988

Newhouse PA, Potter A, Levin ED: Nicotinic system involvement in Alzheimer's and Parkinson's diseases: implications for therapeutics. Drugs Aging 11:206–228, 1997

NIH Consensus Statement: Rehabilitation of Persons With Traumatic Brain Injury, Vol 16, No 1, October 26–28, 1998. Available at: http://consensus.nih.gov/1998/1998TraumaticBrainInjury109html.htm. Accessed January 6, 2007.

O'Sullivan M, Morris RG, Huckstep B, et al: Diffusion tensor MRI correlates with executive dysfunction in patients with ischaemic leukoaraiosis. J Neurol Neurosurg Psychiatry 75:441–447, 2004

Patten BM: The ancient art of memory. Arch Neurol 26:25–31, 1972

Penades R, Boget T, Lomena F, et al: Brain perfusion and neuropsychological changes in schizophrenic patients after cognitive rehabilitation. Psychiatry Res 98:127–132, 2000

Persel CS, Persel CH, Ashley MJ, et al: The use of noncontingent reinforcement and contingent restrain to reduce physical aggression and self-injurious behaviour in a traumatically brain injured adult. Brain Inj 11:751–760, 1997

Posner HI, Rafal RD: Cognitive theories of attention and the rehabilitation of attentional deficits, in Neuropsychological Rehabilitation. Edited by Meier MJ, Benton AL, Diller L. New York, Guilford, 1987, pp 182–201

Prigatano GP: Personality and psychosocial consequences after brain injury, in Neuropsychological Rehabilitation. Edited by Meier MJ, Benton AL, Diller L. New York, Guilford, 1987, pp 355–378

Rapoport MJ, McCullagh S, Shami P, et al: Cognitive impairment associated with major depression following mild and moderate traumatic brain injury. J Neuropsychiatry Clin Neurosci 17:61–65, 2005

Rizzo AA, Buckwalter JG: Virtual reality and cognitive assessment and rehabilitation: the state of the art. Stud Health Technol Inform 44:123–145, 1997

Robertson-Tchabo EA, Hausman CP, Arenberg D: A classical mnemonic for older learners: a trip that works. Educational Gerontologist 1:215–216, 1976

Robinson RG: Neuropsychiatric consequences of stroke. Annu Rev Med 48:217–229, 1997

Rosenthal M: Behavioral sequelae, in Rehabilitation of the Head Injured Adult. Edited by Rosenthal M, Griffith ER, Bond MR, et al. Philadelphia, PA, FA Davis, 1983, pp 297–308

Schacter DL, Glisky EL: Memory rehabilitation: restoration, alleviation, and the acquisition of domain specific knowledge, in Clinical Neuropsychology of Intervention. Edited by Uzzell B, Gross Y. Boston, MA, Martinus Nijhof, 1986, pp 257–287

Schmitter-Edgecombe M, Fahy JF, Whelan JP, et al: Memory remediation after severe closed head injury: notebook training versus supportive therapy. J Consult Clin Psychol 63:484–489, 1995

Schneider WN, Drew-Cates J, Wong TM, et al: Cognitive and behavioural efficacy of amantadine in acute traumatic brain injury: an initial double-blind placebo-controlled study. Brain Inj 13:863–872, 1999

Seron X: Operant procedures and neuropsychological rehabilitation, in Neuropsychological Rehabilitation. Edited by Meier MJ, Benton AL, Diller L. New York, Guilford, 1987, pp 132–161

Sinforiani E, Banchieri L, Zuchella C, et al: Cognitive rehabilitation in Parkinson's disease. Arch Gerontol Geriatr Suppl 9:387–391, 2004

Sivak M, Hill C, Henson D, et al: Improved driving performance following perceptual training of persons with brain damage. Arch Phys Med Rehabil 65:163–167, 1985

Stablum F, Umilta C, Mogentale C, et al: Rehabilitation of executive deficits in closed head injury and anterior communicating artery aneurysm patients. Psychol Res 63:265–278, 2000

Stuss DT, Benson DF: Neuropsychological studies of the frontal lobes. Psychol Bull 95:3–28, 1984

Suslow T, Schonauer K, Arolt V: Attention training in the cognitive rehabilitation of schizophrenic patients: a review of efficacy studies. Acta Psychiatr Scand 103:15–23, 2001

Suzman KB, Morris RD, Morris MK, et al: Cognitive remediation of problem solving deficits in children with acquired brain injury. J Behav Ther Exp Psychiatry 28:203–212, 1997

Wall P, Egger M: Mechanisms of plasticity of new connection following brain damage in adult mammalian nervous systems, in Recovery of Function: Theoretical Considerations for Brain Injury Rehabilitation. Edited by Bach-y-Rita P. Baltimore, MD, University Park Press, 1971, pp 117–129

Walsh JK, Randazzo AC, Stone KL, et al: Modafinil improves alertness, vigilance, and executive function during simulated night shifts. Sleep 27:434–439, 2004

Weddell R, Oddy M, Jenkins D: Social adjustment after rehabilitation: a two year follow up of patients with severe head injury. Psychol Med 10:257–263, 1980

Williams SE, Ris DM, Ayyangar R, et al: Recovery in pediatric brain injury: is psychostimulant medication beneficial? J Head Trauma Rehabil 13:73–81, 1998

Wilson B: Success and failure in memory training following a cerebral vascular accident. Cortex 18:581–594, 1982

Wilson B: Identification and remediation of everyday problems in memory-impaired patients, in Neuropsychology of Alcoholism: Implications for Diagnosis and Treatment. Edited by Parsons GA, Butters N, Nathan PE. New York, Guilford, 1987, pp 322–338

Wood RL: Behavior disorders following severe brain injury: their presentation and psychological management, in Closed Head Injury: Psychological, Social and Family Consequences. Edited by Brooks N. New York, Oxford University Press, 1984, pp 195–219

Wroblewski BA, Joseph AB, Kupfer J, et al: Effectiveness of valproic acid on destructive and aggressive behaviours in patients with acquired brain injury. Brain Inj 11:37–47, 1997

INDEX

Page numbers printed in **boldface** type refer to tables or figures. Page numbers printed in *bold italic* refer to figures within text that are also reproduced in color in the Appendix.

APPENDIX
Reproduction of Color Figures

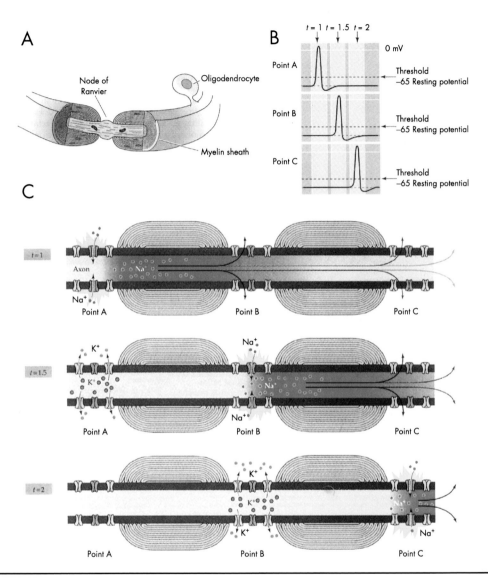

FIGURE 1–2.   Action potential conduction in a myelinated axon.

Panel A. Schematic of a myelinated axon. Oligodendrocytes produce the insulating myelin sheath that surrounds the axon in segments. Myelination restricts current flow to the gaps between myelin segments, the nodes of Ranvier, where Na$^+$ channels are concentrated. The result is a dramatic enhancement of the conduction velocity of the action potential. *Panel B.* Because sodium channels are activated by membrane depolarization and also cause depolarization, they have regenerative properties. This underlies the "all-or-nothing" properties of the action potential and also explains its rapid spread down the axon. The action potential is an electrical wave; as each node of Ranvier is depolarized, it in turn depolarizes the subsequent node. *Panel C.* The Na$^+$ current underlying the action potential is shown in three successive images at 0.5-millisecond intervals and corresponds to the current traces in Panel B. As the action potential (*red shading*) travels to the right, Na$^+$ channels go from closed to open to inactivated to closed. In this way, an action potential initiated at the initial segment of the axon conducts reliably to the axon terminals. Because Na$^+$ channels temporarily inactivate after depolarization, there is a brief refractory period following the action potential that blocks backward spread of the action potential and thus ensures reliable forward conduction.

Source.   Reprinted from Purves D, Augustine GJ, Fitzpatrick D, et al. (eds): *Neuroscience*, 3rd Edition. Sunderland, MA, Sinauer Associates, 2004, p. 64. Used with permission.

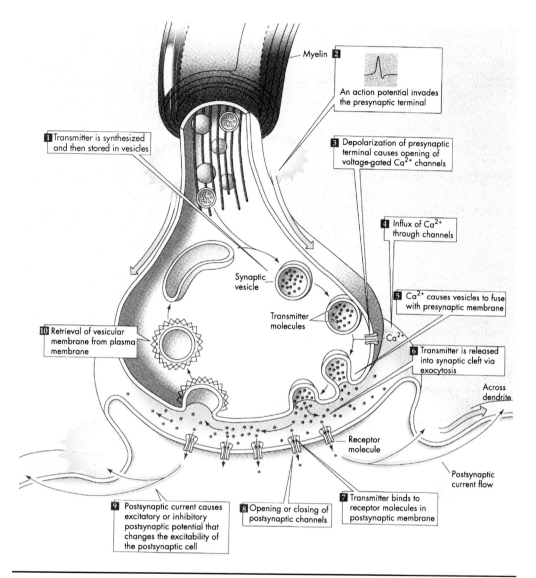

FIGURE 1–5.   Steps in synaptic transmission at a chemical synapse.

Essential steps in the process of synaptic transmission are numbered.

Source.   Reprinted from Purves D, Augustine GJ, Fitzpatrick D, et al. (eds): *Neuroscience*, 3rd Edition. Sunderland, MA, Sinauer Associates, 2004, p. 97. Used with permission.

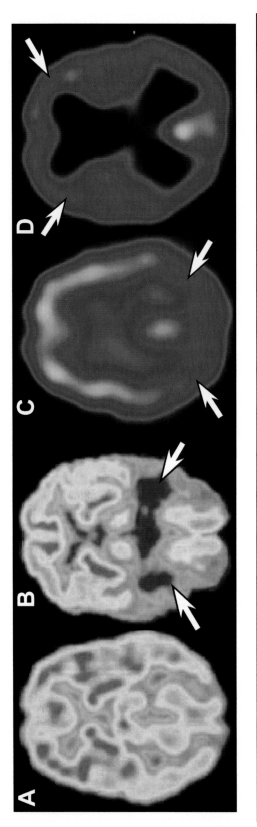

FIGURE 3–4. Diagnostic use of functional imaging in Alzheimer's disease.

Functional imaging is very useful in diagnosis of Alzheimer's disease. Positron emission tomography imaging of cerebral metabolism in normal individual shows high uptake of [^{18}F]-fluorodeoxyglucose (indicated by *orange-red*) throughout the cerebral cortex (*A*). Uptake is reduced (indicated by *blue*) regionally, usually symmetrically (*arrows*), in patients with Alzheimer's disease (*B*) (pictures courtesy of CTI Molecular Imaging, Inc.). Similarly, regional cerebral blood flow, imaged here using single-photon emission computed tomography, is decreased in posterior temporoparietal cortex in early Alzheimer's disease (*C, arrows*). As the disease progresses, frontal lobe involvement is common (*D, arrows*).

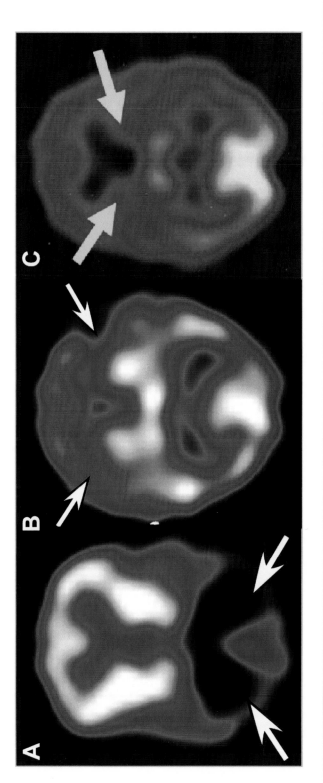

FIGURE 3–5. Functional imaging for differential diagnosis of dementia.

Functional imaging is also useful in differential diagnosis of dementia. A common finding in dementia with Lewy bodies is decreased perfusion in occipital cortex (*A, arrows*). A common finding in frontotemporal dementia (e.g., Pick's disease) is decreased perfusion in frontal and temporal cortex (*B, arrows*). A characteristic finding early in Huntington's disease is decreased perfusion in the basal ganglia, particularly caudate (*C, arrows*). All images are single-photon emission computed tomography.

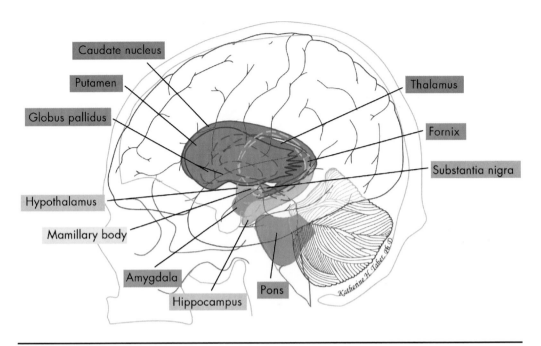

FIGURE 3–6.   This cartoon of a lateral view of the brain and skull shows the approximate positions and configurations of the major subcortical structures.

The colors assigned in this figure are used in the axial atlas (Figures 3–7 through 3–9) to facilitate structure identification.

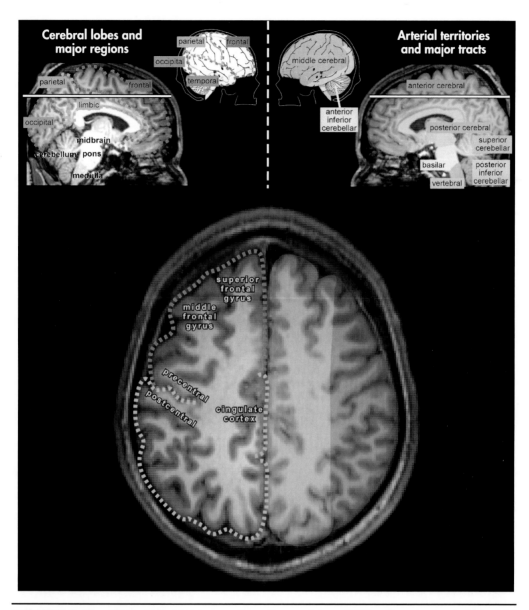

FIGURE 3–7. T1-weighted axial magnetic resonance image (MRI) with major tracts (*right side*) and brain regions (*left side*) labeled.

Major subcortical structures are color-coded to match Figure 3–6. Vascular territories (*right side*) and lobes (*left side*) are color-coded to match the key.

Source. MRI courtesy of Phillips Medical Systems. Atlas section used with permission of Veterans Health Administration Mid-Atlantic Mental Illness Research, Education, and Clinical Center.

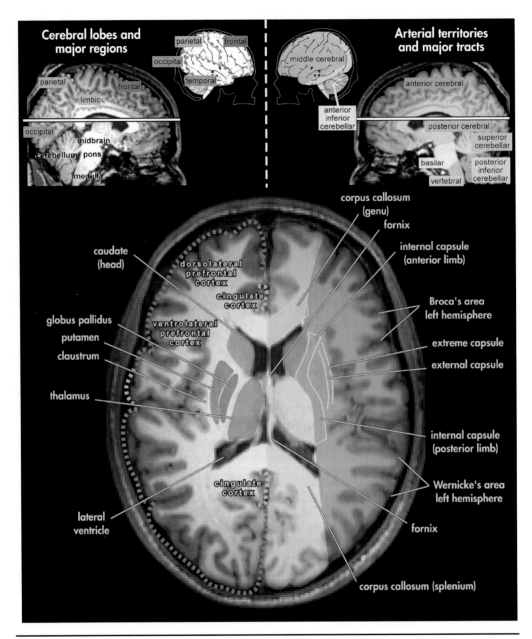

FIGURE 3–8. T1-weighted axial magnetic resonance image (MRI) with major tracts (*right side*) and brain regions (*left side*) labeled.

Major subcortical structures are color-coded to match Figure 3–6. Vascular territories (*right side*) and lobes (*left side*) are color-coded to match the key.

Source. MRI courtesy of Phillips Medical Systems. Atlas section used with permission of Veterans Health Administration Mid-Atlantic Mental Illness Research, Education, and Clinical Center.

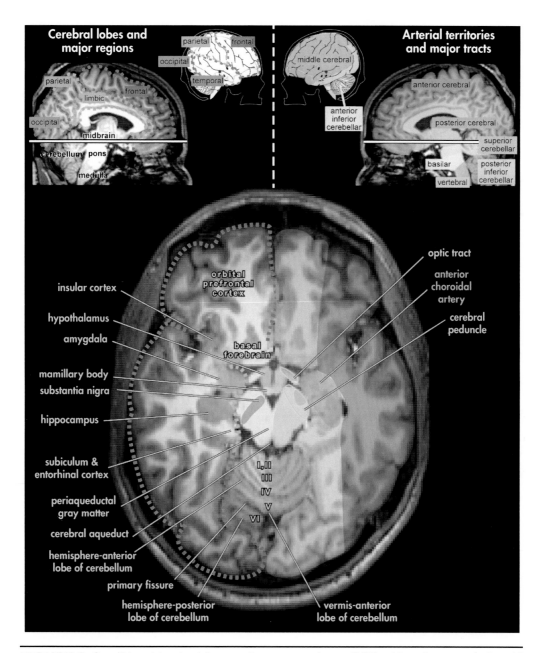

FIGURE 3–9. T1-weighted axial magnetic resonance image (MRI) with major tracts *(right side)* and brain regions *(left side)* labeled.

Major subcortical structures are color-coded to match Figure 3–6. Vascular territories *(right side)* and lobes *(left side)* are color-coded to match the key.

Source. MRI courtesy of Phillips Medical Systems. Atlas section used with permission of Veterans Health Administration Mid-Atlantic Mental Illness Research, Education, and Clinical Center.

SPM, *P*<0.01, *n*=5, 6 minutes

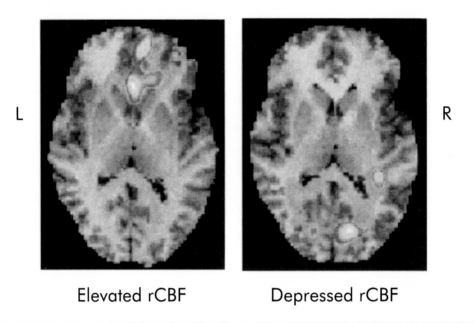

L   R

Elevated rCBF   Depressed rCBF

FIGURE 14–2.   Regional cerebral blood flow (rCBF) localization of ketamine action in schizophrenic brain.

rCBF increases occurred in anterior cingulate gyrus, extending to medial frontal areas (*left scan*); rCBF decreases are apparent in the hippocampus and lingual gyrus (*right scan*). The colored areas indicating significant flow change are plotted onto a magnetic resonance imaging template for ease of localization. SPM = statistical parametric mapping.

Source.   Images contributed by Dr. Henry Holcomb and Dr. Adrienne Lahti.

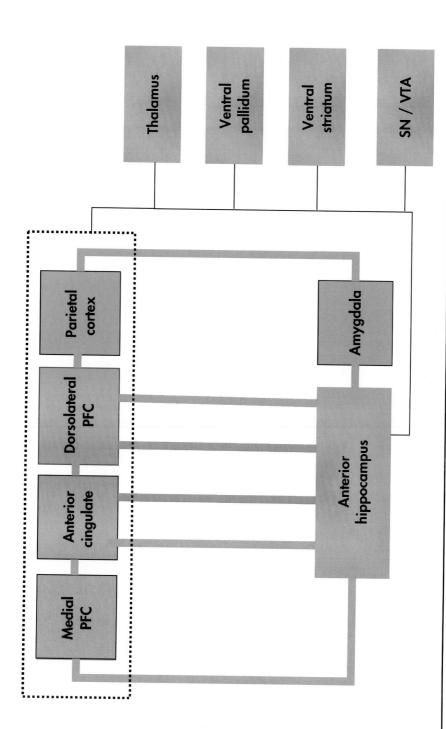

FIGURE 14–3. Hypothetical neural circuits underlying the three symptom domains of schizophrenia.

In this model, a specific neural circuit underlies each of the symptom domains—the psychosis circuit (*blue*), cognitive deficit circuit (*orange*), and negative symptom circuit (*green*). The *dotted line* represents neocortex. Core deficits in the anterior hippocampus can influence functional integrity of each of these circuits. PFC = prefrontal cortex; SN/VTA = substantia nigra/ventral tegmental area.

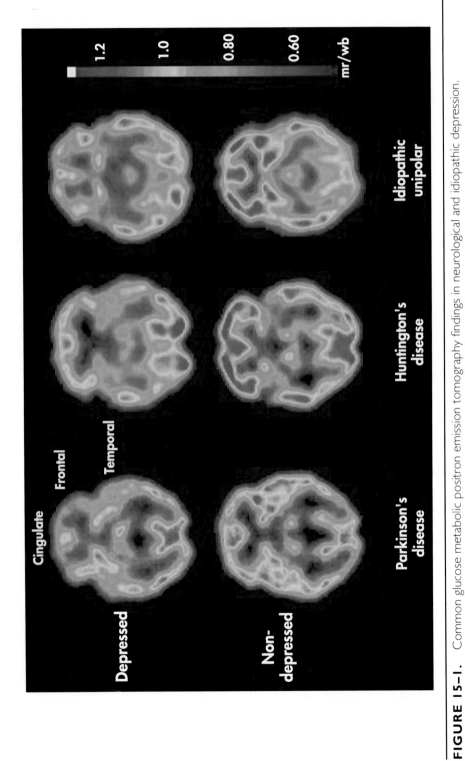

FIGURE 15–1. Common glucose metabolic positron emission tomography findings in neurological and idiopathic depression.

Decreased prefrontal, dorsal cingulate, and temporal cortical metabolism is a common finding across different depressive syndromes, including patients with Parkinson's disease, Huntington's disease, and idiopathic unipolar depression.

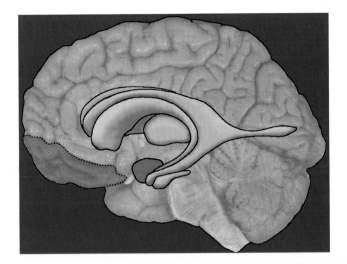

FIGURE 16–1.   Neuroanatomical model of generalized anxiety disorder.

Note the increased activity in temporolimbic areas (Tiihonen et al. 1997b; Wu et al. 1991) as well as in prefrontal areas (Rauch et al. 1997; Wu et al. 1991).

Source.   Reprinted from Stein DJ: *False Alarm! How to Conquer the Anxiety Disorders.* Cape Town, South Africa, University of Stellenbosch, 2000. Used with permission.

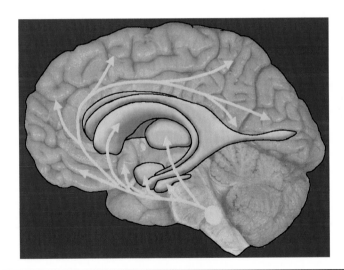

FIGURE 16–2.   Serotonergic circuits project to key regions (prefrontal cortex, orbitofrontal cortex, anterior cingulate, amygdala, hippocampus, basal ganglia, thalamus) involved in the mediation of anxiety disorders.

Source.   Reprinted from Stein DJ: *False Alarm! How to Conquer the Anxiety Disorders.* Cape Town, South Africa, University of Stellenbosch, 2000. Used with permission.

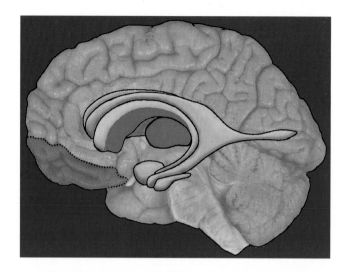

FIGURE 16–3.   Neuroanatomical model of obsessive-compulsive disorder.

Note the increased activity in the ventromedial cortico-striatal-thalamic-cortical circuit (Rauch and Baxter 1998).

Source.   Reprinted from Stein DJ: *False Alarm! How to Conquer the Anxiety Disorders.* Cape Town, South Africa, University of Stellenbosch, 2000. Used with permission.

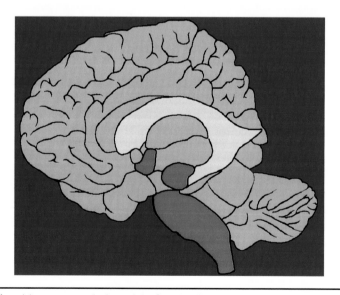

FIGURE 16–4.   Neuroanatomical model of panic disorder.

Note the activation of the amygdala, which has efferents to hypothalamus and brain stem sites (Gorman et al. 2000).

Source.   Reprinted from Stein DJ: *False Alarm! How to Conquer the Anxiety Disorders.* Cape Town, South Africa, University of Stellenbosch, 2000. Used with permission.

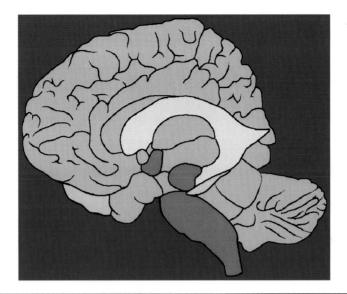

FIGURE 16–5.   Neuroanatomical model of posttraumatic stress disorder.

Note the increased activity in the amygdala and decreased activity in prefrontal areas (not anatomically to scale).

Source.   Reprinted from Stein DJ: *False Alarm! How to Conquer the Anxiety Disorders.* Cape Town, South Africa, University of Stellenbosch, 2000. Used with permission.

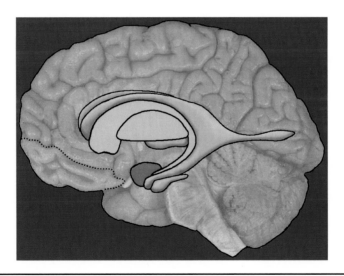

FIGURE 16–6.   Neuroanatomical model of social phobia.

Note the increased temporolimbic activity (van der Linden et al. 2000), decreased basal ganglia dopaminergic activity (Tiihonen et al. 1997a), and perhaps some increased prefrontal activity (Rauch et al. 1997; van der Linden et al. 2000).

Source.   Reprinted from Stein DJ: *False Alarm! How to Conquer the Anxiety Disorders.* Cape Town, South Africa, University of Stellenbosch, 2000. Used with permission.